W9-CNW-859

Overweight and Obesity: Causes, Fallacies, Treatment

Overweight and Obesity: Causes, Fallacies, Treatment

EDITED BY BRENT Q. HAFEN

Department of Health Sciences
Brigham Young University

Brigham Young University Press
Provo, Utah

(Multilith Series)
Library of Congress Catalog Card Number: 74-19000
International Standard Book Number: 0-8425-0263-7
© 1975 by Brigham Young University Press. All rights reserved
Brigham Young University Press, Provo, Utah 84602
Printed in the United States of America
1975   2.5M   4870

Contents

Acknowledgments   ix

Preface   xiii

Part I   Understanding Overweight and Obesity

In Defense of Body Weight   2
Multidisciplinary Approach
   to the Problem of Obesity   7
                      Obesity   13
Newer Concepts of Obesity   17
Do We Dare to Differentiate
Between Obese and Overweight?   27
      When is Fat Excessive?   33
Nature and Nurture in Human Obesity   36
Obesity in an Age of Caloric Anxiety   40
Can We Modify the Number
            of Adipose Cells?   48
Physiology and Natural
            History of Obesity   52
               Hidden Bonds   56
Physiologic Control of Food Intake   63

**Part II   Psychological and Sociological
Aspects of Overweight and Obesity**

Oh How We're Punished
for the Crime of Being Fat   73
      The Stigma of Obesity   77
Negative Mood, Hunger,
   and Weight Classification   81
Psychological Aspects of Obesity   85
Obesity—Understanding the Compulsion   89
Severe Obesity as a Habituation Syndrome   94
            Compulsive Eating   102
Casebook: I Can't Stop Eating   105
               Thin Fat People   108
The Social Psychology of Dieting   112
      Social Factors in Obesity   131

Influence of Social Class on Obesity
and Thinness in Children 137
An Anthropological Approach
to the Problem of Obesity 143
Culture, History, and Adiposity,
or Should Santa Claus Reduce? 152

Part III   **Weight Control Fads and Fallacies**

Diet Madness 158
The Realities of Obesity and Fad Diets 161
The Crash Diet Craze 165
When They Start Telling You
It's Easy to Lose Weight . . . 172
Before You Believe Those Exercise and
Diet Ads Read the Following Report 176
Diet Books That Poison Your Mind
and Harm Your Body 180
The Dangers in Diet Advice 183
Which Diets Work—Which Don't 188
The Truth About the 25 Most Common
Weight Control Myths 191
Ten Common Misconceptions
About Overweight and Dieting 194

Part IV   **Overweight and Obesity
in Childhood and Adolescence**

Fat Babies Grow Into Fat People 199
The Portly, Corpulent, or Obese American 202
Childhood Obesity 209
Obesity in Childhood: A Problem in
Adipose Tissue Cellular Development 216
When to Start Dieting? At Birth 228
Treating Obesity in Growing Children 231
1. General Strategy 231
2. Specific Aspects:
Activity and Diet 235
Food Habits of Obese and
Nonobese Adolescents 240
Obesity in Adolescence 247
Treatment of Obesity in Adolescence 255
Weight Control in a College Situation 259
Obesity Surgery Aids Four Adolescents 264

Part V   **Dynamics of Weight Control**

The Myth of Diet in the
Management of Obesity 267
Management of the Obese Patient 275
A Three-Dimensional Program
for the Treatment of Obesity 286
Treating Obesity: Three Approaches 296
59 Ways to Help Patients Lose Weight 302
Clinical Management of the Obese Adult 309
Etiology of Obesity—the QQF Theory 315

Nutritional Anarchy: A Perspective
on the "Atkins Diet Revolution"   319
Are We Not Now Ready
for a Diet Revolution?   325
A Critique of Low-Carbohydrate Ketogenic
Weight Reduction Regimens   332
The Low-Carbohydrate Diet in the
Treatment of Obesity   337
Rational Diet Construction
for Mild and Grand Obesity   341
An Hour of Exercise vs. a Pound of Flesh   343
So You Think You're Exercising Enough?   346
The Caloric Cost of Running   349
Who Controls Your Eating Habits?   351
Hope for the Obese: Behavior Modification   353
Behavior Therapy in Treating Obesity   355
Treating Obesity with Behavior Modification   360
The Group Way to Weight Loss   367
The Success of TOPS, a Self-Help Group   371
A Therapeutic Coalition for Obesity:
Behavior Modification and Patient Self-Help   376
Overeaters Anonymous—Report on a
Self-Help Group   381
Use of Drugs in the Treatment of Obesity   385
Jejuno-Ileal Surgery: Which Patients Qualify?   389
Intestinal Bypass Operation
for Massive Obesity   394
In Obesity Surgery, Problems are the Rule   400

Index   403

Acknowledgments

I wish to gratefully acknowledge the editors, publishers, and authors of the seventy-six articles appearing in this anthology for their kindness in allowing us to reprint their material. The following is a list of the articles as they appear in the table of contents.

JORDAN, H. A. 1973. In defense of body weight. *J. Amer. Diet. Ass.* 62:17-21.

VAN ITALLIE, T. B., AND CAMPBELL, R. G. 1972. Multidisciplinary approach to the problem of obesity. *J. Amer. Diet. Ass.* 61:385-90.

MAYER, J. 1972. Obesity. *Postgrad. Med.* 51:66-69.

PENICK, S. B., AND STUNKARD, A. J. 1970. Newer concepts of obesity. *Med. Clin. North Amer.* 54:745-54.

CANARY, J. J. August 1973. Do we dare to differentiate between obese and overweight? *Medical Opinion*, pp. 14-22.

Ames/Diagnos. 1972. When is fat excessive? 23:15-17.

CHLOUVERAKIS, C. S. 1974. Nature and nurture in human obesity. *Obes./Bariat. Med.* 3:28-31.

VAN ITALLIE, T. B., AND HASHIM, S. A. 1970. Obesity in an age of caloric anxiety. Reprinted from *Modern Medicine* © The New York Times Media Company, Inc. 38:89-96.

HIRSCH, J. 1972. Can we modify the number of adipose cells? *Postgrad. Med.* 51: 83-86.

NELSON, R. A.; ANDERSON, L. F.; GASTINEAU, C. F.; HAYLES, A. B.; AND STAMNES, C. L. 1973. Physiology and natural history of obesity. *J. Amer. Med. Ass.* 223:627-30.

MAYER, J. 1974. Hidden bonds. *World Health*, pp. 21-27.

HAMILTON, C. L. 1973. Physiologic control of food intake. *J. Amer. Med. Ass.* 62: 35-38.

HARMETZ, A. January 1974. Oh how we're punished for the crime of being fat. *Today's Health*, pp. 21-24.

KALISH, B. J. 1972. The stigma of obesity. *Amer. J. Nurs.* 72:1124-27.

HEWITT, M. I. 1974. Negative mood, hunger, and weight classification. *Obes./Bariat. Med.* 3:24-27.

BRUCH, H. July-August 1973. Psychological aspects of obesity. *Medical Insight*, pp. 23-28.

SALZMAN, L. July 1970. Obesity-understanding the compulsion. *Medical Insight*, pp. 52-62.

Severe obesity as a habituation syndrome. Reprinted from *Archives of General Psychiatry* 22(2):120–27, 1970, Copyright 1970, American Medical Association.

HAREVEN, E. Compulsive eating. In *Man and Woman* 19 (London: Marshall Cavendish): 2114-17.

Casebook—I can't stop eating. In *Man and Woman* 2 (London: Marshall Cavendish): 1224-29.

BRUCH, H. 1973. Thin fat people. In *Eating disorders: obesity, anorexia nervosa, and the person within* (New York: Basic Books), Chapter 11.

MAYER, J.; DWYER, J. T.; AND FELDMAN, J. J. 1970. The social psychology of dieting. *J. Health and Soc. Behav.* 11:269-87.

GOLDBLATT, P. B.; MOORE, M. E.; AND STUNKARD, A. J. 1965. Social factors in obesity. *J. Amer. Med. Ass.* 192:97-100.

STUNKARD, A. J.; D'AQUILI, E.; FOX, S.; AND FILION, R. D. L. 1972. Influence of social class on obesity and thinness in children. *J. Amer. Med. Ass.* 221:579-84.

POWDERMAKER, H. 1960. An anthropological approach to the problem of obesity. *Bull. N.Y. Acad. Med.* 36:75-83.

WEST, K. M. 1974. Culture, history, and adiposity, or should Santa Claus reduce? *Obes./Bariat. Med.* 3:48-52.

TOUFEXIS, A. August 1973. Diet madness. *Physician's World*, pp. 46b-46d.

FINEBERG, S. K. July/August 1972. The realities of obesity and fad diets. *Nutr. Today*, pp. 23-26.

The crash diet craze. Reprinted from *Medical World News*, April 1973, pp. 34-40. Copyright © 1973, McGraw-Hill, Inc.

SINGER, S. November 1972. When they start telling you it's easy to lose weight . . . *Today's Health*, pp. 47-62.

SHERRILL, R. 1971. Before you believe those exercise and diet ads read the following report. *Today's Health* 49:34-36, 68-70.

SCHANCHE, D. A. 1974. Diet books that poison your mind and harm your body. *Today's Health* 52:56-61.

WHITE, P. L., AND RYNEARSON, E. H. 1973. The dangers in diet advice. *Medical Insight* 5:30-34.

Which diets work—which don't. Article by Philip L. White reprinted from *Today's Health*, 49:59-61. Published by the American Medical Association.

Good Housekeeping. 1972. The truth about the 25 most common weight control myths. 175:205-7.

KNOX, G. M., AND BERLAND, T. 1972. Ten common misconceptions about overweight and dieting. Reprinted from *Better Homes and Gardens.* © Copyright Meredith Corporation, 1972. All rights reserved. 50:10-12.

MAYER, J. 1973. Fat babies grow into fat people. *Family Health* 5:24-38.

FLYNN, M. A. 1974. The portly, corpulent or obese American. *Continuing Education* 7:28-33.

WINICK, M. May/June 1974. Childhood obesity. *Nutr. Today*, pp. 6-12.

KNITTLE, J. L. 1972. Obesity in childhood: a problem in adipose tissue cellular development. *J. Pediat.* 81:1048-59.

When to start dieting? At birth. Reprinted from *Medical World News*, September 1973, pp. 31-33. Copyright © 1973, McGraw-Hill, Inc.

DWYER, J. T.; BLONDE, C. V.; AND MAYER, J. 1972. Treating obesity in growing children: general strategy. *Postgrad. Med.* 51:90-94.

———. 1972. Treating obesity in growing children: specific aspects. *Postgrad. Med.* 51:111-15.

HUENEMANN, R. L. May 1972. Food habits of obese and nonobese adolescents. *Postgrad. Med.* 51:99-105.

CARRERA, F., III. 1967. Obesity in adolescence. *Psychosomatics.* 8:342-49.

HEALD, F. P. May 1972. Treatment of obesity in adolescence. *Postgrad. Med.* 51:109-12.

YOUNG, C. M. May 1972. Weight control in a college situation. *Postgrad. Med.* 51:117-120.

Obesity surgery aids four adolescents. Reprinted from *Medical World News*, November 1973, p. 21. Copyright © 1973, McGraw-Hill, Inc.

BRAY, G. A. 1970. The myth of diet in the management of obesity. *Amer. J. Clin. Nutr.* 23:1141-47.

BRAUNSTEIN, J. J. 1971. Management of the obese patient. *Med. Clinics of No. Amer.* 55:391-400.

Behav. Rec. and Therapy. 1971. A three-dimensional program for the treatment of obesity. 9:177-86.

Treating obesity: three approaches. Reprinted from *Medical World News*, August 1972, pp. 20-36. Copyright © 1973, McGraw-Hill, Inc.

Patient Care. 1971. 59 ways to help patients lose weight. 5:114-28.

BRAY, G. A. 1972. Clinical management of the obese adult. *Postgrad. Med.* 51:125-30.

SCHAUF, G. E. 1973. Etiology of obesity—the QQF Theory. *J. Amer. Geriat. Soc.* 21:346-49.

FINEBERG, S. K. February 1974. Nutritional anarchy: a perspective in the "Atkin's Diet." *Medical Counterpoint* 6:12-18.

ATKINS, R. C. February 1974. Are we not now ready for a diet revolution? *Medical Counterpoint* 6:13-24.

J. Amer. Med. Ass. 1973. A critique of low-carbohydrate ketogenic weight reduction regimens. 224:1415-19.

YUDKIN, J. May 1972. The low-carbohydrate diet in the treatment of obesity. *Postgrad. Med.* 51:151-54.

TULLIS, I. F. 1973. Rational diet construction for mild and grand obesity. *J. Amer. Med. Ass.* 226:70-71.

MAYER, J. June 1973. An hour of exercise vs. a pound of flesh. *Family Health*, 5:33-35.

————. July 1973. So you think you're exercising enough? *Family Health*, 5:34-36.

HARGER, B. S.; THOMAS, J. C.; AND MILLER, J. B. 1974. The caloric cost of running. *J. Amer. Med. Ass.* 228:482-83.

KELLY, J. April 1973. Who controls your eating habits? *Family Health* 5:36-37.

STUNKARD, A. J., AND MAHONEY, M. J. 1972. Hope for the obese: behavior modification. *Psychiatry* 35:45,46.

LEVITZ, L. S. 1973. Behavior therapy in treating obesity. *J. Amer. Diet. Ass.* 62:22-26.

BRIGHTWELL, D. R. 1974. Treating obesity with behavior modification. *Postgrad. Med.* 55:52-58.

SHUMWAY, S., AND POWERS, M. 1973. The group way to weight loss. *Amer. J. Nurs.* 73:269-72.

STUNKARD, A. J. May 1972. The success of TOPS, a self-help group. *Postgrad. Med.* 51:143-47.

LEVITZ, L. S., AND STUNKARD, A. J. 1974. A therapeutic coalition for obesity: behavior modification and patient self-help. *American Journal of Psychiatry* 1974, Vol. 131, pp. 423-427. Copyright 1974, The American Psychiatric Association.

LINDNER, P. G. 1974. Overeaters anonymous—report on a self-help group. *Obes./Bariat. Med.* 3:134-37.

GERSHBERG, H. May 1972. Use of drugs in the treatment of obesity. *Postgrad. Med.* 51:135-38.

BUCHWALD, H. August 1973. Jejuno-ileal surgery: which patients qualify? *Medical Opinion*, pp. 40-48.

Postgrad. Med. 1974. Intestinal bypass operation for massive obesity. 55:65-70.

In obesity surgery, problems are the rule. Reprinted from *Medical World News*, September 1973, pp. 34-36. Copyright © 1973, McGraw-Hill, Inc.

Preface

Weight control is a major nutritional concern for 20 to 40 million Americans today. However, the problem of overweight is not a recent one. From the time of Hippocrates and Galen, two early Greek scholars, the problem of obesity has intrigued medical men. Shakespeare mentioned it in one of his plays, *Julius Caesar*. Today it is generally recognized that obesity constitutes a serious health problem for the U. S. population.

The American concern with overweight clogs the public media and the public mind, and often overwhelms the practice time of many physicians. Almost every contemporary magazine offers its readers a new diet to lose weight. Radio and television programs are filled with food advertising extolling the low-calorie virtues of hundreds of food products. The newest fad diet book leaps to the top of the list of best sellers, particularly if it promises weight loss without deletion or limitation of foods eaten for pleasure. Many lay groups such as TOPS and Weight Watchers promote group dieting activities. Public health agencies offer dietary counseling as well as homemaking advice.

Officials of the American Medical Association say the reducing fads cost the public $100 million dollars per year, and investigators in the Post Office Department allege that medical quackery costs the nation more than all crime combined. This is indeed an expensive and dangerous fad. According to the Food and Drug Administration, ten million Americans spend at least half a billion dollars annually on nostrums, useless and unnecessary diet supplements, and books and contrivances to cure their real or imaginary ills. Such beliefs and consequent expenditures cannot be delineated by age or class boundaries since the victims of food faddists have been found concentrated in the older age groups as well as the young, and, surprisingly, in the lower socioeconomic groups.

The dismal prognosis of treatment of overweight and obesity problems by educators, and by clinicians in both the public agencies and private firms, in many respects suggests that perhaps we have done a poor job of educating the little-understood etiology of overweight and obesity. Viewed from another perspective, however, perhaps nutrition educators have done their job too well in some ways. Through a myriad of pamphlets, films, and nutrition programs, the government, food industry sources, and professional groups have sensitized the average American to the important benefits of an adequate diet. However, unscrupulous promoters have capitalized on the public's interest in nutrition as well as the desire to maintain a slim figure.

Obesity is a threat to health, to social and domestic happiness, and to economic security. It is one of our most important problems. The emotional consequences of obesity can be devastating. The idea that all the world loves a fat man is completely erroneous. A fat woman is loved even less. Because of the way society is conditioned against obesity an obese woman, particularly a young woman, sometimes becomes a social, economic, and in many cases, an emotional cripple. Social disapproval is so marked that many fat women develop self-contempt, often commenting, "I hate myself." This is a most unfortunate attitude and limits the success of any reducing program. We try to explain that their obesity is not their fault, but their misfortune. We would do well to remember Plato's remarks to the effect that the human animal consists of a body and a soul, and when one doesn't function well, neither does the other. We can treat obesity with the same compassion we extend to other health problems.

This brings all of us interested in this field into a delicate situation. Are we informed? Do we understand the newest research and treatment programs that are most effective in the area of weight control? Some important questions to ask and ones with which this book deals are: Why do people eat? What is the cause of overweight? What kinds of food do they eat and why? What are some of the psychological and sociological aspects that influence overweight problems? What are the most effective weight control programs? What are the physiological differences in food utilization? These are crucial questions for the nutrition educator as well as for those concerned with the etiology of overweight. Certainly the nutrition educators, health educators, medical and paramedical personnel who are working in any type of educational or treatment program concerning weight control would do well to understand the dynamics of overweight and obesity presented here.

There is no single or simple answer to obesity. Essays included here indicate the complexities of the problem as well as the complexities of people. One goal of the book is to present obesity as a disturbance of the whole person and give due recognition to the importance of the social and psychological

areas of weight control. The readings speak for themselves. They present a diversity of current thought about the problems manifest in overweight and obesity. They range from discussions of the etiology of overweight, the psychological and sociological aspects of overweight, weight control in children and youth, the dynamics of weight control, to the most contemporary diet fads and fallacies.

Although the topic of overweight and obesity is relatively muddled, it is not the purpose of this book to resolve differences and present one particular theory, but rather to present the research and writings of some of the foremost authorities in the United States in the field of weight control and obesity. The essays in this volume have all been selected from reputable health and medical journals, including such varied publications as the *Journal of Pediatrics, Postgraduate Medicine, Journal of Health and Social Behavior, Behavior Research and Therapy, Journal of the American Dietetic Association, Journal of the American Medical Association, Modern Medicine,* and *Medical Clinics of North America.* If obesity is to be approached comprehensively, then the diversity of illustrations in this book should prove helpful to all those who are interested or working in the area of weight control.

Appreciation is extended to the authors and publishers for their permission to reprint the materials selected for this volume.

Part I: Understanding Overweight and Obesity *

Obesity is the presence of excess adipose tissue in contrast to a measure of total body weight which includes bony structure, musculature tissue and body fluids as well as fat tissues.

As crude as the statistical data may be, there is a substantial prevalence of obesity at every age in both sexes, no matter how obesity might be defined.

As recently as 20 years ago, obesity was dealt with clinically as an almost exclusively psychological problem. The rationale was simple: Obesity is due to overeating. Overeating is due either to lack of self-control—that is, gluttony—or to more serious abnormalties of personality.

Fortunately, the intervening years have seen knowledge progress on a wide front. Oversimplifications are no longer tenable to those who are concerned with the problem and its prevention and management. Advances in scientific knowledge have not resulted in any "magic bullet" based on diagnosis of specific neurophysiological or biochemical disturbances. However, the progress witnessed does open avenues for exploration and affords a more comprehensive understanding of the complexities involved.

Obesity, the result of a positive caloric balance, can be the outcome of a number of disturbances. The variations in causes and subsequent manifestations indicate that not all obesity can be considered the same. For this reason, some investigators have come to use the plural term "obesities" rather than "obesity."

Obesity can be classified according to etiology, or underlying causes, or it can be classified according to pathogenesis—changes in the mechanisms involved in the development of obesity, such as the impairment of a physiological or biochemical process. Both classifications are intimately involved in the regulation of food intake.

It is apparent from animal experimentation and from more limited human evidence that the mechanism for regulating food intake is a very complicated one and vulnerable to many neurologic, metabolic and psychologic disturbances. A variety of unrelated events may decrease food intake and similarly, a great number of such unrelated events may increase food intake over the need for maintenance, thus causing overweight and/or obesity.

The diversity of experimental obesities in animals and observations in man illustrate the multiple etiology of obesity.

This section provides a description and definition of overweight and obesity problems as well as an overview with scientific validation for what is presently known concerning the prevalence, causes, and health consequences of overweight and obesity.

*Excerpts from: *Obesity and Health*, U.S. Public Health Service Publication No. 1485.

In Defense of Body Weight

HENRY A. JORDAN, M.D.
Department of Psychiatry,
University of Pennsylvania, and
Philadelphia General Hospital,
Philadelphia

Obesity and reducing are age-old problems,
going back at least to the time of Socrates.
The problem involves equilibrium in energy
balance—which is extremely resistant to
measures to alter it.

The task of discussing obesity is indeed frustrating, whether one considers etiology, epidemiology, or treatment. In spite of the vast literature on all aspects of obesity, our understanding of it remains unclear. A brief glance into history reveals that the confusion surrounding obesity has existed for centuries and that the repetition of statements about it is remarkable. For example, in 399 B.C., Socrates warned overweight persons:

Beware of those foods that tempt you to eat when you are not hungry and those liquors that tempt you to drink when you are not thirsty.

In 1825, Jean Brillat-Savarin, the famous French gourmet, said, (1):

Any cure for obesity must begin with the three following and absolute precepts: discretion in eating, moderation in sleeping, and exercise on foot or on horseback.

Flint, in his textbook of physiology, stated (2) in 1870:

Very little is known concerning the precise mechanism of the production of fat.

In 1883, William Beaumont explained (3):

In the present state of civilized society with the provocation of the culinary art, and the incentive of highly seasoned foods, brandy and wine, the temptation to excess in the indulgences of the table are rather too strong to be resisted by poor human nature.

In 1893, William Osler, noted American physician and teacher, in his text on medicine, reiterated (4) that there were three important factors to be considered in obesity: (a) overeating (b) lack of proper exercise, and (c) excessive intake of alcoholic beverages, especially beer. Very recently, Passmore, a noted British physiologist, restated (5) Beaumont:

The art of our cooks and food chemists stimulate appetite and often make us feed when there is no physiological need for food intake.

All of these statements and variations of them have been made repeatedly throughout history, and, although information about obesity increases continuously, the basic understanding of the mechanisms controlling the excessive deposition of adipose tissue remains elusive.

This paper will not attempt to delineate or discuss

Work supported by Nutrition Foundation Grant No. 384 and Research Scientist Development Aware MH-37224.

the etiology of obesity. Whether the cause is psychologic, physiologic, or metabolic, or a combination of these factors, once an increase in adipose tissue mass occurs, it is extremely difficult to remove this excess. The difficulty and, in most cases, the failure to treat obesity effectively is a prevalent problem independent of the mode of therapy. Whether the treatment involves starvation, diets, drugs, psychotherapy, self-help groups, exercise programs, hormones, and so forth, we have been (a) unable to cause many persons to lose weight and (b) unable to sustain the weight loss for more than a year. A review of medical management of obesity conducted by Stunkard and McLaren-Hume reported (6) that all programs were equally ineffective in their treatment of obesity. Attrition rates in clinics range from 20 to 80 per cent and only 25 per cent who enter therapy lose 20 lb.; only 5 per cent lose as much as 40 lb.

It is interesting, however, that most people, including those who are obese, maintain stable weights unless they are deliberately dieting. Much like the animal with a lesion in the ventromedial hypothalamus who goes through a "dynamic phase" and reaches a new weight plateau, obese persons tend to gain weight and then to stabilize at the new, higher plateau. When the weight stabilizes, one can assume that the energy intake of the organism equals the expenditure. In other words, even though the weight may be abnormally high, an equilibrium in energy balance exists.

Equilibrium in any biologic system is extremely resistant to alteration and, therefore, difficult to change. For example, the regulation of body temperature is rigorously controlled, and any attempt to alter it demands that great stress be placed on the organism. We have performed experiments in which the body temperatures of human subjects have been raised or lowered only a few degrees; immersion in cold or warm water for up to 1 hr. was required to effect any pronounced change. The procedure is uncomfortable, and the physiologic mechanisms resist the change. For example, intense shivering occurs when temperature is lowered, and sweating when it is increased.

Energy equilibrium and control mechanisms

This resistance to alteration of equilibrium apparently controls energy balance involving body weight as well; regardless of the actual weight at which equilibrium occurs, a change in weight is difficult. For example, if a hyperphagic monkey is starved and loses weight, on refeeding, adipose tissue is redeposited and the animal returns to his prestarvation weight (7).

Hamilton's paper which follows (8) shows that regulation of body weight depends on elaborate, but only partially understood, control mechanisms. In his experiments on animals, regulation depends on the control of both input and expenditure or output of energy. When these controls operate effectively, equilibrium is achieved and body weight is regulated. If,

however, the controls are faulty or the usual channels through which they operate are blocked, then the maintenance of equilibrium is disrupted and either gain or loss of weight occurs.

We have been investigating the regulation of energy balance in human subjects in our laboratory, and although normal-weight individuals are capable of maintaining constant weight over long periods, the mechanisms involved remain elusive. For example, when the usual cues, i.e., social, visual, and even gustatory, are removed from the eating situation, normal-weight subjects will continue to consume normal amounts of liquid diet. Even when the subjects voluntarily ingest food intragastrically by stomach tube, they maintain normal patterns of intake (9). We have also challenged subjects with dilution of calories, and although the response to this manipulation is sluggish, sometimes taking three days or more, the subjects increase their dietary intakes and maintain their weights (10). Our work indicates that the human organism is capable of many adjustments in order to maintain energy balance, for, in spite of our experimental manipulations, the equilibrium of caloric intake and body weight resist change.

Other studies further elucidate the resistance of this fine balance to change. Investigators have tried to alter equilibrium in the negative direction by restricting caloric intake and in the positive direction by overfeeding in attempts to produce experimental obesity.

Caloric restriction

First, let me describe the effects of caloric restriction on normal-weight persons. The most detailed exploration of the effects of restricted calories on human subjects was conducted by Keys *et al.* (11) during World War II. They placed thirty-six young male volunteers on an average caloric intake of 1,570 kcal per day for six months. The following effects of semi-starvation were noted: (a) pulse rate dropped; (b) basal metabolic rate dropped; (c) general activity slowed down; (d) libido decreased; (e) weight dropped; at the end of six months, an average decrease of 24 per cent body weight had occurred; (f) tolerance to heat increased; (g) tolerance to cold decreased; and (h) vertigo and giddiness occurred. The first four observations reflect physiologic and metabolic alterations which in one way or another are evidence of the organism's attempts to preserve energy balance by conserving energy. Since the subjects were unable to utilize the responses which would lead to increased intake of energy, the last four changes reflect the organism's failure to maintain equilibrium.

In addition to these effects, numerous psychologic changes were observed, all of which reflected an increased desire for food. Anticipation of eating became exaggerated, craving for food increased, dislikes for certain foods disappeared, preoccupation with food increased, and socially acceptable eating behavior, i.e., table manners, disappeared. In addition, depression, apathy, and general irritability increased. On rehabilitation, it is noteworthy that these changes in behavior and emotions persisted for several months.

Further evidence of the effect of caloric restriction can be seen in the catastrophic events in man's history which dramatically demonstrate the powerful forces that can be evoked to preserve energy balance in normal-weight persons. For example, Salisbury's account (12) of the 900-day siege of Leningrad during World War II is an incredible story of the slow starvation of an entire metropolitan population. During this period, robbery, murder, and, in a few instances, cannibalism occurred.

Caloric restriction in the obese

What happens to the obese person when calories are restricted? Are their responses similar to those of the volunteers in the study by Keys and Brozek? Stunkard reports (13) that there are numerous effects on dieters. They become irritable, preoccupied with food, and in many instances depressed. Furthermore, physiologic and metabolic alterations occur. Bray reported (14) that the basal metabolic rate decreased when obese subjects were placed on a rigid regimen with calories reduced from 3,500 to 450 per day. His subjects experienced an average decrease of 15 per cent in energy expenditure as measured by oxygen consumption. As a result of this altered metabolism, their weight loss did not equal the restriction of calories. It appears, then, that the obese person may be just as resistant to weight loss as the normal person and may suffer as much.

Grinker has been attempting to further characterize the obese person as to taste, perception of food, reactions to weight loss, and so on. Her paper in this issue (15) elaborates on her findings.

Resistance to weight gain

It is apparent that organisms resist change in the negative direction, but do they have the same capacity to resist change in the positive direction? Are there mechanisms for resisting or slowing weight gain? What does the organism do when given an excess of energy? For instance, will excessive food intake in a normal-weight individual lead to obesity? Studies attempting this manipulation are not nearly as numerous as those concerned with caloric restriction, but there have been a few attempts at producing experimental obesity.

Sims and co-workers, at the University of Vermont, attempted to induce excessive weight gain in four normal-weight college students who ingested two or three times their normal caloric intakes each day for three to five months (16). It rapidly became apparent that increasing the weight of these individuals was about as difficult as removing weight, and perhaps more so. At the end of the experimental period, the average weight gain was from 10 to 12 per cent of the starting weight—hardly an obese population. It must be noted, however, that if this gain had been sustained, a marked degree of obesity would have occurred after two or three years.

Following this initial study, Sims et al. moved their research to a prison and repeated the forced feeding with nine inmates. Repeating the above protocol under more controlled circumstances, a 26 per cent increase in body weight occurred, double the amount at double the rate of the earlier study. These workers concluded that the forced gaining of weight was a full-time occupation. Even in the prison study, some subjects did not gain weight, and although the reasons for this are not understood, it was apparent that the level of spontaneous activity was an important factor. For instance, whenever spontaneous activity appeared low, weight increased more rapidly. Perhaps the most striking finding is that when the forced feeding was terminated, weights rapidly returned to pre-experimental levels.

There have been several other experiments in forced feeding.

Passmore et al. compared (17, 18) forced feeding in three thin young men and two obese females, approximately 50 per cent overweight, who previously had been heavier, one by 40 lb. and the other by 57 lb. Observations were made for twenty-three days. For the first nine days (control period), the subjects were given a diet containing 3,390 kcal; during the second nine days, they received 4,490 kcal per day (an excess of approximately 1,100 kcal per day); and for the last five days, 350 kcal per day. Both subjects lost less than 2 lb. during the control period, then gained 6.3 lb. and 5.7 lb. during the overfeeding period. Using a similar protocol, Passmore fed three thin young men, who were approximately 20 per cent under ideal weight, an excess of from 1,400 to 1,800 kcal per day for ten to fourteen days. They gained weight during overfeeding but required almost twice the calories of the obese women to achieve similar weight gains. The thin subjects required an excess of approximately 20,000 kcal to gain 5½ lb., whereas the two obese women gained the same weight on an excess of approximately 10,000 kcal. This difference is partially explained by the excessive water retention of the obese women. Nevertheless, it appears that the thin men were more resistant to weight gain. Studies longer than nine or ten days are clearly needed to clarify the mechanisms involved in weight gain.

In a similar vein, Miller and Mumford conducted experiments (19) in which sixteen normal-weight subjects received an average of 1,400 kcal a day above their usual intakes for four to eight weeks. They were given either high- or low-protein diets, and during this time, weights and metabolic rates were determined for all subjects. The expected weight gain from the excessive calories did not occur. In fact, a subject receiving an excess of 8,000 to 10,000 kcal in a week occasionally lost weight. The most weight gained by any subject during eight weeks was 10 lb.; —an increase of 7 per cent of initial body weight. The basal metabolic rate did not increase during the overeating period, but the 24-hr. consumption of oxygen did. The authors concluded that, as a result of the excess input of calories, changes occurred to increase expenditure of energy and therefore, weight gain was resisted.

Quite clearly, then, the organism resists alterations in energy balance in either direction and defends its body weight. Moreover, similar evidence indicates that the obese individual may be as resistant as the normal person. Is it possible to conclude, then, that the obese person, even though we define his weight as abnormal, is actually in equilibrium but regulating at a different level of body weight? Is this why weight loss is so difficult and is usually followed by a rapid return to pre-diet weight? If the obese person is in equilibrium, then the reasons for our repeated failures at weight reduction become clear. Are we indeed asking the obese person to live in a constant state of semistarvation?

The time element

If the concept of stable, body-weight equilibrium is valid, there must be some mechanism that determines the level of body weight at which equilibrium will occur. At present, these mechanisms are unknown, but it is evident that they must allow the equilibrium to shift to new levels. How long must a new level of weight be maintained before a new equilibrium is reached? Certainly from the work of Keys and coworkers and of Sims *et al.*, six months is not long enough for permanent change to occur; all of the subjects in these experiments rapidly returned to pre-experimental weights. In the study by Keys *et al.*, however, the levels achieved by semistarvation were quite drastic, and it is difficult to assume that a new equilibrium would exist at such a low level of body weight.

Knowledge of the time needed to achieve new equilibrium would certainly have important implications for the treatment of obesity. Perhaps rapid and forceful intervention early in the development of obesity before a new equilibrium is obtained would be effective. The work of Hirsch and Knittle shows (20) critical phases in childhood when fat cell hyperplasia occurs. Prevention of an increase in the number of fat cells in the young child could be enormously important. In the case of adult-onset obesity, it is clear that the number of fat cells does not increase, but the size of fat cells does. Could this be the basis for equilibrium at a high weight level in obesity? We do not know. We do know, however, that the longer a person has been obese, the more difficult weight loss becomes.

If it is true that a long time is required to establish a new equilibrium, then we must devise methods for maintaining disequilibrium for long intervals, even if we do not know the mechanisms at work. While short-term weight losses can be achieved, it is difficult to control both the intake and the output or expenditure of energy for long enough to maintain weight loss and allow equilibrium to occur at a new and lower weight level.

Behavior modification

Recently, psychologists and psychiatrists have applied the techniques of behavior modification to the treatment of obesity, and there is some possibility that this method may provide the long-term control needed. Behavior modification, behavior therapy, and experimental analysis of behavior are techniques which attempt to apply the data and methods of experimental psychology to disorders of human behavior. The underlying philosophy is based on the principles of learning, with the assumption that if a behavior is learned, it can be retrained, or, if unlearned, it can be shaped.

Behavior modification in the treatment of obesity is directed at both the control of ingestive behavior (the when, why, where, and how much) and the control of the activity and energy expenditure of the individual. The concept is that the changes in eating behavior and activity ultimately become permanent, and, therefore, the possibility for long-term alteration of equilibrium is enhanced.

Stunkard has recently reviewed (21) the results of behavior modification in the treatment of eating disorders, so that a detailed discussion of these programs will not be presented here. However, in this issue, Levitz presents (22) the theory and techniques of behavior modification and describes the results of a pilot study involving behavior modification in a self-help group.

Summary

It is clear that obesity is a multifaceted problem, involving both physiologic and psychologic aspects. Regardless of its etiology, perhaps its resistance to our therapeutic efforts is due to the fact that it represents a stable, biologic equilibrium that takes years to build to a high level and similarly may take a long time to return to a lower and more satisfactory level. Future investigations of both animals and man should focus on the long-term psychologic and physiologic aspects of food intake and energy expenditure that operate in defense of body weight.

References

(1) BRILLAT-SAVARIN, J.A.: The Physiology of Taste. (Transl. from French by Fisher, M.F.K.) N.Y.: Alfred A. Knopf, 1971.
(2) FLINT, A., JR.: The Physiology of Man. N.Y.: D. Appleton, 1870.
(3) BEAUMONT, W.: Experiments and Observations on the Gastric Juice and the Physiology of Digestion. N.Y.: Dover Publications, 1959.
(4) OSLER, W.: The Principles and Practice of Medicine. N.Y.: D. Appleton, 1893.

(5) PASSMORE, R.: The regulation of body weight in man. Proc. Nutr. Soc. 30 (Pt. 2): 122, 1971.

(6) STUNKARD, A.J., AND McLAREN-HUME, M.: The results of treatment for obesity. A review of the literature and report of a series. Arch. Intern. Med. 103: 79, 1959.

(7) HAMILTON, C.L., AND BROBECK, J.R.: Hypothalamic hyperphagia in monkeys. J. Comp. Physiol. Psychol. 57: 271, 1964.

(8) HAMILTON, C.L.: Physiologic control of food intake. J. Am. Dietet. A. 62: 35, 1973.

(9) JORDAN, H.A.: Voluntary intragastic feeding: Oral and gastric contributions to food intake and hunger in man. J. Comp. Physiol. Psychol. 68: 498, 1969.

(10) SPIEGEL, T.: The caloric regulation of food intake in man. PH.D. thesis, University of Pennsylvania, 1971.

(11) KEYS, A., BROZEK, J., HENSCHEL, A., MICKELSEN, O., and TAYLOR, H.L.: The Biology of Human Starvation. Vols. 1 & 2. Minneapolis: Univ. of Minnesota Press, 1950.

(12) SALISBURY, H.E.: The 900 Days: The Siege of Leningrad. N.Y.: Harper & Row, 1969.

(13) STUNKARD, A.J.: The "dieting depression": Incidence and clinical characteristics of untoward responses to weight reduction regimens. Am. J. Med. 23: 77, 1957.

(14) BRAY, G.A.: Effect of caloric restriction on energy expenditure in obese patients. Lancet 2: 397, 1969.

(15) GRINKER, J.: Behavioral and metabolic consequences of weight reduction. J. Am. Dietet. A. 62: 30, 1973.

(16) SIMS, E.A.H., GOLDMAN, R.F., GLUCK, C.M., HORTON. E.S., KELLEHER, P.C., AND ROWE, D.W.: Experimental obesity in man. Trans. Assoc. Am. Physicians 81: 153, 1968.

(17) PASSMORE, R., STRONG, J.A., SWINDELLS, Y.E., AND EL DIN, N.: The effect of overfeeding on two fat young women. Brit. J. Nutr. 17: 373, 1963.

(18) PASSMORE, R., MEIKLEJOHN, A.P., DEWAR, A.D., AND THOW, R.K.: Energy utilization in overfed thin young men. Br. J. Nutr. 9: 20, 1955.

(19) MILLER, D.S., AND MUMFORD, P.: Gluttony. 1. An experimental study of overeating low- or high-protein diets. Am. J. Clin. Nutr. 20: 1212, 1967.

(20) HIRSCH, J., AND KNITTLE, J.L.: Cellularity of obese and nonobese human adipose tissue. Fed. Proc. 29: 1516, 1970.

(21) STUNKARD, A.J.: New therapies for the eating disorders: Behavior modification of obesity and anorexia nervosa. Arch. Gen. Psychiatry 76: 391, 1972.

(22) LEVITZ, L.S.: Application of behavioral therapy to obesity. J. Am. Dietet. A. 62: 22, 1973.

Multidisciplinary approach to the problem of obesity[1]

THEODORE B. VAN ITALLIE, M.D.,
and ROBERT G. CAMPBELL, M.D.
*Medical Service, St. Luke's Hospital Center, and Institute
of Human Nutrition, College of Physicians and Surgeons,
Columbia University, New York City; and Monroe Community Hospital, Department of Medicine, School of Medicine
and Dentistry, University of Rochester, Rochester, New York*

*Because of the complex inter-
relationships between regulatory
and metabolic factors that affect
energy balance, the etiology of
obesity remains unclear. An
eclectic approach that uses
methodologies drawn from a
variety of disciplines appears
to offer the best promise of
a solution.*

There are at least two fundamentally different ways of looking at obesity. One is to view the condition as being caused by a disorder of some sort in the body's metabolism which favors increasing triglyceride storage. In its simplest terms, this approach suggests that obesity results because a superfluity of food is pulled into the body, as shown schematically in Figure 1. Alternatively, the accumulation of surplus fat may result from an alteration (not necessarily a derangement) in the central mechanism that normally adapts energy intake to needs. The second approach suggests that an excess of food is "pushed" into the body as indicated in Figure 2. It will be noted that the "push" and "pull" concepts are derived from the more formal classification that divides the obesities under two broad headings, "regulatory" and "metabolic" (see outline on page 386).

This concept of regulatory vs. metabolic obesity, useful as it is, is probably oversimplified. The problem is that metabolic changes within the body are capable of having a direct as well as an indirect effect on the neural centers concerned with regulation of energy balance. One can visualize a "metabolic regulatory" disorder in which, for example, some hormonal imbalance might influence the way the satiety center in the brain responds to postingestion satiety signals or to metabolic information about the organism's nutritional status transmitted from the periphery. Thus, it would seem that the only clear-cut distinction between push and pull would entail separation of psychologic from physiologic factors affecting food intake. Conceivably, lesions involving the regulatory centers could be purely regulatory; however, it is known that such lesions also may have direct metabolic consequences.

Hyperplasia vs. hypertrophy

Within the last few years, attention has been increasingly focused on the organ of obesity, namely, the adipose tissue of obese patients. It has been observed (1) that some obese individuals, notably those whose adiposity developed in infancy or early adolescence, exhibit a vast increase in fat cell number (hyperplasia). This inordinate proliferation of fat cells may represent the body's response to an overgenerous in-

[1]Presented at the 54th Annual Meeting of The American Dietetic Association in Philadelphia, on October 7, 1971.

Tentative grouping of forms of obesity according to mechanism

I. Regulatory obesity (no primary metabolic abnormality)
    A. Psychologic.
        1. Non-neurotic overeating (orientation toward "external" and sensory cues relating to the eating process).
        2. Overeating associated with neurosis.
    B. Physiologic.
        1. Increased energy intake (brain damage).
        2. Decreased energy output (sedentary existence).

II. Metabolic obesity
    A. Enzymatic (?certain forms of genetic obesity).
    B. Hormonal (hyperadrenocorticism).
    C. Neurologic (?certain forms of lipodystrophy).

III. "Constitutional" obesity.
    A. Fat cell hyperplasia.

take of food during certain critical periods of development; however, a genetic predisposition to hypercellularity of adipose tissue also may be involved. In contrast to individuals who suffer from what might be called growth-onset obesity, persons who first become obese in the third decade or later (maturity-onset obesity) appear to have enlarged fat cells (hypertrophy) without a corresponding increase in adipose tissue cellularity.

All obese patients exhibit some enlargement of fat cells, but individuals with marked obesity usually have more cells. In general, individuals with marked obesity first became overweight as children. Hirsch has theorized (2) that a basic defect might involve an inability to limit fat cell size; at appropriate stages of development, this loss of control also could trigger adipocyte hyperplasia.

The number of fat cells appears to be fixed after adolescence; however, the size of the fat cell may vary widely throughout life depending on changes in energy balance. Thus, it is clearly important to attempt to assess all the processes, regulatory and metabolic, that can determine the degree of "fatness" of the adipocyte and, by extension, the degree of obesity.

The metabolic approach

As has been so often pointed out, the kind of questions we ask tend to delimit the potential answers. Thus, research that seeks to account for obesity by identifying suitable biochemical abnormalities will tell us little or nothing about the possible etiologic role of non-physiologic factors. The direction research takes is strongly influenced by the analytic methods available. Indeed, the scientific imagination is conditioned and necessarily restricted by the investigator's grasp of the possibilities of methodology. Accordingly, it is not surprising that early workers sought to explain human obesity in terms of such metabolic concepts as "luxus consumption" and "lipophilia." As we

"PULL" THEORY

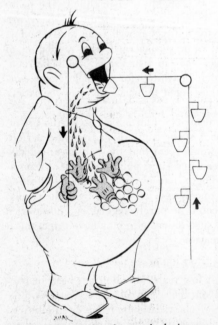

FIG. 1. *The "pull" theory of obesity proposes that a subtle metabolic disorder increases food intake either (a) by affecting hunger-satiety signals transmitted to a "satiety center" or (b) by altering the threshold of the satiety center to such signals.*

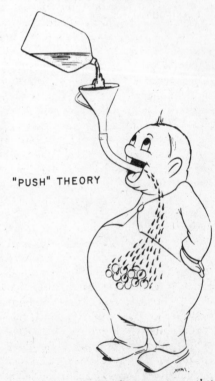

"PUSH" THEORY

FIG. 2. *The "push" theory proposes that the obese person "force-feeds" himself, overeating for non-physiologic reasons.*

know, these efforts proved fruitless, and the more recent and more sophisticated attempts to demonstrate a primary biochemical "lesion" in obese patients at best have yielded equivocal results. However, attempts still are being made, and it would not be wise to foreclose the possibility that, at some point in time, such a lesion will be identified.

For a while, the fact that it was not possible to comprehend the pathogenesis of most human obesity in biochemical terms left the field in a state of scientific bankruptcy. The medical profession, and others, had to be satisfied with the apparent tautologism: "Obesity is caused by overeating."

The very existence of such terms as "exogenous obesity," together with the rather widely held notion that obese persons are that way simply because they "overeat," suggests a tacit acceptance by many observers of the likelihood that regulatory factors are responsible for much of human obesity. However, to a considerable extent, obesity research remained cloistered in the province of metabolically-oriented investigators, most of whom either did not possess or were unaware of the techniques needed to study obesity as a regulatory problem.

The behavioral approach

When new questions finally began to be asked, they were framed in the language of sociology, psychiatry, and experimental psychology. Anliker and Mayer used (3) operant conditioning techniques developed by Skinner (4) to study feeding behavior in normal mice made hyperphagic by administration of gold thioglucose. They learned that the overall rate of feeding of the gold thioglucose-treated mice was much greater than that of the normal controls. Normal mice showed 24-hr. feeding cycles in which there was an initial phase characterized by rapid feeding followed by a second phase in which the rate of feeding decelerated. Such cycling was suppressed in the hyperphagic animals; they ate constantly and gained weight rapidly up to a certain point. Then the 24-hr. cycles reappeared, and the animals' weight curves leveled off as though the mechanism regulating body weight or fat content had been altered to a higher setting.

Miller, a physiologic psychologist, used behavioral measures to study hunger drive in rats with surgically-induced hypothalamic hyperphagia. He found (5) an unexpected discrepancy between the amount of food eaten by the hyperphagic animals and the motivation to eat. For example, the animals with lesions ate much more than the controls, but when they were forced to work to obtain food or if the food was made slightly bitter with quinine, they consumed considerably less than the controls. These observations, together with the results of other studies conducted by Teitelbaum (6), suggested that the hypothalamic-hyperphagic animals continued to overeat because of lack of satiety rather than because of an increased drive

for food. In other words, the lesions did not induce the same general motivational effects as a normal increase of hunger.

Bruch, a child psychiatrist, has pointed out (7) that because of certain experiences in infancy, food and eating can be invested with a special emotional meaning for many obese children and adolescents. Thus, for them, food and eating may serve as surrogates for maternal affection and reassurance. According to Bruch, ". . . the early feeding experience may be too satisfying when both mother and child have a strong interest in food, as often occurs in obese families. Feeding may remain the only situation in which mutual satisfaction is experienced, particularly if the mother is unable to give of herself."

Stunkard and his associates have called attention (8) to the interesting and significant fact that a marked inverse relationship exists between the prevalence of obesity and socio-economic status. One survey showed that the prevalence of obesity among women of lower socio-economic status was 30 per cent, but fell to 16 per cent among those of middle status, and to only 5 per cent in the affluent group. Penick and Stunkard also have pointed out (9) that a distinctive kind of disturbance of body image is one of the very few psychopathologic characteristics specific to obesity.

Recently, Schachter, a social psychologist, and his students have carried out a series of ingenious experiments (10) which have provided increasingly strong support for the concept that obese individuals are relatively insensitive to "internal" (physiologic) cues for hunger and satiety, but are more than normally responsive to "external" and sensory cues related to the eating process. Such cues include the time of day and the sight, appearance, setting, aroma, proximity, and taste of food. In Schachter's view, eating in lean persons is controlled principally by internal signals, being influenced relatively little by external cues. In contrast, obese subjects eat and, indeed, overeat in response to external and sensory cues and appear unable to perceive the physiologic signals that presumably announce hunger and satiety in lean individuals. Schachter's work contains the implication that obesity develops because of a defect in the obese individual's energy regulatory processes that presumably involves a relative insensitivity to internal hunger-satiety cues.

Some new behavioral questions

Although our group could be considered metabolically oriented, we chose to pursue the problem of human obesity by asking behavioral as well as metabolic questions. We wondered how lean and obese subjects would regulate energy intake when they received all of their food as a nutritionally complete liquid diet dispensed on demand by an automatically monitored "feeding machine" (Figure 3). This apparatus has been described in detail elsewhere (11, 12); however, eight years of experience with its use in studying lean

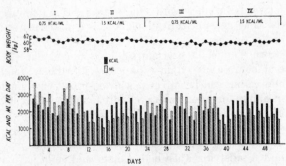

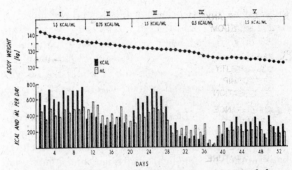

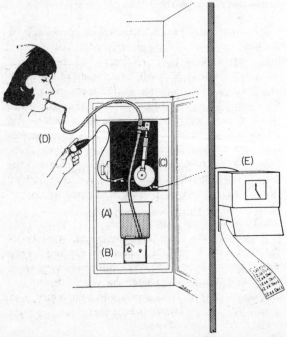

FIG. 3. *Monitored food-dispensing machine. The formula diet (A) is constantly mixed by a magnetic stirrer (B). Tubing from the reservoir leads to a dispensing syringe-type pump (C), which delivers a bolus of formula through the mouthpiece. The entire unit is contained within a refrigerator. The pump is adjusted to respond with a single delivery cycle to the signal of an actuating button (D). Whenever the button is pressed, a predetermined volume of homogenized formula is delivered directly into the subject's mouth by the pump. Each delivery is recorded by a printing timer (E) that records each event, the date and precise time at which it occurred. The timer and recorder are in a room remote from the subject who is unaware of their existence. When the apparatus is in use, the reservoir and pump are covered.*

FIG. 4. *Responses of a lean adult subject to concealed variations in nutritive density. He spontaneously maintained a relatively constant energy intake by making appropriate adjustments in volume of consumption.*

FIG. 5. *Responses of an obese adult patient to concealed variations in nutritive density. He consumed far fewer calories than were needed to maintain body weight and also exhibited no adaptation to the covert changes in caloric density.*

volunteer subjects and obese patients have yielded new information pertinent both to obesity and to the problem of normal food intake regulation.

Briefly, we have observed the following (13): Lean, young adults spontaneously take sufficient calories by machine to maintain their weight at a near constant level for many weeks. In dramatic contrast, grossly obese adults spontaneously take far fewer calories than are needed to maintain energy equilibrium and lose weight rapidly. Lean subjects adapt to concealed changes in the nutritive density of their diet by changing the volume of liquid food ingested so as to maintain a constant caloric intake (Figure 4). Obese subjects fail to show this kind of adjustment to covert changes in caloric concentration (Figure 5). It is important to point out that the subjects have had no way of estimating their energy intake except by counting the mouthfuls of diet swallowed from the dispensing device. Moreover, they have had no way of knowing the number of calories per mouthful and have not been aware that every calorie consumed and the times of consumption were being recorded by a printing timer in another room.

The observation that lean young adults spontaneously regulate their food intake by machine so as to keep weight constant was not unexpected; however, it came as something of a surprise to find that obese adults reduce their energy intake to levels of the order of 20 per cent of the calories needed to maintain energy equilibrium. (When given the opportunity, these same obese individuals consistently consumed quite generous quantities of regular hospital food.)

Why the feeding-machine effect?

Why do the obese subjects consistently reduce their food intake so drastically in the feeding machine situation? Their behavior may be interpreted in several ways. One can postulate that the usual obese subject overeats for non-physiologic reasons. For example, he may use food as an inappropriate means for relieving anxiety or boredom. Or, the hedonistic aspect of eating may be sufficiently reinforcing to overwhelm whatever defenses the body maintains against excessive food intake. Whatever the reason, it is evident that the feeding machine arrangement eliminates most, if not all, of the non-physiologic attractions of food and eating, reducing the former to mere calories and nutrients, and the latter to a monotonous swallowing of mouthfuls of bland liquid.

Under these unappetizing circumstances, the obese individual who was previously "force-feeding" himself with excessive quantities of food (which incidentally also contained excess calories) reverts to a physiologically more normal situation. By "normal,"

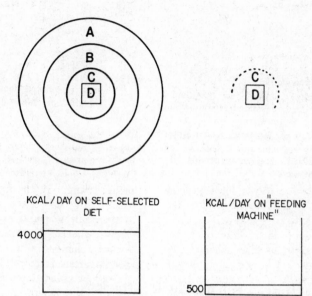

A. RELIEF OF ANXIETY
   AND BOREDOM
   "SECURITY"

B. HABIT
   CONVIVIALITY
   FRIENDSHIP
   CELEBRATION

C. APPEARANCE
   AROMA
   FLAVOR
   TEXTURE
   TEMPERATURE
   VOLUME

D. CALORIES
   NUTRIENTS

KCAL/DAY ON SELF-SELECTED DIET

4000

KCAL/DAY ON "FEEDING MACHINE"

500

FIG. 6. *Some non-nutritive attributes of food believed to affect caloric intake in certain obese individuals. The removal of many of these attributes in the feeding machine situation may help to account for the remarkable reduction in energy intake exhibited by obese subjects who obtain all of their food as liquid homogenate from the monitored dispensing apparatus.*

we mean that one could expect the grossly obese patient to fast spontaneously once the extraphysiologic drive to overeat was turned off. Rats made obese by force-feeding limit food intake spontaneously and lose weight rapidly once the force-feeding has ceased (14). This, in effect, is what our obese patients seem to do under feeding-machine conditions.

One also could argue that our obese subjects, being motivated to lose weight, voluntarily restrict caloric intake while receiving their food from the dispensing apparatus. This possibility has not been completely ruled out; however, there are several reasons why such voluntary abstention is unlikely. First, the phenomenon of spontaneous, dramatic reduction of caloric intake has occurred repeatedly day after day in every obese subject we have studied; second, the subjects could not estimate their intake and had no way of knowing that their input was being monitored; third, they usually ate all of the regular hospital diet offered, even though their motivation to lose weight was presumably ever-present.

Hypotheses

If one accepts Schachter's hypothesis that obese subjects are insensitive to hunger-satiety cues, then it is possible to contend that the machine-feeding situation has removed most of the external cues that drive the obese individual to eat, and that he is unable to perceive the physiologic signals announcing hunger to which lean subjects normally respond. It is also possible that such signals are physiologically attenuated in grossly obese individuals as a normal defense against further overeating. A third possibility is that

satiety signals begin to be perceived by obese individuals when they are no longer "distracted" by external cues. In any case, if the "pull theory" of obesity were correct, it would be difficult to explain the spontaneous fasting of obese patients during machine-feeding. Thus, it seems more likely that the obese individual is, indeed, overeating for non-physiologic reasons and that, as we strip away the non-nutritive epiphenomena of food, namely, appearance, variety, aroma, taste, and so on, we remove the very attributes to which the obese subject is so attracted and leave him instead with the bare bones of nutrition (Figure 6).

Unexplored territories

The new questions, both physiologic and non-physiologic, that have been asked about obesity are beginning to generate new answers; this time they seem more pertinent. However, over the years, obesity has relinquished its mysteries slowly and reluctantly, and we have no way of knowing how many more secrets remain hidden from view.

At first glance, the evidence seems overwhelming that most maturity-onset obesity is non-physiologic in origin and may be considered in large part a psychosomatic disorder. However, the adipose tissue hypercellularity of patients with growth-onset obesity cannot be easily explained in non-physiologic terms, and the apparent "blindness" of obese persons to internal hunger-satiety cues could be the expression of a subtle biochemical or physiologic defect. Thus, the new investigative territories that have been opened up remain largely unexplored and unexploited. For these tasks, the efforts of a number of disciplines, within and outside of conventional clinical nutrition, will be required for a long time.

References

(1) HIRSCH, J., AND KNITTLE, J.L.: Cellularity of obese and nonobese human adipose tissue. Fed. Proc. 29: 1516, 1970.

(2) HIRSCH, J.: Personal communication.

(3) ANLIKER, J., AND MAYER, J.: An operant conditioning technique for studying feeding-fasting patterns in normal and obese mice. J. Appl. Physiol. 8: 667, 1956.

(4) SKINNER, B.F.: Behavior of Organisms. N.Y.: Appleton Co., 1938.

(5) MILLER, N.E., BAILEY, C.J., AND STEVENSON, J.A.F.: Decreased "hunger" but increased food intake resulting from hypothalamic lesions. Science 112: 256, 1950.

(6) TEITELBAUM, P.: Sensory control of hypothalamic hyperphagia. J. Comp. Physiol. Psychol. 48: 156, 1955.

(7) BRUCH, H.: Obesity in childhood. 3. Physiologic and psychologic aspects of the food intake of obese children. Am. J. Dis. Child. 58: 738, 1940.

(8) GOLDBLATT, P.B., MOORE, M.E., AND STUNKARD, A.J.: Social factors in obesity. JAMA 192: 1039, 1965.

(9) PENICK, S.B., AND STUNKARD, A.J.: Newer concepts of obesity. Med. Clin. N. Am. 54: 745, 1970.

(10) SCHACHTER, S.: Obesity and eating. Science 161: 751, 1968.

(11) HASHIM, S.A., AND VAN ITALLIE, T.B.: An automatically monitored food dispensing apparatus for the study of food intake in man. Fed. Proc. 23: 82, 1964.

(12) HASHIM, S.A., AND VAN ITALLIE, T.B.: Studies in normal and obese subjects with a monitored food dispensing device. Ann. N.Y. Acad. Sci. 131: 654, 1965.

(13) CAMPBELL, R.G., HASHIM, S.A., AND VAN ITALLIE, T.B.: Studies of food intake regulation in man. Responses to variations in nutritive density in lean and obese subjects. N. Engl. J. Med. 285, 1402, 1971.

(14) COHN, C., AND JOSEPH, D.: Influences of body weight and fat on appetite of "normal" lean and obese rats. Yale J. Biol. Med. 34, 598, 1962.

Overeating, blood cholesterol, and heart attacks

Just what is the relationship between overeating, atherosclerosis, and heart attacks? At a meeting last November of the American Heart Association in Anaheim, California, Drs. Katti R. Dzoga and Dragoslava Vesselinovitch of the Department of Pathology, University of Chicago reported on work of a team studying the effects of blood fats on aortic tissue culture cells, and the fraction of fat in the blood which is responsible for changes in aortic cells which lead to atherosclerosis.

Working mainly with the aortas of rhesus monkeys, the researchers remove the artery, and the cells are grown from small pieces in a tissue culture system where they are "fed" various lipids. The cells grow if serum from normal animals is given to them. However, with serum from animals fed high-fat diets, the cells grow and divide much faster than with serum from animals on normal diets. This stimulates the growth component of hardening of the arteries. Low-density lipoproteins from animals on high-fat diets are most effective in stimulating cell growth, indicating that high-fat diets are responsible for acceleration of atherosclerosis.

In a man or an animal who overeats, more fat gets into the blood stream. The aortic cells take up this fat and multiply, causing lesions which ultimately lead to hardening of the arteries. Therefore, the more fat on a person's body, the more cholesterol and lipoproteins are in his blood. Blood cholesterol levels usually reflect the amount of low-density lipoproteins circulating and thus the probable development of atherosclerosis in arteries.

Once the arteries take up fat, depending on the type and amount, the cells respond by proliferation, injury, or death. The resulting lesions lead to hardening of the arteries.

The University of Chicago pathologists are studying the components of the lipoproteins in animals fed a high-fat diet which causes the increase in growth of aortic cells. Although serum cholesterol is an index to the cause, they are asking, "Is it actually the real culprit?"—*From HSMHA Health Reports* 86: 131 (February), 1972.

OBESITY

JEAN MAYER, Ph.D., D.Sc.
Professor of nutrition
Harvard University School of Public Health
Consultant in nutrition
Children's Hospital Medical Center
Boston

The ability of the human organism to store large amounts of fat served mankind well when availability of food was seasonal and a continued supply precarious. Under the conditions of life now prevailing in richer countries or among wealthier classes in poorer countries, this accumulation of fat no longer has a *raison d'être*. Because of the penalties to health, comfort and appearance, obesity has become a matter of considerable medical and general concern.

Definition

Obesity used to be defined in relation to height and age. Then it was defined by insurance companies in terms of desirable weight for persons with a small, medium or large frame; however, each type of frame was not characterized. Obesity is properly defined as an excess relative body fat content. The diagnosis is obvious from appearance alone in the very obese person. More moderate obesity is identified by determining subcutaneous fat through skinfold measurement or by calculating body fat through measurement of body density, total body water, body radiopotassium, or other means. The most practical of these definitions is that based on skinfolds, with the most representative skinfold obtained at midtriceps.

The studies leading to the present widespread interest in the relationship of obesity to increased morbidity and mortality were concerned with overweight rather than obesity as such; that is, they defined obesity in terms of excess weight for a given height rather than in terms of fat content. While a very fat (or very heavy) person is both obese and

13

overweight, an individual who is moderately overweight may or may not be obese. Conversely, a sedentary person with poorly developed muscles and an excessive proportion of fat can be obese without being overweight.

Medical Significance

The medical significance of obesity derives essentially from insurance studies. It is useful to consider results of these studies, even though they should be interpreted with reservations. A long-term study of build and blood pressure by the Society of Actuaries showed that among five million insured persons, the mortality in 15 to 69 year old men was one-third greater in those who were 20 percent or more overweight than in those considered "standard risks." Among men 10 percent or more overweight, mortality was one-fifth greater. Overweight women had a somewhat better experience, although the penalty of overweight did increase with weight and with age. (Actually, persons considered standard risks were not necessarily at their most desirable weight. When overweight subjects are compared with men in the weight range with the best experience, the excess mortality is nearly one-half for those 20 percent overweight and is one-third for those 10 percent overweight.)

The excess mortality of men 20 percent or more overweight is associated with the following conditions, in order of frequency: diabetes, diseases of the digestive system, cerebral hemorrhage, heart disease. In women, heart disease replaces diseases of the digestive system in second place.

The effects of overweight are both physical and psychologic. A number of chronic illnesses are made worse by overweight. In arthritis, for example, it leads to greater immobilization, which in turn is likely to make both conditions worse. The condition of the middle-aged diabetic often improves dramatically with weight reduction. Obese people are accident-prone. Surgical procedures are more difficult technically in obese patients.

The "psychology of being obese" is a subject of growing importance. Obese adolescent girls exhibit traits similar to those of minorities subjected to intense prejudice: heightened sensitivity, obsessive concern (with weight), passivity, withdrawal. Being obese during adolescence leads to attitudes (and forms of neuroses) quite different from those observed in persons of normal weight or in persons who become obese during adulthood.

Prevalence

We do not have good data on prevalence of obesity for the population as a whole. Among insured persons, half of the men between 30 and 39 years of age are at least 10 percent overweight and a fourth are at least 20 percent overweight in terms of actual weight compared with weight associated with lowest mortality. These proportions are highest (60 and 33 percent, respectively) in the 50 to 59 year range. Among women the percentages are somewhat lower before age 40, the same at 40 to 49, and greater beyond 49 years. Data for children are sparse. My studies in the Boston suburbs indicate that 10 percent of schoolchildren are overweight.

Longitudinal data permitting a forecast of the evolution of obesity in children are even more meager. In general, studies bearing on this matter emphasize the persistence of childhood obesity. I believe that obesity developing in younger children (before 10 years) or in adolescents (after 16) has a somber prognosis for eventual "spontaneous" weight reduction, whereas obesity developing just before puberty may be an exaggeration of a normal physiologic process and is often self-correcting in a few years.

It has been noted that in the United States obesity is much more prevalent in the lower than in the upper middle and upper socioeconomic classes. A different pattern is seen in poor countries.

Etiology

Ascribing obesity to "overeating" is at worst a tautology, at best an oversimplification. Certainly obesity will not develop unless caloric intake exceeds caloric expenditure. In my experience, normal intake with very low activity is characteristic of the majority of obese children and adolescents in the United States. Obese men tend toward high intake and low activity. Obese women often show both increased intake and low activity.

Detailed descriptions of energy balance do no more than scratch the surface of the problem. For example, before we can describe the pathology of the regulation of food intake, we should know more about the normal mechanism. Our knowledge in this area is still meager.

Regulation of Food Intake

The regulation of food intake appears to be complex, resting on cerebral and extra-cerebral components. An essential component is a pair of centers situated in the ventromedial area of the hypothalamus which act as satiety "brakes" on more lateral symmetric centers that apparently are otherwise constantly activated. The ventromedial area also exerts some measure of control over gastric "hunger contractions." My co-workers and I were the first to suggest that the glucose utilization rate of certain of its cells may activate the ventromedial area. This has been experimentally confirmed in our laboratory and elsewhere. However, this is only part of the overall mechanism; other factors include temperature, osmotic pressure, gastric filling, and conditioning. The role of learning in connection with recognition of such physiologic stimuli is beginning to receive attention.

All in all, it is obvious that the mechanism of regulation of food intake is subject to many possible influences which can bring about an increase in food intake and hence weight accumulation, just as a multiplicity of factors may bring about anorexia and weight loss.

The Obesities

Classification of human obesity is in its infancy, but we know it has a strong familial component, and the evidence suggests that a large component of this familial incidence is genetic. The association of obesity with body types and the possibility that obesity is conditioned by the genetically determined number of body fat cells also emphasize the importance of heredity. Trauma in the form of hypothalamic damage, endocrine disorders, and psychologic stresses also leads to obesity.

Study of the influence of environmental factors has shown that in man, as in animals, reduced physical activity is not followed by a corresponding decrease in food intake. This phenomenon is particularly significant in children and adolescents.

In addition to the above etiologic factors, a distinction between regulatory obesities (hypothalamic, due to conditioning) and metabolic obesities (hereditary obese hyperglycemic syndrome, ACTH tumors) appears to be valid for man. Considerable work needs to be done before specific human obesity syndromes are identified. Until then, efforts at cure or prevention will be directed essentially at influencing the energy balance by reducing intake, increasing activity, and giving psychologic support (motivation to reduce, correction of self-image, and more rarely, correction of a deeper-seated problem underlying "psychogenic" obesity).

Treatment

The general medical case for treatment of obesity, as opposed to the obvious "cosmetic" case, is based on the favorable mortality experience of previously obese groups. Treatment should be based on a thorough knowledge of the evolution of the obesity and of the patient's dietary habits, caloric intake, exercise habits, and energy expenditure in general. Past changes in intake and physical activity should be identified. Family history of overweight, illnesses, and causes of death gives clues to the probable course of the obesity and its likely relation to health and longevity. Determination of the role of obesity in the patient's life situation and of reactions to dieting and weight loss indicates whether the patient should reduce weight.

When the decision to reduce weight is made, the practical task is to take off excess fat at a rate sufficient to be meaningful for a finite period, e.g., six months to a year, yet not so much as to prevent normal function and comfort. A daily deficit of 1000 cal will cause loss of 2 lb a week, a sufficient rate of loss in almost all cases. Half of this rate would still be acceptable. This deficit may be achieved by reducing intake, increasing activity, or both. The diet should be nutritionally acceptable, provide nutrition education, and have sufficient satiety value. For some patients, five snacks a day rather than three meals help to prevent excessive hunger. Amphetamines given to prevent peaks of hunger have proved useful in some cases when diet alone is ineffective.

Increasing physical activity is desirable unless there are strong medical contraindications. Psychologic support is an important part of therapy. A proper psychologic approach is particularly important with children and adolescents. In adolescent girls especially, such dangerous syndromes as anorexia nervosa may sometimes be the result of tactless treatment for obesity.

Newer Concepts of Obesity

SYDNOR B. PENICK, M.D.*

ALBERT J. STUNKARD, M.D.**

Recent research on obesity has done far more than merely advance our understanding of this condition. In distinction to most earlier research in the field, it has provided information upon which it may be possible for the first time to construct effective treatment programs. This is welcome news, for careful study of the results of treatment for obesity have revealed that "most obese persons will not enter treatment; of those who do, most will not lose weight; and of those who lose weight, most will regain it."[19]

The traditional medical view ascribes these failures quite simply to an inability of obese persons to control their food intake—an observation approximately as helpful as that which ascribes alcoholism to an inability to control alcohol intake. And the traditional response of physicians has been similar—frustration and even anger.

Newer research findings have provided support for the concept that obesity is a disease of multiple etiology. Evidence has been developed of (1) the influence of social factors upon the prevalence of obesity, (2) the influence of situational determinants upon overeating, (3) distinctive characteristics of the physiology of adipose tissue, (4) the determinants of disturbance in the body image of some obese persons, and (5) the effectiveness of behavioral measures for the control of obesity.

SOCIAL CLASS AND OBESITY

Within the very recent past a series of studies have documented precisely a heretofore suspected determinant of obesity: social class. To a

From the Department of Psychiatry, University of Pennsylvania, Philadelphia, Pennsylvania

*Resident in Psychiatry; Director of Research, Carrier Clinic Foundation, Belle Mead, New Jersey
**Professor and Chairman of the Department of Psychiatry

Supported in part by a grant (No. MH-15383) from the National Institute of Mental Health, U.S. Public Health Service.

remarkable degree the prevalence of obesity in the general population is under the control of social factors. The most carefully studied is probably socioeconomic status, as defined by education and occupation. In at least three urban populations in the United States and Great Britain, socioeconomic status is inversely related to the prevalence of obesity, particularly in women, and often to a surprising degree.

The first dramatic evidence of the influence of social factors came from the Midtown Manhattan study, a comprehensive survey of the epidemiology of mental illness. Subjects consisted of 1660 adults, between the ages of 20 and 59, selected by stratified random sampling so that their social class distribution approximated that of a far larger area. Subjects were divided into three weight categories, "obese," "normal," and "thin," by measures whose validity seems acceptable. Socioeconomic status was rated through an interview by a simple score based upon occupation, education, weekly income, and monthly rent, and these scores were divided into "low," "medium," and "high."

There was a marked inverse relationship between the prevalence of obesity and socioeconomic status. Figure 1 shows that the prevalence of obesity among women of lower socioeconomic status was 30 per cent, falling to 16 per cent among those of middle status, and to only 5 per cent in the upper status group. The prevalence of obesity in the lower class was thus six times that found in the upper class! And when socioeconomic status was divided into 12 classes, as the richness of the data permitted, the difference between the lowermost and uppermost social classes became even greater, from a low of less than 2 per cent in the uppermost to a high of 37 per cent in the lowermost class.

Among men, the differences between social classes were similar, but of lesser degree. Men of lower socioeconomic status, for example showed a prevalence of obesity of 32 per cent as contrasted with a prevalence of 16 per cent among upper class men.

One notable feature of this study was that it was designed to permit

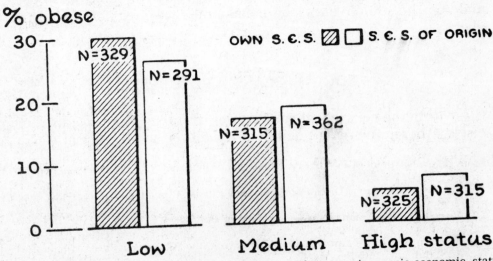

Figure 1. Decreasing prevalence of obesity with increasing socio-economic status (SES). Data exclude one woman about whom no information on the socioeconomic status of origin was available.

causal inferences about the influence of social factors. Earlier studies, which had demonstrated associations between socioeconomic status and psychiatric disorders, had been unable to go beyond these correlations to any statements about cause. The Midtown study, however, ascertained not only the socioeconomic status of the respondent at the time of the study, but also that of his parents when he was 8 years old. Although a subject's schizophrenia, or obesity, might conceivably influence his own social class, his disability in adult life could not have influenced that of his parents. Therefore, associations between the social class of the respondent's parents and his disability can be viewed as causal. And Figure 1 shows that such associations were almost as powerful as those between the social class of the respondents and their obesity!

The influence of socioeconomic status on the prevalence of obesity was confirmed by two recent studies. One, from London, found an inverse relationship between social class and obesity, although the differences were less marked than in Manhattan.[14] The second, carried out by Hinkle et al. on the executives of the Bell Telephone system, was designed to determine the effect of socioeconomic status and social mobility upon the incidence of coronary heart disease. In dramatic contrast to expectations, it was found that socioeconomic status and upward social mobility were *inversely* related to coronary heart disease.[4] These findings were the opposite of the stereotype of coronary disease as the consequence of the drive for achievement and the pressures of responsibility. Examination of the data revealed that obesity was also inversely correlated with status, in part explaining the distribution of coronary heart disease.

SITUATIONAL DETERMINANTS OF OVEREATING

As sociology has demonstrated the impact of environment in a broad sense upon human obesity, experimental social psychology has been able to pinpoint specific situations in which immediate environment exerts an impact. Recent studies have demonstrated the surprising degree to which the eating behavior of obese people is under environmental control.

These studies, by Stanley Schachter and his students,[13] might be said to take their theme from the title of an old paper by Neal Miller,[9] "Decreased hunger and increased food intake in hypothalamic obese rats." In this remarkably prescient study, Miller described for the first time the peculiar feeding behavior of rats made obese by hypothalamic lesions. The cardinal feature of this behavior was that obese rats overate when food was freely available, but when an impediment was placed in the way of their eating, food intake not only decreased, but actually decreased to a far lower level than that of control rats without hypothalamic lesions. Furthermore, it seemed to make little difference what kind of impediment was used. Motivation to work for food was impaired by every task that was devised. These tasks included lifting the covers to food cages, lever pressing for food, accepting the discomfort of crossing an electrified grid, or tolerating dilution of their food with quinine. These studies exploded traditional views of "hunger" as a unitary phenomenon. Hunger as defined by food intake can be quite a different matter from hunger as defined by motivation to work for food.

Study of behavior of hypothalamic obese animals suggests that behavior is characterized by an impairment in the mechanism of satiety, and probably also by an impairment in the drive to eat, as measured in standard experimental situations.[3, 9] This view of the food intake of hypothalamic obese animals has proved congenial to clinicians who have dealt with obese persons. A characteristic complaint is an inability to stop eating once they have started, and it is the exceptional obese person who presents a picture of voracious overeating, or a desire for food which drives him in the way that a desire for narcotics drives the addict, or the need for a drink drives the alcoholic. Until the work of Schachter, however, such characterizations had been based largely upon self reports, and the problem had not been approached experimentally. To a large degree this failure had been based upon the great difficulty in getting obese persons to approximate their usual food intake when they entered a laboratory or, indeed, any controlled environment. Instead, most obese persons undereat and lose weight when they enter a hospital, even when acess to food is unrestricted and when they are encouraged to maintain their body weight temporarily. The "impediment" in this situation is observation of eating behavior by medical personnel. In years of study of obese persons under a variety of conditions, we have observed only one in the act of overeating.

An ingenious experiment by Nisbett[11] assessed in man the behavior described by Miller for hypothalamic obese rats—relative overeating when food was freely available and relative undereating when an impediment was placed in their way. Subjects, who were male university students, were invited to participate in an experiment which was presented to them as an investigation of certain physiological variables. They were told that in order to obtain accurate baselines, it was essential that they not eat after 9:00 A.M. on the day of the test. Appointments were made for early afternoon hours so that the minimum period of food deprivation was 4 hours. Bogus recording electrodes were attached to the subjects, and they performed a monitoring task for approximately 30 minutes. At the end of this period the experimenter announced that the experiment was over, disengaged the subjects from their electrodes, and led them into another room "to fill out some final questionnaires."

The new experimental room contained a refrigerator, a chair, and a table on which were a bottle of soda and either one roast beef sandwich or three roast beef sandwiches. While the subject sat down, the experimenter said casually, "Since you skipped lunch for the experiment, we would like to give you lunch now. You can fill out the questionnaires while you eat. There are dozens more sandwiches in the refrigerator, by the way; have as many as you want." The experimenter asked the subject to check by his office on the way out, and then left, shutting the door behind him.

The procedure was designed to reduce any possible self-consciousness on the part of the overweight subjects in a number of ways. First, the experimenter was absent while the subject ate, and the meal was completely private. The subject could assume that he would not be interrupted because he was to go to the experimenter's office when he was through. Second, the subject was told that there were dozens of sandwiches in the refrigerator and could assume that if he were to take one or two they would not be missed. Third, the subject was given no reason to believe that the experimenter had any interest in how many sandwiches he ate.

Food intake of the obese persons paralleled that of the obese rats. When provided relatively unlimited access to food (under the three-sandwich condition), the obese persons ate considerably more than did their normal weight controls. When the impediment of taking additional food from the refrigerator was introduced in the one-sandwich condition, however, the food intake of the obese subjects fell considerably below that of the controls. This simple and striking experiment is probably the first direct demonstration in man of a kind of eating behavior characteristic of a wide variety of experimentally obese animals.

PHYSIOLOGIC STUDIES OF ADIPOSE TISSUE

A series of classic studies by Hirsch and his colleagues have established that the fundamental characteristics of adipose tissue are determined early in life.[5, 6, 12] The state of nutrition of a rat during its first 3 weeks of life, for example, determines the subsequent character of its adipose tissue and even its future size. Overfeeding during this critical period produces a highly cellular adipose tissue, whereas undernutrition results in tissue with an abnormally low number of adipose tissue cells. With increasing age, adipose tissue progressively loses its ability to grow by cellular hyperplasia, and by adult life, any increase in body fat is accomplished by an increase in cell size, not by an increase in cell number (Fig. 2). The marked obesity produced in adult rats by hypothalamic lesions, for example, was achieved solely by increased cell size, with no change in the number of adipose tissue cells.

The development of a convenient needle biopsy of human adipose tissue has permitted the extension of these studies to human obesity. Results are entirely consistent with those from lower animals. For example, there was little difference in the metabolism of fat samples obtained from obese and nonobese subjects. Furthermore, serial studies of obese subjects during weight reduction revealed that the loss in body fat resulted entirely from a decrease in the size of adipose tissue cells, and not from a decrease in the number of these cells.

The latter findings may explain the carbohydrate intolerance of obese persons, and the restoration of carbohydrate tolerance following weight loss, for the in vitro insulin sensitivity of adipose tissue depends upon the size of the cells and not upon their number. In any given sample of adipose tissue, the larger the cells, the less responsive the sample is to insulin. And it is precisely the size of cells and not their number which is decreased in weight reduction.

This work has important implications for our understanding of

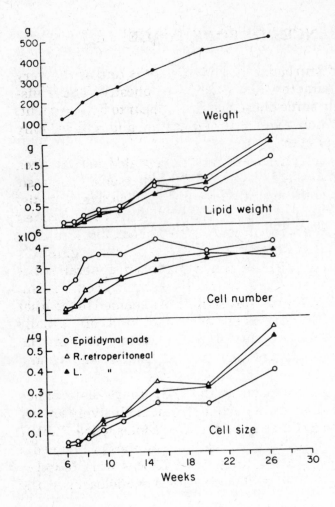

Figure 2. Observations of adipose cellularity at eight different times during growth and development of Sprague-Dawley rats. The large increase in fat accumulation between 19 and 26½ weeks is clearly related to change in cell size rather than to an increase in cell number. In earlier periods, both processes are involved in the growth of the depot.

obesity in man. The fact that cell number does not change in adult life implies a critical period in man, as in the rat, during which the number of adipose tissue cells is established for life. Persons who become obese during this period, perhaps in infancy, perhaps in childhood, may do so through hyperplasia of adipose tissue cells, in contrast to those who become obese in adult life. If this is the case, one would expect them to experience a greater difficulty in weight reduction, for they would be dealing with the double burden of an increased number and an increased size of adipose tissue cells. A person with adult-onset obesity could return to a normal weight simply by emptying his adipose tissue cells of their excessive load of fat. One suffering from juvenile-onset obesity, on the other hand, might be able to achieve a similar degree of weight loss only by decreasing the fat content of his excessive number of adipose tissue cells to an abnormally low concentration.

Clinical experience accords well with these predictions. Juvenile-onset obesity is more resistant to treatment than obesity beginning in adult life. And, as noted below, such persons seem more vulnerable to psychological complications of obesity. Recognition of these factors may help us set more realistic treatment goals for persons with juvenile-onset obesity, decreasing the frustration of the physician and, more importantly, of his patients.

DISTURBANCES IN BODY IMAGE

A distinctive kind of disturbance in body image is one of the very few psychopathological characteristics specific to obesity. These disturbances, which affect only some obese persons, appear to be persistent, unaffected by weight reduction, even of long duration, and relieved only by psychotherapy—often not even then.

A study of 74 randomly selected obese persons revealed disturbances in three aspects of the body image of some of these persons.[18] Interestingly, other obese persons were entirely free of this disorder. The disturbances were noted in (1) view of the self: many patients were revolted by the sight of their bodies and were almost unable to look into a mirror; some avoided activities such as shopping for fear of catching glimpses of themselves in store windows; (2) Self-consciousness in general: many obese persons harbored an intense self-consciousness and even misconceptions of how others viewed them; they sometimes seemed to feel that nothing ever happened to them except in some kind of (usually derogatory) relationship to their weight; (3) Self-consciousness in relation to the opposite sex; these disturbances ranged from avoidance and inhibitions to hateful devaluation of the opposite sex.

One of the most surprising aspects of the body image disturbance was the age of onset. Disturbances occurred almost exclusively among persons who had become obese during childhood or adolescence. Table 1 shows that not one of 40 subjects with adult-onset obesity showed a severe body image disturbance, while such disturbances were found in fully half of those with onset of obesity in childhood or adolescence, the so-called "juvenile obese."

Further study of juvenile obese subjects strongly suggested that adolescence constituted a kind of critical period for the development of these disturbances in body image, and that the disorder was largely confined to persons who were obese during these impressionable years. This presumption strengthens the argument for the prevention of obesity in childhood, and for prompt treatment of children who become obese. The difficulty of this latter task is well documented by a further finding of this study. In a group of nearly 2000 children followed for a period of 30 years, the odds against an obese child becoming a normal weight adult were 4 to 1; for those who did not reduce during adolescence they were more than 28 to 1!

An intriguing experimental study of disturbances in body image of

Table 1. *Degree of Body Image Disturbance According to Age of Onset of Obesity in 74 Persons*

ONSET CATEGORY	SEVERE	MILD	NONE
Juvenile	17	8	9
Adult	0	10	30

$x^2 = 19.44$, df $= 2$, p $< .001$.

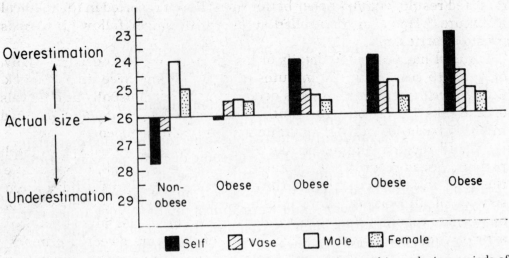

Figure 3. Size estimation of stimuli by obese and nonobese subjects during periods of weight maintenance and weight loss.

obese persons was carried out by means of a projector with a distorting lens which could be manipulated to make pictures of the subjects seem leaner or fatter than they were.[1] Six severely obese adults were studied during a period of several months hospitalization for weight reduction. At the beginning of the study, all six patients slightly underestimated their actual size. As weight loss proceeded, however, they began to overestimate their actual size, and this trend continued throughout the period of weight loss (Fig. 3). Their estimations of the body size of other persons showed no such distortions. These findings suggest that the internalized image of the body size of these patients was relatively fixed, and could not be altered as rapidly as the actual change in body configuration.

IMPLICATIONS FOR TREATMENT

The newer research findings have two implications for therapy. (1) There is a strong probability that obese persons, particularly those with early onset of obesity, suffer from a metabolic disorder. (2) Nevertheless, their food intake is determined to a considerable degree by environmental factors. Appropriate use of these findings could be effective in the control of food intake by obese persons.

The traditional medical model could well be considered an inappropriate use of these findings. This model defines an authoritarian role for the physician, who prescribes a diet and appetite-depressing medication. The patient loses weight, if at all, in large part to please the doctor and to meet his expectations. When the relationship is terminated or attenuated, the patient discontinues the diet and regains weight.

Systematic application of the principles of the new field of the experimental analysis of behavior (behavior therapy) may help the physician design programs more suited to the needs of the obese patient. Recent reviews of the field are commended to the reader.[7, 20] Stuart has reported results which appear better than any yet reported in the medical literature.[16] However, controlled studies with longer follow-up periods must be carried out.

Stuart has published details of his program, which consists, intially, of 12 to 15 sessions of 30 minutes each, occurring three times a week. Subsequent treatment sessions occurred as needed, usually at intervals of 2 weeks for the next 3 months, followed by sessions on a planned monthly basis, as well as "maintenance" sessions as needed.

Daily records of food intake and body weight were kept by each patient. These records were notable for their great detail. For example, the food intake record listed the time, nature, quantity, and circumstances of all food and fluid intake, while the weight record consisted of weights recorded four times a day—before breakfast, after breakfast, after lunch, and before bedtime. Initial efforts were directed primarily toward helping the patient gain control over the time and circumstances of his eating, rather than toward weight loss. For example, a measure introduced early into the treatment consisted of interrupting the meal for a predetermined period of time, usually 2 or 3 minutes, gradually increased to 5 minutes. The patient was instructed to put down his utensils and merely sit in his place at the table for this period of time. The rationale of this maneuver was to give the patient, as early as possible, an experience of control over one aspect of his eating, however small, and to learn that eating was a response which could be broken down into components which could be successfully mastered. Another early device was an attempt to make eating a "pure experience," paired with no other activity such as reading, listening to the radio, watching television, or talking with friends. The rationale of this maneuver was to keep eating separate from any other behavior which might induce eating to continue as a conditioned response to the occurrence of the other behavior. Only after a variety of such techniques of self-control had been mastered did weight loss become a major focus of treatment.

Stuart treated patients individually. The possibility of utilizing group methods for teaching behavioral controls of eating raises the hope of multiplying the effectiveness of a potentially effective technique. Recently evidence has been obtained that group therapy of obesity is superior to individual therapy, under a variety of treatment conditions.[8] Furthermore, there is a strong reason to believe that major assistance in the control of obesity is available from patient self-help groups. Very recently a study of such a group—TOPS ("Take Off Pounds Sensibly")— has revealed that the average results obtained by 22 chapters compare favorably with those achieved by medical management, and that the results of the most effective chapters rank with the very best results in the medical literature.[17]

SUMMARY

Research on obesity has recently produced new evidence for the influence of both metabolic and behavioral factors in its etiology. Both kinds of factors have therapeutic significance. In the metabolic area, evidence that the total fat cell content of adipose tissue may be determined early in life may help to set more realistic goals for the notoriously difficult treatment of persons suffering from juvenile-onset obesity. Recent behavioral discoveries may have more positive therapeutic consequences. Three such discoveries are the marked influence of social factors on the prevalence of obesity, the large effect of situational determinants on the eating behavior of obese persons, and the surprising effectiveness reported by one study on the behavioral management of obesity. These findings give reasonable grounds for hope of improvement in our traditionally poor results of treatment for obesity.

REFERENCES

1. Glucksman, M. L. and Hirsch, J.: The response of obese patients to weight reduction. III. The perception of body size. Psychosom. Med., *31*:1, 1969.
2. Goldblatt, P. B., Moore, M. E., and Stunkard, A. J.: Social factors in obesity. J.A.M.A., *192*:1039, 1965.
3. Graff, H., and Stellar, E.: Hyperphagia, obesity and finickiness. J. Comp. Physiolog. Psychol., *55*:418, 1962.
4. Hinkle, L. E., Jr.: Occupation, education and coronary heart disease. Science, *161*:238, 1968.
5. Hirsch, J., and Knittle, J. L.: Cellularity of obese and nonobese human adipose tissue. Fed. Proc., 1969 (in press).
6. Knittle, J. L., and Hirsch, J.: Effect of early nutrition on the development of rat epididymal fat pads: Cellularity and metabolism. J. Clin. Invest., *47*:2091, 1968.
7. Krasner, L., and Ullmann, L. P., eds.: Research in Behavior Modification. New York, Holt, Rinehart and Winston, 1965.
8. Louden, A. M., and Schreiber, E. D.: A controlled study of the effects of group discussions and an anorexiant in outpatient treatment of obesity with attention to the psychological aspects of dieting. Ann. Int. Med., *65*:80, 1966.
9. Miller, M. E., Bailey, C. J., and Stevenson, J. A. F.: Decreased hunger and increased food intake in hypothalamic obese rats. Science, *112*:256, 1950.
10. Moore, M. E., Stunkard, A. J., and Srole, L.: Obesity, social class, and mental illness. J.A.M.A., *181*:962, 1962.
11. Nisbett, R. E.: Determinants of food intake in obesity. Science, *159*:1254, 1968.
12. Salons, L. B., Knittle, J. L., and Hirsch, J.: Role of adipose cell size and adipose tissue insulin sensitivity in the carbohydrate intolerance of human obesity. J. Clin. Invest., *47*:153, 1968.
13. Schachter, S.: Obesity and eating. Science, *161*:751, 1968.
14. Silverstone, J. T., Gordon, R. P., and Stunkard, A. J.: Social factors in obesity in London. The Practitioner, *202*:682, 1969.
15. Srole, L., et al.: Mental Health in the Metropolis. Midtown Manhattan Study. New York, McGraw-Hill Book Co., Inc., 1962.
16. Stuart, R. B.: Behavioral control of overeating. Behav. Res. Therapy, *5*:357, 1967.
17. Stunkard, A. J., Levine, H., and Fox, S.: A study of a patient self-help group for obesity. Proceedings Eighth International Congress of Nutrition, Prague, 1969 (in press).
18. Stunkard, A. J., and Burt, V.: Obesity and the body image. II. Age at onset of disturbances in the body image. Amer. J. Psychiat., *123*:1443, 1967.
19. Stunkard, A., and McLaren-Hume, M.: Results of treatment for obesity. A review of the literature and report of a series. Arch. Int. Med., *102*:79, 1959.
20. Ullmann, L. P., and Krasner, L., eds.: Case Studies in Behavior Modification. New York, Holt, Rinehart and Winston, 1965.
21. Blohmke, M., Depner, R., Koschorreck, B., and Stelzer, O.: Uebergewichtigkeit bei berufstätigen Frauen in Abhängigkeit ausgewählter biologischer und sozialer Faktoren. Arbeitsmedizin, Sozialmedizin, Arbeitshygeiene, *4*:190, 1969.

Department of Psychiatry
University of Pennsylvania
Philadelphia, Pennsylvania 19104

DO WE DARE TO DIFFERENTIATE BETWEEN OBESE AND OVERWEIGHT?

As many as 30 percent of Americans may be so overweight that they can only be called "obese." For the typical practitioner, many a day's calendar of patients may make this estimate appear highly conservative. Obesity is the commonest nutritional disorder confronting today's clinician.

This ubiquitous problem has produced a sargasso sea of books and articles, research reports and hypotheses—some fact, some fiction, many yet unproven—that entangles clear judgment and obscures the path to effective therapy. Discovery of high insulin levels in proven adult diabetics who are obese; assertions that the quantity of adipose cells is established irrevocably in infancy; all tend to add to the controversy and confusion existing already.

In an effort to sort out the clinical significance of these developments, the editors visited with John J. Canary, M.D., a veteran of more than 20 years of research in endocrinology, metabolism and body composition. Dr. Canary is professor of medicine at Georgetown University School of Medicine in Washington, D.C. The internist is also director of Georgetown's Division of Endocrinology and Metabolism as well as its clinical research unit. Following are excerpts from a recent informal conversation with him.

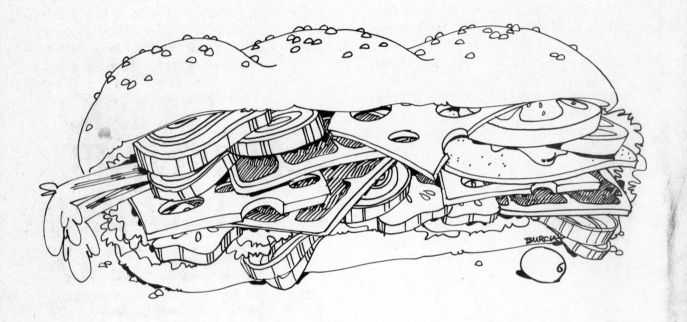

Doctor Canary, about the only thing an outsider can say today with certainty about the field of obesity is that things seem pretty confused. Do you get that impression?

I'm sure that everyone is. For instance, the situation has been tremendously improved by the recent publication in *Nature* of a letter to the editor pointing out, quite rightly, that we do not have really good evidence for what overall nutritional requirements really are in man. The common statement that 70 percent of the world is undernourished, and 30 percent overnourished is probably then somewhat invalid. What happens then when we try to apply these principles to a given individual? There is a lot of work left to do here.

When we go about calculating the appropriate nutritional intake for a given person, we have to recognize that the variables are tremendous. Our bodies have been likened to a metabolic combustion engine, and that analogy is fine—provided we recognize what a highly complex, multi-functional machine we're dealing with. Errors of judgment can be made that could be quite serious. Rest periods, physical activity . . . One person can perform an act of exertion with more efficiency than another. The energy expenditure can vary greatly even for a simple action like climbing the stairs.

Factors of genetics also become extremely important. Our obese patients will tell of members of the family who must eat tremendous amounts to retain their present weight, while others almost literally gain a pound or two passing the table. And yet, when such people are subjected to study, none of the rather gross measurements we can make appear to be abnormal. Yet one person is obviously extremely efficient in use of caloric energy, while the other is quite the opposite. There was an animal study from the Imperial College of London a few years ago which appeared to confirm this. In certain genetically-related animals which were obese, for any given piece of adipose tissue, there was a noticeable difference in heat production, *i.e.,* efficiency of use of energy substrate, when compared with samples from other animals who were not obese.

Well, doesn't this seem to add up to something of a hopeless situation for the everyday practitioner?

No, not at all, because we're talking about a multi-factorial problem, and those may not be the most important factors: What caused the person to become obese in the first place? In the majority of patients, their overweight problem is a shadow of something else. In a number of situations, the underlying disorder, of which obesity is only a symptom, is quite difficult to unearth. A substantial etiologic factor is psychological.

One of my most respected professors, Dr. Chester Keefer, frequently reminded us that: "If you listen to the patient long enough, the patient will tell you what is wrong." Doctors have to take the time to listen to what their patients are saying. It could save a lot of time and expensive tests, although it is expensive in its own right.

Is obesity a diagnosis that can be made with any kind of definition? A 200-pound man isn't necessarily overweight, even if he runs off the life insurance tables.

Most of the people who have worked in body composition define obesity in a rather rigid sense. By and large, women are endowed with slightly greater quantities of fat tissue than are men. Obesity in males would be defined as any proportion of fatty tissue to total body weight that exceeds 20-to-25 percent; while in females it would be more like 25-to-28 percent.

That raises the question: how do you go about determining those numbers? Most of our techniques are not practical for office, home, or clinic work. They involve such techniques as measuring the bodies displacement of water or helium, making adjustments for differences in the density, and a reflection of the composition of the various tissues.

However, you can make use of the insurance tables, particularly the Metropolitan ones. If you read the fine print, as most of us sometimes forget to do, they clearly spell out that the tables are averages of people 25 years of age. But if one takes such tables and estimates a half or three-quarters of a pound more per year for every year above 25, you can get a good approximation of optimum or acceptable body weight. Of course this curve breaks down after the 50th or 55th year, but it's still a good ballpark figure, up to that age.

There are other important techniques, such as the use of skin calipers. But this requires consistent placement, force and multiple site measurements. The most important technique to my mind is looking at the patient. Does he or she *look* obese? It's very helpful to ask patients to bring in some old photographs. You can

often see very quickly from a series of old pictures if the patient has a problem in weight, or in glandular or hormonal control. I can't emphasize how important this can be in terms of time, tests and money saved.

It's also vital to assess whether or not the patients *feel* they have become obese. Their view of their bodies might well differ from the physician's. Sometimes listening to them will go far to explaining the "why's" of this weight gain. For example, the patient may have a peptic ulcer and it happens to be the diet that's the gremlin. Or there may have been a change in housing —from a three-story house with stairs to a one-story ranch style—or a shift in employment that may require a simple diet or exercise modification.

This certainly applies in adults, but we have the recent work of Jules Hirsh and his colleagues at Rockefeller University that has led to the maxim: "Fat babies make fat adults."

This is a very important contribution, but I think there is one aspect that has not been emphasized by the other people who have been interpreting that work. Even if a person has a genetically predetermined number of adipose cells, making it more or less difficult for obesity to occur, it does not automatically follow that the patient must fill them all up. Each one of those cells does not *have* to become hyper-filled with lipid material. It means only that you have the ability, perhaps a little more readily than the next person, to become fat.

This reservoir of pre-existent cells has ramifications for controlling and losing weight. It would be harder for a person with a larger number of fat-laden cells to diet to a point where loss of weight is visible.

We're getting back to nutrition again. A lot of people seem to be putting the blame on the American mother, who might feed her infant too much, or stuff it with whole milk.

It's much too easy these days to blame Mom. It would be ridiculous to suggest that the relationship between child and mother is not a very positive one. But public educational activities that have gone on throughout the world, have pointed out the key aspects of good nutrition. As I said earlier the problem is in defining optimum nutrition. The greatest proportion of serious obesity is found in members of lower socio-economic groups where the low-priced or available foods are higher in their content of fats and carbo-hydrates. The middle-class North American eats a pretty balanced diet, in my experience. Perhaps this is unintentional, but it is no less true.

By the way, our studies have me pretty well convinced that there are some individuals who simply do not need the 1,000-1,200 calories/day called minimal. Some can do quite well on as little as 800 or even 600 daily calories. I emphasize the word "some." These people are frequently accused of "cheating" when they do not lose on 1,000 calories/day on their diets, when on fewer than 1,000 calories they would.

I'm sure you've looked at things like the serum insulin in obese patients. The presence of hyperinsulinemia, even in some diabetics, is extremely puzzling.

Yes, the technique of radio-immunoassay developed by a number of other investigators, has really strengthened our capabilities of looking at these vital substances, which may appear in nanogram or picogram quantities. The late Dr. Berson and his collaborator, Dr. Yalow and a number of others pointed out that, not only do obese persons have abnormally high levels of circulating insulin, but that their circulating growth hormone is abnormally low. This latter derangement, I feel, is very important.

The key question is, would high levels of circulating insulin which has as a basic function the facilitation of fat formation from glucose, have been a cause of the obesity? And by the same token, would the low growth hormone levels be etiologically important? Our studies here clearly indicate that the ordinary stimuli for growth hormone fail to produce the expected elevations in the obese. Would the absence of these surges, which favor the breakdown of fat into its component parts, coupled with the insulin excess, tend to be critical? We think they are.

So there are two biophysical abnormalities, at least, we're dealing with. When an obese person loses weight, insulin falls. What happens to the growth hormone?

The response is very interesting. Although the insulin falls rapidly, the growth hormone suppression may persist for six-to-eight months after the patient has achieved ideal weight. We have the hypothesis that this imbalance is an important factor in the ease with which the obese person often regains the lost weight. They may only have begun to "relax" on their dietary intake, and the weight comes right back. How many times have people told us: "Oh, yes, I've been on successful diets, four or five times."

What I advise is that those who have made the hard fight and succeeded must continue on their strict regimen for at least another year to be on the safe side. I think under such a set of circumstances the chances are much greater for the patient to maintain his ideal body weight.

A very fair question would be, how does the fat tell the pituitary or the hypothalamus that a critical number of pounds of fat has been gained? We don't yet know. But we know it occurs at about the 20- to 30-pound level. Studies in non-obese volunteers who gained weight rapidly by forced feeding have confirmed this.

Obesity certainly occurs in adult-onset diabetes. Yet we said only a moment ago that high insulin levels are also found. Why does this occur?

I can't really say for sure. All obese individuals will produce increased serum insulin levels, apparently to affect sugar metabolism. There is an acquired resistance to the effects of insulin. Work at the Johns Hopkins laboratories seem to favor the theory that the difficulty with insulin's action is within the cell. What these are we don't yet know.

We think that the difference between the obese non-diabetic patient and the obese diabetic is a reflection of an abnormality in insulin production, plus a still mysterious something else. Many of those who are obese and develop maturity-onset diabetes are making an excessive amount of insulin per unit volume of plasma, but still not enough to fulfill their blood sugar needs.

The peripheral problem is that obese patients, diabetic or not, are usually resistant to the effects of insulin. Such patients need two-to-three times the normal amount of insulin to elicit the same reductions in blood sugar such an injection gives in someone with normal weight. Even when near-normal or even normal weight is achieved, a part of this insulin resistance seems to remain.

Our diagnostic tools for diabetes are so poor that I think all the incidence figures published for it are much too low. Perhaps there will be found abnormalities of insulin in those who are obese or diabetic, or both. I can't help believing that the two are somehow related, even though we have to classify the carbohydrate mechanisms of many obese as non-diabetic.

How have you accomplished weight loss in the patients you've studied?

We've concentrated on long-term in-patient metabolic studies on younger and middle-aged patients who were truly disabled by their obesity in terms of their ability to do their jobs or to exist in their family or society. And we've been impressed that dieting, without a sustained exercise program, is not really ideal. And in certain cases it may be dangerous.

Excessive dieting alone, for example, seems to have an adverse effect on heart muscle function. We observed some very disturbing changes in ECG patterns, even in young patients. But in the presence of graded exercises, these did not take place.

In point of fact, those patients who exercised as well as dieted seemed to lose more fat than those who were only restricting caloric intake. These latter sometimes lost more weight, but the extra weight lost was valuable lean tissue in a disturbing proportion. The addition of exercise, I believe, has a great deal to do with the outcome. We certainly don't advocate exercising to exhaustion. The structural abnormalities attending obesity have to be taken into account. For some patients, walking to the end of the hall and back may be all we can safely accomplish until some excess weight has been lost.

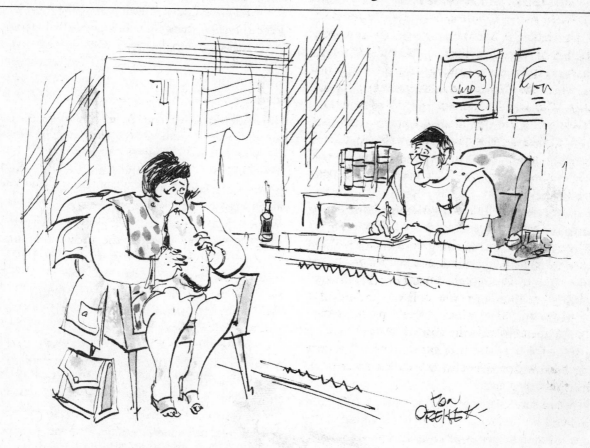

"Frankly, Mrs. Hansen, I'm beginning to wonder if you really want to lose weight."

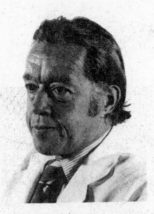

JOHN J. CANARY, M.D.

For many patients it's essential to call in a rehabilitation specialist to advise on the types of exercises patients are capable of doing. The center of gravity of such patients is different; some may have, or can develop, back problems more easily than others, and so forth. You can't just say: "Jog." Exercises must be programmed to fit the patient.

In addition to low-caloric intake and graded exercise, is there anything else the physician should emphasize in a weight-loss program?

Certainly any physiologic or psychologic problems must be taken care of simultaneously if the program is to succeed. No diet will have more than temporary success if the psycho-social problem of which the obesity may be symptomatic is not defined and taken care of. The doctor need not be a psychiatrist, an endocrinologist or a physical therapist to see these things, and neither should they be ignored.

We often find that eliminating the social or physical dysfunction obviates the need for any severe dietary program. Instead, changing a few key habits of exercise, or mild modifications of existing therapeutic diets, may be sufficient. The simple advice to eat a third or a half less than the patient normally eats—not anything special, just less of everything—will frequently suffice. Food restriction is largely by quality and by volume.

There are some patients who do require combined medical and psychological help. And we should be on our guard for these persons all the time.

What about appetite-suppressants and other pharmacologic adjustants?

Sometimes agents that curb appetite are helpful. I tend to use them on a limited basis, where the patient has a serious problem of sticking to a diet on a short-term basis. Something at home or at the job may lead to a resumption of old eating habits.

I do not recommend metabolic acceleration with thyroid hormones. We found that if a person totally starved or used large doses of thyroid, they would lose more weight than with moderate caloric restriction. However, in both circumstances there was a significant loss of lean tissue, not fat; that is, a greater weight loss was of tissue that the patient needed. I also see no reason to encourage the use of low-dose chorionic gonadotropins, now seemingly in vogue again.

Most physicians see obesity on a regular basis, and when they don't they see patients simply overweight. I gather your message here is that they have to consider the whole patient, not just the metabolism of his bodily engine.

That's right. The physician has to see beyond the scales to the patient's environment, family, and circumstances. It's an old saw but still quite true that obesity is frequently a symptom of something else.

Many of the things we've talked about may eventually improve or facilitate therapy. We hope they will. But right now it's important that family doctors listen to their patients, establish communication with them, and find where the underlying problems really are. This is applied psychiatry at a level that any physician should be able to handle.

The refusal of private and public third parties in medicine to accept obesity as a medical problem is another major stumbling block. It is a typical miscarriage of medical judgment.

One final point. I'm not saying, go back to school and learn to measure growth hormone. It might be a useful physiologic adjunct to therapy, but we don't currently have enough of it available. Rapid crash diets, because of their effect on heart function, are hazardous. The use of hormones, such as expensive, inadequate dosages of the gonadotropins cannot be receiving enough FDA supervision. The agency would be much better advised to devote time to such items rather than to the cyclamates.

Right now caloric restriction, a simultaneous exercise program, and regard for the patient are most effective. These are at our disposal. And they work. END

When is fat excessive?

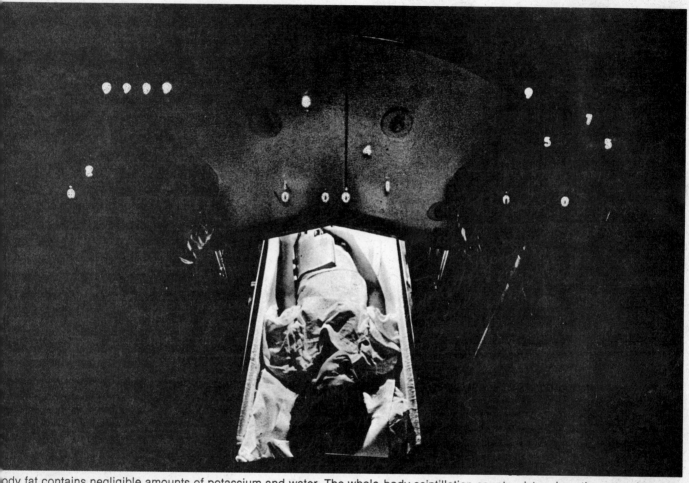

ody fat contains negligible amounts of potassium and water. The whole-body scintillation counter determines the potassium con-
nt of the lean body mass by measuring the emission of the radioisotope K-40, which is 0.119% of naturally occurring potassium.
e glowing lights of the decimal counter are seen superimposed in this photograph taken at St. Luke's Hospital, New York City.

ntil recently the evaluation of over-
eight or obesity was based on simple
servation or reference to standard
eight-weight charts. It is now recog-
zed that obesity in the sense of ex-
ssive fat deposition must be differ-
tiated from overweight as defined
height-weight norms. Football play-
s, weight lifters, and other athletes
ay be overweight according to stan-
rd charts, but they are rarely obese.
nversely, many sedentary middle-
ed individuals may have an exces-
ve proportion of fat to total body
eight yet not be grossly overweight
standard norms.

An increase in weight may result
from increase in lean body mass
(weight of bone, muscle, and organs),
body water, or depot fat. The clinical
implications of weight increase vary,
depending on which body constituents
increase in weight. To clarify the role
of overweight and excessive fat accumulation in morbidity and premature
mortality, ways of measuring the ratio
of fat to total body weight are being
studied.

Methods for evaluating total body
fat include measurement of body density (weight per unit of volume), measurement of body water content (hy-
drometry), and total body radiopotassium content using whole-body scintillation counters.

Densimetric techniques are based on
the fact that fat has the lowest density
of any body constituent. The density of
fat is 0.90; the density of the lean body
mass is 1.10. Therefore, a loss of body
fat results in an increase in specific
gravity in a precise inverse relationship. Body density is usually determined by application of Archimedes'
principle of underwater weighing. Total body water is related to body fat,
presuming fat to be anhydrous and
water to be a relatively constant proportion of lean body mass. Total body
potassium correlates with lean body
mass because potassium is absent or

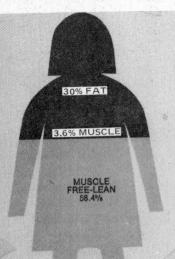

30% FAT

3.6% MUSCLE

MUSCLE
FREE-LEAN
58.4%

WOMAN 50 YEARS

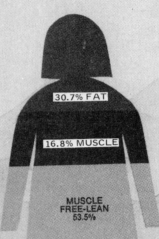

30.7% FAT

16.8% MUSCLE

MUSCLE
FREE-LEAN
53.5%

WOMAN 20 YEARS

26.5% F

19.6% MUS

MUSCL
FREE-LE
53.9%

MAN 50 YE

1.00

1.01

1.02

1.03

DENSITY

1.04

1.05

1.06

1.07

Differences in body composition by age and sex.
(Composition based on data of Anderson;[1] density calculated after Keys and Brožek.[2])

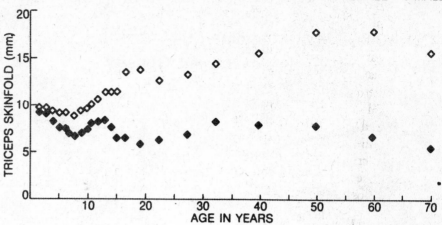

Average triceps skinfold thickness as a function of age and sex (Pett and Ogilvie[3]). Readings significantly greater than these "norms" indicate excessive fat at any point in the life cycle.

13.6% FAT

32.6% MUSCLE

MUSCLE
FREE-LEAN
53.8%

MAN 20 YEARS

present in only trace amounts in fat. Other techniques for estimating lean body mass (the reciprocal of body fat) include anthropometric measurements, creatine excretion, and basal oxygen consumption. These methods are valuable research tools but are not practical for office use.

Measurement of skinfold thickness by a caliper appears the simplest and best method for evaluation of obesity (*i.e.*, caloric overnutrition) in clinical practice. Measurement of skinfold thickness provides a reproducible measurement of subcutaneous fat (about 50 percent of total fat) and an index of total body fat.

Various sites have been used for skinfold measurements but the triceps skinfold thickness is recommended because it is easiest to measure, gives highly reproducible results, and in obese patients gives the highest correlation with body density values obtained by underwater weighing. Also, the triceps skinfold appears to be the most representative of total body fat, regardless of disproportionate distribution of adipose tissue in various areas of the body. The triceps skinfold is measured at the back of the right upper arm exactly midway between the acromion and the olecranon processes. Measurement is made of the doubled thickness of the pinched "folded" skin plus the attached subcutaneous adipose tissue. No advantage is gained by using additional skinfold measurements. The relation of skinfold thickness to body fat content is practically independent of height.

From nine years of age on, women have a higher percentage of body weight as fat than do men. Young women are over two and one-half times as fat as comparable young men; older women are not quite one and one-half times as fat as men of the same age. Body fatness increases with age in both sexes but at a faster rate in males. Women increase 55% in body fatness from the third to seventh decade of life while men increase 187% over approximately the same age span. The body fat represents approximately 28.7% of total body weight for 20-year-old women and 11% of total weight of 20-year-old men. Body fat has increased to 41.9% for women by about age 60 and to 25.8% for men aged 50.5 years.

Individuals less than 30 years of age, whose triceps skinfold exceeds the mean by more than one standard deviation, are designated as obese. It is recommended that the standard established for individuals 30 years old be applied to men and women from 30 to 50 years of age.

Obese patients differ from nonobese individuals in morphologic characteristics other than quantity of fatty tissue. Several studies suggest that obese persons tend to have a typical somatotype, being more endomorphic, somewhat more mesomorphic, and markedly less ectomorphic than the general population. ∎

1. Anderson, E. C.: Ann. N.Y. Acad. Sci. *110*:189, 1963.
2. Keys, A., and Brožek, J.: Physiol. Rev. *33*:245, 1953.
3. Pett, L. V., and Ogilvie, G. F.: Hum. Biol. *28*: 177, 1956.

Controversies in Medicine (II)—
Nature and Nurture in Human Obesity

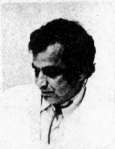

C. S. Chlouverakis, M.D.

DESPITE a respectable number of publications suggesting the involvement of genetic factors in human obesity, the prevailing view considers obesity as due entirely to environmental factors, especially overeating. Thus, obesity is regarded as a self-induced affliction like alcoholism or drug addiction. Furthermore, whereas in the case of alcoholism or drug addiction one may elicit a history of precipitating incidents or factors provoking sympathy or forgiveness, no such excuses are allowed in the case of the obese. Finally, an element of banality is assumed to be involved in the process of becoming obese, and the statement that, "no gentleman ever weighs more than 200 pounds" was made in Congress by not a lesser figure than the Speaker of the House and famous legislator, Thomas B. Reed.

In this paper I will present evidence suggesting that genetic factors may be operative in the development of human obesity. I will propose, however, that the expression of these factors in the developing organism depends on the environment in which this development takes place. Thus, heredity and environment, nature and nurture, rather than being antithetical terms, act hand-in-hand in determing the individual's fatness. Recognition of genetic factors in human obesity would support the concept that each individual has his own ideal body weight. According to this concept, the ideal body weight of individuals being predisposed to obesity might be above the "ideal body weight" as defined by

This work was supported by Grant No. 1 RO1 AM16346-01 MET of the National Institute of Arthritis, Metabolism and Digestive Diseases. I am grateful to Mrs. Linda Knuutila and Mrs. Robbie Billingsley for their valuable help in the preparation of the manuscript.

the author

about

C. S. Chlouverakis, M.D., is director of the Obesity and Lipid Abnormalities Service at the E. J. Meyer Memorial Hospital and an associate professor in the Department of Medicine at the State University of New York at Buffalo. He received his M.D. from the University of Athens in Greece.

the life insurance companies, even if they were exposed to *optimal* environmental influences. To further reduce the body weight of such individuals one would have to *over-optimize* the environment, a manipulation with unknown and potentially harmful consequences.[1]

The Evidence

There have been numerous studies stretching back to the 1930's indicating that the prevalence of overweight is higher among the parents of an obese propositus than among those of a control individual. Similarly, obesity occurs with greater frequency among the offspring of obese parents.[2] These studies, however, are difficult to interpret because of similar cultural patterns(including eating habits) among members of the same family. Furthermore, by treating obesity as an all or none entity, rather than as a continuum of excessive accumulation of adipose tissue, they introduce a considerable amount of error. In an attempt to separate social from genetic inheritance, Withers compared the offspring/parent correlation of body weights in families having at least one adopted child with that observed between natural children and their parents. The weight of natural, but not that of adopted, children correlated with that of their parents. However, analysis of the differences found in the sex-cross correlations, i.e., mother/son and father/daughter led this author to conclude that obesity is inherited but that the expression of obesity is in terms of body build.[3]

Using necropsy material, Bjurulf found that the amount of body fat was correlated with hair growth on the chest and on the proximal phalanges. Since the distribution of hair is genetically determined,[4] the author suggested that the fatty tissue contains some factor not influenced by environmental conditions.[5]

More direct studies on the inheritance of obesity have been performed on identical and fraternal twins. The latter are also called dissimilar, because they are in all respects like non-twin siblings, whereas identical twins, resulting from the fertilization of one ovum by one sperm, have an identical genetic background. Thus any differences observed between identical twins are presumed to be environmental. In classic study of inheritance based on twin-pairs, the mean pair difference in body weight for identical twins was 4.1 pounds compared with 10 pounds for fraternal twins and 10.4 pounds for siblings of like sex.[6] Further insight into the interplay of genetic and environmental factors in obesity was provided by dividing identical twins into those reared in the same or in a different environment. This procedure allowed the authors to express the "heritability" of obesity numerically and compare it with that of other inherited traits. They concluded that obesity is inherited as much as stature and sitting height and more than IQ. The most striking finding of this study, however, was the relative unimportance of environment, since the correlation coefficient between the weights of identical twins reared apart was similar to that of identical twins reared together and significantly higher than that of fraternal twins reared together (Table 1). A similar study which was conducted in Germany in the 1920's had also suggested that body weight is an inherited trait but it also emphasized the importance of environmental factors.[7]

The results of these two studies on twins seem to be at variance with those reported by Osborn and DeGeorge who showed some correlation between the body weight of female but not of male twins.[8] Although it is impossible to offer an accurate explanation for these conflicting findings, the situation may illustrate the point made above, that both genetic and environmental factors are instrumental in determining body weight, and that it is the variable environment which accounts for the differences among these studies. To quote Dobzhansky: "What is inherited is not body weight as such, but the trend of the development of the body, which may result in different weights in different circumstances."[9]

Obesity as Part of Body Build

The possibility that obesity is inherited as part of the total body build has been alluded to already in this paper. Among the many systems used to classify body build (for a review see Keys and Brozek[10]) the most common is that introduced by Sheldon and his colleagues.[11] This taxonomical system is based on 17 measurements made on somatotype photographs of standardized front, side and rear views of the standing nude individual and the reciprocal of ponderal index. Somatotype is a trinomial expression of three basic components rated on a 7-point ordinal scale from minimal (1) to maximal (7) expression. The first component

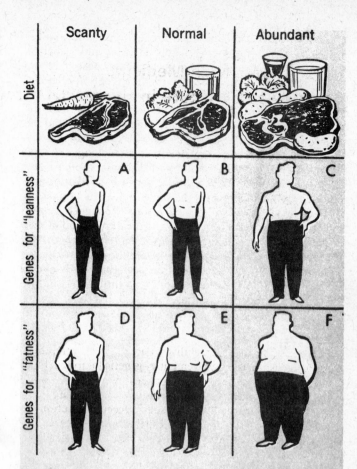

Figure 1: Gene environment interaction. A person who has a gene for "fatness" may actually weigh less than a person with a gene for "leanness", if the former lives on a scanty and the later on an abundant diet.

Adapted from: Dobzhansky, Theodosius: *Mankind Evolving,* Yale University Press, 1962, p. 45.

(endomorphy) rates softness and roundness; endomorphs tend toward obesity with their abdomen overshadowing the thorax and hands and feet being relatively small. The second component (mesomorphy) expresses muscle and bone development. Mesomorphs are muscular and sturdy people. Finally, the third component (ectomorphy) indicates somatic linearity. Ectomorphs tend to be slender and delicate in bone and muscle tissue.

Sheldon regarded somatotype as a permanent endowment of the individual, largely independent of nutrition. He warns for instance that the first component (endomorphy), although often expressed by overt obesity, permeates the whole body, skeleton and muscle. An endomorph when starved will still look like an emaciated endomorph.

Sheldon's somatotyping has been subjected to numerous attacks from many quarters. Hooton considers the first component (endomorphy) as a momentary state of the development of adipose tissue rather than as a permanent or mystical characteristic of the individual.[12] Lasker performed somatotyping measurements on photographs of 34 volunteer conscientious objectors of the Minnesota experiment before and after they were subjected to a European type of famine diet for 24 weeks.[13] He found that

Table 1: Correlation Coefficients(r) and Heritability for Certain Traits in Identical and Fraternal Twins

Trait	Fraternal	Identical Reared Together	Identical Reared Apart	Heritability (Coefficients)
Stature	0.64	0.93	0.97	0.81
Sitting Height	0.50	0.88	0.96	0.76
Weight	0.63	0.92	0.89	0.78
IQ (Binet)	0.63	0.88	0.67	0.68

Adapted from: Newman F, Freeman N and Holzinger KJ: *Twins: A Study of Heredity and Environment,* University of Chicago Press, 1937.

with partial starvation and weight reduction there was a decrease both in endomorphy and mesomorphy whereas ectomorphy increased; all measurements described by Sheldon decreased significantly with the exception of ankle, wrist and head breadths. The author concluded that the criteria of somatotyping are profoundly affected by nutritional factors and even if there is an inheritable aspect of the constitution it can be covered by environmental manipulations.[14] The above criticisms directed against the permanency or stability of human body build are basically valid. There is no permanency since nature is acted upon and modified by nurture. It was the structure of the Minnesota experiment which was responsible for the exaggeration of the importance of environmental and the diminution of that of constitutional factors. Thus, in that experiment the subjects were men of near normal weight subjected to drastic caloric restriction. However, in the case of the overtly obese, dietary manipulations do induce constitutional changes, but certain characteristic features still remain. Thus, despite the artificiality and exaggerations of Sheldon's taxonomical system, one has the feeling that there is a seed of truth in his statement that "endomorphs are usually fat but they are sometimes seen emaciated; in the latter event they do not change into mesomorphs or ectomorphs any more than a starved mastiff would change into a spaniel or a collie. They become simply emaciated endomorphs".[15]

I have seen emaciated obese-hyperglycemic mice and they look like emaciated *obese*-hyperglycemic mice. Also every physician treating obese patients must have noticed that many obese patients, especially those of the gynoid type, still display softness and rotundity around the hips and legs even when their body weight is markedly reduced. This is obviously due to the presence of subcutaneous adipose tissue in these areas, despite weight reduction. It is conceivable that this subcutaneous tissue represents a minimum of attainable adiposity and that this minimum, being genetically determined, is relatively uninfluenced by environmental disturbances. Reduction below this minimum, even if compatible with life, could still be detrimental.

Similar views have been expressed regarding the muscularity of an individual. Thus it has been proposed that the level of maximal and minimal muscularity of an individual as well as the difference between them, is relatively constant, being determined to a large extent by heredity.[16] Were one to accept this view, then the minimum of adiposity or muscularity of an individual, if *set* high enough, would correspond to Sheldon's emaciated endomorph or inactive mesomorph respectively. In simpler terms, one might state that heredity determines the range of fatness, but how fat an individual actually is, or what point he occupies in this range, is determined by environmental factors.

Thus, accepting obesity as being due to both nature and nurture, the controversy between Sheldon and his critics loses much of its fervor. However, it still leaves unresolved the problem of whether obesity is associated with other physical or constitutional characteristics, as Sheldon seemed to believe. If such an association were proven, then obesity would be part of the constitutional makeup of the individual and, as such, might be associated with less visible, and conceivably morbid, traits. This would exonerate obesity as a disease, but not as a sign of a disease.[17] Thus, if obesity were inherited in such a fashion, i. e., as a constitutional package, including morbid traits, treating it would not reduce the risk of increased mortality.

Some evidence suggesting an association of obesity with other physical traits is presented in Table 2 in which an anthropometric comparison is shown between a group of 180 "healthy," white, obese, adolescent girls and a group of 74 non-obese girls.[18] The findings are consistent with the existence of more mesomorphy and less ectomorphy in the obese. Of particular interest, however, is the finding that wrist and ankle breadth, which was uninfluenced by nutrition in Lasker's study and thus probably genetically determined, is significantly greater in the obese girls. To this evidence, one may add that provided by Bjurulf showing an association between obesity and such inherited traits as increased hair growth on the chest and proximal phalanges.[5] This evidence, however scanty it is, is suggestive.

Conclusions

The *nature versus nurture* controversy which has afflicted other areas of anthropological research has been examined in this article with respect to its possible application to human obesity. Evidence has been presented to the effect that heredity is influential in determining how obese an individual may become *in a given set of environmental conditions*. This is shown pictorially in Figure 1 in which two individuals, one having inherited "genes for leanness" and the other "genes for fatness" are subjected to three different environmental settings consisting of scanty, normal and abundant food. The influence of the environment is obvious, as the degree of obesity increases with increasing food. Thus individual C possessing "genes for leanness" but exposed to abundant food is fatter than individual D having "genes for fatness" but exposed to scanty amounts of food. The influence of heredity is also obvious in that in each of the three environmental settings the individual with "genes for fatness" is fatter than the individual with "genes for leanness." Awareness of this predisposition to obesity should prevent individual D from becoming F, by appropriately modifying his own response to his environment. The crucial question is whether the goal of individual F should be to become D or A. In this context, the data of life

Table 2: Anthropometric Comparison Between Obese And "Nonobese" Adolescent Girls

	Obese (180)	Non-Obese (74)	P-value
Age	15.0	15.5	
Weight (lbs)	170.8	120.3	< .01
Stature (cm)	162.0	160.6	
Biacromial Diameter (cm)	36.2	34.8	< .01
Biepicondylar Breadth (mm)	68.7	60.8	< .01
Wrist breadth (mm)	51.7	48.9	< .01
Ankle breadth (mm)	64.2	61.5	< .01
Hand breadth (mm)	73.9	70.7	< .01

Reproduced from:
Seltzer CC and Mayer J: Body build and obesity—who are the obese? *J Amer Med Ass* 189:681, © 1964, American Medical Association.

insurance companies, indicating a more or less continuous fall in mortality rates as obesity decreases, would suggest that the goal of every individual would be to be as thin as possible. I believe that the data of insurance companies are inapplicable in answering this question as they do not take into account the concept of a genetically determined minimum of body fat. This minimum could also be regarded as a physiologic minimum. Assuming that obesity *per se* is indeed associated with increased mortality, then it would not constitute a conceptual leap to consider this physiologic minimum as representing the ideal body weight of the individual. 🔟

REFERENCES

1. Chlouverakis C: Controversies in medicine—Is obesity harmful? *Obesity and Bariatric Med* 2:108, 1973.

2. Mayer J: Genetic factors in human obesity. *Ann NY Acad Sci* 31:412-421, 1965.

3. Withers RFJ: Problems in the genetics of human obesity. *Eugenics Rev* 56:81-90, 1964.

4. Reynolds EL: The appearance of adult patterns of body hair in men. *Ann NY Acad Sci* 53:576-584, 1951.

5. Bjurulf P: Atherosclerosis and body-build with special reference to size and number of subcutaneous fat cells. *Acta Med Scand* 166 (Suppl 349):1-99, 1959.

6. Newman HH, Freeman FN and Holzinger KJ: *Twins: A study of heredity and environment,* University of Chicago Press, Chicago, 1937.

7. Von Verschuer O: Die vererbungsbiologische zwillings-forschung: Ihre licen zweieugen zwillings-und an 2 drillings-parren. *Ergebn Inn Med Kinderheilk* 31:35, 1927.

8. Osborn RH and DeGeorge FV: *Genetic basis of morphological variation,* Harvard University Press, Cambridge, 1959.

9. Dobzhansky T: *Mankind Evolving,* Yale University Press, New Haven, 1962.

10. Keys A and Brozek J: Body fat in adult man. *Physiol Rev* 33:245-325, 1953.

11. Sheldon WH, Stevens SS and Tucker WB: *The varieties of human physique,* Harper and Row, New York, 1940.

12. Hooton EA: Body build in a sample of the US Army Envir Protect Res Div, Hdqs Quartermaster Res and Engrg Command, *Tech Rep EP-102,* Quartermaster Res and Engrg Center, Natick, Mass, 1959.

13. Keys A, et al: *The biology of human starvation,* Univ of Minnesota Press, Minneapolis, 1950.

14. Lasker GW: The effects of partial starvation on somatotype: An analysis of material from the Minnesota starvation experiment. *Amer J Phys Anthropol* 5:323-341, 1947.

15. Sheldon WH: *Varieties of temperament: A psychology of constitutional differences,* Harper, New York, 1942.

16. Lindegard B: Body build and physical activity. *Lunds Universitets Arsskrift* 2:1-17, 1956.

17. Rimm AA: Controversies in medicine—Is obesity harmful?—A rebuttal. *Obesity and Bariatric Med* 2:140, 1973.

18. Seltzer C and Mayer J: Body build and obesity—Who are the obese? *J Amer Med Ass* 189:677-684, 1964.

Obesity in an age of caloric anxiety

THEODORE B. VAN ITALLIE, M.D.

*Director of Medicine,
St. Luke's Hospital Center,
and Clinical Professor of Medicine,
College of Physicians and Surgeons,
Columbia University, New York City*

SAMI A. HASHIM, M.D.

*Director, Division of
Metabolism and Nutrition,
St. Luke's Hospital Center,
and Associate Professor,
Institute of Human Nutrition,
Columbia University, New York City*

■ In the United States and other affluent societies, a growing proportion of citizens live in highly mechanized urban areas where the demands and opportunities for regular physical activity have steadily diminished. In this same environment, a variety of appetizing, calorically rich foods is increasingly available and readily procurable. During the last half century, this trend has shown little sign of relenting. In this setting, obesity has become a serious problem, both for individual patients and for the community.

There is little doubt that even moderate obesity is hazardous to health. Indeed, the increased risks of ill health associated with this disorder are now well recognized. Therefore, this can be considered an age of *caloric* anxiety (Fig. 1) in which the environ-

ment favors a level of food intake in excess of energy expenditure, at the same time generating guilt, shame, and fear in many patients over the consequences of the imbalance.

The physician's role

The responsibility for dealing with obesity and its attendant emotional conflicts usually is laid at the door of the physician. However, the physician's role is

a difficult one because few other medical disorders require the same disciplined and prolonged cooperation from the patient in their treatment. Even under the best of circumstances (in contrast to the successful therapy of acute infection), the results of treatment become manifest rather slowly and the benefits of adequate weight reduction may not become apparent for months or years. These handicaps tend to strain the busy physician's patience and may tempt him to resort to unsound methods of treatment. In his frustration, he may reject the patient for inability to lose weight and may become disillusioned with medical science for failing to provide him with adequate therapeutic tools.

These difficulties must be acknowledged, but they do not make the need for treating obesi-

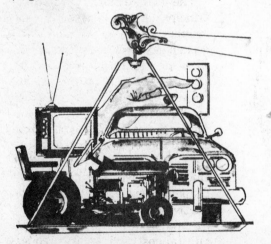

FIG. 1. *The environment favors the displacement of the equilibrium between calorie intake and calorie expenditure in the direction of a positive energy balance.*

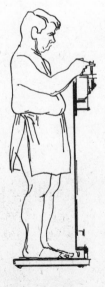

The age of caloric anxiety

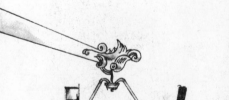

40

ty any less urgent and they should not deter the patient from seeking help or the physician from attempting treatment of suitable patients. However, unless he has a clear understanding of the psychological and physiological problems associated with weight reduction, the physician may be unnecessarily handicapped in his approach to the obese patient.

The problems involved in understanding and treating what appears so simple a disorder cannot be overestimated. But even if the obese patient finds himself unable to adapt to a program of weight reduction, it should be possible for the physician to use his knowledge of the subject for the education of the patient. By increasing the patient's insight into his own problems, the physician can provide reassurance and help relieve feelings of guilt and anxiety which may weigh more

heavily upon the patient than his excess of fat.

Hazards of obesity

The insurance statistics unequivocally relate overweight to a shortened life-span and show an excess mortality that increases in direct proportion to excess weight.[1] Other studies, such as those carried out in Framingham, do not show as dramatic a relationship between moderate obesity and mortality.

The insurance data on the adverse effects of obesity are grim. Excess mortality mounts rapidly with increasing degree of overweight, amounting to 13% in men 10% overweight, 25% for those 20% overweight, and over 40% for those 30% overweight. If mortality among the overweight group is compared with that among the "best weight" group (somewhat below average "normal" weight), men 10% or more

overweight have an excess mortality of one-third; for those 20% or more overweight, the excess is nearly one-half. For women, excess mortality corresponds more precisely to the degree of overweight; for example, in women, 30% overweight is associated with 30% excess mortality.

It is believed that these figures may underrate the excess mortality actually associated with extreme overweight, since the various insurance companies from whose records these data were obtained have been increasingly careful in the selection of overweight risks, particularly among older-age applicants.

It is also important to stress that an "excess mortality" of, say, 100% (double the expected mortality) does not mean a reduction of life expectancy by one-half. Such high ratios reflect a moderate curtailment of longevity but have no simple and direct relationship to length of life.

The relative mortality from the principal causes of death among insured overweight men and women is shown in Figure 2. Diseases of the heart and circulation are the most important because of their preeminent position in the total mortality picture. Among males, the death rate from this group of disorders is about one and one-half times that among so-called "standard risks." Diabetes exhibits the largest relative excess mortality among the major causes, with a death rate almost four times higher than that of standard risks among both men and women. Increased mortality from liver cirrhosis, biliary tract disease, and appendicitis also occurs among over-

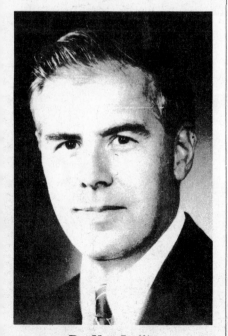

Dr. Van Itallie

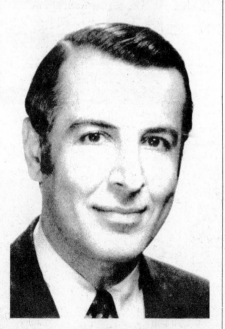

Dr. Hashim

weight persons. Obesity is also generally accepted as a hazard for the pregnant woman and the surgical patient.

The relationship of overweight to diseases of the heart and circulation can be further divided into such principal categories as hypertension, coronary heart disease, renal disease, and cerebrovascular disease.

Obesity, coronary heart disease, and diabetes

Coronary heart disease (CHD) appears to be more common in overweight persons. However, it is not clear whether obesity per se increases the risk of developing coronary heart disease or whether the reported increased risk of CHD associated with obesity is a phenomenon secondary to such risk factors as hypertension, hyperlipidemia, and diabetes mellitus, each of which may have an independent association with obesity. Some observers believe that when these risk factors are taken into account, as in the Framingham study,[2] obesity must be quite marked before it becomes a significant risk factor in its own right.

Obesity is closely associated with diabetes mellitus of the maturity-onset type. This fact is underscored by the use of such terms as "lipoplethoric diabetes" (a designation proposed by Lawrence in England) and "diabète gras," a term coined by L'Abbé in France. Most patients with maturity-onset diabetes are or have been obese. There is evidence that excess accumulation of fat in adipose cells somehow leads to insulin resistance and impaired glucose tolerance. Even in obese patients with normal glucose tolerance, a state of rela-

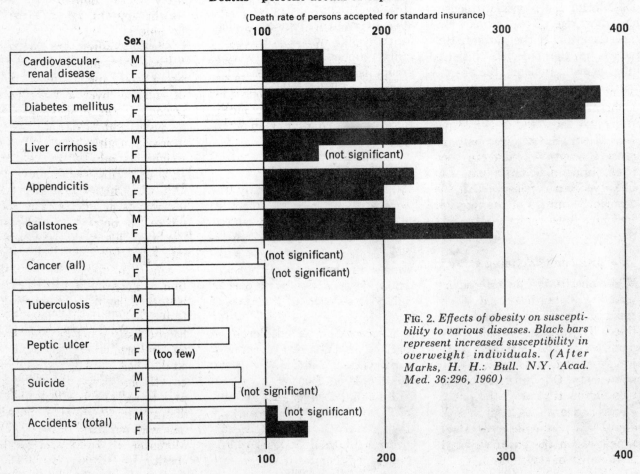

Deaths—percent actual of expected

(Death rate of persons accepted for standard insurance)

FIG. 2. *Effects of obesity on susceptibility to various diseases. Black bars represent increased susceptibility in overweight individuals. (After Marks, H. H.: Bull. N.Y. Acad. Med. 36:296, 1960)*

tive hyperinsulinism may be present, suggesting the existence of latent "compensated" diabetes.

Since diabetes mellitus is often associated with elevated values of serum triglycerides and, to a lesser extent, serum total cholesterol, it may be that some of the risk imposed on the obese subject by the presence of diabetes derives from the hyperlipidemia attendant upon diabetes. Moreover, diabetic patients appear to have widespread small vessel disease involving the basement membranes of capillaries and arterioles. In addition to their association with retinal, neural, and renal damage, such lesions may render the larger arteries somewhat more susceptible to atherosclerotic disease.

Whatever the cause, it is well known that the risk of developing coronary, cerebrovascular, and renal vascular (as well as peripheral vascular) disease is significantly increased in the diabetic patient. Since obese patients are so susceptible to diabetes mellitus, it is not surprising that obesity often carries with it the additional burden of the vascular complications associated with diabetes.

The problem of defining obesity

While obesity is a disorder which usually can be diagnosed by inspection, it is not as easily defined. There is no overall agreement as to the degree of overweight that divides obesity from nonobesity. One arbitrary definition holds that an obese individual is one who is 20% or more above his so-called desirable weight when the extra weight is in the form of stored fat.

Because storage of fat is a normal function of adipose tissue, it is difficult to determine the point at which the quantity of stored fat becomes excessive. It is usually assumed that the "normal" or "best" weight for an individual is achieved between the ages of 18 and 25 years. Hence, any significant positive deviation from this norm could be considered "obesity." Fatness, however, cannot always be predicted on the basis of weight. Height-weight relationships do not necessarily take into consideration an individual's build. For example, there is always the possibility of misinterpreting the significance of weight in heavily muscled people.

The proportion of fat in relation to total body weight increases with age. In one study,[3] approximately 14% of body weight in lean, young adults was fat; in contrast, fat accounted for 25% of body weight in clinically normal but sedentary men of normal weight at age 55.

Growth-onset obesity

Much obesity, particularly the severe form, has its roots in childhood.[4] Children may become obese at any time but this disorder is said to occur most commonly in three phases of childhood: first, in the latter part of infancy; second, at the time of starting school; and third, during adolescence. The incidence of obesity in childhood is not well documented, but in one study conducted in Boston it was reported that 13% of girls and 9% of boys between the ages of 12 and 19 years were sufficiently overweight to be categorized as "obese." Other reports have sug-

gested that between 20 and 30% of the adolescent population is significantly overweight, with girls showing a higher incidence than boys.

One study has reported that the weights of natural children correlated well with those of their parents, while the weights of adopted children showed no correlation with those of the adopting parents. If one of a pair of identical twins is obese, a similar degree of obesity can be anticipated in the other, with notable exceptions. When identical twins are raised in dissimilar environments, the weight difference may be slightly larger, but the primary factor determining body weight appears, nevertheless, to be genetic.

Obese children are likely to become obese adults. In one survey of height and weight in groups of subjects over a twenty-year period, it was found that 86% of overweight boys and 80% of overweight girls remained overweight as adults. In contrast, 42% of normal-weight boys and 18% of normal-weight girls were overweight as adults. The more severe the obesity in childhood, the more likely it is to persist into adult life.

Since an appreciable proportion of overweight adults give a history of having been overweight in childhood, it is clear that childhood obesity must be considered an important determinant of adult obesity. Adults with the growth-onset type of obesity appear to respond less favorably to dietary treatment than individuals with maturity-onset obesity. Moreover, children who develop obesity in infancy are less re-

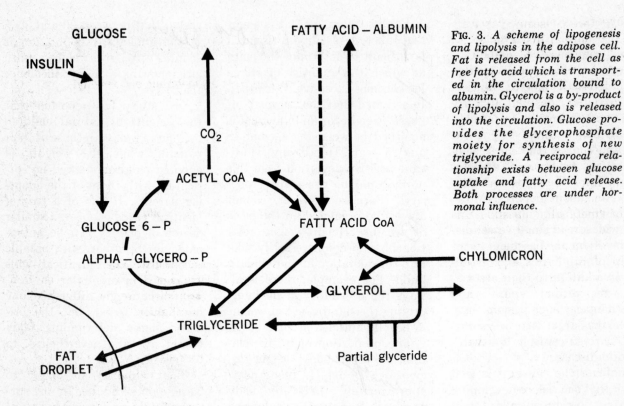

GLUCOSE

INSULIN

FATTY ACID — ALBUMIN

CO₂

ACETYL CoA

GLUCOSE 6 — P

FATTY ACID CoA

ALPHA — GLYCERO — P

CHYLOMICRON

GLYCEROL

TRIGLYCERIDE

FAT DROPLET

Partial glyceride

FIG. 3. *A scheme of lipogenesis and lipolysis in the adipose cell. Fat is released from the cell as free fatty acid which is transported in the circulation bound to albumin. Glycerol is a by-product of lipolysis and also is released into the circulation. Glucose provides the glycerophosphate moiety for synthesis of new triglyceride. A reciprocal relationship exists between glucose uptake and fatty acid release. Both processes are under hormonal influence.*

sponsive to weight-reduction programs than those becoming overweight during puberty. Thus, the time of onset of obesity as well as its severity has some prognostic significance as regards responsiveness to therapy. While the division of obesity into the growth-onset and the adult-onset forms is useful for the physician, it must be remembered that the age of onset within these two broad categories also may influence the chances of therapeutic success.

The adipose cells: behavior, size, and number

Essentially all of the fat that is part of obesity tissue is located inside the fat (or adipose) cells. These cells are not mere reservoirs of fat but are active in the

synthesis of triglyceride from carbohydrate and fatty acids. The degree of "adiposity" or fatness of an individual may reflect both the number of adipose cells in the body and their size.

Whether the number of fat cells in the adult subject is genetically determined is not known; however, there is recent evidence that hyperplasia of these cells may take place early in life in response to a generous calorie intake.[5] Subsequently, the number of fat cells may remain fixed for a given individual, suggesting that change in body fat content after a certain critical phase in development is a function of adipose cell size rather than number. If confirmed, such observations might well have a useful application in the prevention of obesity

later in life, since the number of fat cells in the body would be prone to control by appropriate feeding practices in infancy.

The synthesis and mobilization of fat from adipose cells are processes that are subject to a variety of influences. These are indicated in Figure 3, which also provides a schematic summary of the steps involved in lipogenesis and lipolysis. It is clear that a prolonged imbalance between rates of fat synthesis and mobilization must lead to either depletion or excessive accumulation of triglyceride, depending on the metabolic circumstances.

Thus, one form of imbalance is basically responsible for obesity, and the other must be induced if the treatment of obesity is to be effective. The most common form of obesity would seem to result from a prolonged disturbance in the regulation of food intake ("regulatory" obesity) in which a relative excess of metabolites derived from food is presented to normal adipose cells for further processing and storage. It is also possible that the fat cells themselves could promote obesity by resisting lipolysis while maintaining a normal rate of synthesis (a form of "metabolic" obesity). In earlier textbooks on the subject, this phenomenon was referred to as "lipophilia." At the present time, studies of fat turnover based on the use of radioisotopes suggest that some instances of obesity are indeed of the lipophilic type. If an individual is endowed with an abundance of adipose cells, this cellular overpopulation might be a determinant of obesity, apart from any alterations in the metabolic behavior of the individual adipose cells.

Classification of obesities

From the standpoint of causation, the obesities can be classified under two broad headings, regulatory and metabolic, as shown in the table. Patients with regulatory obesity are those in whom no metabolic abnormality to account for the obesity can be identified. The basis for this type of obesity may be [1] psychological, for example, as the result of neurotic overeating or cultural eating patterns in otherwise normal persons, or [2] physiological, resulting either from a neurological disorder causing increased energy intake or from some form of forced immobilization and reduced energy expenditure. Some patients with immobilizing frac-

Regulatory obesity (no primary metabolic abnormality)
  Psychological
    Neurotic overeating
    Nonneurotic overeating (cultural dietary pattern)

  Physiological
    Increased intake — hypothalamic disorder
    Decreased output — forced immobilization

Metabolic obesity
  Enzymatic
  Hormonal
  Neurological

Tentative grouping of forms of obesity according to mechanism

tures have exhibited this latter phenomenon.

Metabolic obesity results from a "metabolic" disorder in which, for example, fat accumulates more readily than it is mobilized.[6] This form of obesity has been identified in certain experimental animals but the extent of its occurrence in man remains a matter of controversy. The obesity in some patients with insulinoma or with Cushing's syndrome might be considered "metabolic." It is entirely conceivable that as techniques for studying biochemical processes in man improve, other forms of metabolic obesity will be identified.

Clinically, obesity seems most usefully categorized in descriptive terms such as age at onset, degree of severity, presence of an associated pertinent disorder such as diabetes, hypertension, osteoarthritis, or hyperlipidemia, and so forth. Thus, a typical diagnosis might read: regulatory obesity, adult-onset, moderate (associated with diabetes mellitus). While other information concerning the obese patient can well be taken up in the history of the present illness, the age at the onset of the disorder, its degree, and the presence of associated disease would seem of sufficient importance to include in the diagnosis.

Principles of treatment

The reduction of body weight entails restricting calorie intake to a level well below that of energy expenditure. The goals during weight decrease are [1] loss of body fat with a minimal accompanying breakdown of lean tissue, [2] maintenance of physical and emotional fitness during the reducing period, [3] avoidance of untoward reactions to dieting, and [4] establishment of eating and exercise habits that will help the formerly obese patient maintain his weight at the recommended level.

In formulating a reducing diet, a number of factors must be considered. These include the degree of overweight of the patient, his age, his state of physical fitness, his normal level of physical activity, and the presence of associated illness such as hypertension, coronary heart disease, diabetes mellitus, or gastrointestinal disorder. In general, very obese individuals often require diets markedly reduced in calories; otherwise, the time needed to accomplish discernible changes is discouragingly long.

The most drastic reducing diet is one that provides no calories at all. It is now recognized that diets totally devoid of calories must provide sufficient quantities of water, electrolytes (notably potassium), and vitamins to prevent dehydration, excessive muscular weakness, mental confusion, abnormalities of heart function, and other complications. For these reasons, patients who are treated with the "no-calorie" diet should be hospitalized during the period of total calorie starvation. The patient must remain at rest or limit himself to light activity during the fasting period. During the total calorie restriction, fat is burned at an appreciable rate; however, significant quantities of lean tissue are also broken down and lost.

It would seem helpful to define a reference diet that could serve as a "lower limit" in food restriction for ambulatory adult patients. Such a diet would provide enough carbohydrate to reduce or largely prevent ketosis and to minimize wastage of protein and electrolytes. It would contain enough protein to replace wear-and-tear losses and to maintain reasonable reserves. It would provide all other essential nutrients in amounts recommended by the Food and Nutrition Board of the National Research Council.[7]

An example of a suggested lower-limit diet follows:

	gm.	kcal.
Carbohydrate	100	400
Protein	50	200
Fat	22	200
Total		800

Added to this base are all the necessary vitamins and minerals. Water is given in unrestricted amounts. As can be seen, the total number of calories in this lower-limit diet is 800. Because fat makes other foods more palatable and because diets devoid of fat tend to be dry, bulky, and unappetizing, some fat is retained in this diet. Indeed, from a practical standpoint, it is virtually impossible to design an acceptable diet that does not derive at least 25% of its calories from fat.

When the calorie intake is very low, a large proportion of dietary protein is used as a rather inefficient and expensive source of energy. Hence, the intake level of 50 gm. of protein per day is recommended principally because it provides some insurance against protein depletion and because protein-rich foods help to make low-calorie diets more palatable and satisfying.

It will be noted that the lower-limit diet, as described, is "balanced" in the sense that the proportions of carbohydrate, fat, and protein are not too dissimilar from those ordinarily consumed in a calorically adequate diet. In recent years, "unbalanced" diets, particularly diets very low in carbohydrate, have achieved both popularity and notoriety and have been praised by some as being remarkably effective and condemned by others for promoting such side effects as hypercholesterolemia and ketosis. A detailed discussion of the metabolic effects of unbalanced diets is beyond the scope of this paper. It is perhaps sufficient to emphasize that hard evidence is lacking that such diets induce a rate of fat loss greater than can be accounted for by their caloric content. Their supposed anorexic effect probably results from the lack of palatability inherent in any drastically imbalanced diet. Such diets can be sustained for only brief periods and do not appear to provide a realistic basis for the long-term adjustment of food intake needed to maintain the formerly obese individual at his desirable weight.

For the obese individual whose weight is 50% or more above the recommended level (relative weight equals 150 or greater), a lower-limit diet might be appropriate provided that physical activity remains light. If the level of activity is higher, a corresponding increase in the calorie allowance should be made. For the less obese person, a somewhat greater calorie allowance might be appropriate, and calorie levels ranging from 1,000 to 1,800 may be selected depending [1] upon the rapidity of weight loss sought, [2] the ability of the patient to follow the diet without excessive discomfort, and [3] the patient's activity level.

In reviewing principles of weight reduction, it is essential to have an understanding of the caloric equivalence of weight loss. Pure fat has a caloric value of approximately 9 kcal. per gram. Since 1 lb. equals 454 gm., the caloric value of 1 lb. of pure triglyceride is 4,086 kcal. There is evidence that approximately 62% of "obesity tissue" is fat, the remainder being made up of water and other components. Accordingly, it could be reasoned that a patient whose recommended weight is 70 kg. (154 lb.) and whose actual weight is 231 lb., or 105 kg. (relative weight, 150), contains 77×0.62 lb. of triglyceride or 48 lb. of excess fat. To restore this patient to his recommended weight would require a total calorie deficit of approximately $48 \times 454 \times 9$ or 196, 198 kcal. If such a patient were to adhere faithfully to an 800-kcal. diet and have a daily energy expenditure of 3,000 kcal., it would take approximately ninety days to return to the desired weight level. This represents a weight loss of approximately 0.85 lb. per day or 5.7 lb. per week.

Actually, this type of calculation is idealized and inherently inaccurate. For example, an appreciable amount of lean tissue is also lost during a weight-reduction program. The caloric value of hydrated lean tissue is approximately 1 kcal. per gram. Also, as weight is lost, the cost of physical activity diminishes in proportion. Thus, armchair calculations for predicting weight loss are necessarily inexact and have their chief value in providing the patient and his physician with fairly realistic expectations of the quantity of weight that can be lost over a given period of time. Often the patient does not distinguish between weight loss and fat loss, and it is necessary for him to understand that, in terms of accomplishment, water loss is meaningless, while excessive loss of lean tissue is harmful.

It is difficult to formulate a recommended rate of weight loss. Such a rate might be thought of as the maximum rate of fat loss compatible with avoidance of undue protein breakdown, excessive ketosis, and other untoward metabolic responses. Although the patient usually cannot avoid some discomfort while restricting his food intake, the reducing program can be compatible with light physical activity, mental and emotional comfort, and absence of abnormal fatigue. Some patients follow weight-reduction programs far better than others; in rare instances, serious emotional or physical complications may accompany attempts to lose weight. In practice, a desirable and adequate rate of weight loss would appear to be about 0.5 lb. per day. This is the equivalent of approximately 141 gm. of fat and represents a deficit of approximately 1,200 kcal. per day.

Physical activity is a most important part of the usual weight-reduction regime. The extra calories consumed by a given activity are a function of the type of activity, the intensity with which it is carried out, and its duration. In addition, appropriate physical work promotes general health and well-being. There is evidence suggesting that the risk of developing coronary heart disease is accentuated in sedentary individuals. Finally, there is indirect evidence that sedentary persons who increase their daily level of physical activity do not necessarily exhibit a corresponding increase in appetite. Indeed, there may result a paradoxical decrease of food consumption.

Finally, a punitive approach to the problem of obesity is not likely to be productive. Much of the hostility of physicians and dietitians toward the obese patient is likely to result from their own sense of frustration as regards effective treatment. These workers must be understanding and supportive in their attitudes toward the patient. However, it is essential that they explain the problems involved in treatment to the patient in considerable detail and that the difficulties not be minimized.

REFERENCES

1. BUILD AND BLOOD PRESSURE STUDY, 1959. Society of Actuaries, Chicago, 1959.

2. KAGAN, A., DAWBER, T. R., KANNEL, W. B., and REVOTSKIE, N.: The Framingham study: a prospective study of coronary heart disease. Fed. Proc. Vol. 21, Part 2, No. 4, Suppl. 11, 1962, p. 52.

3. BROZEK, J.: Changes of body composition in man during maturity and their nutritional implications. Fed. Proc. 11:784, 1952.

4. WOLFF, O. H.: Obesity in childhood. In: Recent Advances in Pediatrics. Edited by D. Gairdner. Boston: Little, Brown & Co., 1965.

5. KNITTLE, J. L., and HIRSCH, J.: Effect of early nutrition on the development of rat epididymal fat pads: cellularity and metabolism. J. clin. Invest. 47:2091, 1968.

6. MAYER, J.: The physiological basis of obesity and leanness. Parts I and II. Nutr. Abstr. Rev. 25:597, 871, 1955.

7. RECOMMENDED DIETARY ALLOWANCES. 7th revised edition, 1969. National Academy of Sciences, National Research Council, Washington, D.C., 1969.

At present we have only an incomplete answer for the important question of whether we can modify the number of adipose cells. For the rat, one can say yes, we can modify the ultimate number of adipocytes by underfeeding the very young animal. For man, the answer is maybe. Yet it is clearly important to know whether we can modify adipocyte development in man and if such modification could be useful in prevention or early treatment of human obesity. The following is a brief summary of where research in this field stands and what must be done to provide a better answer.

Cell Number in Human Obesity

Obesity is best defined as an increase in the amount of adipose tissue. Other organs or structures may participate in the weight increase of the obese, yet the major and defining abnormality is an increase in adipose tissue. Obviously, this enlargement can come about by an increase in either adipocyte size (hypertrophy) or cell number (hyperplasia).

Technics are available for measuring the numbers of adipocytes in small amounts of tissue removed surgically or by needle aspiration.[1] With these technics, it can be shown that most obese individuals have some increase in adipocyte size, yet in nearly all obese humans, particularly those with obesity of juvenile onset, there is a striking increase in adipocyte number. An average nonobese individual has 25 to 30 $\times$ 10^9 adipocytes. With obesity this number increases 3 to 5 times.[2]

JULES HIRSCH, M.D.

Rockefeller University
New York

Can We Modify the Number of Adipose Cells?

Obesity is a function of both number and fat content of adipocytes. In adults with juvenile-onset obesity, the number of adipocytes is increased in comparison with average nonobese persons. By weight loss, such obese adults can decrease the fat content but not the total number of cells. If the periods of adipocyte multiplication can be pinpointed, prevention or early treatment of obesity may be possible.

Furthermore, the adipocyte number remains fixed in the adult. With weight reduction, as adipose tissue decreases in total size, the number of cells remains constant. Hence, weight loss is achieved by a reduction in cell volume, but the formerly obese individual has a persistent morphologic abnormality with many small adipocytes. As far as we know, this abnormality remains indefinitely after weight reduction.

The situation is quite different when man is made experimentally obese. Sims and coworkers[3] showed that such experimental obesity leads only to filling of adipocytes without a net increase in cell number. In these studies, normal volunteers with no history of disturbance in weight regulation were urged to become obese by increasing food consumption and decreasing energy output. Those who developed sizable increases in adipose tissue stores did so exclusively by filling cells rather than by increasing cell number. Weight reduction occurred spontaneously when overfeeding was discontinued and adipocytes returned to normal size.

Thus, it would appear that garden-variety clinical obesity with hyperplasia of adipocytes is not simply the result of overeating in adult life. Does this hyperplasia occur earlier in life? Are obesity and the filling of these cells a response to the hyperplastic reaction? Some answers are suggested from the study of adipose cellular development and experimental obesity in animals.

Animal Studies

It is simplest to study the development of adipose cellularity in animals with a short life-span that can be sacrificed periodically. The rat has been most extensively studied. This animal is born quite thin, but immediately after birth adipose tissue is deposited rapidly. The ratio of fat to body weight climbs during the early life of the animal. Early in life, fattening is achieved by the appearance of new adipocytes along with adipocyte filling. By 10 to 12 weeks of age, the adult number of adipocytes is achieved and further fattening occurs only by enlargement of cells already present.[4]

Attempts to fatten or thin the animal after the earliest weeks of life lead only to change in cell size. Thus, the overfed or underfed adult rat will expand or shrink adipose tissue but only at the expense of adipocyte volume. Number remains constant. More drastic maneuvers, such as creation of lesions in portions of the brain that control food intake and satiety, lead to extreme obesity in the adult animal but again only by enlarging preexisting cells.[4] In this respect, the experimental obesity in the adult rat and the experimental obesity in man are very much alike.

It was thought that influences acting earlier in life might change adipocyte number. To check this hypothesis, genetic forms

---

Current evidence suggests that most adipose cells are laid down late in gestation, in the first year of life, and in early adolescence.

---

of obesity were examined. A genetic form known as Zucker obesity has been studied in the rat, and a variety of obese mouse strains have been examined. In all these animals the major morphologic change is an increase in cell size very much like that occurring with experimental obesity in adult man or adult animals. In some instances there are also sharp increases in cell number, particularly in the subcutaneous tissue, yet the major morphologic aspect of genetic obesity remains cell stuffing rather than increase of cell number.[5,6]

A most interesting experiment performed some years ago showed that nutritional influences working early in the life of the rat (presumably at a time intermediate between genetic or antenatal influences and adult effects) can and do modify cell number. Numerous rat litters were mixed at birth, artificially providing some rat mothers with large litters (22 or 23) and others with small litters (three to six). The animals reared in large litters were severely deprived nutritionally during the first three weeks of life and were permanently stunted. Although the stunting involved body nitrogen content as well as fat, it was clear from this experiment that stunting was greater in adipose than in other tissues. There was some reduction in adipocyte size but there was also a very marked reduction in cell number. The cell number remained reduced well into the adult life of the animal.[7] This experiment suggests that there may be "critical periods" when nutritional influences can create permanent changes in adipose cellularity.

Development and Modification of Human Cellularity

Developmental studies in man have been too few to give assurance as to what the pattern of cell size and cell number development is throughout infancy and childhood and thus what ages might be critical periods. The data at hand suggest that the newborn human infant has about one-fourth to one-fifth the adult number of cells, with about one-fourth the adult amount of lipid. Thus, a fourfold to fivefold increase in size and number of cells occurs from birth to adulthood. The patterns of fat accretion in man and in the rat are considerably different. The rat deposits fat very rapidly after birth and continues to do so, although at a declining rate, as life progresses. The human infant is born relatively fatter than infants of most other species. Clearly a great deal of fat accumulates in fetal adipose tissue in the last trimester of pregnancy. After the first few months of life there is relatively little further

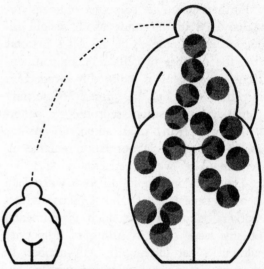

increased number and size of adipose cells

fattening until the adolescent growth spurt begins.

Current evidence would favor the idea that most adipose cells are laid down in the last part of gestation, with some cells added in the first year of life and some in early adolescence. Thus, the period from 1 to 10 years of age may not be a significant time for new adipocyte formation. If nutritional influences can most affect ultimate adipocyte number when cells are appearing, then the critical periods in man are likely to be the last months of gestation, very early in life, and during adolescence.

A few obese infants and children who were studied for adipose cellularity showed increases in cell number even before adolescence,[8] so it is difficult to judge definitively what time in life is best for the treatment and prevention of obesity. If late gestation and adolescence are the important periods, much more attention may have to be focused on maternal feeding and on nutritional practices during the pubertal growth spurt. The latter period would seem to be much more amenable to dietary manipulation.

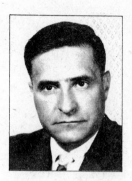

JULES HIRSCH

Dr. Hirsch is professor and senior physician, Rockefeller University, New York.

Unanswered Questions

So much is yet to be learned that it is hard to decide which approaches will be most promising. Nutritional influences on adipose cellularity should be explored in more fundamental terms. Determining adipocyte number during development could be misleading, since some precursor or unfilled adipocytes may escape detection. Studies by Hollenberg, Vost and Patten[9] showed that adipocyte DNA in adult animals incorporates some tritiated thymidine, indicating some turnover of mature adipocytes. New cells may be added as precursor cells fill with fat and join the adipocyte pool. Although turnover may be very small, the DNA kinetics of adipocytes both in precursor tissues and in mature adipocytes must be understood for a full evaluation.

Much more information about the development of normal cell size and number in infants and children is needed. Are some infants hypercellular at birth and thus destined to be obese? Is this hypercellularity the result of maternal feeding practices during gestation, or is it genetically determined? Is it possible to modify the diet of adolescents to control or reduce cell number? Finally, what is the physiologic and regulatory meaning of an increased adipocyte number? In what way might numerous adipocytes signal the central nervous system to promote overfeeding? Could these signals be manipulated to control obesity? These and many other questions may go unanswered for some time, but with what is already known, several recommendations would appear reasonable.

Conclusion

Optimal nutrition for infants and also for adolescents must be redefined. Most often, and with good reason, concern has been focused on undernutrition and inadequate intake of protein, vitamins and minerals. The upper limits must also be defined. It may well be that a restriction of calories, particularly during adolescence, will be of advantage in reducing the incidence of adult obesity.

Again, in an attempt to answer the question posed by the title of this paper, one might say yes, we can modify the number of adipose cells in rats, and in man we should begin making efforts to do so.

REFERENCES

1. Hirsch J, Gallian E: Methods for the determination of adipose cell size in man and animals. J Lipid Res 9:110, 1968
2. Hirsch J, Knittle JL: Cellularity of obese and non-obese human adipose tissue. Fed Proc 29:1516, 1970
3. Sims EA, Goldman RF, Gluck CM, et al: Experimental obesity in man. Trans Assoc Am Physicians 81:153, 1968
4. Hirsch J, Han PW: Cellularity of rat adipose tissue: Effects of growth, starvation and obesity. J Lipid Res 10:77, 1969
5. Johnson PR, Zucker LM, Cruce JA, et al: Cellularity of adipose depots in the genetically obese Zucker rat. J Lipid Res 12:706, 1971
6. Johnson P, Hirsch J: The cellularity of adipose depots in six strains of genetically obese mice. J Lipid Res (in press)
7. Knittle JL, Hirsch J: Effect of early nutrition on the development of rat epididymal fat pads: Cellularity and metabolism. J Clin Invest 47:2091, Sept 1968
8. Knittle JL, Ginsberg-Fellner F: Adipose tissue cellularity and epinephrine stimulated lipolysis in obese and non-obese children. Clin Res 17:387, 1969
9. Hollenberg CH, Vost A, Patten RL: Regulation of adipose mass: Control of fat cell development and lipid content. Recent Progr Horm Res 26:463, 1970

Physiology and Natural History of Obesity

Ralph A. Nelson, MD, PhD; Lorrayne F. Anderson, MS;
Clifford F. Gastineau, MD; Alvin B. Hayles, MD; and Connie L. Stamnes

Physiologic studies reported here show that obese persons use carbohydrate, fat, and protein normally during rest and exercise and are not unusually efficient in the use of these energy substrates. Obese subjects mobilize fat stores for energy as readily as normals. It is not necessary to overeat to become obese; the decrease of basal calorie requirements with age is such that obesity can develop with advancing age while exercise remains constant, even if food intake is reduced to some extent. Subjects tested were persons of various ages whose intake of food ranged from that of hypophagia to that of hyperphagia and whose body weights varied similarly.

The question of why obese persons are obese is as yet unanswered. In this paper, three hypotheses relating to this question are considered.

The first hypothesis states that obese persons are obese because they use calories more economically than do nonobese persons. The second states that the obese have difficulty in releasing body fat for energy needs. The third hypothesis assumes that obese persons are obese because they eat relatively more than nonobese persons. To test these hypotheses, three groups of subjects were studied.

Methods

Group 1.—Since the two largest components of caloric expenditure are basal metabolism and exercise,[1] these two functions were studied in 142 persons having varying amounts of body fat. These persons included those with anorexia nervosa (hypophagic patients), normal and obese children, normal and obese adults, and those hyperphagic children having the Prader-Willi syndrome.[2] The physical features of these subjects are summarized in Table 1.

The basal metabolic rate (BMR) was determined in 82 subjects referred to the obesity clinic. In all patients the weight exceeded the ideal by at least 20%; and in four fifths of them the ideal was exceeded by 40%. All subjects were in the postabsorptive state, none had taken food or water on the morning of the test, and all rested quietly for at least 20 minutes before a ten-minute collection of expired air was obtained. A Haldane analysis was performed on the expired air.

Oxygen consumption and carbon dioxide production were determined under basal conditions and during step exercise in 60 subjects. Subjects studied comprised the following: normal children (14), normal adults (8), obese children (11), obese adults (15), children with the Prader-Willi syndrome (7), and patients with anorexia nervosa (5). The step test consisted of 15 steps per minute for five minutes. For subjects 1.2 meter tall or less, the height of the step was 12.5 cm; for those taller, 22.5 cm. Expired air was collected in Douglas bags during each minute of the last three minutes of exercise. Oxygen and carbon dioxide content of expired air were determined by Haldane analysis. Positive work was calculated from the formula[3]:

$$\text{Work} = \text{body mass (kg)} \times 9.80 \ (\text{m/sec}^2) \times \text{height of step (m)}.$$

Group 2.—In the second portion of the study, the use of fat for metabolic purposes was determined by indirect calorimetry. The normal children and adults and the obese children and adults among the subjects in group 1 collected 24-hour samples of urine for determination of total nitrogen excretion. The collection ended on the morning of the BMR and exercise test. From the 24-hour total urinary nitrogen, and the oxygen consumption and carbon dioxide production at rest and during a steady state of exercise, the consumption (in grams) of protein, carbohydrate, and fat during basal and exercise metabolism was calculated[4] for each subject.

Group 3.—In the third portion of the study, relationships between kilocalorie intake, weight, age, and the decline of BMR associated with aging were studied. For this, 22 case histories were analyzed in the medical

From the Mayo Clinic and Mayo Foundation, Rochester, Minn.

Read in part at the meeting of the Federation of the American Societies for Experimental Biology, Atlantic City, NJ, April 10-14, 1972.

Reprint requests to Mayo Clinic, 200 First St SW, Rochester, Minn 55901 (Dr. Nelson).

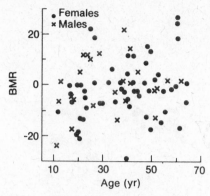

Fig 1.—Basal metabolic rate (BMR) of 82 patients seen in obesity clinic.

record department of the Mayo Clinic. The records of these 22 patients (12 women, 10 men) were chosen for detailed analysis because they represented subjects normal in body weight for their height and sex at the age of 30 years; and they regularly returned to the Mayo Clinic for review and had no significant health problems during the 35-year period of examination. For the purpose of combining and analyzing data, a value of 100 was assigned for their body weight at the age of 30 years. Changes in weight were then determined for the next 30 to 32 years and expressed as a percentage of 100; and from these data, the change in mean body weight of the group at various

ages throughout the 32-year span was calculated. A "reference woman" (1.63 meters [5 ft 5 in], 54.4 kg [120 lb] at age 30) and a "reference man" (1.73 meters [5 ft 9 in], 70 kg [154 lb] at age 30) were chosen as representatives for the group.

Using the food nomogram[5] and assuming that exercise consumed a constant proportion of 35% of the basal metabolic kilocalorie expenditure, the kilocalories necessary for the reference woman and man to eat to describe the mean body weight curve for the group were calculated. The kilocaloric requirements for the reference man and woman at the age of 30 years were assigned a value of 100, and subsequent changes in these requirements were expressed as percentages of that base. The food nomogram takes into account the decline in basal kilocalorie requirements with age and the increase in kilocalorie requirements with an increase in surface area. Nine kilocalories in excess of daily requirements were assumed to be necessary for the reference person to gain 1 gm of fat, though in clinical practice this value is perhaps closer to 8 kcal/gm fat.[6]

Results

Groups 1 and 2.—BASAL METABOLIC RATE.—The mean BMR for the population of obese patients was −0.6% and the standard deviation (SD) was ±10.6% (BMR for normals: mean, 0; SD ±9.7%). The BMRs of 53 (65%) of the obese subjects were within the range of ±10%, usually cited as being normal; the BMRs of 22 (27%) of the obese subjects ranged between ±10 to ± 20; and the BMR was outside the ± 20 range in seven (Fig 1). Thus, the obese subjects demonstrated remarkably normal BMRs.

Among the subjects exercised, the obese children were as tall as normal children but weighed about twice as much (Table 1). The mean height of children with the Prader-Willi syndrome was 27.25 cm (11 inches) less than that of the normal children; the mean weights were similar. Of the adults, the obese were about twice as heavy and the patients with anorexia nervosa were one half as heavy as normal subjects. The BMRs were normal in all but the patients with anorexia nervosa: the mean BMR of the latter group was −22% (range, −14 to −44%).

RESPIRATORY QUOTIENT.—During mild step exercise, in all subjects, the oxygen consumed (Fig 2) and carbon dioxide produced (Fig 3) were directly related to the positive work performed. Even in patients with anorexia nervosa, oxygen consumption was related to work performed, despite their low BMRs.

Obese children and obese adults tended to use more fat in basal metabolism than normal children and adults (Table 2); the difference was almost statistically significant (P between .1 and .05). Between normal and obese persons, the nonprotein respiratory quotient (NPRQ) was not statistically different, the relative proportion of fat to carbohydrate used thus being similar in all groups of subjects at rest.

During exercise, obese subjects used as much fat as normals, even though utilization of carbohydrate was significantly increased (Table 2). Differences in exercise NPRQ values were again borderline in their significance.

Group 3.—The detailed analysis of medical records revealed that 67% of the women and 70% of the men were overweight at some time during the 32 years of follow-up study; 50% of both groups were overweight at the

Fig 2.—Positive work (step exercise) and oxygen consumption in normal and obese children and adults, children with Prader-Willi syndrome, and patients with anorexia nervosa.

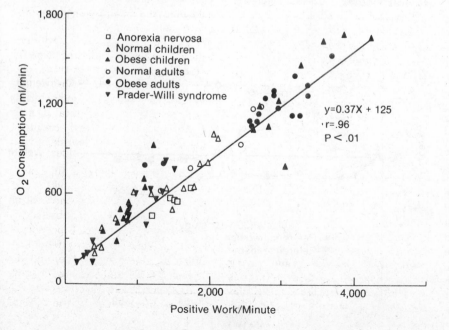

$y = 0.37X + 125$
$r = .96$
$P < .01$

age of 62 years. Approximately one third of the group became obese, but only 17% of the women and 10% of the men were obese at the age of 62 years. The mean body weight of the group of 22 patients gradually increased and these patients became overweight at 50 years of age (Fig 4). Between the ages of 42 and 62 years, there was a slight increase and subsequent decrease, but essentially, the mean value for the group remained in the overweight category for 20 years. The kilocalorie intake of the men would have had to decrease by almost 5% in order to describe the body weight curve (Fig 4). The kilocalorie intake of the women must have increased by almost 5% for the first 12 years, but then it too had to be reduced by almost 6% over the next 20 years to describe the body weight curve of the group. Between the ages of 30 and 54 years for the men, and between the ages of 42 and 54 years for the women, caloric intake was decreasing, although both sexes were gaining weight. To have remained at ideal body weight, men would have had to have decreased kilocalorie intake by 11% and women by 5% over the entire 30-year period. A man weighing 70 kg (154 lb), eating 2,400 kcal, and expending 2,400 kcal at the age of 30 years would weigh 91 kg (201 lb) at age 62 if no changes were made in either food intake or exercise.

Comment

The results from the first portion of the study (group 1) showed that the obese population used calories for basal metabolism normally. The mean BMR and variability about the mean were nearly identical with normal population groups.[7] Our data also confirm the earlier finding of Boothby and Sandiford[8] that the BMR in obese subjects is normal. We conclude that an abnormally low BMR is not an etiologic factor in obesity. Since the BMR is computed on the basis of surface area, it follows that the obese person is actually using more oxygen and burning more fuel than his lean counterpart of similar age, sex, and height. In fact, if the BMR of the obese person were computed on the basis of the surface area of his lean counterpart, he would have a BMR of perhaps plus 20 or plus 30. In this re-

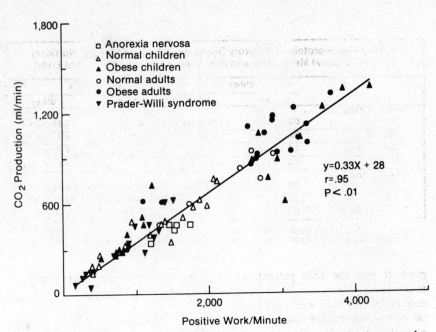

Fig 3.—Positive work (step exercise) and carbon dioxide production in normal and obese children and adults, children with Prader-Willi syndrome, and patients with anorexia nervosa.

Table 1.—Means (and Ranges) of Age, Height, and Weight of Exercised Subjects

	Age, yr	Height, Meters	Weight, kg
Children			
Normal (N = 14)	11 (6-17)	1.5 (1.2-1.8)	40.4 (21.3-62.7)
Obese (N = 11)	10 (4-17)	1.5 (1.2-1.7)	75.2 (34.0-125.6)
Prader-Willi			
(N = 7)	8 (5-16)	1.2 (1.0-1.4)	40.8 (20.9-80.7)
Adults			
Normal (N = 8)	44 (25-55)	1.7 (1.5-1.9)	63.5 (39.5-85.7)
Obese (N = 14)	37 (19-69)	1.7 (1.4-1.8)	108.8 (67.6-204.5)
Anorexia nervosa			
(N = 5)	20 (15-29)	1.6 (1.6-1.8)	39.9 (32.7-48.5)

Fig 4.—Body weight changes associated with age in normal aging population (open circles) and kilocalorie intake of women (closed squares) and men (closed circles) necessary to describe the body weight curve assuming no change in rate of daily exercise.

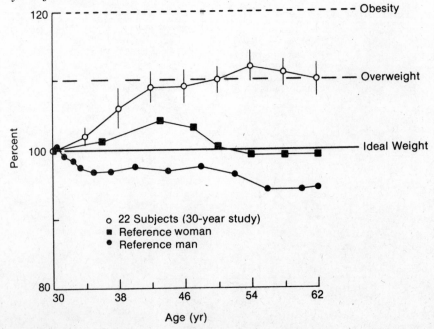

Table 2.—Nonprotein Respiratory Quotients (NPRQ) and Use of Nutrients (gm/hr) in Basal Metabolism and Step Exercise (Mean ± Standard Error)

	Children		Adults	
	Normal	Obese	Normal	Obese
Basal Metabolism				
NPRQ	0.83 ± 0.01	0.81 ± 0.03	0.79 ± 0.02	0.76 ± 0.02
Fat	3.2 ± 0.3	4.1 ± 0.6	4.4 ± 0.5	6.3 ± 0.7
Carbohydrate	5.0 ± 0.8	4.9 ± 1.3	2.8 ± 0.6	2.2 ± 0.9
Protein	2.2 ± 0.2	3.0 ± 0.4	2.9 ± 0.3	3.5 ± 0.3
Step Exercise				
NPRQ	0.73 ± 0.02	0.80 ± 0.03*	0.77 ± 0.03	0.84 ± 0.02
Fat	14.2 ± 2.0	18.9 ± 3.0	19.8 ± 4.0	24.0 ± 4.0
Carbohydrate	6.7 ± 2.0	22.0 ± 6.0*	21.0 ± 6.0	57.0 ± 10.0†

*Significantly different from normals, when $P < .05$.
†Significantly different from normals, when $P < .02$.

gard, it was the thin patient with anorexia nervosa who appeared more economical in kilocalories used for basal metabolism rather than the obese subject.

There was also no indication that obese subjects were more economical in use of calories during exercise; both oxygen consumption and carbon dioxide production were related only to the work performed. From the most thin to the most obese, the amount of work determined the caloric output. Of some interest was the normal increase in use of oxygen during exercise in anorexic subjects despite the extremely low BMR in this group.

The obese subjects in our studies demonstrated no difficulty in mobilizing fat stores as a source for energy. In fact, they tended to use more fat than normals for the energy requirements of basal metabolism and exercise. In no way could our data implicate a decreased ability to mobilize fat for energy needs as an etiologic factor in obesity.

The data derived from medical histories and the food nomogram[5] show that, although the BMR is normal in obese people, its decline with age is of such magnitude that obesity and overweight can be produced in subjects of normal weight as they grow older by not changing exercise or eating habits. In fact, our analysis shows that both women and men reduced kilocalorie intake, yet became overweight and obese. We assumed daily exercise of the group to be constant; since it ordinarily tends to decrease with age, decreases of kilocalories consumed were probably even greater than we had calculated. Because decreased kilocalorie requirements with age can produce weight gain despite some decrease in kilocalorie intake, daily exercise, in addition to decreasing food consumption, becomes important as a measure to counterbalance the decrease in basal requirements. There may be some truth to the often heard statement, "Doctor, I don't eat as much as I used to, but I have gained weight."

References

1. Johnson OC: Present knowledge of calories, in *Present Knowledge in Nutrition*, ed 3. New York, The Nutrition Foundation, Inc, 1967, pp 1-5.
2. Zellweger H, Schneider HJ: Syndrome of hypotonia-hypomentia-hypogonadism-obesity (HHHO) or Prader-Willi syndrome. *Am J Dis Child* 115:588-598, 1968.
3. Williams JE, et al: *Modern Physics.* New York, Holt, Rinehart & Winston Inc, 1968, p 124.
4. Consolazio CF, Johnson RE, Pecora LJ: *Physiologic Measurements of Metabolic Functions in Man.* New York, McGraw-Hill Book Co Inc, 1963, pp 313-317.
5. *Mayo Clinic Diet Manual*, ed 4. Committee on Dietetics of the Mayo Clinic. Philadelphia, WB Saunders Co, 1971, p 160.
6. Davidson S, Passmore R: *Human Nutrition and Dietetics*, ed 4. Baltimore, Williams & Wilkins Co, 1969, pp 106-107.
7. Boothby WM, Berkson J, Plummer WA: The variability of basal metabolism: Some observations concerning its application in conditions of health and disease. *Ann Intern Med* 11:1014-1023, 1937.
8. Boothby WM, Sandiford I: Summary of the basal metabolism data on 8,614 subjects with especial reference to the normal standards for the estimation of the basal metabolic rate. *J Biol Chem* 54:783-803, 1922.

OBESITY, HEREDITY AND HUNGER

hidden bonds

by Professor Jean MAYER
Harvard School of Public Health, USA

Overeating leads to obesity; yet more important than the large amount of food may be the small amount of exercise. In other words, if you want to eat a lot, take a lot of exercise. In some cases of obesity, heredity may also be a factor. (Photos WHO/P. Almasy)

Systematic study of the mechanisms by which the intake of food is controlled did not start until the early forties, but some facts basic to our understanding of hunger had been established before that time. Haller, the Swiss biologist, had suggested in 1777 that hunger was a complex of gastric sensations which localize in the stomach. For over a century the idea that hunger sensations were due to the excitation of stomach nerves remained the most generally accepted theory. Finally, in 1912, it was tested experimentally by Walter Cannon, who, using a rubber balloon linked by a thin tube to an outside pressure gauge, showed that hunger sensations appeared whenever the empty stomach contracted vigorously. A Chicago physiologist, Anton Carlson, found that during a prolonged fast the tension of the empty stomach and the frequency and intensity of its contractions became progressively more pronounced. Carlson hypothesized that the vagus nerves were the main pathway for gastric impulses travelling from the abdomen to the brain and that the "primary hunger centre" must be in the medulla, the posterior part of the brain, from which these nerves arise.

Before World War I, two French pathologists, Camus and Roussy, conducting autopsies on very obese patients, found that some had brain lesions situated in or impinging on the hypothalamus, a part of the brain located on the floor of the brain hemisphere, just above the pituitary. (The hypothalamus has since been shown to play a part in the control of water intake, body temperature, reproduction, and other basic functions.) Experiments on both sides of the Atlantic then showed that if two small centrally located areas of the hypothalamus of rats, the "ventromedial areas", are destroyed, the rats overeat and become obese. I myself was able, in the early fifties, to demonstrate that by making minute symmetrical surgical lesions in the hypothalamus of the mouse, overeating can be induced even in an animal which already has a food intake 30 times greater per unit weight than man.

The actual role of the ventromedial areas was elucidated by the use of behavioural techniques. Miller and his associates, working at Yale, showed that while animals with lesions in these areas overate (we say, in the Greek-derived jargon of medical science, that they are "hyperphagic"), they would not work as hard for food as normal animals and might, in fact, be less hungry. My associates and I, using special cages, trained "hypothalamic hyperphagic" mice as well as normal mice to press a lever to obtain

56

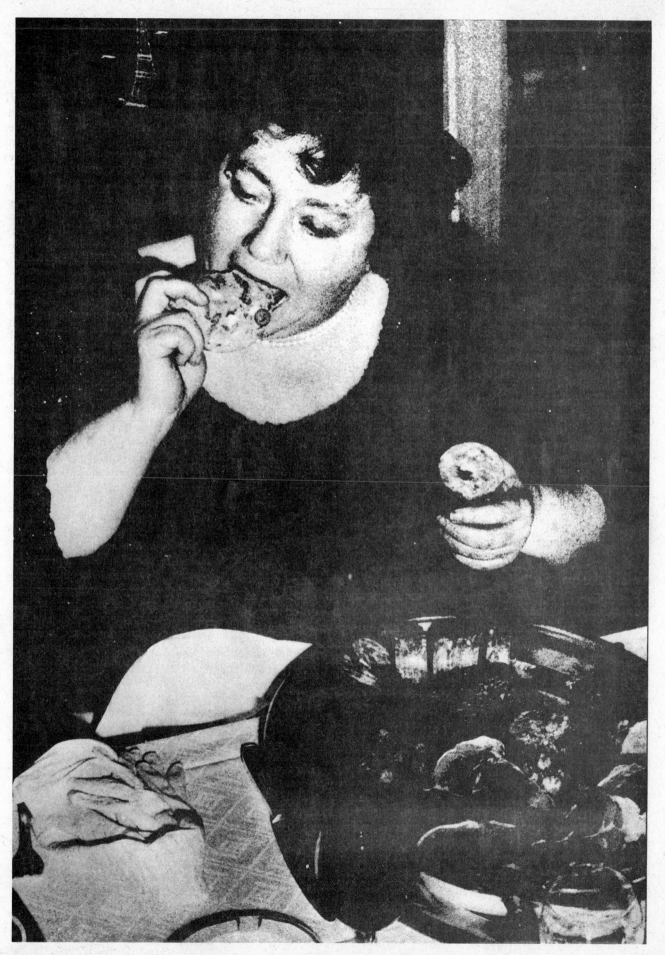

57

57

obesity, heredity, hunger

Studies on small rodents often pave the way to observations on human subjects. Mice and rats have been used extensively in the laboratory by the author and other investigators in their research into obesity. (Photo WHO) →

small pellets of food. The rate at which the animals press the lever is a measure of hunger. When satiety supervenes, the animals slow down and stop. We found hunger unaffected after hypothalamic lesions, but satiety periods shortened. In other words, it appeared that the ventromedial areas are "satiety centres", brakes on an otherwise constantly activated feeding mechanism.

That the feeding mechanism may also be controlled by the hypothalamus was indicated when an Indian physiologist, Bal K. Anand, showed that the destruction of small "lateral areas" right and left of the satiety centres caused animals to stop eating and drinking. Scoras Morrison and I demonstrated that the cessation of eating in animals with these lesions was not a consequence of the cessation of drinking and the resultant dehydration of the animal. Keeping the supply of body water normal through tube feeding did not automatically restore the eating. This brought support to the idea that the ventromedial areas ("satiety centres") act at various times as a brake on the lateral areas ("feeding centres"), which otherwise keep the animals stimulated to eat. In 1967 Edward Arees and I, using a recently developed technique for tracing fibres in the brain, were able actually to trace the fibres going from the "satiety" centres to the "feeding"

centres, thus giving a solid anatomical basis to the idea that the two centres are closely related and that what is regulated is not hunger but satiety.

With at least part of the brain mechanism identified, the next problem was: to what does the satiety centre respond? What activates it? In other words, what determines satiety?

The most accepted view today is based on experiments demonstrating that the satiety centres contain cells particularly sensitive to blood glucose (we call them glucoreceptors) and to the action of hormones (such as insulin), to which the rest of the brain does not respond. This view has been supported by a great many different experiments: in man one can show that, while the utilization of blood sugar is in progress, hunger (and the contractions of the stomach) is absent (and vice versa). Experiments in animals show that substances which decrease the rate of glucose absorption by cells increase food intake, as do substances which cause the loss of glucose through the kidney or cause low blood glucose through other means. If the glucoreceptors are destroyed by attaching heavy metals to glucose, the animals overeat permanently and get fat. Anand demonstrated that as glucose gets taken up by the satiety centres, the satiety centres are electrically

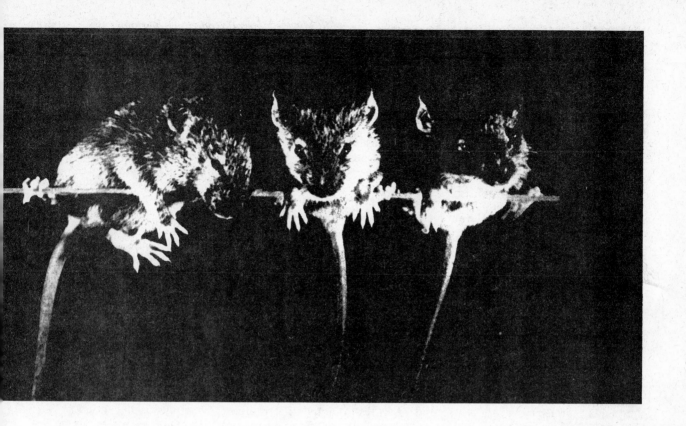

very active and the feeding centres very quiet, while by contrast, in the absence of this glucose uptake, the satiety centres are electrically inactive while the feeding centres are very active. On the basis of this "gluco-static mechanism" we were able to follow the way in which the satiety centres, acting through a group of nerve fibres called Schutz' Bundle (their role had been unknown until then), control the nucleus of the vagus nerve and through it, the stomach (hunger) contractions and the secretion of hydrochloric acid in the stomach.

We thus are beginning to understand what goes on at the brain level in the hunger mechanism. We have also begun to learn what goes on in the tissues. In particular, in the past few years we have learned that the adipose tissue—the fat cells and the blood vessels and other cells which give the fat cells nourishment and structure—is very active and does not simply register whether intake is greater than output or vice versa, but actively competes for blood nutrients, glucose in particular, and thus influences food intake. In experimental animals we thus find two kinds of obesity. One kind is those obesities due to something gone wrong in the brain mechanism which regulates the intake of food (as when the satiety centres are destroyed surgically or chemi-

cally). These have been called "regulatory obesities". The other kind is those obesities where there is something wrong biochemically with the animal's metabolism, so that its adipose tissue (fat cells) makes too much fat or does not burn it readily enough. These obesities I have called "metabolic obesities". Obviously in both kinds of obesity the animal has eaten more than he has expended; but, while the law of conservation of energy cannot be challenged, it does not by itself explain obesity.

Many obesities in experimental animals are genetic in origin. For example, "obese-hyperglycaemic" mice, an example of metabolic obesity, are characterized by a greater number of fat cells, by high blood glucose, a high level of blood insulin and a curious abnormality in the metabolism of the fat cells which we feel we have finally unravelled. In man there is also good evidence that genetics is very important. The number of fat cells seems predetermined (except perhaps for some increase during the first year under the influence of overabundant nutrition). Obesity runs in families: in the Boston area thin parents have, on the average, 7 per cent children obese at high-school age. If one parent is overweight, the rate is 40 per cent; if both parents are overweight, the rate is 80 per cent. Children adopted from birth do not show this association with the weight of their parents, showing that heredity, not family food habits, is the crucial factor (a finding confirmed by a large-scale study in England).

While it is obvious that in many cases obese individuals have an extremely large food intake, there are many cases where the appetite and food intake of the obese are quite normal; in some cases even below average. To understand how such individuals can still be in positive energy balance, let us look at the relation between overweight and exercise, a problem long confused by erroneous ideas which have survived tenaciously in popular literature.

The first erroneous view is that exercise requires relatively little caloric expenditure. Were this true, it would follow that even high levels of physical activity could be of only small importance in the balance between calories ingested and calories expended; this balance, of course, determines the development of overweight. The second false idea is that, *at any level of caloric intake*, an increase in physical activity is automatically followed by an increase in appetite and is, therefore, self-defeating as a weight control measure. Too often, these misstatements have been popularized by clinicians and nutritionists who, though well and extensively informed on other matters, have never tested the validity of these particular propositions. Let us look at the evidence available on both points.

The first misconception, minimizing the cost of physical activity, could be avoided by anyone who has carefully perused a table of "recommended dietary allowances" or "caloric requirements" such as have been elaborated by the League of Nations, the US National Research Council, or, more recently, by the Food and Agriculture Organization of the United Nations and WHO. For example, the daily allowance for men recommended by the National Research Council varies from 2,400 calories for "sedentary" men to 4,500 calories for "very active" men. Nor does the latter figure represent an upper limit. Labourers, soldiers and athletes are advised by the NRC that they may require up to (and occasionally more than) 6,000 calories. Surely a factor which can more than double daily energy expenditure is not one to be casually ruled out as of no great importance in determining caloric balance! In fact, the cost of walking (in terms of caloric expenditure over the cost of sitting) varies from 200 to 350 calories per hour, depending on the speed, for a

150-pound man; swimming will consume twice as much. The peaks reached in athletic competition may approach 1,200 calories per hour, a rate that untrained persons would not reach and which even trained athletes could not maintain. Forgetting such extremes, a caloric expenditure rate of the order of 500 to 600 calories per hour represents a degree of physical activity which can be comfortably endured for at least half an hour by an average healthy adult, even if he is out of condition. A trained man should feel all the better after a full hour or more of such exercise. For those for whom translation into foods means more than caloric counts, the expenditure corresponding to 30 minutes of this type of exercise is equivalent to an average size piece of apple-pie decorated by a standard scoop of ice cream. You can eat your cake and not have it with you always, if you substitute regular exercise for regular deprivation.

Even more important, it has already been noted that the cost of activity is dependent on the subject's size. In exercises where no heavy object outside the body is moved, the cost of exercise increases proportionately to bodyweight. If excess bodyweight be such that it impairs body movement, the cost of exercise will actually increase faster than does bodyweight. An overweight person will thus burn a greater amount of body fat for the same amount of exercise than will a person of normal weight.

Let us now examine the second major argument against exercising to control weight—namely, that it is a self-defeating practice. The idea that an increase in appetite normally follows an increase in activity is true if the subject was reasonably active to start with. The mechanism of regulation of appetite adjusts caloric intake to expenditure, so that the body will not burn away its substance if called upon to perform a suddenly increased amount of work. This relation does not hold, however, if the subject was inactive to start with; decreasing activity below a certain limit will no longer be accompanied by a decrease in appetite. This new finding explains why "underexercising" rather than "overeating" as such may well be the most important cause of the prevalence of overweight today.

As happens so frequently, studies on small rodents paved the way for observations on human subjects. The Nutrition Department at Harvard studied the way the food intake of white rats varied when their exercise was varied. We used a motor-driven treadmill and accustomed a large group of rats to running on it. Then we divided the large

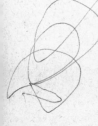

group into a number of smaller groups, which were exercised, respectively, for one, two, three and up to 10 hours daily; we measured their food intake during a few weeks of regimen and followed the changes in their weight. We compared them with similar animals left unexercised in their cages.

We found that rats exercised one or two hours daily did not eat more than did the unexercised rats; indeed, they ate somewhat less. But the animals with restricted activity slowly accumulated weight. From two hours daily onward, increasing durations of exercise were accompanied by increasing food intake up to a duration of eight hours of exercise, which represented the peak the rats could endure. The weight of the active animals stabilized at a lower level than that characteristic of the sedentary rats. Swimming the animals gave the same result. Below the range of "normal activity", where the adjustment of intake to appetite is very accurate, there is a "sedentary range" where appetite is stuck at a "minimum" value higher than expenditures.

This can be illustrated even more dramatically. Dwight Ingle showed that if rats were prevented from moving at all by placing them in a small tunnel-like cage, they became extremely fat. The genetically obese mice which have been studied in our laboratory are at least 10 times less active than their non-afflicted brothers and sisters; inactivity precedes the development of obesity. Exercising these young obese mice or breeding into the obese group the "waltzing gene" (which produces locomotor troubles) will considerably slow down the accumulation of excess weight: appetite will not increase correspondingly. Similarly, farmers have always known that if you want to obtain the fattest possible steer, hog, or fowl, you should prevent any form of movement on the part of these producers of tallow, lard or foie gras. Decreasing the activity of the animals by tethering, penning or cooping them up will not depress the appetite correspondingly, and a more satisfactory degree of obesity will be reached.

These findings are not confined to animals. A number of years ago I studied an industrial population group in the jute mill area south of Calcutta. The range of physical work there was much greater than what one could encounter in the United States. At one end of the scale there were physically inactive accountants and bazaar merchants, who did little but sit during their waking hours. At the other extreme, labourers carried loads as heavy as their own bodies for eight or nine hours a day. Between these two groups could be found a multiplicity of more or less active occupations. The diet, based essentially on rice and lentils, was fairly uniform, and monotonous. The relationship of food intake, bodyweight and physical work in this population was found to be strikingly like that previously seen in experimental animals. The sedentary merchants and clerks ate a little more than did the more active electricians, mechanics and drivers, and were about two stones (or 6.35 kg) heavier. The lower limit of the "normal activity" range was reached by the latter group. From there on, with an increase in physical work, weavers, bale-carriers, cutters, firemen, and so on showed an increasing food intake, not an increase in weight. Similar studies have consistently yielded similar results.

The role of decreased activity seems particularly important in childhood obesity. In general, the large amount of psychiatric literature dealing with this vexing problem has tried to explain why obese children overeat: as an escape from tensions at home, as a substitute for the affection of one parent or both, as a result of parental neglect or oversolicitousness, because of a desire for size and recognition, as a protection in excessive shyness, and so on. But although a particularly observant child psychiatrist, Hilde Bruch, has noted that obese children were often inactive, it is only recently that the basic assumption has been questioned: do all obese children eat excessively as compared to normal weight children, or could some of them get their caloric supplement from underexercising?

A study we conducted on high school girls first showed that inactivity is indeed the major factor in perpetuating obesity in many, if not most, overweight youngsters. Examination of the dietary intake and of the schedule of equal groups of overweight and normal weight girls, matched for age and height, showed that the obese students fell into two groups. One group, and by far the larger, contained girls who ate no more than the normal weight girls but who exercised considerably less. All the "sitting" activities were emphasized at the expense of walking and active sports. Television-watching consumed four times as many hours in this groups as it did in the normal weight group. The second group (the existence of which emphasized the fact that there is more than one cause of obesity) ate more than the normal and exercised normally. These were of the red-cheeked, cheerful type, and while "overweight," they appeared less "overfat" than the inactive group. Other studies indicate that the same situation prevails with boys as well.

More recently we have used a film technique to quantify this phenomenon. Every three minutes a camera takes a three-second shot of the activity of obese or non-obese subjects engaged in a given sport or activity. Beverly Bullen and I have recently analyzed 29,000 such shots: they show that obese youngsters playing volleyball are immobile 80 to 90 per cent of the time (as compared to 50 per cent for the non-obese); playing singles tennis, 60 per cent (as compared to less than 20 per cent for the non-obese). While non-obese youngsters swimming expend five or more calories per minute above basal, most of the obese youngsters expend no more than one—they float, sit or stand in the water. *Why* the obese are so inactive— whether it antedates or follows obesity—is under study in our laboratory. At any rate, there is little doubt that this inactivity is one of the main factors which makes the obesity self-perpetuating.

The fact that a tendency to inactivity (and to overweight) appears very early in life is demonstrated by a recent study I conducted with a paediatrician, Hedwig Rose, on infants. Following 31 infants from birth to 15 months, we found that fat babies tended to be inactive babies with a very moderate appetite, while active babies ate much more but were thinner and lighter.

Obesity thus appears to be in many instances a "disease of civilization". Mechanizations of work and of transportation combine to decrease physical exercise. For many of us, particularly in economically developed countries, physical activity has been so decreased by our mode of life that we no longer respond to a further decrease in exercise by a further decrease in appetite. Excess calories accordingly accumulate as fat. If we want to avoid this, we must either exercise more or feel hungry all our lives. ■

Physiologic control of food intake

C.L. HAMILTON, PH.D.
Research Psychologist,
Veterans Administration Hospital, and
Departments of Physiology and Psychiatry,
University of Pennsylvania, Philadelphia

Three regulatory systems are believed to be involved in controlling food intake, two of which include body supplies of carbohydrate and fat. Adjustments are made via the nervous system, primarily through the hypothalamus.

The study of physiology is the study of control and regulation. Basically, this is a simple concept that was expounded in the nineteenth century by Claude Bernard, who introduced the idea that much of the body's work is oriented toward maintaining a fairly constant state of internal affairs (1). Cannon elaborated (2) this theme and wrote of homeostatic mechanisms involved in maintaining mean values for physiologic parameters. Homeostasis for Cannon was a dynamic state wherein physiologic parameters might deviate from the norm or "set point" but control mechanisms capable of correcting this error were available. In a regulated system, certain variables are maintained close to the "set point," and others are controlled in appreciation of that regulation. For example, considering levels of blood glucose as *regulated*, insulin release is *controlled* as a consequence of that regulation.

Control systems

One enters another level of sophistication when the concept of control is introduced. Control implies two types of feedback systems—positive and negative. In a positive feedback system, if the regulated variable strays from the "set point," the control mechanisms operate to increase the error in the same direction. In negative feedback systems, any deviation from the homeostatic value initiates control mechanisms that operate to reduce the error and return the system to the "set point." A simple example of this process is the automatic volume control (AVC) on the modern radio. A negative feedback system operates to maintain the level of sound established when the control is set. Radio station signals vary in intensity; when they are too high, the AVC of the receiver reduces the intensity so that the preset level is maintained. If the radio operated with positive feedback, the louder the signal from the station, the louder the output of the set, since the control would increase the degree of error. One can see that positive feedback systems are generally undesirable and, in some cases, could cause the system to self-destruct. When man determines the "set points" in machinery and designs the control circuits, the analysis of the systems is relatively simple.

In biology, we cannot often agree on the physiologic parameters that have "set points," let alone the design of the control circuits.

For most physiologists, homeostatic mechanisms refer to internal and external secretions, adjustments of vascular tone, and so forth. It was Richter who first expressed (3) the idea that overt behavior was also involved in physiologic regulations. It is surprising that it took so long for us to recognize this, since much of our everyday behavior is homeostatically derived. When we feel chilly, we turn up the thermostat if indoors or put on more clothing if outdoors. Both behaviors are adjustments that tend to reduce heat loss and help to maintain the regulated body temperature.

Superimposed on the control and regulatory systems is the concept of priorities and compromises best elucidated by Adolph (4), who reminded us that under certain circumstances, one regulatory system may be compromised in deference to the needs of another. Thus, in the desert even without drinking water, man still loses body water through perspiration, even though he is threatened with dehydration. In this instance, regulation of body temperature has a higher priority than body water content, presumably because heat stroke is a more acute threat to life than dehydration. It is within this complex system that we consider food intake as a variable controlled in appreciation cf pertinent regulatory systems.

Feeding controls
Feeding in mammals has been variously attributed to sensation originating in the stomach, to conditions of glucose utilization, to levels of circulating amino acids, to mass of adipose tissue, and to conditions of body temperature regulation. While there is little doubt that all of these mechanisms are involved in some manner, there are divergent opinions regarding the interactions of the various systems under the circumstances of living.

Whatever parameter is to be regulated, the body must in some manner be sensitive to its "set point" and also to any degree of deviation. In essence, in the physiologic negative feedback systems, we consider that there must be an error detector which in turn initiates effector activity to reduce the error. Most investigators agree that the brain serves this purpose. While we have made significant progress in elucidating the function of the brain in the control of feeding, much more information is needed before we can present a reasonably inclusive model. Available information is based primarily on animal experiments and the clinic. To summarize: at the highest level of the nervous system, we know that infants born without a cerebral cortex show sucking behavior and control food intake reasonably well. The role of the cortex in adult animals has not been adequately studied. Data from animal experiments on the role of the limbic system in feeding have been contradictory and not de-

finitive enough to be included in an overall scheme of the control of feeding. The most dramatic effects on feeding result from lesions placed in the hypothalamus. In general, we can say that bilateral ablation of the ventromedial portion of the hypothalamus is followed by hyperphagia and obesity. Ablations of the adjacent areas of the hypothalamus, several millimeters lateral, are followed by aphagia, and, if the animals are not force fed, starvation results. In rats with such lesions, if proper procedures are followed, feeding behavior is restored, especially if a highly palatable food is presented (5).

With successful lesions of the ventromedial area, animals may show a threefold increase in food intake along with a dramatic reduction in spontaneous activity, the combination of which leads to eventual obesity. Other effects of lesions of the hypothalamus on feeding will be covered in greater detail when we consider specific regulatory systems.

Oral sensations and feeding
Feeding begins with the oral cavity and taste sensations. It is common experience that the palatability of food influences the amount consumed. The "Thanksgiving effect" is real, i.e., no matter how full one may feel, he can usually be enticed to eat a little more if a favorite food is offered. Regardless of the common-sense nature of such an observation, we have little experimental evidence to support it.

Le Magnen has shown (6) that in the rat trained to eat its 24-hr. ration in 2 hr., food intake is increased when different flavored diets are presented every half hour. The texture of a diet also is an important influence on intake. Rats show a preference for a greasy diet compared with dry chow, even when the food is made greasy by adding petrolatum (7).

In general, the mouth is important, not only because it is the normal port of entry of food, but because of the taste sensations aroused and the feel of the food. It is believed that these factors modify food intake but are not major contributors to the maintenance of energy balance.

Gastrointestinal tract and feeding
Gastric contractions and stomach distension and their relation to feeding are involved in perhaps the oldest theory of the control of food intake. Cannon and Washburn (8) and Carlson (9) were the first to collect experimental evidence on this point. The fact that it has been shown subsequently that patients with stomachs removed also experience feelings of hunger and satiety suggests that sensations from the stomach might be useful when present but expendable in the overall control of feeding.

More recent experiments have demonstrated a neural link between the gut and the hypothalamus. Anand and his associates have shown (10) that artificial distension of the cat's stomach by balloon is accompanied by increased electrical activity of the ventromedial hypothalamus. They found no change in the electrical activity of the lateral or ventromedial hypothalamus during "hunger contractions," indicating a satiety function for the ventromedial hypothalamus related to stomach distension.

Mayer's work (11), using the hormone glucagon with rats, provides further evidence of the interaction between the stomach and the hypothalamus. Glucagon produces hyperglycemia apparently by stimulating hepatic glucogenolysis, increases metabolic rate, and decreases gastric motility. Anand *et al.* had reported that glucagon injections in the cat were followed by increased electrical activitiy of the ventromedial area with a concurrent inhibition of gastric contractions. Mayer's work with glucagon showed that in rats with lesions of the ventromedial hypothalamus, glucagon did not inhibit gastric contractions. Such data lead us to believe that the hypothalamus is in some manner involved with feeding via the stomach, but the evidence is not convincing enough to conclude that such a link can account for the hyperphagia seen after ventromedial ablation.

Presently, we may postulate that neural impulses arising from gut filling are afferent to the central nervous system and thus serve to inform the controlling mechanisms of the extent of the stomach distension. In this manner, one may consider the system a safety device that prevents overfilling. However, the influence of gastric filling seems at times to be influenced by the physiologic priorities of the organism. For example, with cold stress, rats can double their food intake overnight. In this case, either the gut-filling feedback is ignored, its sensitivity altered, or gastric motility enhanced. Whether one or a combination of these adjustments is made is not known at present.

Thermostatic control of feeding

The thermostatic theory of the control of food intake as proposed by Brobeck (12) states that under certain circumstances, food intake is controlled as part of the system of body temperature regulation. The basic observation supporting this hypothesis is that in most homeotherms studied so far, food intake is increased in the cold and reduced in the heat. In the rat, food intake may range from 126 kcal per day at an environmental temperature of 7°C. to 18 kcal per day at 35°C. Furthermore, if the animals are force fed in the heat, they suffer heat stroke and die (13). In response to temperature stress, rats and most mammals appear to make feeding adjustments compatible with survival.

Evidence for the role of the brain in these feeding accommodations has been gathered from studies of the effects of ablation of the thermosensitive area of the brain. This area lies just dorsal to the optic chiasma and ventral to the anterior commissure and is referred to as the preoptic anterior hypothalamus (POAH). In the rat, ablation of this area is followed by labile regulation of body temperature; the animals

are hypothermic in the cold and hyperthermic in the heat. Feeding behavior in such situations is not adjusted to environmental thermal stress; the animals overeat in the heat and undereat in the cold (14).

Additional evidence for the role of these thermosensitive neurones in the control of feeding has been presented by Spector *et al.* (15). They showed that artificial heating of the POAH in the rat was accompanied by increased food intake; conversely, cooling the area resulted in a depression of feeding. Although these data presented evidence for direct interaction of feeding and temperature regulation, they posed a dilemma for the thermostatic theory. Brain-heated rats appear to be heat stressed, and normally one would expect food intake to be depressed. Since the opposite effect occurred, we are still without an explanation of the phenomenon.

Even so, there is little doubt that at times, feeding and temperature regulation are part of the same system. Within the context of priorities and compromises of the organism, temperature regulation is second only to regulation of P_{o2} and P_{co2}. Heat-stressed animals sacrifice water for evaporative heat loss, although water may not be readily available. They also reduce food intake to avoid further stress that results when the body is obligated to dissipate the extra load.

Data on the relationship of feeding and thermal stress in man are difficult to evaluate, since man has more control over his micro-environment than the lower animals. However, if you are giving a dinner party in hot weather and want to save on the food bill, it is not a bad idea to turn off the air conditioner.

The glucostatic theory

Most physiologists would agree that blood glucose levels are regulated. Feeding must obviously be a part of that system, since all glucose is derived eventually from exogenous sources. The minute-to-minute regulation of blood glucose is the result of ingestion, absorption, storage, synthesis, utilization, and excretion. These processes are influenced by many hormones. Insulin, the best known of these, lowers blood glucose —by enhancing the deposition of glycogen in liver and muscle and by increasing the rate of fat formation—and provides one of the most potent control circuits in the body.

The primary and perhaps sufficient stimulus for the release of insulin is the level of blood glucose perfusing the pancreas. The higher the level of glucose, the more insulin released. In maturity-onset diabetes, blood glucose levels may be very high, either because insufficient insulin is available or its action is in some manner inhibited. In either case, the kidney excretes as much of the excess glucose as possible and a gross control is maintained. Another hormone produced by the pancreas, glucagon, has a hyperglycemic effect, the action of which we have already mentioned. Epinephrine, another hyperglycemic hormone, is activated primarily by increasing the rate of glycogen breakdown by the liver. The glucocorticoids of the adrenal cortex are also hyperglycemic in action and thus antagonistic to insulin in that they increase gluconeogenesis and mobilize fats from adipose tissue. From the pituitary gland, two hormones are important in blood glucose regulation, ACTH by its action on the adrenal cortex and growth hormone with its apparent inhibitory effect on the peripheral utilization of glucose. Even a cursory review reveals the complexity of the regulation of blood glucose, and consideration of feeding within the system has not added much clarification.

In many animals, with the exception of ruminants, hypoglycemia induced by insulin injection results in increased feeding (16), whereas induced hyperglycemia by intravenous injection of glucose does not suppress food intake (17). A more subtle hypothesis relating feeding to blood glucose, called "the glucostatic theory," had been proposed earlier by Mayer (18). This theory proposes that feeding is related to the rate of utilization and not the absolute levels of blood glucose. Feeding is enhanced when the rate of utilization of glucose is low and inhibited when it is high. Theoretically, after a meal, the rate of glucose utilization is elevated, as determined by the arterial-venous (A-V) differences. During periods of deprivation, when body stores of fat are being used for energy, the A-V differences are small and feeding is enhanced. The experimental data for this position have been contradictory. A-V blood glucose differences do rise after a high-carbohydrate meal but not after a meal high in protein, although in both cases feelings of satiety are present.

Experimental production of low rates of glucose utilization can be accomplished by using the glucose analogue, 2-deoxy-D-glucose (2DG), which inhibits glycolysis and glucose utilization in a variety of tissues, including the brain, by competitive antagonism of the phosphohexose isomerase reaction. In addition, injection of 2DG is followed by hyperglycemia, resulting in a preparation with high circulating levels of glucose and a brain relatively deprived of glucose. Smith and Epstein have demonstrated (19) that injection of 2DG increases food intake in rats and monkeys. These data lead one to believe that 2DG glucose privation is similar to induced hypoglycemia in its effects on feeding, since it may make no difference to the system controlling feeding whether the glucose is in short supply or is not available metabolically.

In a later paper, Smith *et al.* perhaps summarized (20) the status of the glucostatic theory for the present, concluding that although glucose privation to the degree seen with injection of 2DG is an unusual and expendable stimulus for ordinary feeding, the results do not exclude a minor, facilitating role for the glucostatic hypothesis in the initiation of feeding.

The lipostatic hypothesis

Considering all the social pressures that surround feeding in man, it is remarkable that, aside from any known pathology, an adult's body weight remains fairly constant. This relative constancy has led some to propose that body weight is a regulated variable and food intake is controlled as a consequence. Kennedy was the first to postulate formally (21) that the cumulative balance between energy intake and energy loss involved a regulation of body fat. The regulation was thought to be maintained by some as yet unknown metabolite, directly related to the mass of adipose tissue and sensed by the central nervous system which, in turn, affected the mechanisms controlling feeding. No solid experimental evidence has been reported in support of this hypothesis. There is circumstantial evidence, however, supporting the concept that body weight is regulated and that each individual may have his own "set point." Cohn and Joseph have shown (22) that rats tube fed calories in excess of their normal intake so that they became obese relative to their controls ate little food after cessation of forced feeding. Food intake returned to normal only after the animals had lost the extra body weight gained during forced feeding.

Hoebel and Teitelbaum have presented (23) similar evidence for rats with ventromedial hypothalamic lesions. They showed that animals made obese by daily insulin injections (increasing food intake) did not exhibit hyperphagia after lesioning. Not until they were fasted to a lower body weight did they overeat and regain their prefast obesity. Such evidence led these authors to propose that the effect of the hypothalamic lesions of the ventromedial area was to elevate the "set point" for body weight. Additional evidence for this position is the well known fact that hypothalamic, hyperphagic rats are hyperphagic only until they reach some stable body weight; after they become obese, their food intake returns to close-to-normal levels. An obvious conclusion from such evidence is that the ventromedial hypothalamus is in some manner related to the system controlling body weight and acts as a brake on excess weight gain.

Inherent in systems of control and regulation is the concept of checks and balances. Powell and Keesy reasoned (24) that if one area of the hypothalamus is ablated and the "set point" for body weight elevated, then ablation of another area of the hypothalamus might result in a lower "set point." The lateral hypothalamus was a natural area for exploring this idea, since lesions there are followed by aphagia. In the Powell and Keesy study, rats were placed on a restricted diet until their body weights were considerably below that of controls; then the lateral hypothalamus was lesioned bilaterally. Under these conditions, the animals did not exhibit the aphagia usually seen with such lesions. When the animals were force fed to the controls' body weights, they became aphagic. The tentative conclusion was that the lateral hypothalamic lesions had lowered the "set point" around which body weight was regulated.

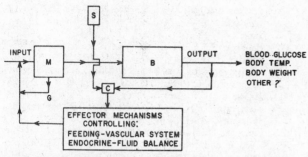

FIG. 1. *Oversimplified model of regulatory systems controlling food intake. S indicates the "set point"; C, the comparator; M, flow of the system; and B, biochemical portion of the flow system. For further explanation, see text.*

This is a provocative proposition and one that deserves more investigation. It has been shown that ventromedial hypothalamic lesions lead to greater amounts of adipose tissue in rats, even when they are not permitted to overeat (25). Perhaps lateral lesions are followed by a reduction in the mass of adipose tissue in animals maintained on isocaloric amounts of food. In this manner, body weight could be regulated, as Kennedy suggested (21), by control of the size of fat depots.

However, not all experiments support the hypothesis that body weight is regulated; arguments against this theory have centered on the evidence that body weight can be altered in a predictable manner. Corbit and Stellar (26) and Mu *et al.* (27) have shown that the degree of obesity in hypothalamic, hyperphagic rats can be enhanced by feeding a highly palatable diet. Mayer has shown (28) that in normal rats, body weight can be increased if their activity is restricted and that in hot environments, body weights of rats are maintained at lower-than-normal levels (29). Shifts in body weight under all of these conditions may merely represent a re-ordering of priorities with body weight compromised.

Anecdotal evidence strongly favors the hypothesis that body weight is regulated, if for no other reason than it is so difficult to reduce. Weight reduction has been an obsession in the United States, as evidenced by the many diets proposed and the reducing fads perpetrated on the public. In a world where malnutrition is a major health problem, it seems ironic to suggest that the secret of reducing body weight is to learn to live with hunger.

Other factors related to feeding

Three regulatory systems believed to be involved in controlling food intake have been discussed. Two of these included body supplies of carbohydrate and fat. The possibility remains that the body supply of protein may also be regulated, although experiments so far have generated paradoxical results.

If rats are presented a 5 per cent protein diet (22 to 25 per cent is optimal) and are maintained at a room temperature of 25°C., they become anorexic and die within forty-five days. However, if given the 5 per cent diet and maintained at 8°C., they increase food intake and survive. Furthermore, rats maintained at room temperature (25°C.) on the low-protein diet and exercised on a treadmill also increase food intake and survive (30, 31).

Only when rats are forced by other priorities (cold stress and exercise) to increase caloric intake do they cover their minimal protein requirements and survive. Such evidence indicates a predominant role for caloric control over protein regulation.

The anorexia of protein malnutrition is unexplained, but it occurs in rats placed on diets lacking a single essential amino acid (32). There is evidence that under such conditions, the anorexia is protective, for if these animals are force fed the deficient diet, they develop pathologic lesions and die. While the mechanism of this adjustment is not clear, the reduction in food intake appears to be a compromise that prevents the occurrence of more acute conditions.

In cafeteria-style experiments, the data are more encouraging for an interpretation of protein regulation. Rats select diets with approximately 25 per cent protein over those with higher or lower protein content and diets with a normal complement of amino acids over an amino acid deficiency (32).

In general, the evidence for the regulation of protein and amino acid content of the body is suggestive, but not substantial enough to place it within the systems controlling feeding. However, relatively little attention has been focused on the problem.

There is an intimate relationship between the system regulating body fluid content and food intake. Animals deprived of water reduce food intake and, conversely, fasting animals reduce water intake. On ingestion of food, the flow of water into the gastrointestinal tract results in a relative dehydration and a demand for water. This is the phenomenon of postprandial thirst. It appears that when water is not readily available, food intake is reduced to prevent further dehydration. In the hierarchy of priorities, regulation of body fluids appears to rank above control of the intake of nutrients.

Summary

The basic requirement of a simple model of the regulatory systems controlling food intake is depicted in Figure 1. This is a closed-loop system with negative feedback. The value of whatever might be regulated by the system is determined by the "set point" (s). "Set point" information is supplied the comparator (c) which, in addition, receives information from the output. The comparator continuously monitors the output information, determines the direction and the magnitude of any discrepancy, and initiates the appropriate effector activity to accomplish needed corrections. We assume that these adjustments are made via the nervous system, with the central components primarily in the hypothalamus. Presently, it appears that within the hypothalamus, the information is conducted by neurotransmitters activating alpha and beta receptors (33).

The flow of the system is at first mechanical (M) in nature—seeking food, mastication, swallowing, and stretch of the stomach. There is a short feedback loop from the stomach via the stretch receptors which can affect the input independent of the "set point-comparator" loop. The second portion of the flow system is biochemical (B) and is most intimately involved with the output. The effector mechanisms are many, and we have included only a few of the more general ones.

Inherent in the entire scheme is the concept of motivation. By this we mean that the organism is driven physiologically and behaviorally toward the maintenance of "set point" values. Assuming, for example, that body weight is regulated, then any reduction from the "set point" is followed by an increased urge to eat. Similarly, when body weight is in excess of the "set point," there is an urge to reduce food intake. We are reminded that it is as difficult to add body weight purposefully as it is to reduce.

References

(1) BERNARD, C.: An Introduction to the Study of Experimental Medicine. (Transl. from French by Greene, H.C.). N.Y.: Henry Schuman, 1949.

(2) CANNON, W.B.: The Wisdom of the Body. Rev. N.Y.: W.W. Norton, 1939.

(3) RICHTER, C.P.: Animal behavior and internal drives. Q. Rev. Biol. 2: 307, 1927.

(4) ADOLPH, E.F.: Physiological Regulations. Lancaster, Pa.: Jacques Cattell, 1943.

(5) TEITELBAUM, P., AND EPSTEIN, A.: The lateral hypothalamic syndrome. Psychol. Rev. 69: 74, 1962.

(6) LE MAGNEN, J.: Habits and food intake. In Code, C.F., ED.: Handbook of Physiology, Sec. 6, Alimentary Canal. Vol. 1 Baltimore: Williams and Wilkins, 1967.

(7) HAMILTON, C.L.: Rat's preference for high fat diets. J. Comp. Physiol. Psychol. 58: 459, 1964.

(8) CANNON, W.B., AND WASHBURN, A.L.: An explanation of hunger. Am. J. Physiol. 29: 441, 1912.

(9) CARLSON, A.J.: The Control of Hunger in Health and Disease. Chicago: Univ. of Chicago Press, 1916.

(10) ANAND, B.: Nervous regulation of food intake. Physiol. Rev. 41: 677, 1961.

(11) MAYER, J.: The hypothalamic control of gastric hunger contractions as a component of the mechanism of regulation of food intake. Am. J. Clin. Nutr. 8: 547, 1960.

(12) BROBECK, J.R.: Food intake as a mechanism of temperature regulation. Yale J. Biol. Med. 20: 545, 1948.

(13) HAMILTON, C.L., AND BROBECK, J.R.: Temperature response of tube-fed rats. Am. J. Physiol. 203: 383, 1962.

(14) HAMILTON, C.L., AND BROBECK, J.R.: Food intake and temperature regulation in rats with rostral hypothalamic lesions. Am. J. Physiol. 207: 291, 1964.

(15) SPECTOR, N.H., BROBECK, J.R., AND HAMILTON, C.L.: Feeding and core temperature in albino rats: Changes induced by preoptic heating and cooling. Science 161: 286, 1968.

(16) EPSTEIN, A., AND TEITELBAUM, P.: Specific loss of the hypoglycemic control of feeding in recovered lateral rats. Am. J. Physiol. 213: 1159, 1967.

(17) BAILE, C.A., ZINN, W., AND MAYER, J.: Feeding behavior of monkeys: Glucose utilization rate and site of glucose entry. Physiol. Behav. 6: 537, 1971.

(18) MAYER, J.: Glucostatic mechanisms of regulation of food intake. N. Engl. J. Med. 249: 13, 1953.

(19) SMITH, G.P., AND EPSTEIN, A.: Increased feeding in response to decreased glucose utilization in the rat and monkey. Am. J. Physiol. 217: 1083, 1969.

(20) SMITH, G.P., GIBBS, J., STROHMAYER, A.J., AND STOKES, P.E.: Threshold doses of 2-deoxy-D-glucose for hyperglycemia and feeding in rats and monkeys. Am. J. Physiol. 222: 77, 1972.

(21) KENNEDY, G.C.: The role of depot fat in the hypothalamic control of food intake in the rat. Proc. Royal Soc. Lond. (Biol.) 140: 578, 1953.

(22) COHN, C., AND JOSEPH, D.: Influence of body weight and fat on appetite of "normal," lean and obese rats. Yale J. Biol. Med. 34: 598, 1962.

(23) HOEBEL, B.G., AND TEITELBAUM, P.: Weight regulation in normal and hypothalamic hyperphagic rats. J. Comp. Physiol. Psychol. 61: 189, 1966.

(24) POWELL, T.L., AND KEESY, R.E.: Relationship of body weight to the lateral hypothalamic feeding syndrome. J. Comp. Physiol. Psychol. 70: 25, 1970.

(25) HAN, P.W.: Hypothalamic obesity in rats without hyperphagia. Trans. N.Y. Acad. Sci. 30: 229, 1967.

(26) CORBIT, R.L., AND STELLAR, E.: Palatability, food intake and obesity in normal and hyperphagic rats. J. Comp. Physiol. Psychol. 58: 63, 1964.

(27) MU, J.Y., YIN, T.H., HAMILTON, C.L., AND BROBECK, J.R.: Variability of body fat in hyperphagic rats. Yale J. Biol. Med. 41: 133, 1968.

(28) MAYER, J., MARSHALL, N.B., VITALE, J.J., CHRISTENSEN, J., MASHAYEKHI, M., AND STARE, F.: Exercise, food intake and body weight in normal rats and genetically obese adult mice. Am. J. Physiol. 177: 544, 1954.

(29) HAMILTON, C.L.: Interactions of food intake and temperature regulation in the rat. J. Comp. Physiol. Psychol. 56: 476, 1963.

(30) ANDIK, I., DONHOFFER, S., FARKAS, M., AND SCHMIDT, P.: Ambient temperature and survival on a protein-deficient diet. Brit. J. Nutr. 17: 257, 1963.

(31) MEYER, J.H., AND HARGUS, W.A.: Factors influencing food intake in rats fed low-protein rations. Am. J. Physiol. 197: 1350, 1959.

(32) HARPER, A.E.: Effects of dietary protein content and amino acid pattern on food intake and preference. In CODE, C.F., ED.: Handbook of Physiology, Sec. 6, Alimentary Canal, Vol. 1. Baltimore: Williams and Wilkins, 1967.

(33) HOEBEL, B.G.: Feeding: Neural control of intake. Ann. Rev. Physiol. 33: 533, 1971.

Part II: Psychological and Sociological Aspects of Overweight and Obesity *

The many psychological and sociological disturbances that are frequently found and reported in obese patients pose a special problem in any discussion of the health implications of obesity.

In many of the published reports the groups studied have not been truly representative of the general obese population. The obese individuals who are most likely to consult a psychiatrist are usually those who are emotionally disturbed also. In general, the fat people examined by psychiatrists are the fat people who present overtly neurotic symptoms. As a consequence, any deductions made from such studies about the frequency and type of psychological disturbances in obesity should be carefully examined before applying the findings to the total population of fat people.

Similarly, psychological studies based on observations of fat people in special settings are also biased by the very factors that led the individuals to congregate in the first place. Any conclusions that may be drawn about the prevalence and severity of psychological abnormalities in such populations can be erroneous and may therefore not be generally applicable.

The foregoing comments are not meant to indicate that psychological disturbances have not often been responsible for the overeating that causes many patients to become and to remain obese. It is difficult to determine, however, which type of psychological disturbance produces overeating, whether a single disturbance, or many, and whether the disturbance and the severity of the overeating are proportional. It is likewise difficult to determine to what extent these disturbances contribute to the obesity of varying individual cases.

Regardless of what psychological factors may have led to obesity, additional disturbances may be created by attempts at weight reduction, or the existing disturbances may be aggravated. Food is a general source of comfort for most people regardless of weight status. Careful evaluation is needed to be certain that food restriction in some patients will not result in psychological manifestations. Many people thus need psychological help during dieting, but the need may be transient (only for the period of active dieting) and may be fulfilled by many measures other than formal psychotherapy.

Psychological disturbances that are an effect of obesity rather than a cause constitute a separate problem. For example, it has been suggested that social pressures on the obese adolescent girl cause such psychological symptoms as obsessive concern with body image, passivity, withdrawal and expectation of rejection.

In dealing with fat people—as in almost any other clinical problem—physicians observe a spectrum of human behavior. The patients may vary considerably in the degree of addiction to food, in the time of eating, in their familial, occupational, and personal relationships and in all other aspects of the panorama of human life. No single concept provides the explanation for either the cause, the treatment, or the psychic manifestations of a problem that is so complex. When psychiatric treatment is clearly necessary, it can be prescribed. In other situations, however, physicians should keep in mind that the patient's problem may be one neither of psyche nor soma but rather a conflict with the standards of society.

Eating and dieting are American preoccupations. We have the most bountiful food supply in the world and for many medical, social, and psychological reasons we have arrived at body weight ideals that are not compatible with the atmosphere of plenty. The number of people who are or who have been on diets cannot even be estimated. A woman will diet for a week or more before a special party to look her best or to fit into a gown. Some people will diet for a few weeks before a vacation in order to feel more comfortable in a bathing suit or even to be able to eat more heartily on the "American Plan." In short, there are people who diet for special temporary reasons or as a kind of postponement of eating—and with the conscious intent of eating more later. Many others sporadically pursue diets in commercial establishments such as diet salons, milk farms, and luxury diet resorts.

We have no knowledge of the weight loss in these situations, nor of the psychological effects of dieting, nor of failure to diet successfully. Our only sources of information on the psychological effects of dieting are the studies reported in the medical literature. They have been neither as numerous nor as well designed or controlled as one could wish.

The question naturally arises whether the emotional results of dieting can be considered apart from success or failure in terms of weight loss. It has been thought by some that dieting is fraught with serious emotional consequences; for example, conversion symptoms, depression, suicide or psychosis.

One investigator has reported: "For a large number of overweight persons, the mechanical prescription of reducing diets has had unfortunate consequences, for a smaller number it has been disastrous." He has stated that 51 percent of the obese women in a nutrition clinic reported untoward responses to previous attempts at weight reduction and "a more detailed investigation of 25 women revealed that nine had suffered emotional disturbances of psychotic intensity during present and past attempts at weight reduction." Other investigators have reported similar complications.

Not all investigators, however, agree that dieting may be responsible for severe emotional upsets. Some believe the obese have an "automatic safety valve" that causes them to abandon the diet before they get into serious trouble, and that the incidence of depression in patients who are dieting is no greater than the incidence in the general population.

The anxiety and depression levels of more than 150 unselected dieters were followed by the use of brief but valid psychological tests. About 15 percent of the dieters were found initially to be significantly anxious or depressed. Many of these failed to appear for a second appointment. During the diet about 12 percent of the total either continued to be upset or became so. These generally lost little or no weight. During the diet, no psychiatric emergencies occurred although two patients who had been previously institutionalized were found at the first visit to require hospitalization.

Of interest in the foregoing study is the finding that a few patients who lost no weight had rising levels of anxiety during the diet. In general, of the individuals who pursued the diet for any length of time, those who were anxious at the onset became more so as the diet went on, regardless of the presence or absence of weight changes. During the diet, the depression levels did not change in any statistically significant way. Interestingly, the most successful weight losers showed less anxiety and depression at the end of the diet than at the beginning. This study did not confirm the common belief that significant depression often results from or accompanies dieting. It was the authors' opinion that biased sampling resulting from psychiatric referrals for difficult or disturbed patients may produce erroneous conclusions. There is no doubt, however, that starvation diets and diets enforced on unstable personalities do produce serious psychological consequences.

A discussion of the psychological effects of dieting would be incomplete without a brief mention of the predieting personalities of the obese. One study has found "obese patients who were highly neurotic and others who were impressively stable." About 20 percent were free of "diagnosable pathology . . . the same proportion found in the general population." According to one report, the obese, on the average, scored higher on the Taylor Manifest Anxiety Scale than a large sample of nonobese. Another study of over 100 obese dieters matched with an equal number of "normals" for age, sex, and socioeconomic and marital status demonstrated that "while private and clinic patients showed some slight differences in anxiety and depression means, neither obese group was significantly more anxious or depressed than the normal sample with which they were matched." Other recent studies have revealed no significant personality differences between the obese and the matched "normals."

Studies have reported that more of the obese than the nonobese tend to be poor, single, divorced, separated, or widowed. When study samples are composed principally of such subjects, or when patients in the study are tremendously overweight or are already emotionally disturbed, more alarming psychic effects are seen from dieting.

There is little doubt that dieting for an emotionally unstable person can and does have disastrous results—neurotic symptoms, depression, suicide, or psychosis, to name a few. Obviously then, diets should not be promiscuously or casually prescribed. As in all forms of medical practice, an evaluation of the total physical and emotional state should be made before any significant alteration in the patient's life is attempted. All sorts of activities, including eating, may be used as defenses against psychological pathology. If we deprive a person of such defensive gratifications, we are obliged to replace them constructively.

One author believes that dieting is not likely to be successful and that difficulties may arise if the onset of obesity was before adolescence, or if previous attempts at dieting led to depression or other psychological problems. The same author also anticipates difficulties when the patient's goals appear to be unrealistic or if the eating pattern is deviant—of the kind characterized, for example, by the night-eating syndrome or by binge eating. Others have reported that levels of anxiety and depression, as revealed by specially constructed psychological tests, are predictive of dieting success: The more anxious and depressed personalities achieve poor results with dieting, and the obese who are better adjusted are able to diet more successfully.

One should hesitate to generalize about the psychological results of dieting. This hesitancy is further advised since many who diet successfully do not maintain the weight loss. We are really talking about the large numbers of people who "diet" with no significant weight loss or the smaller number who soon regain their weight, or an even smaller number who lose weight and maintain the loss—about whom we know very little. Again, we should also remember that the reports from which we draw our conclusions do not necessarily describe a fair sample of dieters. Many successes occur which are never reported in the literature.

Some attempts have been made to classify the obese in various ways and to correlate the psychological effects of dieting with the type of obesity. There appears to be insufficient evidence at this time for any definitive conclusion. It may well be that the advancing weight of the middle-aged sedentary person presents a quite different problem from that of the truly obese individual. The former may lose weight more easily and with less distress since the excess weight he carries is less meaningful, that is, it may be less well integrated into the personality and therefore less tenaciously held.

Obesity is not an accidental accompaniment to overeating, nor can it be resolved by firm commands to eat less or by threats of dire consequences. It is clear that obesity is an integrated process, not an alien aspect of the body or psyche, and as such is part of an equilibrium. It cannot easily or for any length of time be altered without the establishment of a new equilibrium.

The psychological and sociological consequences of dieting must be considered within the context of the problem of obesity. Obesity must be considered as a kind of steady state, albeit an undesirable one, at least from the point of view of general health and longevity. Dieting is an attack on this equilibrium which will be resisted unconsciously (and sometimes consciously) even in the presence of ego pressures for weight reduction. The remarkably poor results in dieting, the frequent minor emotional difficulties, and the occasional major mental disorders all attest to the tremendous ambivalence that surrounds dieting efforts. This ambivalence seems to derive from conflicts which are of internal sources, although occasionally the conflict may be between internal and external forces (especially in children). It is mainly the internal conflict which is pertinent to the lack of success in dieting as well as to the emotional difficulties encountered. The conflict seems to be between the ego-centered hopes and wishes and the more basically and tenaciously held fantasies regarding body weight and size. Until this conflict is individually resolved, it may be that many very obese people will not be able to lose permanently a significant amount of weight. This does not mean that lesser goals for such people are not attainable or desirable.

This section is a vital overview of psychological, sociological and anthropological factors that have a significant impact not only on the development of overweight problems but also on the dietary process itself. Too often in our attempts to treat and prevent weight problems we ignore the social stigmas that operate as precursors to the eventual development of compulsive eating.

*Excerpts from: *Obesity and Health*, U.S. Public Health Service Publication No. 1485.

Oh, How We're Punished For The Crime Of Being Fat

The writer, now at a respectable weight, recounts the pain she has absorbed—from the outside world and from within—for being obviously overweight. The memory and consequences are pressed indelibly into her soul...with self-acceptance, recently acquired, her salvation.

By Aljean Harmetz

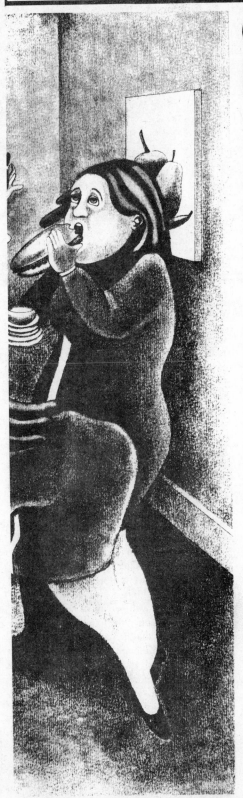

The photograph of me in the album is inexplicable. Frail and solemn, I stare out from the summerhouse—five-year-old eyes unblinking, fragile bones covered by a white dress that blows in a wind now more than 30 years dead.

As often as I turn to that page, I cannot recognize myself in the thin and untroubled child standing beneath a pine tree.

I have other images of myself.

I close my eyes and see the fat fifth grader, flushed with shame, standing in line for the required weigh-in at the school nurse's office. In my mind's ear, I hear her announce once more, "112 pounds"; and my long-since adult body cringes at the memory.

My mind is an album of shameful photographs. Fat thighs bulging beneath gym shorts so tight that they cut the flesh, I lumber down a hockey field or lunge to block a shot by my basketball opponent. Despite my weight, I am a surprisingly good athlete, but the pleasure of competing is always muted by the nakedness of white shirt and maroon shorts. Off the field, away from the court, I wear a heavy navy blue pea jacket, tightly buttoned on even the hottest summer day to hide my body from the outside world. When I was six years old, a swimming coach thought I was worth training seriously, but—by the time I am 12—I have stopped swimming almost completely. Alone in the water, I am too unprotected.

From what do I need protection?

From ridicule. From laughter. From the casual, unintended insult. From my own, unsought images of myself. By the time I am 12, the patterns are set—patterns that it will take 25 years to break. It is as though I have cut out a grotesquely misproportioned paper doll—50 extra pounds of hips and thighs—and then cast it in unbreakable concrete. Even during the thin times—the weeks and months when I balance precariously at a proper, normal weight—I am weighted down by the concrete image, encased in it.

The old, they say, do not think of themselves as old but are constantly surprised by the parody of their youthful face that they see in the mirror. The fat have a double burden. At their thinnest, they are aware of being fat. At their fattest, they yearn for the world to recognize their thin and fragile souls.

For a fat child, it begins early, that abrasive contact with the external world that rubs the soul raw just as the thick thighs chafe the flesh between them. When I was eight years old, I was not chosen to play "Peaseblossom," "Moth," "Cobweb," or "Mustardseed" in *A Midsummer Night's Dream*, although I was the most accomplished actress among the younger girls at the expensive boarding school which I attended. Those four were the only speaking parts available to the third, fourth, fifth, and sixth graders; and they were given to thin and delicate girls who mumbled the words.

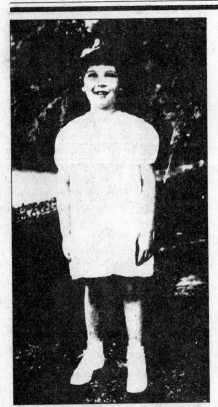

Aljean Harmetz, at five, thin and untroubled (above); at the age of 15, 40 pounds overweight (right, top); and today, at normal weight, with daughter Elizabeth (right, bottom).

Fat children early learn to become injustice collectors. There is always the unbought party dress that "makes you look too fat"; the years of wearing brown and navy blue because "in that color, you don't look fat at all"; the whispered conversations with teacher or summer counselor by a parent intent on justifying us to a normal-sized world; the cups of hot chocolate withheld from us alone; the public embarrassment of hard-boiled eggs and celery sticks when we are surrounded by the chocolate cupcakes of our friends.

It is for our own good, they tell us, our parents and caretakers, as they lock the refrigerator. We will feel better when we are not fat, they say. We will be happier. We can buy pretty clothes, and people will think we are beautiful. All true, of course.

And all false.

I was a secret eater by the time I was 10, wolfing down candy bars in the darkness of a Saturday matinee after first walking three blocks out of my way to buy the candy in a drugstore where nobody knew me. I ate the Milky Ways and Three Musketeers, the Almond Joys and Butterfingers too quickly to enjoy them —afraid, always, that the lights would go on before I had finished, impaling me before I had managed to wipe the chocolate

from my hands and throw the wrappers under a seat half a row away.

I hid candy then—under my underwear, on the shelf of my closet—and I hide it still. I no longer eat the hidden candy, but I feel uneasy unless it is there, a constant reminder that no one will ever deprive me again. Fat children grow up deprived of more than food for their bloated bodies. They are deprived of approval, of success, of smiles they should have won, of honors they deserved. Twenty extra pounds make the world step back in distaste from the ugly child in front of it. Each step the world takes backwards means another hamburger, another bag of French fries, to assuage the pain of being unloved. Then what a tangled web we weave of jelly beans and chocolate syrup, of lemon frosting and thickly buttered bread. And what angry, frightened spiders we are, trapped in the web we have woven.

The sticky fibers cling to our souls. My husband insists that he has never thought of me as fat, although there have been moments in our 14 years of marriage when I was as much as 45 pounds overweight. His insistence has no validity to me. Nearly everything in my life has been tainted by the knowledge that I acquired before I was 10 years old. I was fat at 10. In some corner of my soul, I will be fat forever.

Even my memories are tinged by that perception, as a colored filter over the

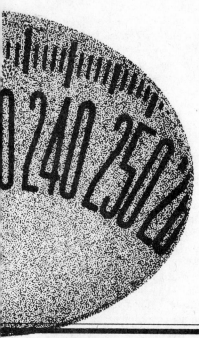

camera lens tinges each photograph. I was 15 pounds overweight at my wedding, and I wore a navy blue going-away dress to make myself look thinner. I weighed 221 pounds the September after my graduation from college. For six months of my junior year in high school, I was thin. I wore pink dresses embroidered with red apples and could pass a mirror without averting my eyes. Gorging myself on licorice and Hershey's chocolate the morning after my first child was born, I wore a size 12 nightgown. In nine months of pregnancy, I had kept myself from gaining more than eight pounds.

It was only a year ago that it first occurred to me to wonder why fat people should be ashamed. (What is there in our loss of control that frightens the people around us and makes them respond by shaming us?) Stuffing our bodies with unnecessary food is private poulticing of a private wound. Mildly self-destructive. On a par with compulsive cigarette smoking. But leagues below alcoholism, barbiturate dependence, drug addiction, suicide. Yet I became ashamed of my body so long ago that I no longer remember when or how it happened.

The photograph album includes a picture of me, at the age of 15, standing in front of the Statue of Liberty. The blue pea jacket is buttoned to my chin, while my New York cousins gaze serenely at the camera in their seersucker shirt-waists and cotton halters. But, years before that New York trip, I would refuse food in public only to stuff chocolate drops into my mouth in private; and I was already an expert at hiding in the shadows of the ladies' room of the Beverly Theater, waiting for the lights to go out and the picture to begin before running to my seat in the safe darkness.

The feeling of shame starts early. I had my first basal metabolism test at the age of eight, the first unnecessary thyroid pills when I was nine. If we cannot control ourselves, doctors and loving parents will impose controls on us. My body was the mirror of my mother's failure to cope with me, and that forced her to take sides against me.

It is unhealthy to be fat, our parents say, in vindication of themselves. And it is, of course. So they treat the symptom rather than the cause. Attacking our weight is easier than facing the problems buried beneath our mounds of fat.

(There is no one, all-purpose *problem*. Fat children and adults eat to fill unexplainable voids; the ugly, overfilled body is easier to endure than emptiness. We eat to avert the future or recapture the past, to stuff ourselves with the love we have missed or defend ourselves against the rage we cannot admit. We punish— or reward—ourselves with every unnecessary mouthful. Would I have been fat if my father had not left my mother and me when I was two? Would I have swol-

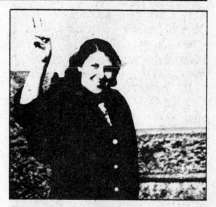

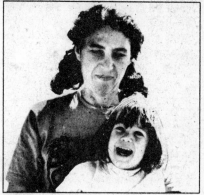

len like a poison toad if I had not been sent to my first boarding school before I was six? Would I have needed to weight my angers down with food if I had had a brother or sister to share the burden of being the focus of my mother's life?)

Our parents respond to our excessive weight by taking our bodies away from us. They are injected with drugs to help control our weight, fed small portions of drab food, weighed and measured and weighed again. We are objects to be made as attractive as possible. Packaged in slenderizing clothes and hairdos, we are coaxed and bribed and punished into making our bodies conform to the external demands of others.

And they do conform. For a while, at least. We lose the weight that has been demanded of us. But, as soon as possible, we gain it back again. Spitefully. Helplessly. Without intending to, except in some layer of our minds far below the surface. Then the roller-coaster ride begins again.

It can last for decades, that unceasing movement up and down the scales, until we are dizzy with the climbs and plunges, nauseous from the continual rounds of starvation and overeating. If we have any pride at all, we struggle down from the mountainous peaks of our obesity, whipping our bodies into making the descent. But sometimes, pride is lost. Then we ride the tide of our rising weight, strapped into a driverless car on some garish midway. *Thin* is too far away, an unreachable goal.

I did that once—got steadily bigger, like some helium-filled balloon, until I reached the immensity of 221 pounds. Ninety pounds overweight, I grasped some thread-thin strand of sanity and rode it down. I spooned, into the vast reservoir of my body, two last hot-fudge sundaes, on an October night, and started on a diet that was to last 11 months. I am amazed, still, that I was able to understand the danger that threatened me, to reach for control at the moment when it was almost forever out of my reach.

Ninety pounds overweight is monstrous. Twenty pounds shoveled away from that mountain of fat—30 pounds, 40 pounds—mean nothing. Half a year of starvation, and we are still grotesquely fat. We are defeated before we begin.

I managed to lose 90 pounds because I was lucky enough to have no other obligations. I spent that year, after my graduation from college, dieting—as someone else might spend a year taking a secretarial course or as a speech therapist. For the first four months, I slept 16 hours a day—willing my body into suspended animation. I woke at four in the afternoon for my solitary meal of lettuce, cucumber, and two ounces of rabbit thigh and then plunged back to sleep as soon as possible. I read, listened to the radio, ate my measured 350 calories a day, and never stepped beyond the boundary of my own backyard.

We are strange creatures, we compulsive eaters. We wrap ourselves in magic rituals. We are paradoxically frail as we waddle down the street. A piece of chocolate cake, three pancakes with maple syrup, and our diet is broken; it cannot be mended. We have failed, and any failure must be soothed with food. For four months I defended myself against that failure by locking the outside world away.

When I reached 175 pounds, the months of charts and measurements began. Each day was neatly graphed in black ink—65 calories in a piece of dry toast, 30 calories worth of strawberries. I weighed myself compulsively each day —stepping on and off the scale a dozen times until I was standing lightly enough to slave another quarter of a pound. Hips, thighs, waist, bust were encircled by a tape measure and the results recorded. Each new dot was charted and connected to the dot before, so that eventually I had vast star charts of my internal progress.

I haunted supermarkets during those months, surfeiting my eyes with the food I would not allow myself to eat. The food I did not eat filled my imagination, hundreds of thousands of calories spilling and splashing over in my head. My life was centered around food as fully as if I had spent my days devouring it.

I lost 90 pounds that year. When did the climb upward start again? Within six months, I think. (The journey downward is, often, a mystical trip. When we are no longer fat, we think we will be beautiful, successful, well loved. But losing weight does not automatically change everything else. The reality of the end of the journey is often more than we can endure.) But never again did I allow myself to get so close to losing control. Some safety valve in my brain stopped the reckless eating after 30 or 40 pounds.

I was a fat child. I have been, for most of my life, a fat adult. My weight falls within the normal range on those life-insurance charts against which I have always matched myself and found myself wanting. I will never be the slender, hipless model of my fantasies, but I do not think I will ever be fat again. Yet, I cannot really answer for tomorrow, next week, next year. I do not even know with absolute certainty why I was fat—what lost love I found in food, what devastating angers I buried between the layers of cake, among the ears of corn. I only know that, nearly 30 years after I ceased being a child, I could no longer tolerate the childishness of centering my life around food. And I was tired of self-imposed self-hatred.

I am still a compulsive eater. I cannot manage a single day without the taste of something sweet. But, I have built boundaries within which I seem to be able to live. A piece of hard candy dims the need for boysenberry pie. Half an English muffin, spread with jelly, blocks more dangerous desires.

Life at a normal weight will never be easy for me. When you stay fat long enough, your weight becomes the central focus of your world. You cannot look beyond it or around it. It blocks, distorts your vision—an invisible, self-imposed wall. I have stepped beyond my wall, but I am not comfortable in the sunlight. A world where all the clothes fit is almost embarrassing to me. (I never felt that I deserved nice clothes when I was fat.) Meeting someone I have not seen for a long time, there is still the frantic attempt to remember how much I weighed when they last saw me. Are they awed at a weight loss of 44 pounds or mildly approving of a loss of 15?

I still cannot eat freely and joyously. Overindulgence is punished by shame. Nor can I eat carelessly. I lurch and jerk between eating austerely and plunging into food as I might into a swimming pool. My body is much too eager to break free of the restraints which I have imposed on it; and perhaps it always will be. But I can look in the mirror now. What I see there is flawed. The hips will always be too big, the thighs painful to observe. But I can live with the pain I have, at last, grown beyond the need for perfection.　TH

The Stigma of Obesity

It's not enough for a nurse to tell an overweight patient to lose weight, she must understand the pressures—physical, emotional, and societal— the patient has to contend with and offer a relationship the patient can trust.

BEATRICE J. KALISCH

Society stigmatizes people with any characteristic it considers undesirable. The characteristic may be labeled a handicap, shortcoming, failing, disgrace, weakness, or, in the words of a leading authority on the theory of stigma, a "spoiled identity"(1). While the degree of undesirability may vary extensively, the common factor in such characteristics is lack of full social acceptance. The afflicted person is deprived of his right to be evaluated according to his unique personality.

In our society, the obese are invariably subjected to stigmatizing attitudes. Obesity has most commonly been considered completely physical or psychological, or both in origin; however, it must also be viewed as a social phenomenon. The ways that various cultures and even subgroups within the same culture define it in terms of beauty and ugliness gives weight to this.

DR. KALISCH is associate professor in the School of Nursing, University of Southern Mississippi, Hattiesburg. She earned her B.S. degree from the University of Nebraska in Omaha, her M.S. from the University of Maryland in Baltimore, and her Ed.D. in Human Development with a minor in nursing from the University of Maryland, College Park.

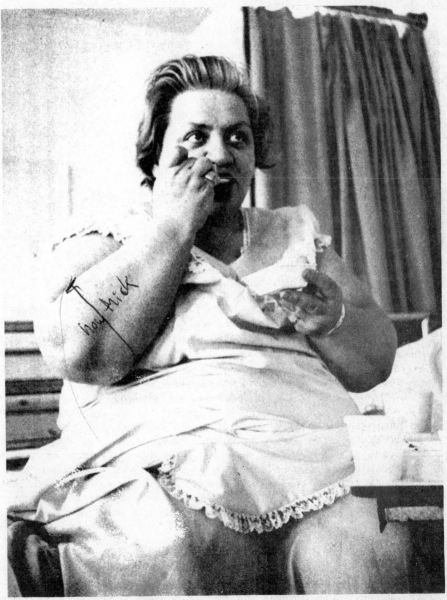

In our society, the fat person is often barred from attaining the privileges, opportunities, and status accorded to others.

One has only to look at Renaissance art to discover that plumper body types were favored at that time. In some cultures where food is scarce, a high status is accorded to those who weigh more because this indicates financial success.

Social class has also a potent influence on weight in our society. A study of the residents of a central area in New York City showed that extreme overweight was seven times more frequent among women of the lower socioeconomic class than those of a higher class. In men, the same relationship existed, but to a lesser degree(2).

The fact that obesity is a social phenomenon within our culture is seen also in dieting patterns. Wyden notes that even though only 11 percent of the total United States population falls in the upper- or upper-middle classes, these classes contain 24 percent of all dieters(3).

Women diet more than men and teen-agers more than adults(4,5). That obesity is a greater social disadvantage for a woman than a man in our society may account for this difference between the sexes. The obese woman finds it more difficult to move up the social ladder, relate to others, and obtain a suitable marriage partner than does the obese man. Moreover, the self-concept of American women is connected with physical desirability. The appearance of men is important, but financial status, educational achievement, and occupation affect his value more.

Another cultural influence is that the shape of men's clothing conceals body form and thus can hide bulges, while women's clothing is designed to reveal the configuration of the body. Adolescents diet more than adults probably because physical appearance is of great importance at that period of life and teen-agers tend to regard any type of deviation from the peer group norm as negative.

Why We Stigmatize

What causes a person to stigmatize another? It stems from our self-concept. Upon seeing a distortion, we feel threatened, probably because it reminds us of our own unearned good luck and our vulnerability. Stigmatizing attitudes increase our feelings of well-being, safety, and superiority. In other words, this mechanism allows us to dissociate or deny our common condition of vulnerability with the afflicted. Those with strong egos have less need to reject than those with weak ones.

Degree of Stigma

Studies have been directed to finding out how serious is the stigma attached to obesity in the United States. Richardson and his associates investigated how 650 boys and girls, 10 and 11 years of age, reacted to the physical disabilities of other children.

The children were shown six, black-and-white line drawings of a child with no physical handicap, a child with crutches and a brace on one leg, a child sitting in a wheelchair with a blanket covering both legs, a child with one hand missing, a child with a disfigurement on one side of the mouth, and an obese child. The results showed that, almost unanimously, the normal child was the most preferred and the obese child the least desirable(6).

Using this same ordering task of the six drawings, Maddox and others conducted a study with various adult groups, including persons they defined as most likely to be indifferent to the societal preference for leanness (elderly persons, Negro men, low-income persons). These groups, too, considered the picture of the obese child to be the least desirable and likable(7).

Obese applicants to colleges were found to be less likely to be accepted than the nonobese, even though there was no measurable difference in academic achievement, social class, and motivation(8).

Physicians have also been found to have negative attitudes toward the obese whom they described to be more "weak-willed," "ugly," and "awkward" than other patients(9).

Reasons Given for Stigmatizing the Obese

One justification frequently given for the negative connotation fatness carries in our society is that success depends to a great degree on physical attractiveness. Another reason given is that excess weight is detrimental to health, and health is a valued measure of status and security. A relationship between thinness and length of life has been reported frequently with reports indicating the obese are more prone to diabetes mellitus, cardiovascular, digestive and renal diseases.

Some interpretations of these relationships have recently been criticized for oversimplification. Formerly the weight-height tables used by the insurance companies disregarded the influence of body type and composition. Later they added modifications for frame size, without precise definitions of frames. Using the standards of height, age, and sex, today overweight refers to heaviness, while obesity refers to excessive amounts of body fat. It is possible to be overweight and not overfat and vice versa. Body type determines how much of excessive weight may be due to muscles, bones, fluids, and fats.

The Build and Blood Pressure Study, 1959 by the Society of Actuaries has largely influenced the belief that excess weight is associated with poor health(10). The findings, which revealed a consistent gradient advance in mortality with increasing degrees of overweight, have propagated the notion that all degrees of excess weight constitute a risk to longevity and health. A 1966 reevaluation of the 1959 study demonstrated that there was no significant excess in actual over expected mortality until the level of extreme obesity was reached. At this point, the mortality ratio rose in a very steep progression(11). The source book on *Obesity and Health* states that "The association of body fat and mortality below the level of frank obesity is not clear" (12).

Obesity is regarded as more than a beauty and health issue in our society, however. Many look upon excessive weight gain as immoral. Historically, the Protestant ethic emphasized impulse control and thus, in this case, abstinence from overeating. And gluttony, of course, is one of the seven deadly sins. Fat-

"To mention weight control to a person before a relationship based on genuine acceptance is established, is one way to doom the efforts to failure."

ness is not necessarily due to eating large amounts of food. Many Americans may be obese due to the sedentary lives they live. Yet, people associate the handicap with gluttony and self-indulgence(13). Under controlled, hospitalized conditions some persons find it most difficult to lose weight and numerous physiologic factors affect the process(14).

However, society continues to place the blame on the individual. Maddox found that, while the obese were held responsible for their own condition, people with other handicaps were not so blamed(15). And Goffman points out that whenever the stigmatized are believed to be the cause of their condition, the irrational, prejudicial attitudes are exaggerated(1).

Results of Stigmatizing Attitudes

An obese person finds his condition a constant barrier to attaining the privileges, opportunities, and status accorded to others. Physical and bodily discomfort that stems from obesity seems to be of less significance to him than the suffering imposed by the socially derogatory attitudes held by those around him. Fat people are ridiculed, despised, and often avoided.

When an obese person seeks

medical care, his personal tragedy may equal or exceed that of patients with more socially accepted physical diseases. The suffering and frustration associated with the obesity, however, may go beyond that of other physical ailments.

For an overweight person, hospitalization often mandates exposure of his overweight condition. On admission the routine weigh in may humiliate him; he realizes the results will become part of his chart for the hospital staff to see. A hospital gown may not fit and, even if it does, gives little protection from exposure. His body is exposed for treatments, bathing, and other procedures, and his food intake is monitored. Even though the nurse may not be critical of him, he may feel that she is.

As Goffman points out, the worst result of stigmatizing attitudes is that the afflicted come to accept the negative evaluations of the society(1).

In a study of high-school girls, for example, such personality traits as withdrawal, passivity, expectation of rejection, and extraordinary concern with self-image were found to characterize the obese(16). The obese, then, tend to live up to the expectations that others have of them, accepting a tremendous

amount of blame for their predicament—a typical, unfortunate example of the self-fulfilling prophecy.

An examination of physicians' attitudes revealed that they thought that obesity was either incurable or only slightly amenable to help(17).

One cannot help but wonder if the reported low success rate in the treatment of these individuals is related to the expectations of failure by physicians, nurses, and other helpers.

Combating the Stigma

Before a nurse can build a relationship with an obese patient which will help him strengthen his self-concept she must first examine her own feelings about obesity. She may well hold many of the unwarranted prejudices of the general public and might find it useful to separate myths from reality.

Most stigmatizing attitudes stem from erroneous assumptions, and when rational understanding is achieved the stigma is eradicated. However, achievement is not easy, because it must be preceded by the difficult and painful process of becoming self-aware.

Unconditional acceptance of the person is the key to helping the obese. Cahnman concludes from his

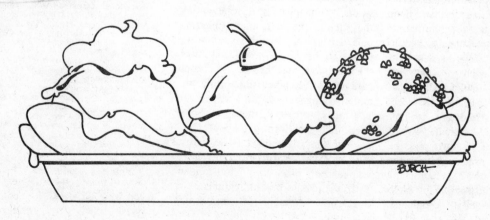

study of obese adolescents that acceptance of the individual must come *before* the weight reduction (18). To mention weight control to a person before a relationship based on genuine acceptance is developed, is one way to doom the efforts to failure. Because of the shame and guilt many obese persons experience, it may be difficult for them to talk about their true feelings and concerns.

Often, persons who have succeeded in reducing their weight to the normal range are unable to eradicate the self-hate and inadequacy they felt when they were overweight. Because we humans strive for self-consistency, if a formerly fat person does not revise his self-concept, he will most likely be unable to retain the weight loss. The nurse can help the patient adjust to his new identity, to help him retain his weight loss.

A typical response when normal individuals interact with the stigmatized is to pretend that the stigmatizing condition such as obesity does not exist. The person is aware that he is not genuinely accepted. In such a relationship, if a nurse advises or lectures the patient, he may build defenses to ward off anxiety. A common coping mechanism is denial. This defense interferes with his losing weight or adjusting in other positive ways.

Beyond assisting the patient to work through his problems by accepting him, the nurse can help him deal with the negative societal reactions. He should be helped to become aware of, and resistant to, stigmatizing attitudes rather than returned "cold" to the community. An understanding of why people react in the way they do will help the overweight person to cope with pressures he will undoubtedly face.

Goffman demonstrates that because the stigmatized are cut off from society, they associate with a group of persons, known as the 'own' group who share the stigma(1). With these persons, the obese can gain "instruction in tricks of the trade" as well as acceptance.

This may account for the epidemic spread of the "Weight Watchers" and other reducing clubs. It may be appropriate for the nurse to encourage certain patients to join clubs of this type so that they will have a subgroup to relate to and thus gain moral support.

It is important to start with the assumption that people don't want to hurt others. In hospital or other institutional settings, group sessions in which the staff can talk out their feelings and concerns about the obese would likely be helpful. A change in attitudes, however, is not likely to occur overnight. If any staff member continues to stigmatize obese patients, or for that matter any patient, the nursing leader must make the situations unrewarding for him either by reprimanding or dismissing him. This should be an established policy rather than an occasional informal action.

Helping the people abandon stereotypes and helping the stigmatized reconstitute their self-images are two sides of the same rehabilitative coin. All too often, however, the nurse neglects her responsibility for education of the public.

In the expanding role of the nurse, it seems imperative that she assume responsibility, along with other health professionals, for such programs.

Health education is still a largely unstudied field and outcomes of programs may be unexpected. For example, in York and Reading, Pennsylvania, a one-year campaign to decrease the negative, stigmatizing attitudes toward epilepsy was instituted. But instead of eradicating the stigma, the campaign tended to polarize attitudes and many were found to be more prejudiced after the campaign than before(19). Thus care must be taken in setting up and carrying out such a program. It is a fairly well established fact, however, that dwelling on the differentness of the stigmatized is an error. The most successful programs have emphasized how the handicapped person is like normal individuals.

Effective nursing of the over-

weight patient requires that both the nurse and patient focus on an obesity destigmatization process. Above all the patient should be appropriately involved in an assessment of his strengths and limitations in relation to his condition so that he does not feel manipulated and misunderstood. With acceptance from others as he is, the individual is then more likely to be able to deal realistically with his feelings and excessive weight. A corollary is to work with other health personnel and the public to develop accepting and empathic attitudes toward the obese.

References

1. GOFFMAN, ERVING. *Stigma; Notes on the Management of Spoiled Identity.* Englewood Cliffs, N.J., Prentice-Hall, 1963.
2. MOORE, M. E., AND OTHERS. Obesity, social class, and mental illness. *JAMA* 181:962-966, Sept. 15, 1962.
3. WYDEN, PETER. *The Overweight Society.* New York, William C. Morrow and Co., 1965, p. 8.
4. DWYER, J. T., AND MAYER, J. Potential dieters; who are they? *J.Am.Diet.Assoc.* 56:510-514, June 1970.
5. ———, AND OTHERS. Body image in adolescents; attitudes toward weight and perception of appearance. *J.Nutr.Educ.* 1:14-19, Fall 1969.
6. RICHARDSON, S. N., AND OTHERS. Cultural uniformity and reaction to physical disability. *Am.Sociol.Rev.* 26:241-247, Apr. 1961.
7. MADDOX, G. L., AND OTHERS. Overweight as social deviance and disability. *J.Health Soc.Behav.* 9:287-298, Dec. 1968.
8. CANNING, H., AND MAYER, J. Obesity—its possible effect on college acceptance. *N. Engl.J.Med.* 275:1172-1174, Nov. 24, 1966.
9. MADDOX, G. L., AND LIEDERMAN, V. Overweight as a social disability with medical implications. *J.Med.Educ.* 44:214-220, Mar. 1969.
10. THE SOCIETY OF ACTUARIES. *Build and Blood Pressure Study. Volume I.* Chicago, The Society, 1959.
11. SELTZER. C. C. Some re-evaluations of the build and blood pressure study, 1959, as related to ponderal index, somatotype, and mortality. *N.Engl.J.Med.* 274:254-259, Feb. 3, 1966.
12. U.S. PUBLIC HEALTH SERVICE, DIVISION OF CHRONIC DISEASES. *Obesity and Health.* (Publication No. 1485) Washington, D.C., U.S. Government Printing Office, 1966, p. 6.
13. DWYER, J. T., AND OTHERS. Social psychology of dieting. *J.Health Soc.Behav.* 11:269-287, Dec. 1970.
14. GORDON, E. S., AND OTHERS. New concept in the treatment of obesity. *JAMA* 186:50-60, Oct. 5, 1963.
15. MADDOX, AND OTHERS. *op. cit.* pp. 296-297.
16. MONELLO, L. F., AND MAYER, J. Obese adolescent girls, an unrecognized "minority" group? *Am.J.Clin.Nutr.* 13:35-39, July 1963.
17. MADDOX, G. L., AND OTHERS. Overweight as a problem of medical management in a public outpatient clinic. *Am.J.Med.Sci.* 252:394-403, Oct. 1966.
18. CAHNMAN. W. L. Stigma of obesity. *Sociol. Q.* 9:283-299, Summer 1968.
19. LEONARD WOOD MEMORIAL. *Combating Stigma Resulting from Deformity and Disease.* New York, The Memorial, 1969.

Negative Mood, Hunger And Weight Classification

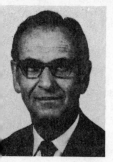

Mark I. Hewitt, M.D.

Questionnaires completed by 747 respondents documented changes in mood with hunger and satiety. Generally speaking, negative mood correlated with hunger and positive mood with satiety. Negative mood, sensed more often by women, may further the weight problem and may explain in part the desire for patients with a weight problem to have mood-elevating medication.

THE degree to which emotions play a role in the cause or continuation of a given patient's obesity remains obscure. Yet, attempts to link some aspect of psychopathology to obesity have been the subject of numerous publications.[1-9] Conclusions among the authors have varied.

Through the administration of a highly structured, hunger-satiety questionnaire to men, women, boys, and girls, Mayer and associates[10-13] were able to detect changes in mood as hunger sensations changed in severity and again as satiety approached. In general, they described these mood variants either as "negative" (depressed/apathetic, irritable,

The author wishes to acknowledge his sincere appreciation for the excellent guidance and statistical review provided by Mr. Kenneth D. Kotnour and for the editorial assistance of Ms. Bonnie Olinger.

about the author . . .

Mark I. Hewitt, M.D., is Director of Regulatory Affairs for the 3M Company. Dr. Hewitt received his medical degree from the Indiana University School of Medicine. He is a frequent abstractor for *Obesity & Bariatric Medicine*.

nervous/tense) or "positive" (cheerful, calm/relaxed, contented). Satiety, according to these investigators, appeared to be associated with changes in mood, i.e., as the urge to eat began to wane, a positive mood tended to supplant a negative one.

It appeared of interest to investigate, by means of such a questionnaire, whether or not changes in mood during the transition from hunger to satiety was the same when groups having varying degrees of weight-control were compared. The design of the questionnaire afforded the opportunity to evaluate mood in respect to hunger and satiety among such groups.

Method

Approximately 1000 questionnaires,[14] modified slightly from that used originally by Mayer et al.,[11] were distributed randomly over a period of about 15 months throughout the United States, among professional medical product and pharmaceutical sales representatives and their wives, administrative office personnel, members of two groups of subjects interested in weight reduction, and to undergraduate nurses in the Saint Paul, Minnesota area. Distribution of the questionnaire was intentionally made by third parties, e.g., national sales managers, nonmedical or paramedical personnel, and a director in nursing education.

In brief, this questionnaire was designed: to explore, in depth, hunger and satiety under various circumstances; to dwell in detail upon certain meal-related items such as food preoccupation, meal-skipping, beverage ingestion, and snacking; and to relate these events to meals. Each questionnaire was accompanied by full instructions for its completion as well as an explanation of its purpose—to obtain as much information as possible about hunger and satiety sensations. The questionnaire, highly structured and consisting of 00 multiple-choice questions, was to be filled out without interruption after an evening meal. About 30 to 45 minutes were required for its completion. The one modification pertinent to this report consisted of having each respondent identify with one of the three following weight-problem categories:

1) "I've always been able to eat anything I want and have no weight problem;"
2) "What weight problem I have I can control myself by watching what I eat without having to go on a special diet or seeing my doctor;" or
3) "I am unable by myself to control my weight and have tried diets with or without my doctor's supervision. My weight has tended to go up unless I diet and I've had several ups and downs."

Respondents were also asked to classify themselves either as being underweight, overweight, or of satisfactory weight.

Among the 100 questions were 6 questions that asked each respondent to choose one or more given adjectives expressing either a negative mood (depressed/apathetic, irritable, nervous/tense) or a positive mood (cheerful, calm/relaxed, contented) in the following situations;

A) with extreme hunger (the hungriest the respondent had ever felt);
B) at two hours before the main meal;
C) at 30 minutes before the main meal;
D) on sitting down to eat but *before* actually eating;
E) after a few bites of food; and
F) at the *end* of the meal.

The selection of one or more negative or positive adjectives was sufficient to classify the respondents' predominant mood as either negative or positive in relation to these specified situations.

Data were tabulated and contingency table analyses were performed through the use of a computer. Statistically significant differences were evaluated at a risk level of P .05 using the Chi square distribution.

Results

Of all questionnaires distributed, a total of 747 were completed by 302 males (40%) and 445 females (60%). All respondents self-classified their current weight as either underweight (UWT), satisfactory (SAT) or overweight (OWT) of these, 719 of the 747 respondents (96%), 286 males (40%) and 433 females (60%), self-classified their weight-control problem as either no weight problem (NWP), self-controlled weight problem (SC), or no weight control (NWC). These results by categories are shown in Table 1. It can be seen that among these respondents the number of males and females in either the underweight (UWT) or no weight problem (NWP) categories is about the same. However, in the satisfactory weight (SAT) or self-controlled (SC) weight problem categories the number of females showed a relative increase over males. This trend continued into the overweight (OWT) or no weight control (NWC) categories where in the former there were about 50 percent more females than males (283 vs 180) and in the later, two and one-half times more females than males (150 vs 60).

Sex more than age determined distribution into weight-problem groups. However, younger females fell significantly more often into NWP and SC groups and the older, into NWC group.

Table 1: Weight Categories Of Respondents

Self-Classified Weight

Sex	UWT	%	SAT	%	OWT	%
Male	22	3	100	13	180	24
Female	30	4	132	18	283	38

Self-Classified Weight Problem

Sex	NWP	%	SC	%	NWC	%
Male	77	10	149	21	60	8
Female	86	12	197	28	150	21

Figure 1 compares the percentage of negative mood responses between men and women when grouped as NWP, SC, and NWC. Similarly, Figure 2 compares the prevalence of negative mood among men and women when each is grouped according to self-classified weight (UWT, SAT, or OWT). Statistically significant group differences, when present, for each of the periods A to F are noted in each Figure.

The profound ability of hunger to incite a negative mood among these subjects was apparent. The markedly pervasive "tranquilizing" effect surrounding the eating process was also seen particularly at certain intervals, i.e., sitting down to eat but before actually eating (D); after a few bites of food (E); and at the end of the meal (F). Statistically significant male-female differences have been noted in Table 2. Data for the underweight subjects were limited and insufficient to determine statistical differences. Significant male-female differences existed in self-control (SC), and in satisfactory and overweight categories, especially in the anticipatory intervals (A, B and C). In these groups with few exceptions the percentage of negative mood responses was significantly higher in women than in men. There is a general increase in prevalence of negative mood in women as either the weight problem or self-classified weight increases.

Physicians treating patients having a weight problem recognize that while emotional aberrations often are present the extent to which emotions are causal is not readily apparent. Although it is not possible to be certain that the population sampled in this study is representative of the general population, it is tempting to extrapolate from these results to the general population. Whether or not the predominance of a negative mood as related to over-all hunger and satiety sensations is a cause, an accompaniment, or one of the sequelae of the weight problem cannot be answered by these data. However, the relationship, even if inexplicable appears to exist and should be recognized in management of these patients.

From these observations it became apparent that negativity of mood was present to some degree in all respondents, irrespective of their weight or their type of weight-control problem. While with most of us the depression, the apathy, the irritability may lie at a subconscious or barely conscious level with extreme hunger or before meals, perhaps it is reasonable to speculate that

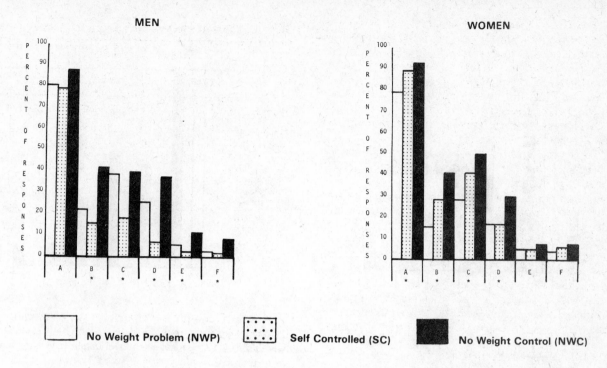

MEN   WOMEN

No Weight Problem (NWP)   Self Controlled (SC)   No Weight Control (NWC)

*—Indicates one or more groups are significantly different from one another at any given time (P <.05)

FIGURE 1: COMPARATIVE PREVALENCE OF NEGATIVE MOOD—WEIGHT PROBLEM GROUPS

negativity of mood more often reaches a conscious level in those with a weight problem. That it may be allied either to the observed greater incidence of overweight in women or possibly to a greater emotional lability in women may deserve consideration. Militating against this view is the increase in negative mood seen in both males and females among those unable to control their weight.

These data lead one to speculate that negativity of mood is not the sole explanation for obesity. At times it was

Table 2: Comparative Percentage Of Negative Mood Responses Among Male and Female Respondents

Period	Sex	Weight Problem Groups			Self-Classified Weight Groups		
		NWP	SC	NWC	UWT†	SAT	OWT
A	Male	81	79	88	79	82	80
	Female	79	89*	93	87	91*	92*
B	Male	22	16	43	46	17	27
	Female	16	28*	41	21	25*	48*
C	Male	39	18	40	62	25	17
	Female	28	41*	50	41	35*	54*
D	Male	26	7	38	30	15	17
	Female	17*	17	30	18	17	33*
E	Male	6	3	12	17	7	3
	Female	5	5	7	10	4	11*
F	Male	3	2	9	15	4	4
	Female	4	6*	7	7	4	9

* Denotes statistically significant male-female differences (P= < .05)

† Denotes limited data.

relatively marked in those having no weight problem. The underweight, particularly the males, appear to have shown this same tendency with the limited data available. More sampling of this type of individual would be needed to show if this trend is significant. Whether or not some of the underweight respondents who demonstrated considerable negative mood may later fall victim to a weight-control problem is open to conjecture. Too, concern in itself about a potential weight problem may help explain the increased negative mood in some of the underweight respondents.

In view of these observations, it is tempting to speculate on the surreptitious role negative mood may play in and the degree to which it may affect management of patients with a weight-control problem. Because negativity of mood among these respondents appeared to be so effectively assuaged at mealtime, this relationship may serve as a potent force to initiate, perpetuate, or worsen a weight-control problem. Further, one may consider the mood-lifting quality of some anorexigenic agents to have played an even greater role in their total efficacy than heretofore assigned it. Conversely, the absence of this mood-lifting quality may have accounted in part for the relative ineffectiveness of some agents that have not had this attribute. Also, coffee, often drunk in large amounts by those with a weight-control problem, may be used not only as a substitute for snacks but also to provide some stimulation sought by those sufficiently hypersensitive to caffeine. Also, the decreased use of alcohol by those respondents admitting to a weight-control problem, which was documented in this study but not detailed here, may in part represent the unwitting avoidance of an agent that pharmacologically is a depressant.

It was also observed that the negative mood in all respondents, except in males self-classified either as no weight control (NWC) or overweight (OWT), became

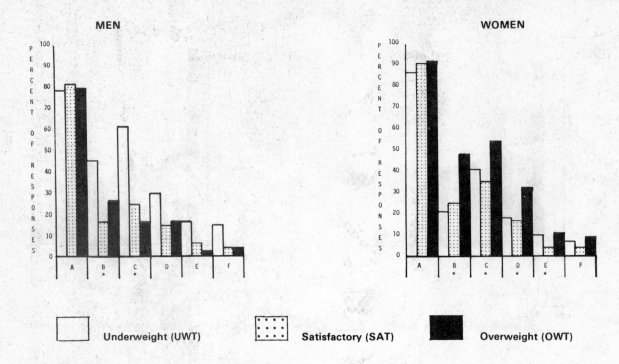

MEN   WOMEN

☐ Underweight (UWT) ⦂ Satisfactory (SAT) ■ Overweight (OWT)

*—Indicates One Or More Groups Are Significantly Different From One Another At Any Given Time (P < .05)

FIGURE 2: COMPARATIVE PREVALENCE OF NEGATIVE MOOD—SELF-CLASSIFIED WEIGHT GROUPS

heightened 30 minutes before the main meal, a level exceeded only by that accompanying extreme hunger. No explanation is apparent for the disparate mood response of the male with a weight problem at this specific interval. The observation of a heightened negative mood at interval C is consistent with the long-held belief that a person with an "empty stomach" may be less receptive and amenable to decision making than one with a "full stomach."

Conclusions

Data received from 747 respondents who completed a highly structured questionnaire have been reviewed specifically in respect to the incidence of negative mood accompanying hunger and satiety and the following conclusions drawn:

1) In general, negative mood was a normal accompaniment of hunger and positive mood, of satiety.

2) Negative mood was often more prevalent in those respondents self-classifying themselves as having either a weight-control problem or being overweight; however, it also was sensed by some who admitted having no weight-control problem.

3) With one exception, whenever there was a significant statistical sex difference in negative mood associated with hunger, women were more negative in their response.

4) The prevalence of negative mood with hunger may explain partly the desire of those on a weight reduction program for medication to lift a mood usually ameliorated instead by the ingestion of food or stimulant beverages.

5) Negative mood conceivably may further the weight-control problem, especially in the overweight. ⓜ

REFERENCES

1. Rennie TAC: Obesity as a manifestation of personality disturbance. *Dis Nerv Syst* 1:238, 1940.

2. Bruch H: Obesity in Childhood and personality development. *Amer J Orthopsychiatry* 11:467, 1941.

3. Hamburger WW: Emotional aspects of obesity. *Med Clin N Amer* 35:483, 1951.

4. Bruch H: Psychological aspects of reducing. *Psychosom Med* 14:337, 1952.

5. Young CM, Berresford K, Moore NS: Psychologic factors in weight control *Amer J Clin Nutr* 5:186, 1957.

6. Suczek RF: The personality of obese women. *Amer J Clin Nutr* 5:197, 1957.

7. Salzman L: Obesity, understanding the compulsion. *Med Insight* 2:52, 1970.

8. Rotman M, Becker D: Traumatic situation in obesity. *Psychother Psychosom* 18:372, 1970.

9. Holland J, Masling J, Copley D: Mental illness in lower class normal, obese and hyperobese women. *Psychosom Med* 35:351, 1970.

10. Monello LF, Seltzer CC, Mayer J: Hunger and satiety sensations in men, women, boys and girls; a preliminary report. *Ann NY Acad Sci* 131:593, 1965.

11. Mayer J, Monello LF, Seltzer CC: Hunger and satiety sensations in man. *Postgrad Med* 37:A97, 1965.

12. Mayer J, Thomas DW: Regulation of food intake and obesity. *Science* 156:328, 1967.

13. Monello LF, Mayer J: Hunger and satiety sensations in men, women, boys and girls. *Amer J Clin Nutr* 20:253, 1967.

14. Hewitt MI: Respondents self-appraisal of weight control. A preliminary report. Presented at the annual meeting, American Society of Bariatric Physicians, Las Vegas, October 5, 1972.

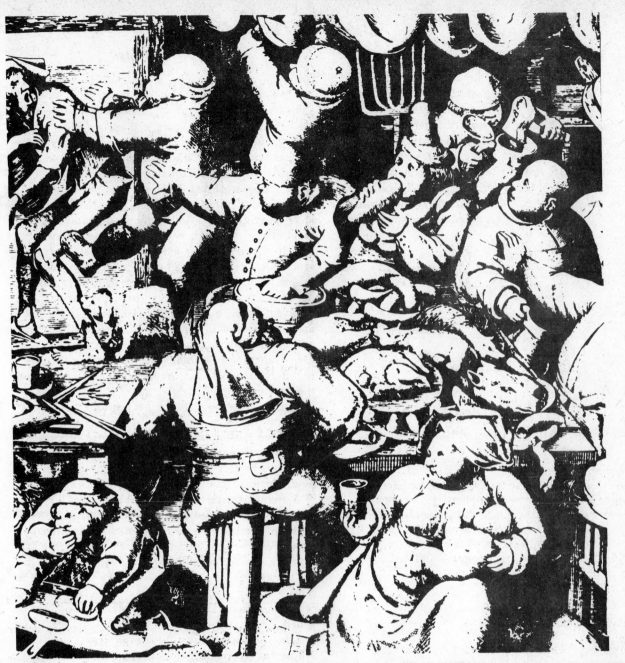

Psychological Aspects Of Obesity

By HILDE BRUCH, M.D.

The trouble with obesity and even more its treatment is the bewildering fact that logic doesn't seem to work. It has been known since the time of antiquity that reduction of food intake and increased exercise will accomplish a predictable loss of weight. Being cautious about what they eat does work for the millions and millions who have made dieting a national preoccupation and work constantly at watching their weight. How to stay slim is everybody's preoccupation and supports multi-million dollar businesses for many non-medical agencies.

The physician is left to treat those in whom the obvious doesn't seem to work, and he must face the fact

Treating the uncooperative obese patient requires more than a diet calculated to correct the energy imbalance responsible for the overweight. The physician must understand the how and why of the underlying physiological, regulatory and psychological disturbances.

continued

that however appropriate the diet he calculates, it cannot be effective unless the person for whom it has been prescribed adheres to it. Understanding the uncooperative fat patient takes a distinctly different conceptional and operational approach than calculating a diet to correct the energy imbalance responsible for the overweight. It requires, instead, an understanding of the how and why of the underlying physiological, regulatory and psychological disturbances. We have made much progress during the past decade in our knowledge

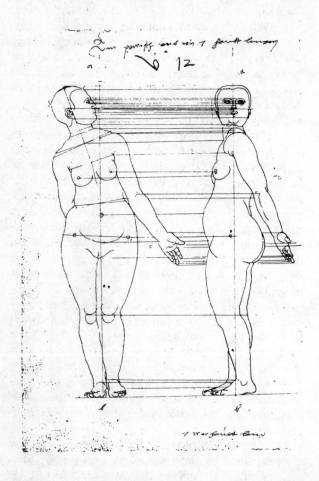

of the various physiological aspects of weight regulation and its disturbances. My discussion here will be on the psychological implications of obesity.

No psychological diagnoses are applicable, of course, to all of the millions of people who are too fat. Those who come to psychiatric attention are in a way a self-selected group who ask for help after conventional treatment approaches, including repeated reducing regimens, have failed. Often they had reacted with renewed weight increase or had suffered emotional upheavals during their efforts. Whether such people represent a large or small percentage of the enormous number of overweight people is not known. They constitute the problem cases who keep physicians and nutritionists puzzled and dissatisfied with their efforts.

Often these patients are discounted in reports of

treatment results because they are "uncooperative." But in talking about obesity, whatever other subdivisions one chooses to apply, it is necessary to differentiate between two basic groups: those who can reduce and function well while doing so, and those who encounter serious difficulties while dieting and find it intolerable. In extended contact with such troublesome cases, we have learned that in spite of the handicap of overweight there are people who function better at a level of weight that is above the so-called average. In them obesity, through a faulty adaptation, may serve as a protection against more severe illness; it represents an effort to stay well or to be less sick. For such people reducing is not the cure of their problems. At best, as the underlying problems are clarified and resolved, dieting may become possible—a sign that they are now capable of handling life problems in a more rational and appropriate way.

In evaluating psychological problems it is necessary to differentiate between the factors that play a role in the development of obesity, those that are created in the obese person by a culture that is hostile and derogatory towards even mild degrees of overweight, and finally the tension and conflicts that are precipitated by efforts at reducing. The picture is further complicated by the fact that in each phase physiologic and psychological factors interact and influence each other.

A frequent assertion states that the psychological problems of obese people are due to the rejecting social attitude. These insults are real enough, and condemnation of overweight appears to be on the increase. Yet intimate contact reveals that those most hurt by this are individuals who suffer from severe self-doubt and have a poor body image and inadequate self-concept, with consequent extreme dependence on the opinion of others, in all areas of living—not only in regard to weight and appearance. Obese adolescents, and adults whose excess weight goes back to early life, are particularly vulnerable because they consider themselves ugly, and despise and loathe their body and its large size. Yet when they try to reduce they feel diminished and empty and become even more unhappy. People who grow heavy after they have reached adulthood usually do not express such self-derogation, nor do

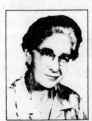

Dr. Bruch is professor of psychiatry, Baylor College of Medicine, Houston, Tex.; and has recently published a book, *Eating Disorders: Obesity, Anorexia Nervosa and the Person Within* (Basic Books, Inc.).

they expect that they would set everything right and change their whole unhappy life by losing weight.

This negative self-concept is often attributed to the condemning cultural attitude. This is not so; at best it is only a part of the problem. A large group of fat children who were seen in a pediatric clinic during the 1930s and whose development was followed into adulthood showed wide differences in their self-concept and overall adjustment. Those who had been accepted and encouraged by their families developed a good self-concept and had a positive body image. They were not particularly affected by the negative cultural attitude but had made a healthy adjustment which included the ability to maintain control over their weight,

Abnormal weight must be evaluated in relation to whole development

though often at a level somewhat above the average. In contrast, those with early signs of emotional disturbances associated with severe intrafamilial problems and conflicts did poorly in regard to both weight and adjustment. They were the ones who suffered excessively from the hostile cultural attitude and experienced it as a personal rejection. It seems that those who eventually become psychiatric patients and whose psychological problems are closely interwoven with the factors that make for obesity come from this second group, those with early signs of inner trouble. If excess weight alone is taken as the starting point, without regard for other developmental aspects, the delineation of the psychological problems in obesity remains vague and contradictory.

To differentiate between various patterns of psychological reactions it is necessary to evaluate for each patient the functional significance of his abnormal weight in relation to his whole development. Three main groups emerge with this approach. The largest group is comprised of overweight people whose moderate and fairly stable weight excess developed after adolescence and who, like people of normal weight, may encounter all kinds of psychological difficulties which are not, however, related to their weight problem. Much of the confusion about the psychological factors in obesity is due to the fact that observations on such ordinary overweight people are not separated from those made on patients in whom the weight disturbance and psychological difficulties are closely intermingled.

Even these latter patients do not present a uniform picture. Psychological factors were first recognized in people who grew obese following some traumatic event (reactive obesity). This was described as "paradoxical obesity" by German and French authors after World Wars I and II, seen then in women whose obesity developed after severe mental shock, such as bombing, evacuation, or the loss of a beloved person. The precipitating event is not always so dramatic. Obesity may develop under various circumstances where other people might react with a depression: separation from home, fear of desertion and loneliness. Often this aspect is not recognized until a manifest depression develops when reducing is attempted.

In developmental obesity the weight disturbance is intrinsically interwoven with the whole development, and is often associated with severe personality disturbances. Some fat children do not suffer from it; their excess weight is an expression of their constitutional make-up or a family tradition of abundant eating. But in the majority of fat children, and adults whose obesity goes back to early life, these constitutional factors are intermingled with severe emotional disturbances. Such individuals grow up in families which fail to respect their need to be recognized as individuals and express themselves. Though the manifest clinical picture may vary, such fat youngsters have certain basic features in common. The most important is the feeling of not being in control of their own sensations and actions, even of not owning their own body. They have failed to organize discriminating awareness of the signals of bodily urges, in particular awareness of hunger as a signal of nutritional need; they also lack conviction of emotional and interpersonal effectiveness.

We have reconstructed the early life experiences of such patients from detailed observations of their interactions with their families, and they reveal definite abnormal patterns. Though these children were generally well cared for, their own expressions of need were disregarded; instead, the mother superimposed what she felt the child needed and when, according to her own concepts and impulses. This was expressed in every detail of the child's physical and psychological care. Thus the developing child was deprived of an important learning experience: recognizing the relationship between felt discomfort, appropriate response and felt satisfaction. What is clinically apparent is a deficit in the regulation of food intake. It appears now that the old reproach of obese people having no will power describes an important functional deficit, namely that "hunger awareness" has not been programmed properly.

This deficit is perceptual, and conceptual awareness

of hunger is a prerequisite for the misuse of eating in the service of various non-nutritional needs which have widely different symbolic meanings. Whatever emotional tension or frustration they experience, such people will react with the feeling of needing to eat; either they are helpless in controlling these impulses, or they become anxious and depressed when attempting to do so. This inaccuracy in hunger awareness and the dependence on outer stimuli also explains the paradox that obese people often reduce successfully under strictly controlled conditions, such as in a hospital or reducing institution where they will adhere to a drastic

Weight loss alone will not solve the underlying problems of living

regimen, only to regain the weight as soon as they are back in their old surroundings. In the sterile atmosphere of a hospital where no food is in sight except what is served on the plate, it is relatively easy to abstain from eating (even though there, too, cheating does occur). The most tempting place is the ordinary home where food is readily available whenever the impulse to eat, for whatever reason, comes up.

People with these deficits often complain about feeling empty, and act and behave as if their center of gravity is not within themselves but somewhere in the outside world, controlled by someone else. They bemoan their fate of being too fat, use the obese state as an alibi for all their handicaps, and yet feel helpless to change the sad state of affairs. They are usually awkward and tense in social contacts and are described as withdrawn and seclusive, and this is "explained" as being due to the obesity.

Though obesity is a serious social and psychological handicap, weight loss alone is unable to solve the underlying problems of living. Attempts at reducing often increase the psychological difficulties. For people who reduce before they have experienced the inner emotional changes which make a better adjustment possible, there are three potential outcomes. The great majority will try and try, will lose some weight, and then suddenly give up and regain or exceed their former weight. For others the stress of starving themselves, the loss of their large size, and the new real or imagined expectations may prove too much, and seri-

ous emotional disturbances, even frank psychotic behavior, may break through. A third group succeeds in becoming and staying thin, but their conflicts are far from solved by having lost weight. On the contrary, their difficulties now have a chance to flourish, since the ugliness of being fat no longer prevents them from putting their unrealistic dreams to the test. Such people, though they no longer look obese, are far from cured; they still resemble fat people with all their unsolved problems, conflicts and exaggerated expectations. Only they no longer show their fat. They have become *thin fat* people, who impress the casual observer, their friends and acquaintances as enviably slim, attractive and interesting, though they themselves know how unhappy they are and what price they pay for their artificial slimness.

They show many similarities to those in whom the wish to be thinner and the refusal of food results in anorexia nervosa, a condition that may be conceived of as a caricature of what happens when the common recommendation that reducing will make you slim, beautiful and happy is taken too literally and carried to the extreme. Yet there are also definite differences between thin fat people and anorexics, since anorexia nervosa patients continue on the downhill course and aim at a body weight far below normal. Their thought distortions concerning weight, food and why they must deny themselves are truly delusional. Anorexia nervosa is a rare disease, the end state of the unrealistic preoccupation with weight and size. Just as only a few of the numerous shy and withdrawn obese adolescents develop into full-blown schizophrenics, so only a few of the many thin fat people will progress to the malignant state of anorexia nervosa.

The relative frequency of this tragic course of events, an obese adolescent developing anorexia nervosa or schizophrenia, is probably low but not unique. The possibility of a malignant development should be kept in mind when dealing with an obese young person who has unusual difficulties following a reducing regimen while simultaneously complaining violently about the abnormal weight and feelings of social inferiority. In my observations, most of the fat patients who become overtly schizophrenic have been in treatment for obesity at one time or another. In some, psychological difficulties had been recognized but the potential for schizophrenic development had usually been overlooked. Developmental obesity is not only a problem of weight and calories, but an expression of serious personality disturbances, and tampering with the weight of such an obese youngster carries with it the danger of exposing the schizophrenic core of his development. Before weight control can be successful, he needs to become aware of the conflicts and circumstances from which he has tried to escape by excessive eating, and he needs help in growing beyond his basic sense of incompetence and helplessness. □

Like drug or alcohol
addicts, many excessive eaters
are compulsively driven
to eat — to the point of illness — by inner
drives that they can neither
understand nor control

By LEON SALZMAN, M.D.

OBESITY—
UNDERSTANDING
THE COMPULSION

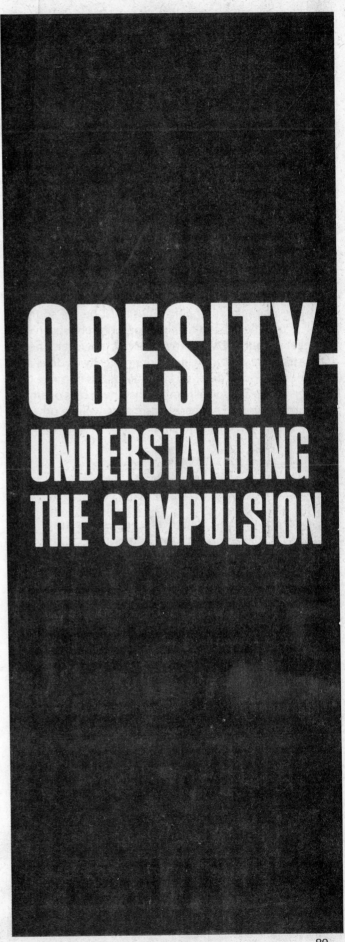

Obesity has long been recognized as a psychological problem as well as a physiological one.[1-19] But the vision of a pill or a magic potion that will allow an individual to eat whatever and whenever he pleases without any concern over accumulation of fat still remains as an obstacle to the adequate control of the obesity problem. Both psychological and physiological issues, including genetics, biochemistry, energy output, and caloric intake[20] must be considered in the effort to fully comprehend this disorder. The tendency to emphasize the physiological factors, however, derives not only from the failure of physician and patient to acknowledge the psychological issues, but also from the nature of the obese person's character structure which encourages denial and assumes an omnipotent capacity to be exempt from the consequences of cause and effect.

A great many persons overeat in the context of their metabolic capacity or diminished activity and therefore slowly gain weight, and though this serious problem affects a large number of Americans and people in other affluent countries, such weight gain is controllable within reasonable limits. I shall focus not on such moderate overweight, but upon the extreme type of obesity, where excessive fat is immediately obvious and where the problem is mainly a psychological one. This type of obesity is qualitatively as well as quantitatively different from the minor overweight problems which are more closely related to cultural preferences and personal esteem than to disease states. Analogous to the distinction between the social drinker and the alcoholic, I shall be referring not to the social eater, but to the food addict. Like alcoholism, the addiction to eating which leads to extreme obesity has definable characteristics and psychological roots which can be identified.

The analogy to alcohol continues even to the severity of the withdrawal symptoms which accompany extreme obesity when dietary restrictions are imposed.

the obsessive-compulsive syndrome—"complete control or no control"

Like many alcoholics, eating addicts are often "secret eaters" who publicly eat little and privately gorge on fantastic amounts of food. This often leads others to assume that glandular difficulties must be the source of the trouble, since the individual is rarely observed to eat too much. Overeating does not, however, affect the structure of family life as dramatically as does alcoholism, nor do its severe manifestations impinge on others in the antisocial manner that the excess of alcohol intake does. For these reasons, as well as others, I feel it is often more difficult to treat than alcoholism.

Food plays many complicated roles necessary for action besides supplying the nutrition necessary for life. In his early years, man requires the assistance of other persons when he eats; in later years the presence of other persons adds particular zest and pleasure to eating. In addition to fulfilling man's needs for fellowship and intimacy, the giving and receiving of food are dramatic ways of conveying interest, affection, and desire to care for another human being, and food is often used as a substitute, literally and symbolically, for the physical manifestations of tenderness and love. Many authors have established the significant role of the oral area in the depressive disorders as well as in other characterological disorders. No one could ever doubt the intimate and potent relationship between food and personality development if they could observe the drama of the anxious mother trying to force food on her child, or the effect on the child when nutritional requirements receive no interest or attention from his environment.

The obese individual, however, is still reluctant to recognize the intimate relationship between his eating habits and his emotional state. The recognition of this is often confused by the oversimplified notion that overeating is directly related to tension, and that therefore anxiety should be manifest in each eating

bout. The failure to discover such a relationship enables the already skeptical observer to discard any further consideration of psychological principles and return to his search for the magic potion.

Case studies seem to indicate that extreme obesity is intimately related to the obsessive-compulsive syndrome, a disorder in which the individual is compelled to act out certain rituals in order to achieve a feeling of control over his environment. The individual attempts to achieve perfection or infallibility and thereby to guarantee his existence. The obsessive devices — procrastination, isolation of affect, indecision, distraction, and displacement — are all attempts to establish such guarantees and to avoid commitments which may lead to future danger. All the maneuvers are performed to achieve and exert control over oneself and others; the obsessional person is therefore rigid and controlled, particularly in those areas of his living which involve his emotional life and are not entirely under voluntary control. Since absolute control is impossible, he often tries to "control" by total avoidance of control of any kind. He is totally organized, or completely disorganized; meticulously clean or sloppily indifferent to cleanliness. Thus the obsessive-compulsive syndrome is essentially concerned with always being in control either by active attempts at control, or by abandoning all efforts to exert any degree of control. This description applies with equal validity to the compulsive drinker, gambler, drugtaker, and masturbator, as well as to the compulsive eater.

Even though eating is a very familiar activity, as a compulsion it is no different from more bizarre phenomena such as ritualistic handwashing. However, excessive eating has always been heavily loaded with moralistic and derogatory connotations and the victims were labelled pigs, gluttons, and sinners. The overeating was labelled as "abuse to one's person" and was considered to be one of the cardinal sins.

While obesity in females did not always carry moral or social censure, it was generally considered esthetically undesirable. Though other compulsions such as handwashing rituals were early recognized as a medical problem, the compulsion of overeating was not. It was for a long time considered to be the consequence of weakness, sinfulness, or inadequate self-control, rather than a medical condition. The moralistic attitudes toward obesity have clouded the obsessional factors and served to interfere with their proper handling for a long time.

Like drug or alcohol addicts, excessive eaters are compulsively driven to eat, not through taste or hunger — for they often stuff and gorge, without any enjoyment, to the point of illness — but by inner drives that they can neither understand nor control. Often they eat alone and in secret, following a ritualistic pattern such as reading while eating to avoid recognizing the excessive intake, or eating in a particular order or fashion. The secrecy also permits them to maintain the illusion of eating sparsely, since they do not eat much in the presence of others. Often they repress or simply forget the eating binges which take place at odd times, such as during the night. At times their denial is so extreme as to suggest a schizophrenic dissociation process, and sometimes the compulsive tendencies of such people do go to the point of psychotic disorganization, including delusions of grandiosity.

The loneliness and emptiness of the compulsive eater are suggested by his symbolic attempt to swallow everything in order to fill his own emptiness. Nothing can be left in the refrigerator or on the table, since it might not be there tomorrow. **Like a squirrel storing nuts for the winter, he cannot leave anything behind.** Coupled with this is the attitude of being entitled to get all that is going around, and the fear of being cheated unless he takes in all he possibly can. This feeling of entitlement often derives from early deprived experiences, but more frequently it relates to grandiose expectations and claims in which he sees himself as being omniscient and omnipotent, worthy of all attention and fulfillment. Often eating binges take place in an atmosphere of rebellion, where the person feels entitled to special rewards for having been previously denied. The rebelliousness may be in response to praise, if the person interprets the praise as insufficient, phony, or manipulative. One 280-pound lady would regularly overeat when her husband told her that she looked fine and seemed to be losing weight. She knew that she was still overeating, and therefore felt his remarks were phony and designed to mislead her.

The capacity for self-deception and the delusional distortions of the self-image are striking phenomena in the compulsive eater. They are most dramatically seen in the notion that calories will not affect him if nobody else is aware of the excessive intake. One patient who weighed 350 pounds would regularly stand nude before a full-length mirror, openly admiring her figure, which she thought looked slim and graceful. She ate very little at mealtime and could not entirely understand why she was overweight. Her husband was convinced that she overate only on infrequent occasions when he would waken early in the morning and inadvertently find her gorging on huge sandwiches, soft drinks, cakes, and candies. He was quite unaware of how frequently these bouts took place.

Denial may reach psychotic proportions in many compulsive overeaters. They feel that they live prudent and only mildly uncontrolled lives, do not acknowledge the secret eating, and claim that their weight increase is a mysterious development unrelated to food intake. Bruch notes in her classic studies

Dr. Salzman is Professor of Psychiatry, Director of Psychoanalytic Medicine at Tulane University School of Medicine. He is also past President of the Academy of Psychoanalysis.

there can be "opposing" compulsions

on obesity that the self-image of the obese person is often that of a thin person who will starve unless he continues to eat. It is the converse of the anorexia nervosa patient who is extraordinarily thin but refuses to eat because he sees himself as an obese person who will become even more gross and ugly unless he controls his food intake. At times the obese person may have delusions of being denied nourishment by a hostile world, or of being invaded by worms which will destroy him unless he eats enough to satisfy them.

The overall problem of control which is manifested in compulsive inability to stop eating appears in other areas of living as well. Obsessive-compulsive patients are pressured by their uncertainties and feelings of impotence, caught up in attempts at perfection and invulnerability, and need to control all their actions and also those of others. One moderately obese compulsive eater refused to acknowledge her approaching menopause. She said she was not ready for it and hadn't decided she wanted it yet. She was desperately searching for approval, and while her entire activity was directed at the control of others, she tried to justify her behavior by insisting that she was just a puppet in the hands of her husband and others and couldn't exert enough self-control to stop eating — even though her capacity for controlling herself and others was far beyond the ordinary. She denied her overeating, except in rare moments of self-awareness when such an admission fitted into her conception of her own superiority. In addition, she considered herself above the usual laws of digestion and caloric issues, and insisted that she should be able to eat as much of whatever she pleased without having it affect her whatsoever. Her phobias, somatic preoccupations, and communication difficulties were all classically obsessional.

This same syndrome was strikingly demonstrated in another 285-pound woman whose compulsive eating was complicated by increasingly severe kleptomania. Most of her eating was done in secret, between meals or in the evening, and because she was extremely re-strained in the presence of her family, she managed to engage their sympathy and support. She was extremely rigid, stubborn, and rebellious. To avoid being taken advantage of, she would refuse to budge an inch once she had made up her mind; at other times she refused to make a decision for fear that she might have to change it. Often she firmly believed that she was not fat and had a beautiful figure. Every positive comment from her husband was translated into an affirmation of her attractive figure, but since his compliments were not freely given she used them as justification for a new eating binge. Her belief that she was entitled to anything she wanted, on her own terms and without any cost whatever, her evasions and her denial of reality, were evident in both her obesity and her kleptomania, in her feelings of immunity from the natural laws of biology and the social laws of property.

The coexistence of these two compulsions raises the question of why some compulsions direct the individual to antisocial acts while others produce actions that are destructive only to the individual involved. The compulsion itself is amoral, and is the result of a defensive process. The direction of the compulsion and its acceptability to the culture are determined by the particular ethos and values of that culture. Such actions as voyeurism or the compulsion to expose one's genitalia may have severe consequences in one culture and be relatively unnoticed in another. The individual may not regard his compulsion as an immoral act even when the society does; on the other hand, some compulsions which may not antagonize the culture may be entirely unacceptable to the individual himself. The ability to treat some compulsions successfully is sometimes thwarted by the legal consequences of the behavior, which may override the psychiatric considerations. But the com-

effective
treatment requires specifics,
not sermons

pulsion, while involved in moral issues, must be understood outside the question of values or cultural prejudices.

These two cases emphasize the significance of understanding compulsive behavior in the recognition and treatment of obesity. Demonstrated here in extreme cases, this understanding is necessary in the treatment of even mild obesity and will perhaps discourage the prevalent notion that an obese person is perfectly able, through resolve and determination, to overcome his obesity. If it is a compulsion, treatment requires more than sermons, commands, entreaties, or resolutions. It demands understanding, growth, and maturing before such resolve can be effective, and a recognition and identification of all the devices and techniques that are present and which invariably cause a breakdown of the resolution to lose weight. Emphasizing to the patient his continued failure only leads to further despair, a greater feeling of hopelessness, and a greater need to eat. This becomes a widening, vicious circle.

Psychotherapy alone can rarely do the task, since the resolution of many neurotic disorders, particularly the obsessive-compulsive disorders, requires more than insight. The patient needs action in the form of assistance towards change. The therapist must use encouragement, support, pressure, and guidance, and often drugs and advice, in order to propel change. Understanding is the prelude to change, not change itself. In the long run, the treatment of obesity must use the same modalities as the treatment of other addictive disorders. □

SUGGESTED READING

1. Bruch, H.: The Froelich syndrome, *Am. J. Dis. Child.* 58: 1283, 1939.

2. Bruch, H.: Obesity in childhood: 3. Physiologic and psychologic aspects of food intake of obese children, *Am. J. Dis. Child.* 58: 738, 1940.

3. Bruch, H.: Obesity in childhood: 4. Energy expenditure of obese children, *Am. J. Dis. Child.* 60: 1082, 1940.

4. Bruch, H. and Touraine, G.: Obesity in childhood: 5. The family frame of obese children, *Psychosom. Med.* 2: 141, 1940.

5. Bruch, H.: Obesity in childhood and personality development, *Am. J. Orthopsych.* 11: 467, 1941.

6. Bruch, H.: Puberty and adolescence: Psychologic considerations, *Advances in Ped.* 3: 219, 1948.

7. Bruch, H.: Psychological aspects of reducing, *Psychosom. Med.* 14: 337, 1952.

8. Bruch, H.: Fat children grown-up, The Johns Hopkins Medical and Surgical Association, Baltimore, Maryland, Feb. 25, 1955.

9. Bruch, H.: Role of emotions in hunger and appetite, *Am. N.Y. Acad. Science* 63: 68, 1955.

10. Bruch, H.: The emotional significance of the preferred weight, Symposium on Nutrition and Behavior, *Am. J. Clin. Nutrition,* 5: 192, 1957.

11. Bruch, H.: Psychopathology of hunger and appetite, in changing concepts of psychoanalytic medicine, New York, Grune & Stratton, 1956.

12. Bruch, H.: The Importance of Overweight, New York, W. W. Norton, 1957.

13. Bruch, H.: Developmental obesity and schizophrenia, *Psychiatry,* 21: 65, 1958.

14. Johnson, M. L. et al: Relative importance of inactivity and overeating in the energy balance of obese high school girls, *Am. J. Clin. Nutr.* 4: 37, 1956.

15. Mayer, J.: The physiologic basis of obesity and leanness, *Nutr. Abstr. and Reviews:* 25: 597, 1955, and 25: 871, 1955.

16. Snapper, I.: Food Preferences in Man: Special Cravings and Aversions, *Ann. N.Y. Academy of Science.* 63: 92 (July 15) 1955

17. Stunkard, A. J. et al.: The night-eating syndrome, *Am. J. Med.* 19: 78, 1955.

18. Stunkard, A. J.: The dieting depression: untoward responses to weight reduction among certain obese persons, *Am. J. Med.* (in press).

19. Stunkard, A. J. and Dorris, R. J.: Physical activity: performance and attitude of a group of obese women, *Am. J. Med. Sci.* 233: 622, 1957.

20. Gordon, E. S., Goldberg, E. M., Brandabur, J. J., Gee, J.B.L., Rankin, J. Abnormal energy metabolism in obesity. *Tr. A. Am. Physicians* 75: 118, 1962.

Severe Obesity as a Habituation Syndrome

Evidence During
a Starvation Study

David W. Swanson, MD, and
Frank A. Dinello, PhD, Chicago

Reprinted from ARCHIVES OF GENERAL PSYCHIATRY 22(2):
120-27, 1970, Copyright 1970, American Medical Association.

IT IS estimated that 20% of the population of the United States, or approximately 40 million adults and children, are overweight. Gordon et al[1] have pointed out that obesity of such widespread proportions is a problem of affluent societies, occurring when an abundance of food is available to great masses of people. Presumably, many in this overweight population are what they are because of the mere availability of food. For

Submitted for publication July 17, 1969.
From the Department of Psychiatry, Loyola University of Chicago Stritch School of Medicine (Dr. Swanson), and the Department of Psychology, DePaul University (Dr. Dinello), Chicago.
Reprint requests to Department of Psychiatry, Loyola University of Chicago Stritch School of Medicine, 2160 S First Ave, Maywood, Ill 60153 (Dr. Swanson).

some, however, the reasons for excessive food intake are less obvious; the severely obese person so exceeds his caloric needs that his fatness threatens his own physical and social wellbeing.

Although emotional factors are apparently of importance in such obesity, Stunkard[2] points out that this assumption is based on two very general findings: first, that obese persons admit they eat when they are upset and, secondly, that such persons manifest more neurotic traits than their nonobese counterparts. Similarly, Kaplan and Kaplan,[3] in their review of the diverse emotional constellations found in the obese person, could not relate fatness to a specific psychological problem. These cautious conclusions emphasize that psychological causes of obesity are certainly nonspecific and incompletely documented.

At this time obesity is still best viewed as having multiple causes—metabolic, neurological, psychological, and socioeconomic. In this respect it is like many other disorders in medicine and especially those in psychiatry; an exact cause-and-effect relationship and pathophysiology are unknown. Nevertheless, the clinician must somehow conceptualize the relationship between his obese patient and food. The fact is that if this patient properly controls his caloric intake no physical harm results and he ultimately achieves an acceptable weight. Unfortunately, such control is not routinely within the capacity of the obese patient, perhaps because of organic factors or psychological limitations, or a combination. The result for patient and physician is behavior typical of a habituation syndrome with food as the substance that is used uncontrollably. To illustrate such an observation this report presents the addictive behavior of 25 severely obese subjects before, during, and after extensive dietary restriction, including prolonged therapeutic starvation for periods up to 85 days.

The World Health Organization suggests that:

Drug addiction is a state of periodic or chronic intoxication, detrimental to the individual and society produced by the repeated consumption of a drug. . . . Its characteristics include: (1) an overpowering desire or need (compulsion) to continue taking a drug and to obtain it by any means, (2) a tendency to increase the dose and (3) a psychic (psychological) and sometimes a physical dependence on the effects of the drug.[4]

Habituation or psychological dependence refers to compulsive use of a drug because of the relief or pleasure it affords but without the development of physical dependence, severe intoxication, or of those other effects usually considered detrimental to the individual or society.[5,6]

Habituation and a habit-forming substance are considered more benign than addiction; a habit-forming substance may, however, be so abused as to become an addicting one except that it does not produce physical dependence. A majority of the public probably is mildly habituated to caffeine, nicotine, or alcohol and it is of little clinical significance. Some, however, are addicted to alcohol because of the intoxication produced, the overpowering desire for it, the increasing amounts consumed, the detrimental effects associated with it, and the possibility of a tolerance-withdrawal component. Contrariwise, narcotics are clearly addicting drugs, yet in the pain-wracked terminal cancer patient they may produce a physical dependence and a resulting need to take the drug but a genuine psychological dependence does not exist. The habituation-addiction differentiation is, thus, rather ambiguous. Most important to the clinician are the patient's compulsive use of the drug, psychological dependence, and the destructive effects produced, irrespective of the habit-forming or addicting substance used.

Although food is not considered a drug and eating is surely something besides a habit, the observations to follow suggest that the severely obese person can be accurately viewed as a clinically habituated person. Food is used to such excess that it produces sedation, there is a compulsion to use it to excess, a tendency to continually increase the amount, a psychological dependence, detrimental effects on the person and his family, and behavioral changes when the customary intake of food is restricted.

At least three compulsive patterns of eating have been described previously. Stunkard[7] has noted a "night-eating syndrome" in 10% of obese persons. In such cases evening hyperphagia and insomnia are precipitated by stressful life situations and usually recur until alleviation of the stress. He noted another pattern termed "the binge eating syndrome" in approximately 5% of obese persons. In this instance there is a sudden, compulsive, large ingestion of food in reaction to stress such as a frustrating experience. It is associated with self-condemnation, drastic dieting, and recurrent eating binges. He termed a third pattern "eating-without-satiation" in which a subject with a history of encephalitis could not stop eating despite the absence of hunger. This syndrome was unrelated to stress.

This Study

Method.—Subjects were selected on the basis of a body weight exceeding an ideal weight by at least 50%, and in fact, most patients weighed over 300 lb (136.1 kg). Subjects had to be motivated for severe dietary restriction and receptive to hospitalization on a metabolic research unit for a minimum of two months. They did not undergo formal psychological evaluation although a judgment of motivation and cooperativeness was made by the senior metabolic investigator and a research nurse before acceptance into the program. Thus, patients with overt psychosis or severe personality disorder were excluded. After acceptance into the study subjects were maintained on a moderately restricted caloric intake for approximately ten days prior to complete starvation while physical status and metabolic baseline values were established. The starvation regime was carefully explained to the patient but no exact length of starvation was established.

The starvation technique consisted of total elimination of caloric intake. A prescribed daily intake of fluids, B-complex vitamins, and potassium bicarbonate was required. Physical activity in the hospital was not restricted but excessive perspiration was discouraged. Extensive physiological and metabolic monitoring was done on a rigid schedule (body weight, fluid intakes, urine output, vital signs, serum electrolytes, liver function studies, renal function studies). Observations of behavior were made prior to, during, and after starvation. Twelve subjects were seen by the senior author for formal psychiatric evaluation prior to starvation and twice weekly for the duration of hospitalization. Three additional subjects were interviewed in retrospect about starvation. In all 25 subjects the medical chart, daily nursing observations, social history, and available psychological testing were reviewed.

General Observations.—Twenty-five subjects (24 men and one woman) were studied. Age and weight data are presented in the Table. Age range was from 23 to 55 with an average of 39 years. Weights prior to starvation were from 198 to 473 lb (89.8 to 214.5 kg) (average 315 lb [142.8 kg]) and weight loss was from 22 to 124 lb (10.0 to 56.2 kg) (average 67 lb [30.4 kg]). This weight loss included prestarvation and poststarvation observation periods of varying lengths during which the subjects were on restricted caloric intake. All subjects lost weight even on diets up to 2,000 calories. Complete starvation continued for 8 to 85 days (average 38 days). During starvation the average per day weight loss was approximately one pound.

Metabolic correlates of starvation in these subjects have been reported in detail by Spencer et al.[8,9] Of particular psychological interest is the consistent loss of appetite in all subjects paralleling the metabolic acidosis caused by breakdown of fats. The acidosis reached a nearly maximal value in 48 hours and physical sensations of hunger were usually absent thereafter. Although other metabolic changes accompany starvation, none of the subjects experienced any sustained physical ill effects. The minor physical discomforts experienced by some subjects were light-headedness, mild headache, abdominal cramping early in starvation, and a later occurring unpleasant taste.

Observation Prior to Starvation.—In this population of superobese subjects 14 (56%) were grossly overweight prior to age 16, and 15 (60%) reported significant obesity in one to five members of their immediate family. Ten (40%) were unmarried.

For all subjects food was the focus of daily life. Although they often minimized their food intake, like the alcoholic rationalizes his drinking, most eventually admitted their excessive eating. Food was the source of greatest pleasure and this included not only eating it but working with it. Nine subjects were employed as cooks and five more prepared the meals in their own household. Two other men spent several hours a day in favorite restaurants where they not only ate excessively but also socialized. Some subjects described workdays where they ate little but experienced an increasing anticipation of the time when they could go home and spend four to eight hours preparing large quantities of food and eating it. Some admitted consuming 6,000 to 10,000 calorie meals during these periods. The evening would begin with extensive preparation of the meal with consumption to the point of physical discomfort (distention, nausea, vomiting), drowsiness, and finally sleep. The desire to spend the evening in this manner caused avoidance of social contacts. Yet another illustration of the intense desire to eat was noted in the subject who after work had only enough money for either two sandwiches or his bus fare; he chose the former and walked three miles to his home.

Most subjects reported specific foods which had intense appeal; once they began consumption there was no stopping. For one this was pork chops—he would begin with one and did not stop until he had eaten the ten he had purchased. For others it was cheese, stew, hamburgers, chocolate chip cookies, cake, etc. During diet efforts some specifically avoided these foods for fear they would not stop eating. Two subjects admitted to extensive nocturnal eating. One regularly awakened three times a night, would get up to urinate, and then proceed directly to the kitchen. Some variety of episodic eating characterized most subjects although it was modified in the chefs who often ate continuously.

Besides the intense pleasurable affect produced by eating—which was unanimous in these 25 subjects—most were convinced they obtained some relief from anxiety and frustration by eating. After experiencing what they felt was unreasonableness of their customers, bosses, or wives they found privacy and food soothing. Yet, as severe fatness produced shame, guilt, and isolation, the subjects complained of unhappiness and loneliness. In fact, this feeling of sloppiness and being unlike other people was the principle stated motivation for starvation. All believed that if they lost 50 to 150 lb (22.7 to 68.0 kg) and again looked like normal people that the happiness and productivity resulting would allow them to control their obesity in the future.

Sixteen (64%) had intermittently consumed moderate to large quantities of alcohol. This was usually beer. Some, in an effort to control this, had switched to soft drinks and two regularly drank 12 to 15 bottles of this daily. Only one subject was considered an alcoholic at the time of hospital admission.

All subjects had attempted diets. They had typically gained, lost, and regained hundreds of pounds. The ability to diet and lose weight had convinced some subjects they could control their obesity if absolutely necessary. Most admitted that after losing poundage they felt they could relax the diet for a day or so, only they never returned to it. Many reasons were given for dieting, eg, ridicule, dislike of physical appearance, threat to health, threa'ened loss of job, or marital unhappiness. When the subjects applied for starvation all had physical complications due to obesity. Hypertension, latent diabetes, dyspnea, chest pain, and sleepiness were the most common ones.

Prior to starvation none of the 25 subjects had overt psychotic or neurotic disorder. Ten (40%) subjects had diagnosable personality disorder (passive-aggressive, 7; antisocial, 2; hysterical, 1) based on history, mental status examination, and prestarvation ward observations. These disorders were ingrained maladaptive patterns that had moderately disrupted social, occupational, or interpersonal functioning. They included as manifestations alcoholism, criminal behavior, prolonged unemployment, and sexual deviation. In those subjects not diagnosable a variety of personality trends were noted (compulsive, 6; dependent, 5; extroverted-cyclothymic, 4). Prior to starvation these superobese people were not problems in the hospital setting for they were generally compliant, self-doubting, optimistic about what others could do for them, and desirous of finding an answer to their weight problem.

Observations During Starvation.—Although the physical sensations of hunger were present for 48 to 72 hours this period was tolerated well. In fact, only two subjects dropped out of the program before two weeks. Initially the subjects seemed pleased with their self-denial and weight loss.

The first evidences of a stressed state were efforts by the fasting subjects to excessively structure their time beyond the already extensive routines demanded by the research metabolic setting. Most patients established elaborate schedules involving gym work, walking, occupational therapy, reading, painting by number, and keeping elaborate weight charts. Additional evidence of stress was an increasing preoccupation with food. They talked in detail of favorite dishes and the majority collected recipes and pictures of food. Dreams about food were common. Two subjects had their wives bring in pastry and insisted on watching families and staff eat it. "Cheating" was also indicative of stress. All subjects thought of it but the exact incidence is unknown. Three men admitted it. One reported such feelings of tension one evening that he left his bed, went to a vending machine area and ate several sandwiches. Despite the staff's warning that the metabolic studies would expose anyone going off starvation, several subjects insisted they had devised a timing of caloric intake which escaped detection. When violation of starvation was suspected subjects would deny it, become indignant, or give excuses to explain a weight change.

Dependence on the staff and manipulativeness increased as starvation progressed. Subjects would request exceptions in the rules or prolonged explanations of common procedures. The level of cooperation gradu-

Weight Loss

Subject	Age	Weight Prior to Starvation lb	Weight Prior to Starvation kg	Days Starved	Weight Lost lb	Weight Lost kg
1	33	337	152.8	85	102	46.3
2	45	286	129.7	18	33	15.0
3	32	326	147.9	8	22	10.0
4	46	271	122.9	33	49	22.2
5	55	198	89.8	41	44	20.0
6	38	370	167.8	42	124	56.2
7	43	337	152.8	61	77	34.9
8	37	242	109.8	27	24	10.9
9	23	323	146.5	38	61	27.7
10	43	290	131.5	74	74	33.6
11	40	341	154.7	45	66	29.9
12	42	304	137.9	71	104	47.2
13	45	330	149.7	20	59	26.8
14	33	473	214.5	46	103	46.7
15	36	304	137.9	48	71	32.2
16	30	332	150.6	44	53	24.0
17	32	334	151.5	41	66	29.9
18	42	306	138.8	32	51	23.1
19	31	315	142.8	35	66	29.9
20	43	306	138.8	39	90	40.8
21	35	271	122.9	24	73	33.1
22	48	297	134.7	25	53	24.0
23	42	297	134.7	10	57	25.9
24	43	341	154.7	24	97	44.0
25	45	337	152.8	27	80	36.8

ally diminished. Some subjects produced uncertainty about when to terminate starvation. Although unhappy and wanting to eat they would, at the same time, insist on prolonging starvation. They vascilated and if medical-psychiatric reasons were given for termination they were disgruntled.

Overt psychopathology—other than the personality patterns noted on admission—was observed during starvation in 17 (68%) of the subjects. The disorder was often mild, did not require treatment, and was most significant because it represented a change from admission. The psychopathology was of four types: paranoid trends, 7 (28%); characterological trends, 4 (16%); depressive trends, 4 (16%); and anxiety, 2 (8%).

The most obvious clinical signs were in the subjects with paranoid trends. These persons usually went through a period of increasing concern and apprehension about their physical condition, family, or finances.

Then they brooded and attributed their problems to staff inefficiency. Suspicions, accusations, and angry threats were made; one subject was physically abusive. Some subjects used ideas of reference to justify hostility while others confessed an awareness of their anger. One man asked for help after discharge because he was so angry when in traffic that he feared he would kill any aggravator by smashing his car into them.

CASE 1.—An example of definite paranoid disorder was a 36-year-old single man (subject No. 15) who weighed 350 lb (158.7 kg) on admission, 304 lb (137.9 kg) at the beginning of starvation, and 233 lb (105.7 kg) at discharge. Initially he was an extroverted, pleasant, humorous man who was very candid about his uncontrolled eating. He was ashamed of his appearance and also of his past record which included nine years of criminal activity and imprisonment during which his weight never exceeded 230 lb (104.3 kg). In the last five years he had "gone straight," worked regularly, and also gained 150 lb (68.0 kg). Early in starvation he was jovial and helpful to another fasting subject but talked regularly about food. On day 14 of starvation he was angry at a staff member and another patient and threw his urinal to the floor. He apologized for the tantrum but soon complained of insomnia and obsessive thinking. By day 25 he accused everyone of being phony and was belligerent and suspicious. He decided after recommendation to stop starvation but later pleaded for permission to continue. After this he showed alternating and less severe periods of belligerence and depression until day 45 when he apparently cheated on the fast, denied it, and became very restless and dependent. On day 49 he was re-fed on a 600-calorie diet. During the next week he was intermittently cooperative and belligerent. He increasingly criticized the hospital staff and accused them of racial prejudice, homosexuality, and intentional persecution of him. He made physical threats, kicked a door, and left the hospital against medical advice.

This man had a long history of aggressive-criminal behavior during which he was heavy but not excessively obese. During five years of rapid weight gain he had worked and conformed to society. During prolonged dietary restriction he manifested mistrust, anger, assaultiveness, and psychotic paranoid thinking.

Although at least 12 subjects manifested depressive features during starvation, only four had this as a prominent finding. These persons, like those with paranoid features, usually experienced a period of apprehension and concern about themselves or their family. They would try more than most subjects to be good patients, especially by working harder on ward projects. Feelings of hopelessness were expressed and helplessness was evident in their request for attention. Two subjects felt they were unattractive when thin and described feeling hollow or appearing "skinny," although both were still obese. One questioned, "What's the use if you can't enjoy a good meal?" None were psychotically depressed.

Two subjects developed severe anxiety disorder, terminated starvation, and felt it urgent that they leave the hospital. They admitted to increasing tension and alternately pleaded to eat or to be helped in remaining on starvation. They denied physical hunger but finally explained they must eat or go "crazy."

CASE 2.—Subject No. 19 was a 31-year-old single man who was physically fragile, phobic, and enuretic until age 14. By age 15 he weighed 200 lb (90.7 kg) and his enuresis had improved. He weighed 325 lb (147.4 kg) on admission, 315 lb (142.8 kg) at starvation, and 249 lb (112.9 kg) at discharge. He owned his own business and felt stressed by demanding customers. At night he relaxed by eating. He was a shy, conscientious man who admitted to a huge food intake. He did not like controversy, was self-depreciatory, and moderately apprehensive. He showed increased attention to detail and controlled most conversations with this technique. He was very helpful and well-liked. After starvation began he did many number paintings and collected a drawer full of recipes. This subject's starvation period was interrupted by one week on a 600-calorie diet. During his second fast he complained more of worry about business and was restless and bored. His dependency on the staff increased and a favorite request was for advice on whether to stop starvation. On day 33 he felt so tense he wanted to run away from the hospital. On day 35 he broke starvation by eating, which he admitted, although he was promised that starvation would be terminated anyway in two days.

This man had evidence of neurosis in childhood but his symptoms abated somewhat concomitant with his becoming obese and entering adulthood. Anxiety, compulsivity, and obsessiveness were marked during the latter phase of starvation.

The subjects with changing character patterns during starvation did not often complain of subjective discomfort. Perhaps more than other subjects these patients experienced a sense of well-being during starvation. They became more ambitious, articulate, and confident. One man who was distinctly passive and phlegmatic on admission delighted in this increased confidence but as starvation progressed he admitted to concern over some impulsive ideas which he was entertaining. In some plans he did not care if others were hurt by his actions—he sensed a feeling of recklessness in himself. Another subject engaged in increasing amounts of provocation against the staff. He was confident he could break the rules without detection and said he did this; then he would flaunt this by nearly exposing his actions to those he had deceived or would confidentially tell certain personnel members. When manipulation was impossible he appeared dejected or brooded.

Starvation was terminated according to plan or for medical reasons in 15 subjects. In the remaining subjects termination was requested or resulted from other psychological factors resulting in a 40% incidence of withdrawal in highly motivated obese persons.

Follow-up Observations.—The subjects were re-fed on strict diets (600 to 1,200 calories) designed to continue weight reduction. Most were confident they could continue successful dieting after discharge; none, however, did. A follow-up[10] revealed that all the subjects regained weight. In fact, within a year, all except four were at a weight equal to or exceeding that upon admission; these four achieved partial success by utilizing intermittent starvation, self-prescribed amphetamines, diuretics, or psychotherapy but were continually troubled by personal and occupational problems.

After starvation a typical pattern was to follow prescribed diets for a short time, but then at some point justify excessive eating because of life stresses or the fact they were safely 50 to 150 lb (22.7 to 68.0 kg) below a top weight. They did not, however, return to regular dieting. Weight was regained slowly at first, but later at rates of 20 lb (9.1 kg) per month. When again grossly overweight the subjects had fewer unwanted feelings. They were dismayed with their fatness but felt they could not diet in the face of work or family demands. In their estimation so much concentration on weight control resulted in insufficient energy for other demands.

Comment

These superobese subjects used food uncontrollably. Although food does not produce a state of intoxication it did, as consumed by these people, regularly produce sluggishness and drowsiness. Although sedation was not the professed goal of these subjects when they ate, they were aware of food's effectiveness in modifying their tensions and frustrations. Besides these conscious factors, however, the subjects described eating automatically and without reason, for they were often not even hungry. They ate compulsively despite an understanding of obesity's threat to physical well-being and social functioning. Food intake could be curtailed but only temporarily, except in the hospital. There was a specificity in the use of food, for though some subjects intermittently substituted alcohol for excessive food they consistently preferred the latter.

Another similarity to a habituation pattern is noted when food was severely restricted. While this was not withdrawal in any physical sense, the fantasies of food, diet violations, rationalizations for terminating treatment, tension increase, and developing psychiatric disorder illustrate unwanted feelings associated with food restriction. There is a need to escape such restriction and return to a large food intake.

Observations from other starvation studies, in general, support the findings in this report of increased psychological difficulties when food is restricted; these manifestations are, however, nonspecific in type and severity. For example, Crumpton et al[11] found little evidence that starvation was a threat to psychological health, but they did note increases in irritability, immaturity, tension, and depression. Similarly, Kollar and Atkinson[12] concluded that starvation itself was not psychologically harmful, but they too noted increases in stubbornness, hostility, anxiety, depression (including a suicidal attempt), and covert eating in all of their subjects. This was attributed by the authors to interpersonal problems and not solely to the fasting. Rowland[13] noted more marked evidence of psychological stress. All of his subjects prior to starvation showed marked characterological disorder but no overt neurotic or psychotic patterns. During fasting, resentment, aggressiveness, and depression were noted in all subjects and two of six displayed psychotic features.

Of course, a possible explanation for these symptoms associated with food restriction is that starvation will produce psychological changes in any subject—obese or nonobese. The stress of marked food restriction in persons of normal weight is documented; psychological changes are reported in experimental studies and in accounts of unintended starvation (famine, concentration camp, and geographical isolation).[11-13] In these instances, however, the starved persons had some caloric intake and, thus, an appetite. Such physical sensations of hunger are a stress not present in the total starvation regime used in the current study. Furthermore, in the instance of unintended starvation the victims were facing a life-threatening situation—external threat from a hostile environment and internal threat from a weakened physique with disordered metabolic functions. The obese subjects were starved under supportive conditions and their metabolic functions were sustained by their own enormous caloric reserve and by supplements. They had no physiological need for food but, nevertheless, manifested the behavior of a stressed person.

There are thus several clinical, if not etiological, parallels between superobesity and a habituation-addiction disorder such as alcoholism. A common pattern of social and physical discomfort develops which initially motivates some persons to treatment. Upon admission both types of patients manifest a variety of characterological or underlying psychiatric problems, but these are nonspecific. Motivation for restriction of the food or alcohol is initially good and control of intake is possible, especially in the supportive environment of a hospital. With prolonged restriction, however, a certain number in both groups will evidence an increase in personality or psychiatric problems. In some subjects before discharge, and in the majority afterwards, there is a return to secretive and excessive use of food or alcohol. Despite logic, resolution, and adequate caloric supply, adherence to a diet is exceedingly difficult. The patients are ashamed when they regain weight, minimize their intake, and miss appointments, as does the alcoholic in each instance.

The excessive use of food is a pattern established early in superobese persons; the severest obesity tends to occur in the individual who early uses food to produce pleasure or reduce psychological or physical disequilibrium or both. It remains unclear what causes this early and persistently excessive need for food. The following have been posed: overactive appetite center, impaired satiety center, disordered glucostatic mechanisms, alteration of fat enzymes, conditioned behavior, symbolic satisfaction of unfulfilled wants, anxiety, depression, desire for isolation, and socioeconomic frustration. What-ever the basic cause, it ultimately produces subjective unrest for the obese person, either directly or by conflict with the environment. It appears that the afflicted person may be handling the unrest by using food as a drug. Until an exact etiology is found, the clinician treating severe obesity can profitably regard the condition as a habituation syndrome. This places the difficulty of treatment in perspective and emphasizes the necessity of using the multiple therapeutic approaches now utilized in other addictions.

Summary

Twenty-five superobese subjects were studied before, during, and after prolonged dietary restriction. Clinically they manifested a habituation syndrome. Food was used to such excess that it produced sedation, there was a compulsion to use it to excess, a tendency to continually increase the amount, a psychological dependence, and behavioral changes when the customary intake of food was restricted. Although the etiology of obesity remains unclear, both treatment approaches and prognosis are clarified when the habituation features are recognized.

Dr. Herta Spencer and the staff of the Metabolic Research Ward, Veterans Administration Hospital, Hines, Ill, assisted in this study.

References

1. Gordon, E.S.; Goldberg, M.; and Chosy, G.J.: A New Concept in the Treatment of Obesity, *JAMA* 186:50-60 (Oct 5) 1963.

2. Stunkard, A.J.: "Obesity", in Freedman, A.M., and Kaplan, H.I. (eds.): *Comprehensive Textbook of Psychiatry*, Baltimore: Williams & Wilkins Co., 1967, p 1060.

3. Kaplan, H.I., and Kaplan, H.S.: The Psychosomatic Concept of Obesity, *J Nerv Ment Dis* 125:181-201 (April-June) 1957.

4. Expert Committee on Drugs Liable to Produce Addiction, *WHO Techn Rep Ser No. 59*, p 9.

5. Gregory, I.: *Fundamentals of Psychiatry*, Philadelphia: W.B. Saunders Co., 1968, p 551.

6. Kolb, L.: *Noyes Modern Clinical Psychiatry*, ed 7, Philadelphia: W.B. Saunders Co., 1968, p 516.

7. Stunkard, A.J.: Eating Patterns and Obesity, *Psychiat Quart* 33:284-295 (April) 1959.

8. Spencer, H.; Lewin, I.; and Samachson, J.: Changes in Metabolism in Obese Persons During Starvation, *Amer J Med* 40:27-37 (Jan) 1966.

9. Scheck, J., et al: Mineral and Protein Loss During Starvation, *J Amer Diet Assoc* 49:211-214 (Sept) 1966.

10. Swanson, D.W., and Dinello, F.A.: Follow-up of Patients Starved for Obesity, to be published.

11. Crumpton, E.; Wine, D.B.; and Drenick, E.J.: Starvation: Stress of Satisfaction? *JAMA* 196:394-396 (May 2) 1966.

12. Kollar, E.J., and Atkinson, R.M.: Responses of Extremely Obese Patients to Starvation, *Psychosom Med* 28:227-246 (May-June) 1966.

13. Rowland, C.V.: Psychotherapy of Six Hyperobese Adults During Total Starvation, *Arch Gen Psychiat* 18:541-548 (May) 1968.

14. Keys, A., et al: *The Biology of Human Starvation*, Minneapolis: The University of Minnesota Press, 1950, vol 2.

15. Schiele, B.C., and Brazek, J.: Experimental Neurosis Resulting From Semi-starvation in Man, *Psychosom Med* 10:31-50, 1948.

16. Meerloo, J.A.M., and Klauber, L.D.: Clinical Significance of Starvation and Oral Deprivation, *Psychosom Med* 14:491-497 (Nov-Dec) 1952.

Compulsive eating

Overeating and obesity are often symptoms of emotional and psychological problems. What are the underlying causes and how can the compulsive eater recognize them and stop overeating?

The problem of overweight attracts much attention and concern in modern Western society. In nearly all cases obesity is the result of overeating. Although this is generally recognized, the problem still persists and is quite rightly the cause for some alarm — for obesity, as well as causing distress to the fat person, can lead to diabetes and heart disease.

In spite of this awareness and the concern it has brought, little impact has been made on the proportion of people affected. A study has shown that one person in 10 in Britain is significantly overweight, the majority of these being women. The greatest incidence is in working-class women who are experiencing the menopause — 50 percent of this group were found to be severely overweight.

Biologically, food is essential for survival, providing the body with necessary energy. Yet food has much more significance to people than meeting this need. It has meanings of symbolic kinds for the individual and the significance of these varies from person to person. Apart from this personal relationship between the individual and eating, food has additional meanings in terms of the relationship between individuals and in terms of the structure of culture and society.

In an industrialized society, where food supplies are predictable and well organized, it might be thought that people could afford to relegate their involvement with food to a secondary place in their lives. The fact that this has not come about is a reflection of the complex meanings food has come to have for the individual and society. Eating has social significance. It brings individuals, families, and acquaintances together around the table at mealtime, and provides the occasion for social gatherings. Thus the individual who prefers to eat alone is regarded as anti-social.

Eating together can serve not only to provide mutual enjoyment but also as a means of communication. The tea break and the coffee break are familiar institutions and provide an opportunity for people working together to communicate and interact. Such communication is important not only for the individual but often for the efficiency or work which involves a combined effort of individuals. In the same way, the passing round of food at parties draws people together and provides an opportunity for communica-

tion. People tend to take these social and cultural aspects for granted, for they are almost universal.

For most people, eating has a straightforward function overlaid with meanings of individual and social significance. How then does compulsive eating arise? How does a person's eating become excessive, and so give rise to obesity?

A tendency to obesity can be de mined very early in life, starting eve the womb. If the mother overeats gains excessive weight during pegna she may have a heavy baby, and o weight babies tend to remain overwe

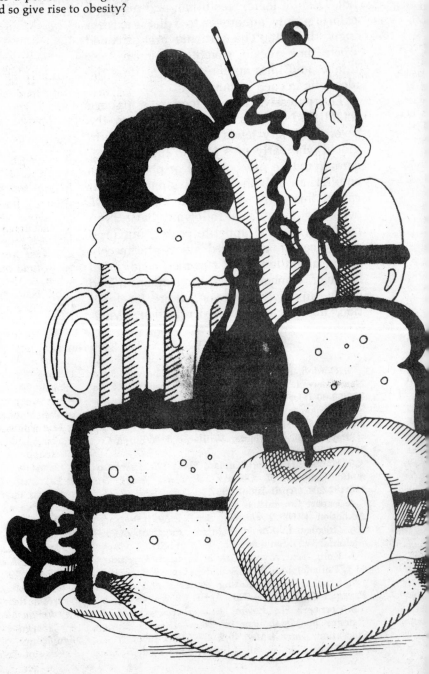

roughout life—conversely thin babies rely become very fat. The number cells in the body which store fat is ed early in life and from then onwards e number does not vary. They may, however, remain full of fat or they may be pty. If these constitutional factors were ore widely recognized, the fattest baby uld not continue to be regarded as the nniest.

During infancy, the most significant ntact between mother and child is ough the breast, or its substitute the ttle, at feeding time. Not only may the int be comforted by feeding when he is ngry but sometimes when he is distressed other ways. Through this sort of contact h the mother, food can come to have portant meanings for the child to do h love, rejection, security, and unity. us the mother and child feeding relanship can set a pattern for later life which eating can allay unpleasant feels quite apart from hunger.

he comforting effect of food may not ays be due to psychological defence chanisms alone but can also be related to effects of food itself. Food is a drug, , like all drugs which promote a sense vell-being, it may be abused. Abusers of d might be regarded as 'food addicts' er than 'compulsive eaters'. Food acts a sedative and may be used by some ple for this purpose. Most people are re of the feeling of sleepiness after eavy meal. Research into the link veen nutrition and sleep suggests that ohydrate is a very effective sleep-ucer—and food addicts primarily select ohydrate for their overeating bouts. also the most fattening type of food weight for weight, it contains more ries than protein and is less filling fat.

ne of the commonest situations that es a tendency to overeat is associated loneliness. The housewife who is at e alone all day may not be able to stop ling and will eat high-carbohydrate ks instead of proper meals, claiming that not worth cooking just for herself.

is situation occurs most often, however with single girls who are alone in the ings and take to eating chocolates, ts, and biscuits after supper. In this tion, the girl often feels hungry in the instance and starts eating. Hunger is allayed but eating continues, and a d or two of chocolates may be umed, before the girl, feeling bloated auseated, finally stops. She then may ercome by feelings of remorse, guilt, shame. Eating in this way helps orarily to relieve feelings of boredom, ation, social isolation, and rejection, ften gives rise to obesity as well as

guilt. Because she becomes fat, the girl will then feel unattractive and will become even more withdrawn.

People who are suffering from depression are inclined to overeat in order to comfort themselves. This leads to weight gain, which is made worse by the inactivity which often accompanies depression. The fatter the person grows, the more inactive he or she becomes and so a vicious circle is set up. A worsening of his or her self-image also develops and the depressed person again turns to food for comfort.

A depressive state is frequently related to disturbance in personal relationships. It is, for example, common among wives who suspect their husbands of infidelity or who just sense a lack of attention from them. In these circumstances the remedy to the problem lies in resolving the underlying interpersonal conflict. If this can be done, the depression, food addiction, and obesity resolve themselves.

A person involved in a relationship with a partner who has started overeating should attempt some soul-searching and the partners should examine the relationship together to determine whether there are any stress factors which might contribute to the overeating. The partner of the food addict should try to react with understanding, reassurance, and encouragement and not with threats, insults, and rejection.

When, as is common, a wife overeats, a positive and supportive attitude on the part of the husband is most helpful, although this can be combined with a degree of firmness. The husband can help by encouraging his wife to eat the right foods and by not asking her to provide such things as cakes, biscuits, and crisps for him. It will be easier for her if such tempting, carbohydrate foods are not kept in the house. Instead of giving her boxes of chocolates, he should offer her flowers.

Because compulsive eating is often a secret and solitary activity, the wife should avoid pastimes such as watching late-night television alone. The husband should encourage his wife to go to bed when he does. In such circumstances, where both the woman and her partner react together positively to resolve the problem, the chances of success are good. The overeating itself, and not the resultant obesity, is the defence against emotional distress.

In other instances the obesity itself can come to serve as a defence for the individual. Overeating in adolescent girls, for example, is fairly common. The teen-age girl who is shy and sensitive may have profound conflicts over her emerging sexuality, which she perceives as tempting yet threatening. She may be fearful of contact with boys and, as a result of her loneliness, she may overeat. She may then

welcome her obesity because it helps to protect her from close contact with boys. Furthermore, her own sexual feelings may actually diminish. Because excess carbohydrate acts as a sedative this can, in some people, reduce sexual activity.

In such a case, food addiction and obesity are a way of dealing with severe emotional insecurity. The girl will cling strongly to her defence and give it up only when the underlying conflicts have been resolved. In many cases, as the teenage girl gradually matures and gains in self-confidence, she sheds her defence.

This kind of overeating can occur within a marital relationship as a means of avoiding sexual contact. A woman who feels that her husband makes excessive sexual demands may overeat so that she will become fat and therefore undesirable. Another woman who is tempted to have extra-marital affairs may overeat so that her obesity will deter any would-be seducer and remove the temptation. In some cases the husband even encourages his wife's over-indulgence in food.

Margaret, a middle-aged woman who had been married for many years, was concerned about her own sexual feelings and promiscuous behaviour. Her husband, Jim, was aware that he himself had a low sex drive, and consequently he felt threatened by his wife's behaviour. When Margaret started to indulge in bouts of overeating, Jim actively encouraged her. He plied her with chocolates and special treats such as cream cakes. Her obesity and resultant lethargy led to a lessening of interest in sex.

When she sought medical advice for her obesity her doctor found that she was also suffering from depression. She was referred to a psychiatrist and taken into hospital. During this time Jim refused to co-operate in her treatment.

The treatment was successful and Margaret was released from hospital—slimmer, and with her former libido. After her return home and renewed contact with Jim, however, she began to overeat and put on weight again.

In such a case, medical treatment can achieve permanent success only if the partner and family co-operate. There can be tremendous pressure from the family for the individual to retain her state of overeating and obesity, and any attempts she makes to change are strongly resisted.

Joan, who was 26 years old, lived with her parents and two younger brothers. Harry, her father, worked for a biscuit company and frequently brought home packets of biscuits from work, which he offered to the family. Both Joan and her mother enjoyed eating and had always been plump. On the death of the grandmother, to whom Joan had been close, she did not mourn but comforted herself with food. Her weight gradually increased over the next five years and she was eventually admitted to hospital weighing 336 pounds. Joan stayed in hospital for some months, during which time she lost 112 pounds in weight. When her parents visited her, they frequently brought chocolates which they gave to the patient in the next bed. They often tried to get Joan to discharge herself and finally Harry threatened to deprive her of her room at home.

When Joan did leave hospital she went to live in a hostel and her father became depressed. During her time in hospital, other members of her family, and her mother in particular, had put on weight themselves. In this case, food and obesity had complex symbolic meanings within the family which were threatened by Joan's desire for treatment. When there is such massive resistance to change among those closest to the patient, the outlook must be bleak for the individual.

Most obesity is the result of overeating and only rarely is it a symptom of an underlying glandular disorder. It may sometimes, however, be a symptom of mental illness such as depression. More often depression is associated with weight loss and insomnia but in some cases over-eating and excessive sleeping may occur. The condition may involve profound sadness, loss of energy and interest, and sometimes feelings of worthlessness and hopelessness. When the depression is treated, the sufferer's weight returns to normal.

Overeating can also occur in *anorexia nervosa*, a rare, potentially serious adolescent weight disorder, usually affecting girls. The condition begins with dieting which then becomes excessive and results in profound loss of weight. The girl becomes increasingly terrified of returning to her normal weight. In this state, as she loses further weight, the girl often becomes increasingly ravenous. She may give in to this impulse in episodes of overeating that involve the consumption of loaves of bread and pounds of cakes. In common with the obese nibbler, the girl is likely to feel ashamed, guilty, and disgusted by her behaviour. Medical treatment should be sought for this condition.

The majority of instances of overeating are not associated with serious illness and the individual can take several simple measures to combat obesity. If there is an underlying conflict in a relationship, it may be possible for the partners to discuss their feelings and come to a better understanding. Where the conflict is severe and deep-seated, they may need to seek professional help.

If overeating takes the form of bouts of massive food consumption in secret, associated with guilt and shame, relief can come if the sufferer is able to overcome her secrecy and remorse and to discuss her feelings with her partner. In the case of a single girl living at home, she should confide in her mother and enlist her support. The mother can help considerably by preparing nutritious, low-carbohydrate meals and by making sure that sweets and biscuits are not left around. Encouragement and support in dieting is always helpful. Group pressures can be even more effective than individual support and slimming groups work on this principle.

The compulsive eater should avoid drastic diets because they create a ravenous appetite. The most popular diets are those containing reduced quantities of carbohydrates. The dieter should select a diet which it is easy to adhere to—the goals should be realistic. More weight can be lost by eating smaller meals at more frequent intervals than by eating the same quantity of food taken in one or two meals a day.

Foods forbidden by the diet should not be kept in the house. When the person does have an uncontrollable urge to nibble, she should eat a carrot or celery rather than biscuits, nuts, or cakes. She should try to think in terms of 'What can I do?' rather than 'What can I eat?' Boredom and inactivity are the worst enemies of the compulsive eater, so it is important to keep the mind occupied, to allow no opportunity to think about food. She should also try to do something which needs both hands—such as knitting or sewing—so that she cannot almost unconsciously pick up something to eat. She should also undertake some form of regular exercise. If this can be done with a group, such as a tennis club or health club, there will be greater incentive. Not only will the exercise help the person to slim, it will also improve the general health and hence the morale.

If the compulsive eater can find other activities and interests, food becomes less significant and eventually is relegated to its proper place. Eating becomes once again a social and individual pleasure—not a compulsion.   EDWARD HAREVEN

CASEBOOK
can't stop eating

...ase can you help me,' Maureen had ...ten in her letter. 'I am desperate. I ...very fat and I look awful. Sometimes ...te my looks so much that I don't want ...o on living. I am 21. I've tried slimming ...years but nothing seems to work. I just ...'t stop eating. Please could you see me ...n?'

...offered Maureen an early appointment ...she arrived well on time. She was ...ed very fat, although I did not think ...t she 'looked awful'. She had long, ...k hair and she was quite pretty. There ...something babyish about her face ...ch made one want to relate to her as if ...were a child rather than a young woman. ...was wearing a short, tight dress ...ch accentuated her size. She sat down, ...ng to pull her dress over her knees.

...thought I was going to be late,' she ...'. 'I had an awful job trying to decide ...t I should wear. I wanted to look as ...e as possible. But whatever I put on ...de me look terrible.' Maureen's eyes ...d with tears. She searched in her hand-... 'Do you have a handkerchief?' she ...ed, her voice trembling.

...offered her a box of paper handker-...efs.

...I was cross with myself for getting into ...h a state before I came here.' She ...bed at her eyes. 'But perhaps it's just ...well. You can see how desperate I feel ...ut everything.'

...Tell me about it.'

...Well, this morning was typical. As soon ...I woke up I felt terribly depressed. ...anted to close my eyes and go back to ...ep. I often get to the office late—I'm a ...ist—because I can't bear getting up. ...always in trouble for it. And then ...at also makes me late is never being ...e to decide what to wear. This morning ...s worse than usual.'

...Why?'

...I don't know. It was almost as bad as ...ting ready for a party. The office is ...ryday life, although even on an ordinary ...rning I hate facing the mirror. But ...ng to a party, or coming to you, is a ...t of challenge.'

'What is the challenge about?'

'Well, at a party one wants to be popular.' Maureen paused. 'Of course, what one really wants is to find a boy friend.'

'I notice that you said, "what one wants", not "what I want".'

'I suppose it's because I'm scared. I do want a boy friend, but I'm frightened that no boy will want me.'

'Have no boys ever wanted you?'

'There have been some. But they've never gone on wanting me.'

'Why was that?'

'It was my fault, I think. I'm so awkward. I can never forget how fat I am. I know that boys notice and it puts them off. It frightens them away.'

'But you say there were some boys who were interested in you.'

'Yes, but there have been so many false starts. I remember one boy I met at a party who really liked me. He was so nice to me that I felt wonderful. For a whole evening I forgot about my size.'

'So when life is good you do forget about your weight.'

'Yes. But then it caught up with me again. We made a date for the following Saturday and I kept imagining how marvellous it would be and what a good-looking fellow he was. I knew I had to make a success of it.

'And then I began to doubt whether I could. I got myself into such a state by the Saturday that I could hardly say anything. I think he was very disappointed with me. At the party I'd sparkled—as much as I can, anyway. I'd been witty and made him laugh. But on the Saturday I was tense and tongue-tied. I knew he'd never ask me out again—and he didn't. I was miserable for weeks afterwards. I didn't feel like going anywhere or doing anything and I ate and ate.'

'So you overeat when you are desperate, when you feel hopeless. But tell me more about your boy friends. Has there been anyone else?'

'Well, there was Terry. We went out together for about six months. I found it easier to be with him. We could really talk to each other. I could tell him how ghastly it was to be fat. He told me about his problems, too. He was brought up in an orphanage. He has had a rather sad life. He always thought too little of himself and somehow we seemed to understand each other.

'But even then I was anxious. I never believed that he could really care for me. However much we saw each other was never enough for me. I kept thinking he was looking at other girls, and on the evenings I didn't see him I wondered whether he was with someone else. I wanted to see him all the time.'

Maureen, at 21, had already spent many years trying to lose weight. It was not until she had lost her boy friend and almost all hope of ever being slim that she began to understand the connection between food, greed—and love.

'It sounds as if you were as greedy for his company as you are greedy for food. You can't get enough of it and it doesn't satisfy you.'

'Yes, that's just what he said: "You're never satisfied." It upset him. He said it made him feel as if he were nothing—as if he had nothing of any use to give me—because he couldn't make me happy for any length of time. Gradually he started to make excuses for not seeing me and I heard from a friend of mine that he had found another girl friend. They didn't stay together long. And then he moved up to the Midlands. I've had several letters from him. In the last one he said he might come down and see me soon.'

'How do you feel about that?'

'I'm afraid to start hoping. If we did start going out again it might end in the same painful and confusing way, like it did before.'

'You mean your greed might destroy it again?'

'Yes. I always start with good intentions but then they come to nothing.'

'Like your attempts at losing weight?'

'Yes.'

'Can you tell me about them?'

'I've started slimming countless times. Once I went to my doctor and he put me on a diet. Another time I joined a club for girls who wanted to lose weight. Often I see a diet in a magazine which seems just right for me. I dash out and buy all the right

Compulsive eating is neither enjoyable nor satisfying. But it can become a habit which is hard to break and harder to understand.

food and for a few days I really stick to it. I get a great kick out of eating properly. I look at myself in the mirror and suddenly I feel hopeful. I even start doing exercises every morning.

'But then something happens. Sometimes I feel like the alcoholic behind a bar. I'm surrounded by food—in the fridge at home, on the breakfast table, in the bakery shop I pass on the way to work—and it's all too tempting. I always expect I'm going to lose masses of weight very quickly, and when I don't I'm very disappointed. Or I catch sight of my reflection in a shop-window and it disgusts me. Or I go to a party and nobody takes any notice of me. Or someone at the office teases me, and I suddenly feel desperate. And before I know what I'm doing I'm out buying chips or currant buns or a box of chocolates which I take up to my room at home and eat in secret. And then I'm even more disgusted with myself.

'The crazy thing is that I've never quite given up hope. I wouldn't torture myself so much over my clothes if I had. I do still care how I look. I care desperately.' Maureen had begun to cry again. 'You can't imagine what I feel when I go shopping. I'm sure that everyone stares at me and sniggers about my size. I feel like an elephant.' She blew her nose. 'Now I

sound like one, too, don't I?' She laughed and dried her eyes.

'I'm sorry I keep on crying. But it's such a relief. In the stores I'm always so embarrassed about asking for the largest size. Some of the shop assistants feel sorry for me. Others are snooty and tell me it's very difficult to suit someone with a figure like mine. And I never know whether to dress like other girls of my age or like an older woman. All the outsize shops are so conservative. Anyway, eventually I go and have tea and a bun and I am angry and disgusted with myself. And I buy some material and a pattern and make the dress or the skirt myself. But it always looks a bit amateur. I don't know why I bother.'

'But you do bother—which is a good thing.'

'Yes, I suppose so. I did so want to wear the right thing to see you.'

'What would have been the right thing?'

'I didn't know. That was the problem. I had no idea what you would expect.'

'And you felt you had to fit in with my expectations?'

'Yes.'

'Why, I wonder?'

'I suppose I wanted to please you so that you would be nice to me and not just send me away saying you couldn't help.'

'As if you were a hopeless case?'

'Yes.'

'I have an idea that being "hopeless" means more to you than just being too fat. It goes further than that, doesn't it?'

'Yes, although it's so closely tied up with my being fat that I don't know what comes first.' Maureen searched for words. 'I often feel hopeless, a dead loss, impossible. I hate myself for being the way I am. I'm always in the way.'

'How do you mean?'

'Well, as long as I can remember, I always felt I was one too many at home. I've got two sisters and a brother, all older than me. I was always pushed around.'

'In what way?'

'I was the youngest and I was always the slowest and clumsiest. The others teased me. I didn't like it very much, even though I knew it was all in fun. My sister, who is only 18 months older than I, always made trouble for me. She'd put the blame

on me when toys were broken or the [c] was let out. But whenever I started to c[ry] and I went to my mother she'd say, "N[ot] again, I'm sick of tears and running noses[.]" And she'd send me out of the room.'

'But I did not do that to you when y[ou] burst into tears.'

'No. That's why it was such a reli[ef.] I felt you were accepting me. Of cour[se] there is a difference. Mother was oft[en] tired and overworked. We have a ve[ry] old-fashioned house and there was nev[er] much money. Things are a bit easier n[ow] because my eldest brother and sister ha[ve] left home, and both my other sister an[d I] contribute towards our keep.

'But four children are a lot for [one] family.' Maureen stared down at her han[ds] looking young and vulnerable. 'I do[n't] know whether I'm imagining things, [but] I'm almost sure my parents hadn't plan[ned] to have me. I was one too many. Th[ree] children would have been quite enou[gh] for them.'

There was a silence. Then Maure[en] went on, almost if she were talking to h[er]self, 'Last week, I suddenly remember[ed] that feeling of not being wanted. My b[est] school friend got married last year. She [has] just had a baby girl. I went over to g[ive] Sheila a gift and see the baby. As I ra[ng] the doorbell I could hear the baby cryi[ng.] It sounded terrible. I couldn't stand it[, it] went right through me.'

'Perhaps it affected you so much beca[use] you know from your early experie[nce] what it feels like to be a hungry ba[by.] These things remain in feeling, if no[t in] memory.'

'Yes. Mother says I used to cry a [lot] when I was a baby—much more than [the] others ever did. I don't remember hea[ring] the sound for years. But there was She[ila] offering this tiny creature a bottle and [the] baby was crying and crying. It wa[s an] exasperating sound, full of anger [and] helplessness and despair. Sheila see[med] nervous and tense, as if she wanted to pl[ease] the child, but didn't know how. And [the] baby—well, even when she took the bo[ttle] she seemed too angry and greedy for [the] food to enjoy it.'

It was the concept of enjoyment [with] which Maureen and I began our dis[cus]sion the following week. I suggested

hough Maureen was desperately greedy
 the food she ate, she gulped it down
thout getting much pleasure from it. The
re depressed she was the less she ened it, and the more guilty and empty
 felt afterwards.

 asked her to give me details of her
ly diet. A heavy breakfast and evening
al were both cooked by Maureen's
ther.

'Mother still thinks I'm a "growing
l",' Maureen told me ruefully. 'It's ab-
d, isn't it? She's so used to my size
t it's almost as if she doesn't want me
be any thinner.' Maureen paused. 'But,
course, it's unfair to put the blame on
. I don't help myself—that is what's
portant. I nibble in the office, I eat
eets at my desk, I don't bother to walk
 swim or do exercises. Feeling angry
h my mother doesn't really get me
ywhere, does it?'

'That depends on whether you have fully
derstood why you are angry. The anger
u felt towards your mother when you
re a baby was because she did not pro-
le food as soon as you wanted it. She had
 power to give and to withhold food—
d love. Then you are angry with your-
f for being so greedy and ravenous.

'Somehow, you think, it must be all your
lt. You were angry with your mother,
you must be bad and not worthy of love.
od, as you know, stands for love and
ving. It is not just a simple problem to
 with a more sensible diet or running
und the park every morning.'

'Yes, I see what you mean. I have often
ought about the ways in which I'm still
ry tied to Mother. My feelings towards
r are so mixed, so intense. I imagine
at most other people of my age, even if
 times they feel warm or angry towards
eir mothers, don't get swept away
 their feelings quite as much.

'And I do see the connection between
od and love. When I feel good, when I
ink that people like me, I don't eat
arly as much as when I'm depressed. It's
lled comfort-eating, isn't it? I've read
ts of books about why people overeat.

Only the trouble is that eating like that is
no comfort at all.'

'It sounds more like hunger that wants
to destroy and devour. It makes me think
of violent anger which leaves a desert of
emptiness in its wake.'

'Yes, that's really right. Afterwards I
feel heavy and horribly full, but with an
overpowering feeling of emptiness.

'I grew up with the feeling of being an
unwanted child and that Mother wasn't
ever particularly fond of me. But when you
were talking about love, I remembered
that she was sometimes very nice to me.
She'd take me on her lap and cuddle me
and tell me stories. But it was never for
long. I never had enough of her. And I always suspected that she was cuddling me
from a sense of duty. Then, as I got fatter
and the children at school started to tease
me, I was sure that I was so ugly that nobody would ever want me on their lap.'

'That links up with your fear that boys
won't want you and the way you are afraid
to get involved with Terry again. Although you had several happy months with
him, you couldn't believe that he wanted
you. You gulped down his affection for you
and eliminated it again, just as you do with
food, so that it left you empty.'

I saw Maureen every week for six
months. Gradually she started to lose
weight. There was no startling change, but
by the end of that time she looked altogether more confident. She had bought a
long dress which suited her colouring and
successfully hid her curves, and she had
begun to wear accessories which drew
the eye to her face and accentuated her
prettiness.

More important, she had moved away
from home to share a flat with some friends.

'It means I'm more in control of the food I
eat,' Maureen explained. 'I don't bother
to cook potatoes so they are never on the
table. My flatmates are very strict with me,
which helps. I go to see my family once a
week. I try to avoid having a meal with
them. But Mother still tries to ply me
with food! It's easier to refuse, now. I feel
so much more grown up.

'And I get several letters a week from
Terry. He's coming down to work in
London again. So I'm really trying to look
nice for him when he arrives.'

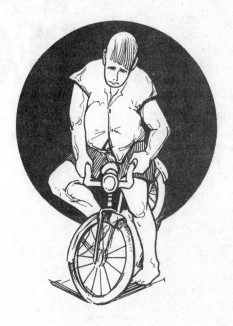

Saul Bellow's brief sketch of Angela, Mr. Sammler's niece, (*Mr. Sammler's Planet*) could easily be applied to countless American women. Her appearance and behavior sound familiar to us, though it impressed her uncle as strange.

"Angela was in her thirties now, independently wealthy, with ruddy skin, gold-whitish hair, big lips. She was afraid of obesity. She either fasted or ate like a stevedore. She trained in a fashionable gym. She wore the odd stylish things which Sammler noted with detached and purified dryness, as if from a different part of the universe. What were those, white-kid buskins? What were those tights—sheer, opaque? Where did they lead? That effect of the hair called frosting, that color under the lioness's muzzle, that swagger to enhance the natural power of the bust! Her plastic coat inspired by cubists or Mondrians, geometrical black and white forms; her trousers by Courrèges and Pucci."

In spite of her up-to-date, mod appearance and well-controlled figure, Angela was not happy. She was always getting involved in wild schemes to improve herself and the world, and she found solace in going to a psychiatrist. This, too, has a familiar ring. My own knowledge about the seemingly successful but desperate fight against obesity comes from many patients who came for psychiatric treatment for a variety of reasons, and who on first contact did not seem concerned with their weight at all.

Fat people are apt to blame all their difficulties on being fat and they hope for a new lease on life after they get thin. Many begin reducing confident of finding the pot of gold at the end of the rainbow. Few reach the goal; otherwise we would not be so concerned about fat people's inability to stick to a diet. But there are some who follow through, who can deny their desire for food and achieve the beautiful slim figure that is supposed to be the magic key to the doorway to success and happiness. And it may be that there are many for whom things work out this way; it so happens that I am not familiar with this course of events. People who are successful and stay reduced and are relaxed about it do not go to physicians with their weight problems; they certainly will not come to a psychiatrist.

From my observations there are three outcomes for people who reduce with the unrealistic goal of expecting a changed life before they have experienced the inner emotional changes which make these new adjustments possible. The majority will try and try, will lose some weight and then, suddenly they will give up and regain and often overshoot their former weight. For others the stress of starving themselves, the loss of their size, the new real or imagined expectations may prove too much, and serious emotional disturbances, even frank psychotic behavior, may break through.

There is a third group of people who succeed in becoming and staying thin, but whose conflicts are far from solved by having lost weight. On the contrary their difficulties now have a chance to flourish, since the ugliness of being fat no longer pre-

Extensive weight loss won't always cure obesity. Achieving thinness can complicate emotional problems.

HILDE BRUCH, M.D.

THIN FAT PEOPLE

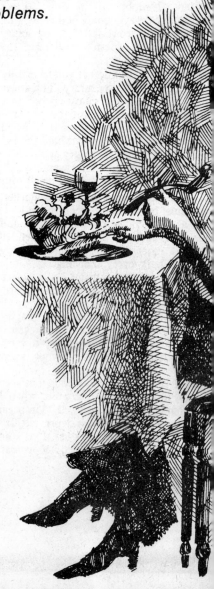

ts them from putting their un-istic dreams to the test. Such ple, though they no longer look se, are far from cured; they still mble fat people with all their un-ed problems, conflicts, and exag-ated expectations. Only they no ger *show* their fat. It is to this up that I wish to apply the term *n Fat People*, an expression I rowed from F. Heckel, who stated 911 in *Les grandes et petites obé-s* that we cannot consider a fat son cured, even though he has his weight, unless all the other ctional symptoms have also dis-eared. Loss of weight alone rep-

resents a pseudo-cure. The patient becomes "un obèse amaigri; mais il est toujours un obèse." The charac-teristics of a good cure, Heckel says, are that it should be lasting and that it should not make unreasonable de-mands on the patient.

Problems become more severe for those who have a tendency to be obese, or who use overeating to amel-iorate serious emotional tension. I am most familiar with this pseudo-thinness from my contact with the relatives of fat young people. When-ever one hears a thin, even scrawny-looking mother speak with particular vehemence and disgust about the fat-

ness of her child it is not a far-fetched guess (and one easily confirmed) that this mother owes her fashionable figure to eternal vigilance and con-scientious, semistarvation dieting. Fathers are not exempt from this rule. It seems to me that the hostile emo-tional overcharge is related to envy in the parent about the child's dar-ing to satisfy his appetite and im-pulses. The parent's rage reveals their shame that the child's fatness exposes the despised family endowment. It is in families with this intense hostil-ity that I have most often seen a ma-lignant development of childhood obesity, with schizophrenic or *anor-exia nervosa* as the outcome.

Many women make a fetish of be-ing thin and follow reducing diets without awareness of or regard for the fact that they can do so only at the price of continuous strain and tension and some degree of ill health. There are millions of young girls and women who starve themselves in order to look like these envied models for whom slimness is a well-paid pro-fessional pose. Ordinary young wom-en do not get paid for being slim. When they become young mothers they will complain continuously about fatigue, about their children's problems, and about their own irri-tability. Little attention has been paid to the fact that their attempt to ful-fill fashion's demands to be skinny is directly related to these problems. Having grown up with the concept that thinness is identical with beauty and attractiveness and is desirable for its own sake, they have become used to living on a semistarvation diet, never eating more than their bony figures show. Never having permit-ted themselves to eat adequately, they are unaware of how much of their tension, bad disposition, irritability, and inability to pursue an educational or professional goal is the direct re-

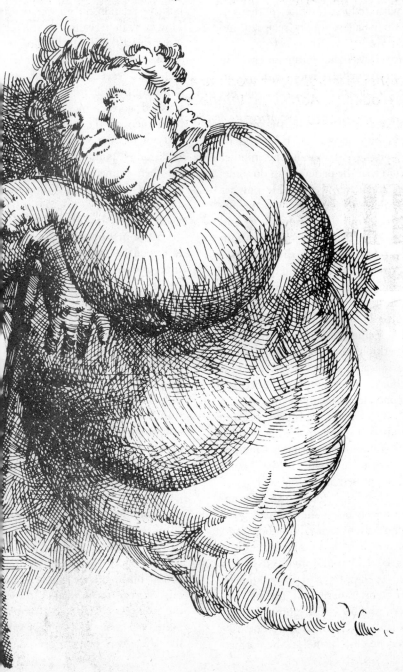

From Eating Disorders *by Hilde Bruch, M.D.,* ©*Basic Books, Inc., Publishers, New York,* 1973.

Reprinted from *Medical Opinion,* vol. 2, No. 10, October, 1973, pp. 50-56.

sult of chronic undernutrition.

It is impossible to assess the cost in serenity, relaxation, and efficiency of this abnormal, overslim, fashionable appearance. It produces serious psychological tensions to feel compelled to be thinner than one's natural make-up and style of living demand. There is a great deal of talk about the weakness and self-indulgence of overweight people who eat "too much." Very little is said about the selfishness and self-indulgence involved in a life which makes one's appearance the center of all values, and subordinates all other considerations to it. I do not know how often people are aware of the emotional sacrifice of staying slim. An English writer, Clemence Dane, expressed it succinctly: "Staying slim is like being witty—it is beastly hard work."

Chronic malnutrition based on abnormal preoccupation with weight is common, but not readily recognized as abnormal because it appears under the guise of desirable slimness. These chronic reducers, the "thin fat people," are likely to escape correct diagnosis because our slimness-conscious culture will admire their starved appearance instead of offering them needed help. They come to medical attention only when the weight preoccupation interferes with their living, or when malnutrition gives rise to complaints of fatigue, listlessness, irritability, difficulties in concentration, or chronic depression. It has become customary to prescribe tranquilizers for them; three square meals a day would be a more logical treatment, but one that is equally unacceptable to physicians and patients who share the conviction that being slim is good and healthy in itself.

Frequently these people come to the attention of psychiatrists. Though successful in controlling their weight, they have remained unhappy and dissatisfied, and this theme, with endless variations, runs through their many complaints. Just as food never satisfied them, never gave them what they

really wanted, so they are now dissatisfied with their new slim figure and disappointed in what it has achieved for them.

Not infrequently parents, and also physicians and psychiatrists, reinforce a fat person's unrealistic expectation about what he should weigh. Ingrid, aged 20 years, was referred for consultation by her psychiatrist, who mentioned in the referring letter how "stunning" she had looked when she had brought her weight down to a very low level. She had been successful with reducing while in therapy, but then had suddenly relapsed and was now heavier than before.

Ingrid was the youngest child in a wealthy, achievement- and appearance-conscious family; her mother and older sister were small-boned, slim, and well-dressed. In contrast, Ingrid had been a fat baby and by the time she was a toddler her mother insisted that the pediatrician do something about her weight. He put her on a diet and gave her appetite depressants. Ingrid remained large and heavy as a child, but was continuously pressured to be slimmer; several times she was hospitalized to force her weight down. Like her older siblings she did well in school, but at 10 or 11 she had refused to work at all, feeling unable to endure the competition. From then on there were repeated efforts to get her into psychiatric treatment, but she refused to cooperate with any plan.

With adolescence Ingrid became severely preoccupied with her weight. She began to demand that her mother keep no extra food in the house. Gorging herself alternated with bouts of faddish and unrealistic dieting, all to no purpose. She retained good social relations with both boys and girls, but there was no dating. When 16 or 17 she became involved with a group of hippies and drug addicts. After a brief period of feeling "accepted" she became frightened about their activities. At this point she asked for psychiatric help. She formed

a good relationship with her therap and quite early in therapy said th she had put herself on a diet, th she had heard people ate as a su stitute for love; she felt she was lov and therefore did not need to stu herself. Whatever the dynamics, the end of about the first year of trea ment she had lost 90 pounds, dow from nearly 225 to 135 pounds, an she was beautifully slim. This fi weight loss was a relatively slow a complishment and it was felt at t time to be related to her firm an positive relationship to her therapi However, in reevaluating this perio it appeared that even this first redu ing was associated with rather faddi diets and excessive use of amph tamine pills. But Ingrid was still n satisfied at reaching this weight an from then on there were many u and downs. She would gain as muc as 30 or 40 pounds in a few week but then immediately reduce agai The last impetus for losing was stay at a famous seaside resort by th whole family. Ingrid wanted to loo attractive in a bikini bathing suit an lost about 30 pounds in a very sho time, and lost some more while at t resort. When she returned home sh was at her lowest weight, nearly 1 pounds. She looked strikingly beau ful and people stared at her on t street. She also received boundle praise from her parents and fro her therapist who noted, howeve that during this period of force thinness she was tense and anxiou almost manic. During her hipp period, she had dropped out of schoo now she decided to take courses f a high school diploma, and also b gan ballet dancing and yoga exe cises. Suddenly she had many dat

Ingrid maintained her low weig for a few months, but then launche herself upon the most compulsi eating binge of her whole life. Jea ousy seemed to be related to the ea ing problem. Her older sister e pected her first child and even befo the baby was born Ingrid resente that it might receive more attention than she. She would eat constantly, day and night, and during frequent nocturnal icebox raids would eat absolutely everything edible in the house.

Ingrid continued in therapy but now was angry at her therapist for not having cured her. She appeared frightened and severely depressed by the sudden awareness that she did not want to be thin, though consciously she insisted that she wanted to lose weight. There was rapid increase in weight and by the time she came for consultation she looked as though she weighed more than 200 pounds; she absolutely refused to go near a scale. However, she did not look as monstrous and grotesque as her parents' and therapist's description had suggested. Ingrid was tall and broadly built; she looked massive and too heavy for her frame, but her high weight was not as abnormal as the weight she demanded. She had said that she could not possibly be happy unless she weighed 115 pounds and kept it at that figure.

In reviewing her life story and her previous treatment experiences, Ingrid felt she had always been under mother's domination, overcontrolled and forced to do things; her only way of asserting herself was saying No. During the consultation she was quite responsive and we focused on the deficits in her concepts of control, psychologically and biologically, and

on the futility of trying to achieve a better self-concept through the manipulation of her weight. She had proven to herself repeatedly that she could reduce but the effort and tension made it impossible to maintain the weight loss. The same applied to her other efforts to achieve something worthwhile.

Progress in long-standing, fluctuating adolescent obesity cannot be measured in terms of weight, but only in terms of overall competence. Better weight regulation becomes possible as a result of better adjustment; it is not a precondition for it. Ingrid absolutely rejected a treatment approach in which weight was not the first consideration. But with such a phobic compulsive preoccupation with weight, the first treatment goal must be correction of the unrealistic expectation. Weight regulation must be seen as a positive achievement after other aspects of coping have been mastered.

The observations reported here run counter to the whole campaign against overweight which, in fact, says exactly the opposite: That reducing is necessary to improve one's physical health, social position, and emotional outlook. These arguments are used daily to convince fat people that they should reduce. It seems to me necessary to point out that a mechanical approach to overweight carries grave mental health hazards. The road of propagating scientific standards of nutrition is littered with landmarks of overly zealous errors and failures. It is my impression that the overeager propaganda about reducing diets, even though obesity is an abnormal state of nutrition, overlooks a basic human problem, the need for satisfaction of vital needs. "The best women are rich and thin" may be a good slogan for the jet set; it is potentially dangerous for the ordinary overweight person.   END

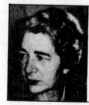

Hilde Bruch, M.D. (*University of Freiburg, 1929), is Professor of Psychiatry at Baylor College of Medicine, and has written over 150 articles and four books on the subject of eating disorders, including* The Importance of Overweight. *She is also a Diplomat of the Board of Child Psychiatry.*

The Social Psychology of Dieting

JOHANNA T. DWYER   JACOB J. FELDMAN   JEAN MAYER

Harvard School of Public Health

This article reviews relevant epidemiological data on the prevalence of medically defined weight problems and of weight control efforts in the United States. It explores factors that may influence people to engage in weight control behavior in the first place and to choose dieting over other methods of reducing. It advances explanations to account for differences in the prevalence of dieting phenomena among various age and sex groups. Finally, it suggests several ways of improving the effectiveness and coverage of weight control programs.

INTRODUCTION

THE prevalence of excess weight in the American population as a whole is high—so high, in fact, that in some segments of the population it has reached epidemic proportions. Excess weight is a serious health problem because it is associated with respiratory, arthritic, gall bladder, and cardiovascular diseases (U.S. Public Service, 1966). Certain types of coronary heart disease, namely angina pectoris and myocardial infarctions, are more common in obese persons and frequently lead to sudden death (Seltzer, 1969). The significance of excess weight on the public's health may therefore be considerable.

Dieting is a popular American avocation. Because the reduction to or maintenance of weight at normal levels can result in decreased risk and severity of certain chronic diseases, successful weight control has great medical significance, and health reasons cause many persons to diet. However, since social factors are equally, if not more, important in motivating weight control behavior, one must understand the social psychology of dieting.

DEFINITIONS

Overweight. It is important at the outset to define what health professionals mean when they speak of overweight and obesity. Overweight is defined as body

weight in excess of an ideal weight, based on height- and sex-specific standards. Overweight can result from excesses of bone, muscle, fat, or, more rarely, fluid. Almost everyone who is more than 20 per cent overweight is also overfat, or obese. However, not all people who are heavy are excessively fat. The relative contributions to overweight of bone, muscle, and fat vary from person to person, and it is often hard to recognize these differences. The component that actually causes weight in excess of normal is less than clear when overweight is in the more moderate range, (i.e., less than 20 per cent over ideal weight), and this brings diagnostic difficulties if weight alone serves as the criteria for overfatness. This brings us to the definition of a second term: obesity.

Obesity. Obesity is defined as body fatness in excess of an age and sex specific standard. Body weights grossly in excess of standards are indicative of obesity. Moderate overweight sometimes, but not always, is due to obesity. Some people whose weights are normal are also obese. Thus, overweight (heaviness) and obesity (excessive fatness) are not necessarily synonymous, and weight deviations give only imprecise estimates of obesity. Football players, for example, may be overweight because of their massive bone and muscle structure, yet not be overfat at all.

Body type. Body types, or somatotypes, which describe differences in physical conformation and structure between persons, are important in the study of weight deviations. These variations in outward appearance are due, at least in part, to

* The studies from our laboratories reported in this review were supported in part by a grant-in-aid from the National Institute of Arthritis and Metabolic Diseases (AM 02839), National Institutes of Health, Public Health Service, Bethesda, Maryland.

underlying anatomical differences in the amount, distribution, or conformation of fat, muscle, and bony tissue, which are reflected in body form. These variations have been precisely defined and described systematically by Sheldon et al. (1963); his system contains three major components: (1) endomorphy, which is characterized by softness and roundness of appearance; (2) mesomorphy, characterized by a combination of bone and muscle development; and (3) ectomorphy, characterized by linearity, fragility, and attenuation of body build. The most common somatotypes in the population combine all three of these components to varying degrees.

Most obese persons are not simply thin persons with an excessive body burden of fat; their body types have been found to differ in other aspects as well. The majority of the obese tend to be somewhat larger in their bone and muscle components as well as fatter than their nonobese counterparts (Seltzer and Mayer, 1964; 1969). Different weight goals are thus necessary for persons of different body types to allow for the fact that they vary in relative contribution of the nonfat components to their weights.

Dieting. The world "dieting" covers a multitude of different types of eating behavior. Some persons believe that they are dieting when they substitute noncaloric sweeteners for sugar, while others consider they are doing so only when they are subjecting themselves to a total fast. In most of the studies reviewed in this article, few attempts were made to identify the types of changes in eating habits that were categorized as dieting. Thus, all that can be inferred from statements that respondents were "on diets" is that these persons reported changing their usual food intake in some way in order to lose weight, however effective or ineffective, extensive or limited, their efforts may have been.

PREVALENCE OF OBESITY

Obesity is the major health factor that motivates people to diet; therefore, the epidemiology of obesity in this country needs scrutiny. The prevalence of obesity varies with age, sex, probably socioeconomic class, and perhaps ethnic variables such as race. The percentage of persons who are obese (that is, 20 per cent or more above ideal weight) generally rises with age from early childhood until late in life, so that far more adults than children or adolescents are obese (see National Center for Health Statistics, 1966). Sex differences in the prevalence of obesity do not appear until adulthood. Men gain more weight with age during their early 20's than do women, and by the end of their 20's and 30's more men are obese or overweight than women (see U.S. Public Health Service, 1966; Hathaway and Foard, 1960). Women achieve their maximum weights about two decades later than men and have a greater relative gain with age, however, so that by early middle age the proportion of obese women exceeds that of men. By late middle age many more women are obese than men. This may be due in part to obese men dying in proportionally greater numbers than obese women or nonobese men.

The prevalence of obesity also apparently varies somewhat by socioeconomic class. In their study of whites in midtown Manhattan, Moore et al. (1962) found that as social class rose, the prevalence of obesity decreased, particularly among women. In adolescents, associations between obesity and social class appear to be weaker: Huenemann et al. (1966a) found that higher mean income of the home census tracts of California adolescent subjects was associated with deceased prevalence of obesity, but Canning and Mayer (1966), working in New England, found no relationship between the educational levels or occupations of the adolescents' fathers and the prevalence of obesity in their sample.

Occasionally racial differences in the prevalence of obesity have been mentioned (Hathaway and Foard, 1960), suggesting that the prevalence of obesity among Negro women is higher than among white women. Differences among men are not as pronounced and suggest a slightly higher prevalence among white men. However, racial differences are usually confounded with socioeconomic class variations, so that it is difficult to say from presently available evidence whether racial differences would exist if class were held constant.

PREVALENCE OF CONCERN ABOUT WEIGHT AND DIETING BEHAVIOR

Age. Excessive weight deviations tend to be more common and severe among adults than adolescents, yet adults are much less concerned about their weights and less apt to take remedial measures than teenagers. An opinion poll conducted in 1964 on a national stratified sample (Wyden 1965:1) revealed that over 30 per cent of those adults who had a weight problem were not even concerned about their weights. Only about 10 per cent of the adults with weight problems were dieting to lose weight, about 20 per cent were watching their weights so that they would stop gaining, and the rest were concerned but took no action against overweight. Another poll done in the early 1960's (Wyden 1965:66) showed that concern with weight in adults rarely led to dieting; if any action was taken, it was more likely to cut out food regarded as "fattening" to prevent future gains, rather than to attempt to remove excess weight which had already accumulated. The "wishful dieters," as those adults who were concerned about their weights but doing nothing to lower them were called, gave as their main reasons for failure to diet lack of will power, enjoyment of eating, and procrastination.

In contrast, the studies of Huenemann et al. (1966a, 1966b) and Dwyer et al. (1969) indicate that almost all obese and many nonobese adolescents are concerned about weight, and that they engage in remedial efforts more often than adults.

Sex. Sex differences in the prevalence of concern about weight clearly favor females, although the prevalence of obesity is not always higher and, in some age groups, may be lower than in males. Dwyer and Mayer's (1970) analysis of several national public opinion polls revealed that concerns about weight and dieting behavior were much more common among adult women than among men. Polls taken in 1956 found that 45 per cent of the women and 22 per cent of the men wanted to lose weight, and that 14 per cent of the women and 7 per cent of the men were currently on diets to do so. Polls in 1966 showed that 42 per cent of the women and 35 per cent of the men interviewed felt that they were over their best weights, and 14 per cent of the women and 6 per cent of the men claimed that they were doing something to lose weight. While concern with weight appeared to be rising among the men over time, dieting behavior was not.

Weight was perceived as much more of a problem by teenage girls than by boys in the surveys of health concerns of adolescents done by Deisher and Mills (1963) and Adams (1966). Huenemann et al. (1966a, 1966b) investigated concerns about weight in senior high school students. On the basis of physical measurements, about 25 per cent of both the boys and the girls were classified as being obese or somewhat obese. Almost 50 per cent of the girls and somewhat less than 25 per cent of the boys expressed concern about their overweight and described themselves as being too fat. Concerns about overweight and obesity were present in many nonobese girls. A large proportion of the girls and a much smaller proportion of the boys were trying to lose weight or change their body proportions. Dieting was the most popular method of doing this.

Dwyer et al. (1969) studied attitudes of high school seniors toward their weights. Sixteen per cent of the girls and 19 per cent of the boys had triceps skinfolds that would be classified as obese. Over 80 per cent of the girls but less than 20 per cent of the boys wanted to weigh less than they did. Among the twelfth-grade, upper-middle-class New England girls they studied, over 60 per cent of all the girls had dieted by the time they were seniors in high school. Thirty per cent were on reducing diets on the day they were questioned. Only 16 per cent of all the girls were obese, and virtually all these girls had dieted, and many leaner girls as well. Of the boys in the same high schools, only 24 per cent of all the boys had ever dieted, and only 6 per cent were on reducing diets on the day they were questioned. Nineteen per cent of these boys were obese, but only a small proportion even of this group was on a reducing diet.

Weight Status. Heavier people in general tend to be more concerned about weight than lighter people. Almost all of the studies relevant to this point have been done on adolescents, however; little work has been done on adults. Hinton et al. (1963), Dwyer et al. (1969), and Huenemann et al. (1966a, 1966b) found that overweight or obese adolescents were more likely to be concerned about their weights and dieting to change them than nonobese adolescents.

Social class and ethnicity. Dieting and concern with overweight seem to be somewhat more prevalent among upper- than lower-class adults, although there are fewer obese persons in the upper classes than in the rest of the population. Only 11 per cent of the population falls in the upper- or upper-middle-class brackets, but they contain 24 per cent of all dieters (see Wyden, 1965:8). Dwyer and Mayer's (1970) analyses of opinion polls showed that concern with weight and dieting behavior increased slightly with occupational status but not educational level in men, and with both education and occupation in women. Newman (1957) found that a greater proportion of overweight upper-class women saw themselves as overweight and attempted to lose than did lower-class women.

The associations between obesity and social class are not as strong in adolescents as they are in adults. No data are available on the relationship of dieting to social class in adolescents. Little information also is available to indicate whether the prevalence of dieting varies by ethnic variables such as race, religion, or national origin.

THE CHAIN OF DECISIONS LEADING TO DIETING

Regarding dieting as the logical terminal behavior resulting from a stepwise choice of a certain set of options makes it easier to understand the social psychology of dieting. The sequence of events that may result in dieting are (1) recognition of a weight problem; (2) decision to remedy it; (3) choice of source of treatment; and (4) choice of method of treatment. Each of these steps offers several options, so that the decisions and actions of the people involved may vary considerably at each step in the process. Let us turn now to a closer examination of the factors which come into play at each step.

I. *The decision that one is too fat.* Before he is likely to engage in dieting behavior, the potential dieter must realize that he has a weight problem. Equally obese people often differ in their opinions as to their body weights. Some are convinced that they are too fat, others are not, and still others have no opinion at all. One reason for the diversity of opinions is their salience. Membership in social and cultural groups may cause people to vary the attention and importance they place on body weight. Individuals within a particular sociocultural group differ in their exposure to various professional and lay persons and other sources of information that might make them perceive that they are too fat. In addition, individuals vary in their own inherent interest and concern about fatness and appearance.

Differences in opinion may also evolve from the type of prevailing standards or norms that are used. Various types of standards are used as criteria for diagnosing obesity; health professionals and laymen often differ in their assessments of fatness status, since their standards are based on different considerations.

The standards most universally used by physicians, other health workers, and many laymen to diagnose obesity are the tables of ideal or desirable weights for each height, frame, and sex. These have been derived by insurance companies (Metropolitan Life Insurance Company of New York, 1959) from actuarial studies and are based on health considerations. However, these tables have rather severe shortcomings (see Seltzer and Mayer, 1965; Seltzer, 1965). The problem most germane to the current discussion is the fact that no clear specifications are given of what is meant by frame.

If overweight that may be due to large amounts of bone and muscle is mistaken for obesity—which is due to overfat alone—this may lead to misdirected and fruitless dieting efforts or unrealistic goals for body weight. While diets and exercises make it possible to reduce the weight due to extra fat, it is impossible to reduce the bone and muscle components of weight by these measures. Conversely, if overweight due to excessive fatness is wrongly identified as being due to a large build, no action may be taken against obesity. Thus, the distinctions of build are important ones to make. Moreover, ideal weights for persons of certain builds, particularly for those with large endowments of muscle and bone, may be unrealistically low as weight goals for the general population (see Seltzer, 1965). Norms of obesity more valid and precise than weight alone are available.

One simple way of assessing body fatness is to measure the size of the triceps skinfold, the subcutaneous fat depot over the triceps muscle on the back of the upper arm. This measurement allows a reasonably satisfactory estimate of the total body burden of fat to be made, and standards for obesity based on this measurement have been established (Seltzer and Mayer, 1965). A slightly more complicated method of estimating body fatness is the "body envelope method" of Behnke (1961), which is based on a number of physical measurements, including several fat depots. Many of the studies reported here use one of these two measurements for the objective assessment of obesity.

Many laymen rely on standards based on appearance or social acceptability as well as weight tables to evaluate their weight or fatness status. But is there any regularity or consistency in aspects of physical appearance related to weight that are aspired to? If so, how stable are they? Obviously, if ideas of what is "too fat" or "too thin" change either as the individual progresses through the life cycle or from year to year like fashions in dress, judgments about what is "too fat" or "too thin" may also change.

Fairly uniform, implicit norms for the appearance of the body do appear to exist in this country. While they vary somewhat from person to person because of their strong roots in individual opinions and attitudes, these norms are on the whole quite consistent. They are probably based on collective observation by the population of what is common in the community or in society in general, coupled with an unconscious judgment about what is to be regarded as normal. Norms for certain aspects of appearance are regarded as unattainable for some; for example, if the norm is that American women should be about 5'6" tall, a 5'1" woman can never attain the norm and will always be regarded as short. Other norms for physical appearance, such as lack of obesity, are generally regarded as attainable by all. While aberrations or striking deviations from these norms may not be regarded as abnormal or pathological from a medical standpoint, society's judgment or the opinion of influential members of society that they are not "normal," or deviant, may generate concern and discomfort in the unfortunate individuals who happen to possess these characteristics.

Homogenous ideals for these aspects of physical appearance also exist within this country. Ideals arise from man's attempts to visualize and classify not what is common or normal, as is true in the case of standards or norms, but what is perfect, that which is uncommon and desirable for that reason.

Just as fashions in clothes vary, norms and ideals for bodily appearance change from culture to culture and over time. Arabs, for example, esteem different, plumper body types than do Americans. During the late Renaissance, a young woman who had wide hips and an ample expanse of abdomen regarded herself as beautiful, while her twentieth-century American counterpart abhors these very characteristics in herself. Thus, since norms and ideals do change, there is no reason to assume that the current ones will last forever. Slimness may remain in vogue, or it may be replaced by a more amply padded figure. Such shifts could have striking effects on the prevalence of concern over weight and on dieting efforts.

Almost no work has been done on adult norms or ideals for weight, although a few studies have been done on adolescents. Their weight aspirations appear to vary with sex, body fatness, weight, and perhaps race. Dwyer et al. (1969) explored weight goals among high school seniors in a New England suburb. Among the girls, means for the weights they thought were the best for themselves on the basis of health decreased with decreasing body fatness and were always lower than their actual weights, except for the leanest girls, who felt that they should weigh a few pounds more than they did. When the same girls were asked what they wished to weigh, taking all considerations (health, appearance, etc.) into account, weights were even lower. The situation was quite different for the boys: Both weight goals were higher than actual weights. Huenemann et al. (1966a, 1966b) reported racial as well as sex differences in desires for body weights for high school sophomores. Caucasian girls wanted to lose more weight than Negroes or Orientals, although Negro girls were heavier. In contrast to the girls, boys of all races wanted to weigh more than they actually did and also wanted to be taller. Oriental boys were the lightest and shortest and also those who wished the greatest increases in weight and height.

Within each sex adolescents have fairly uniform ideals for the relative size of body parts, and these may influence their weight goals. Many adolescents appear to believe that appearances closer to their ideals in body parts can be brought about by a change in body weight. The studies of Huenemann et al. (1966a) and Dwyer et al. (1969) suggest that boys wish to gain weight and to be larger in almost all dimensions, especially in those that might signify strength or athletic prowess, such as the upper torso or arms. Girls, on the other hand, want to be smaller in almost all dimensions and to lose weight, although they are content about their

heights. Girls also have very different concerns about their bodies; they wish to be smaller, especially in their torsos (with the exception of the busts) and thighs. Huenemann et al. (1966a) suggested that while adolescent girls attribute their overweight to overfatness and regard it as undesirable, boys attribute their overweight to build components other than fat and regard it as desirable.

Uniform ideals of body type that may affect weight aspirations also exist. In Dwyer et al.'s (1969) study, adolescents were asked to choose among six female silhouettes (ranging from extreme ectomorphs to extreme endomorphs), first, the silhouette they considered to be their ideal, and second, that which was regarded by them as the most feminine. A majority of both sexes picked the female silhouette representing a mesomorphic ectomorph as being their ideal and also the most feminine figure. A substantial portion of the girls chose the extreme ectomorph, while the boys did not, suggesting that the girls' ideals were more ectomorphic than those of the boys. When male silhouettes were rated, the silhouette representing the extreme mesomorph was chosen by an overwhelming majority of the boys and a majority of the girls as their ideal and as the most masculine. Girls showed a wider range of responses, suggesting that the boys' ideals for masculinity were more mesomorphic than those of the girls.

A great deal of confusion seems to exist between what are attainable norms or realistic expectations and what are virtually unattainable ideals and unrealistic with regard to physical appearance. Time spent attempting to alter aspects of appearance that cannot be changed is wasted, while that spent striving toward attainable norms is time well spent. It is thus of crucial importance to ascertain how realistic weight-related norms are and how much hope of fulfillment they offer before people are urged to aspire to attain them. Clearly, both the feminine ideal of a slender, full-bosomed fashion model's build and the masculine ideal of the barrel-chested, muscle-bound football player are only realizable for a small percentage of the population, since such body builds occur only rarely in actuality.

II. *The decision to lose weight.* Even after the potential dieter has realized that he is too fat, he must be motivated to undertake a weight control program. It is abundantly clear that the factors encouraging people to follow through involve more than health motivations, even among those with the greatest health risk from their obesity.

Among adults, fear of poor health is the primary, but not the only, reason given by men who undertake reducing diets (see Wyden, 1965:7). Other reasons such as appearance appear to be equally if not more important in motivating women to lose weight. In adolescent girls, the desire to change certain aspects of appearance or become more attractive is almost universally the primary reason for dieting behavior (see Dwyer et al., 1967). On the other hand, Dwyer et al. (1969) found that boys embarked on reducing diets primarily to improve their physical fitness and sports ability. Huenemann et al. (1966b) also found that the adolescent boys and girls they studied undertook diets for appearance rather than for health reasons most of the time.

Many Americans decide to lose weight because of the pervasive negative attitudes toward obesity that permeate the social climate. Obesity is regarded as more than solely a health issue, not only by the afflicted individuals themselves, but even by physicians and other members of society. Obesity evokes negative stereotypes about behavior and personality traits as well as appearance, although these generalizations may not correspond to actuality. Maddox et al. (1968) recently showed that most Americans regard obesity as a socially deviant form of physical disability. The subjects in their study blamed the obese for being fat, but felt that persons with other physical handicaps should not be blamed because they were not responsible for their conditions. The authors of the study expected certain groups, notably low-income subjects, Negro males, and elderly persons to be indifferent to the standard American preference for leanness and to value fatness instead. However, the negative attitudes toward obesity ran so deep that even members of these groups considered fat persons less likeable than nonfat ones. Some members of society are even more extreme and look upon obesity as downright immoral. They apparently base such judgments on the belief that it arises from either or both of the sins of gluttony and sloth.

An obese appearance evokes negative and stereotyped attitudes as early as childhood. Staffieri (1967) asked boys from four to ten years of age to assign various behavior or personality traits to silhouettes representing extremely endomorphic, mesomorphic, and ectomorphic body types. He found that stereotyped responses began to appear between the ages of four and five, and that differences had become apparent by the age of seven. At age seven, all adjectives assigned to the endomorph with a significantly greater frequency than to the other silhouettes were socially unfavorable (for example: fights, cheats, mean, lazy, etc.). All of those assigned to the mesomorphic silhouette were favorable (for example: strong, best friend, clean, etc.), and those assigned to the ectomorph were personally unfavorable or indicative of social submissiveness (for example: sneaky, afraid, quiet, etc.). The children liked the mesomorph better consistently after the age of seven, and after this age they were also able to classify their own body types fairly accurately. Hassan (1968) also noted that stereotyped ideas of the character traits and behavior of persons with different body types existed in grade-school children of both sexes, and that those whose body types were less favored had less self-regard and less accurate self-concepts.

Professional persons, such as physicians, who are trained to regard all sorts of physical problems dispassionately, might be expected to be free from such stereotyped beliefs about the obese. However, a study by Maddox and Liederman (1969) revealed that a negative evaluation and characterization of obese persons extended to doctors' attitudes as well. Obese patients were described by their doctors as being more weak-willed, ugly, and awkward than their other patients. The obese have also been noted to appear to accept more blame and feel more guilt about their condition than those with other types of physical disabilities. Perhaps this is due in part to physicians' attitudes toward them.

Obesity may affect interpersonal relationships even in childhood. Matthews and Westie (1966) reported that grade-school children indicated the greatest social distance from overweight children in their classes. Among the children he studied, Staffieri (1967) found that mesomorphic boys received the highest number of "best friend" choices, and endomorphs the fewest, from their peers.

Obese children, especially girls, have particular social problems when they reach adolescence and heterosexual interest picks up. Bullen et al. (1963) found that extremely obese girls had significantly fewer dates than nonobese girls. The obese were in fewer nonsport clubs, organizations, and groups in and outside of school than the nonobese. They did not participate as actively in those groups of which they were members as did the nonobese.

Canning and Mayer (1966) presented evidence that unconscious prejudices of high-school teachers in writing recommendations or among college interviewers against obese adolescents may hinder their chances of being accepted by the colleges of their choice. Application rates and academic qualifications among the obese were equal to those among nonobese twelfth graders in the schools they studied, yet acceptance rates into high-ranking colleges were lower for obese students, especially for girls. Canning and Mayer (1967) also found that obesity did not have any effect on high school performance as measured by IQ scores, PSAT or SAT scores (achievement tests), absences, or enrollment in extracurricular activities. Thus it appears that the extreme concern of the obese with weight and their own and teachers' negative evalu-

ations of obese adolescents do not prevent them from performing well or even excelling in many areas.

Our own self-regard largely reflects what others think of us. Other factors being equal, persons with an attractive appearance tend to develop high self-regard, while those whose appearance is regarded as unattractive tend to have lower self-regard, and may strive to change this appearance. Therefore, it is not surprising to find that obese children and adolescents have extremely negative self-images. In a study of high-school girls at a summer camp in New England, Monello and Mayer (1963) found that the obese girls showed personality characteristics such as passivity, obsessive concern with self-image, expectation of rejection, and progressive withdrawal—all strikingly similar to the traits of ethnic and racial minority groups due to their status as victims of prejudice. They also accepted the dominant negative values toward obesity prevalent in our society. Canning and Mayer (1968) demonstrated that the obsession with their weights was so great that nonrelated areas became involved in the issue. In sentence-completion tests dealing with interpersonal situations, obese girls were more apt to give responses indicating concern about weight, while the responses of normal-weight controls were related to other normal concerns and reactions of adolescents. The obese girls persisted in interjecting concern with wishes or things in their lives that generated anxiety. Direct questions about weight and appearance also brought significantly higher response from the obese than the nonobese.

Alexander (1968), in working with female college freshmen, found that endomorphs were significantly less accepting of themselves than were ectomorphs or mesomorphs. Maddox et al. (1968) found that the disvaluation of fatness and denial of identification with the obese extended not only to the general public but to people who were themselves obese. When obese subjects were asked to compare themselves to their ideal selves and to fat people for various characteristics, their answers revealed that they felt they were less like their ideal selves but also less like obese people than did normal-weight subjects.

The early and prolonged exposure to negative sociocultural attitudes toward obesity encountered by those whose obesity begins in childhood appears more detrimental to self-image than does obesity of adult onset. Stunkard and Mendelson's (1961) study indicates that adults afflicted with obesity of the latter type do not approve of their overweight, but do not loathe their bodies or hate themselves because of it. Tarini (1962) has shown that many of them deny their fatness. In contrast, the Stunkard and Mendelson (1961) study found that certain obese adults, most of whom had been obese since childhood or adolescence, looked upon themselves as grotesque and ugly; they tended to blame their weights for far-removed troubles, to divide the world into fat and nonfat, and to disregard factors such as talent, intelligence, and wealth in favor of appearance in judging others. Stunkard and Burt (1967) confirmed these findings on another sample of obese adults and again found that disturbances in body image clustered in persons obese since childhood or adolescence. Bruch (1958) observed that many persons obese since early life who later successfully reduced their weights still felt that they were ugly and fat.

Thus, from many standpoints—conformity to current standards and ideals for appearance, self-regard, social acceptability, and health—obesity is detrimental. Many obese persons undoubtedly undertake weight control behavior to escape some of this social and moral opprobrium as well as to decrease health risks.

III. *Source of treatment*. The potential dieter must now decide whom to consult for help in losing weight. He may seek advice from a health professional, a lay practitioner, or he may choose to treat himself. This choice is probably largely determined by the individual's perceptions and opinions on the cause and severity of his condition. If he believes that his obesity is connected to a pathological physical or psychological condition, he is likely to seek medical or psychiatric help; if he believes that he is well and that his obesity is uncomplicated from the medical standpoint, he will probably treat himself or engage the services of a lay practitioner, such as the leader of a diet club. However, other variables may also influence his decision. In terms of the economy of money, time, and effort involved in arranging for treatment and access to treatment, the self-administered methods rate the highest. However, if we examine the adequacy of medical supervision and the amount of psychological support they provide some of the methods employed by lay practitioners and health professionals are superior. Further, persons whose obesity is severe (or who regard it as such, even if it is not) are more likely to choose these sources. Those whose obesity is complicated by some other physical or emotional problem often seek medical help. In addition, many other related variables that involve the perception of illness and of health-motivated behavior may determine the source of treatment.

IV. *Choice of method*. The next decision confronting the individual who wishes to lose weight is the method. There are three basic popular methods that can be used either alone or in combination to bring about weight loss: (1) dietary modifications, (2) increased physical activity, and (3) medications. Dietary modifications accomplish the objective by decreasing caloric intake, increased physical activity by raising caloric output. Medications vary in their action; some act as appetite depressants, others as laxatives or diuretics, and a few, such as thyroid extract, increase metabolic rate and therefore energy expenditure. Psychiatric treatment for obesity is based on the premise that solving the patient's emotional problems will motivate him to lose weight. These last two treatments are usually coupled with or result in changes in food intake or energy expenditure as well.

The source of treatment chosen to some extent dictates the methods and techniques available for losing weight. For example, lay practitioners are usually involved in managing diet clubs and health spas, while health professionals are the only ones who can prescribe most medications or refer patients to dietitians for diet therapy. However, choice of method is also influenced by several other interrelated factors: (1) the individual's views on the cause of his obesity (2) cost and availability of the method, and (3) compatability of the method with the individual's life style.

Views on the causation and proper treatment for obesity. Mayer (1968) has recently reviewed and summarized current scientific opinion on the etiology and pathogenesis of obesity. The most common type of obesity in this country today is generally agreed to be environmental in origin, arising from inactivity rather than from excessively large food intakes on the part of the obese versus the nonobese. Only a small percentage of cases appears caused by pre-existing pathological conditions, either physical or psychiatric. Thus, most competent physicians treat most of their obese patients through reducing diets or increased physical activity, and they are extremely conservative in using medications. The more potent medications such as thyroid extract or "rainbow diet pills" (consisting of thyroid extract, diuretics, digitalis, and amphetamines) in combination with extremely rigid diets have in the past few years been misused by some disreputable "diet doctors." Their patients have paid dearly in money and may also have jeopardized their health by their patronage.

Lay and medical opinion on the cause and proper treatment for obesity vary. Lay opinion stresses overeating rather than inactivity as the major cause of obesity, and perhaps these views lead to the high value placed on the efficacy of dieting. For example, in Huenemann et al.'s (1966a) study of knowledge in high school students of the causes of obesity, over half of the freshman boys and even more of the girls believed that fatness was due chiefly to overeating. Modifications in diet greatly overshadowed changes in activity levels among both boys and girls. Less than half of both sexes realized that the obese did not exercise as much as the

nonobese. By the time these students had reached the twelfth grade, boys had begun to adopt the opinion that obesity was due to underactivity, while girls remained committed to their earlier beliefs. Boys had also become more partial to exercise than girls. Dwyer et al. (1967) also found that twelfth-grade boys were more likely to incorporate greater physical activity into their weight control efforts than were girls. Bullen et al. (1963) similarly found that the obese adolescent girls they interviewed thought they were fat primarily because they ate more, had greater appetites, and snacked more than their nonobese friends.

Unfortunately, no work has been reported on the opinions of adults on the causes of obesity, but it is likely that their beliefs are similar to those of adolescents. Given the public's general conviction that food and overeating are the major cause factors operating in obesity, it is easy to understand why reducing diets are so popular.

Cost and availability. Self-administered methods are the easiest to employ. Dietary modifications and increased physical activity can be undertaken by anyone who chooses to do so without any contact with a physician, although they are often more effective under a physician or dietitian's direction. Psychiatric treatment with some weight-loss technique is available only from physicians. The more potent medications are available only by prescription, and access to them therefore entails seeing a physician. Some of the less powerful drugs, such as certain appetite-depressants, weak diuretics, bulk producers, laxatives, and other nostrums can be obtained over-the-counter in drugstores without prescription, but these are usually used in conjunction with dieting.

Compatability of method with life style. The ease with which weight loss can be fitted into one's normal life is vitally important in determining choice of reducing method. Most people acknowledge the value and stress the beneficial effects of exercise and activity, and they may be partial to reducing drugs in controlling weight when discussing it or advising others, but when it comes down to their actual weight-control efforts, in practice they rely chiefly, if not exclusively, on dietary methods. The difficulty of obtaining diet pills and the inconvenience involved in taking them probably account for their rather limited use.

However, the unpopularity of physical activity has a more complex explanation. People seem to think that dieting is an easier method of curing obesity than burning off calories by increasing exercise and physical activity. Considering the relative amounts of disruption to established habits and life style in general that go along with each type of modification, they are probably right. The constraints imposed by life style on activity levels seem to be even greater than those on eating habits. Patterns of inactivity probably have an even stronger hold and are more difficult to overcome than habits of overeating. In addition, increased physical activity usually requires a greater rather than a lesser time input, which busy people are loathe to make, while the skipped meals and eating less that are often involved in dieting patterns require no time expenditures and may even save time. Special facilities, such as swimming pools, are required for many of the types of exercise people like best; other sports require several teammates or other players for a game. Further, many simple activities, such as walking, which seem to face none of the above obstacles, are difficult in many areas where streets are unsafe. Finally, the disinclination to increase activity as a means of controlling weight is due partly to the widely held but mistaken, belief of most Americans that they are not inactive or sedentary. The great majority of Americans do lead sedentary lives; they do not perform much physical labor that involves substantial energy expenditures. Inactivity and the sedentary life are apparently confused in many peoples' minds with sloth—laziness, sluggishness, idleness, or indolence. To say that a person is sedentary has no moral overtones. Americans are sedentary, but this does not mean that they do not engage in a great deal of tiring activity; it simply means that most of this activity does not involve large caloric outputs.

Another widespread belief that works against the adoption of activity as a means of losing weight is that exercise must be violent and unpleasant, such as calisthenics, jogging, or weight.lifting, in order to contribute substantially to weight loss. While this is not true, it undoubtedly discourages many persons from engaging in greater physical activity. In terms of all of these variables that affect life style, the easiest, most pleasant, and most popular method of losing weight seems to be dieting.

At last the potential dieter has become an actual dieter and has embarked on his diet. This, of course, gives no assurance that he will actually lost weight. The efficacy of the dietary treatment will depend on the soundness of the regimen itself, the zeal with which it is followed, and its duration. Unfortunately, very little has been written on the psychological factors that influence these variables, and more intense study is needed in this area.

POSSIBLE EXPLANATIONS OF THE GREATER RATE OF DIETING AMONG FEMALES THAN MALES

On the basis of evidence that has been presented, several plausible reasons can be suggested for the greater rate of dieting among females than among males:

First, weight deviations are more of a social liability for females than for males. If their weights are excessive, females are at a greater social disadvantage both in their relationships with other females and in their relationships with males. Their social mobility is also inhibited to a greater extent. Successful men are often overweight or obese; successful career women and the wives of famous men rarely are.

Second, weight-related aspects of appearance are more intertwined with the self-concept in females than in males. The sensitivity of the self-images of females to weight problems may encourage them to undertake corrective efforts. It is little wonder that, since women know the importance of their physical appearance particularly in determining how the male half of the human race will regard them as well as in influencing other females' opinions of them, appearance becomes so tightly bound up with self-image. Men have always desired physical attractiveness in their mates and have valued it highly. Although appearance is certainly an important factor in how females assess the eligibility of their male partners, other considerations, such as the prospective husband's potential as protector and provider, tend to rank higher among the criteria important to their selection. Extra pounds pose a powerful threat to a female's appearance, and hence generate greater concern and ego involvement in females than in males. Men's concerns with respect to their bodies seem largely tied to functional aspects of appearance that suggest physical or sexual prowess. Obesity and leanness must be severe before they become real detriments or imply deficits in the area of physical performance to others. The self-concepts of females, on the other hand, are more intimately involved with myriad aspects of body appearance other than those suggesting physical prowess, and their body images are adversely affected by much smaller deviations. As soon as many women gain a few pounds they feel obese, even though the level of fatness is not sufficient to be noticed by others, and certainly not enough to affect physical performance. Thus, similar deviations in pounds of excess weight above normal that might be merely annoying to a male are devastating to a female's concept of herself.

These differences in the salience of weight status to the individual are illustrated in the accuracy of self-reporting of weight. Huenemann et al. (1966b) found that sixteen-year-old girls reported their weights much more accurately than did boys of the same age. They attributed this to the boys' lack of awareness of their weights. Dwyer et al. (1969) found that boys weighed themselves less frequently than girls, which might indicate that they were less interested in their weights. Girls, particularly the fatter girls, showed a striking tendency to report weights on questionnaires that were markedly less than their actual weights,

while boys reported their weights quite accurately. Perhaps girls knew what they weighed but were embarrassed and sensitive about reporting it, resorting to intentional underreporting.

A third reason for the heightened concern of females about weight is rooted in physiology: Obesity is more visible in females than in males. Normal, young, mature females have almost twice as much fat on their bodies as do males. Furthermore, fat on females is distributed more conspicuously; women tend to have more fat on the extremities, hips, and chest, while men have most of their fat on their torsos and are leaner in the extremities. Females thus add extra fat at highly visible or interesting points, and attention is called to it automatically.

A fourth reason that may explain the zeal of females to lose weight and the relative torpor of males to do so may be due to differences between the sexes in the prevalent mistaken notions about body composition and weight loss. Males tend to overestimate the contributions of build to weight and consequently are often uninterested in lowering their weights. Many males seem to believe that reducing diets will result in muscle as well as fat loss. For example, Glucksman and Hirsch (1968) observed men who were undergoing weight reduction and found that they were obsessed with the thought that their loss of weight was causing the physical disintegration by affecting their strength and virility. Some adolescent boys believe that dieting will stunt their growth. Loss of strength and size is very threatening to males, and perhaps because of these beliefs they shy away from dieting. When males do diet, they seem partial to high-protein diets in combination with increased physical activity similar to the types used by athletes in training. This form of dieting, which might be labeled the "training-table mystique," appeals to them for several reasons. It has a virile aura about it, is in line with males' convictions that underactivity is an important cause of obesity, and conforms to cultural beliefs that males should be physically active. Unfortunately, the physical activity aspect often degenerates into only perfunctory efforts to do push ups, or, in the case of adult men, an occasional sauna bath and massage to ease the conscience and provide the illusion of fitness. Thus, the relative disinclination of males to lose weight by dieting and their propensity to do so only if it is coupled with physical activity are probably rooted in their aspirations to appear larger and more mesomorphic.

Underestimation of the contribution to weight of build components other than fat is common in girls and women and can lead to dieting or other weight-loss behavior when it is not called for. For example, Dwyer et al. (1967) found that a large number of adolescent girls were dieting because they mistakenly attributed their relative largeness and heaviness to fatness rather than to the other components of build that were truly responsible. They were on diets because they thought they were obese, although they were really below average in body fatness as measured by the triceps skinfold. Similarly, Goldman et al. (1963) found several girls at a special summer camp for treatment of obesity who, although far from obese, believed that they were. Casual observation of the members of "Weight Watchers" and similar dieting clubs suggests that many adult women labor under similar misconceptions. Cultural stereotypes that females should be dainty eaters and less physically active than males also encourage dieting. The desire of girls to lose weight probably reflects their desires to be smaller and more ectomorphic as well.

A fifth reason for the predominance of female dieting is fashion. Since the dawn of history, clothes designs have been influenced by three principles: seduction, the attraction of persons of the opposite sex; hierarchy, the expression of personal or social superiority through clothing; and utility, the protection of the body. Male fashions in dress have generally been dominated by hierarchy and modified by utility, with very little emphasis on the seduction principle. Thus, most men's clothes are shapeless enough to conceal large amounts of fat and all but the most deviant body conformations. What little male fashion is present is found largely among young unmarried men. Female fashions, on the other hand, have been largely under control of the seduction principle, modified by utility and hierarchy. They are designed to call attention to the erotic potential of the body. Until modern times, modish dress was the prerogative of the unmarried young girl and the not-quite-respectable older woman of the world. Traditionally the married female had very little concern for her attractiveness, and her seclusion in the home and devotion to her family gave little incentive and few opportunities for the display of attire. However, over the past 50 years fashion has become important for almost all American women, and today, women of all ages and matrimonial states follow it to some extent. It has been theorized that female fashions change periodically to direct attention to a new area of the body that has remained hidden in the recent past and thus become erotically interesting. For some reason, at any rate, areas given particular emphasis do change; the breasts are emphasized during one decade, the legs in another.

Clothes tend to be designed with an ideal female body type in mind. These ideals change, as do fashions and hemlines, but more slowly. Since early in this century the somewhat ample, mature figure favored by the Victorians and Edwardians has been out of fashion. The slight frame has been the ideal, although emphasis has shifted from the legs to the bosom and back again. For the past several decades, fashions have been tailored for the very tall and slim, or, alternatively, for the tall, narrow-hipped, rather wide-shouldered female figure. Women who are short, stout, or wide hipped with narrow shoulders have difficulty dressing à la mode. Women with more ample endowments are at a disadvantage and often take steps to bring their figures more in line with current ideals. Male body ideals, like male fashions, are relatively static and do not change so dramatically.

POSSIBLE EXPLANATIONS FOR DIFFERENCES IN DIETING PREVALENCE BETWEEN ADOLESCENTS AND ADULTS

Adolescence is a period that is particularly favorable for dieting and other weight reduction efforts for several reasons:

First, adolescents are more self-conscious about their bodies than are adults. This may be due in part to their recent experience with the dramatic physical changes, brought about by the accelerated growth of puberty, which confer a virtually new appearance. The heterogeneous nature of adolescent growth patterns accentuates physical differences and makes them extremely noticeable. Adolescent girls mature about two years sooner than boys, so that by late high school they have reached their fully-mature size and are likely to become concerned if the weights at which they have stabilized seem to be too high. On the other hand, many boys of the same age are still growing. Even obese boys may convince themselves that their weight problems are only temporary and that they will grow out of them, although this is unlikely to actually be the case. Concerns about underweight are extremely common among adolescents who are late maturers and who, because of this, are shorter and lighter than their peers. Asynchronism, or lack of coordination in development, is also often present during adolescent growth. A common asynchronism is rapid weight gain with height gain lagging behind. It may cause embarrassment and generate weight-control efforts in afflicted adolescents. All of these physical changes occur at the very time in life when social and cultural pressures are the strongest for homogeneity and conformity in matters of appearance as well as in many other aspects of life. Dwyer and Mayer (1967a, 1967b, 1968) have shown that failure to attain appearance ideals can cause a great deal of discontent and unhappiness among adolescents, especially among those more noticeably deviant from them. These wounds may still smart among some adults.

Adults, whose adolescent growth is far behind them, have had more or less constant physiques for years, and have had time to become accustomed to and accept their bodies, imperfections and all. Accordingly, obesity of adult onset usually has less severe and detrimental effects on self-image than does obesity of juvenile onset and is less likely to impel the afflicted individual to diet.

Second, recent experience with extensive body alterations during the adolescent growth spurt may make teenagers receptive to the idea that changes in weight are possible and encourage their optimism about the probable success of their weight-control efforts. By comparison, adults are used to their bodies as they are and know from experience that weight changes are difficult to achieve.

Third, adolescents are more physically active than adults. Thus, their physical performance is more hindered by the effects of extreme obesity. However, there are some sports in which sheer crushing power is important, and for these a slight degree of overweight may be an advantage.

Fourth, the desire to conform to others and to ideals in weight, appearance, and many other aspects of life is particularly strong during adolescence, probably stronger than it is in adult life. Teenagers tend to regard being different from their peers as tantamount to being inferior. These feelings often lead to attempts to change body weight and to bring it back into line with the norms for the group. Adults are less likely to feel the need to conform in these respects.

Fifth, adolescent desires to demonstrate their independence or to rebel against their parents may sometimes lead them to alter their eating habits, especially if their parents are opposed to the idea or manner in which they do it.

A final factor is that weight deviations among adolescents are more likely to be diagnosed and treated early. Teenagers are almost universally given yearly school medical exams, and those who are obese are urged to take action against it. School health personnel are usually advocates of preventive medicine and encourage adolescent weight-control efforts. Conversely, adults often go for years without any physical examination, and their weight deviations are thus likely to be more severe, established, and difficult to reverse by the time they are finally diagnosed. Even then, as Maddox et al. (1966) have revealed, many obese adults are not urged to take action against it because of their physicians' disinterest in preventive medicine or dismal experience in past efforts to treat obese adults.

VARIATIONS IN DIETING PREVALENCE BETWEEN DIFFERENT SOCIOECONOMIC GROUPS

Little evidence is available on variations in the perception of obesity by socioeconomic status, race, or ethnicity. Goldblatt et al. (1965) have suggested that perhaps lower-class persons do not regard obesity as culturally undesirable as do those of higher social status, because their experiences with deprivation may have led them to connect obesity with well-being and prosperity. With respect to this, it would not be surprising to find that variations by social class existed in views toward obesity. People in different social classes vary in the types of lives they lead and in their behavior toward many problems, particularly health problems. Therefore, they would not be expected to exhibit homogeneous behavior in dealing with obesity. On the whole, however, the similarities between social classes are more impressive than class differences with regard to concern about weight and dieting. Every social class contains many persons who are obese, concerned about their weights, and dieting to correct them. Perhaps this is due to the fact that all are exposed to the same mass media, schools, and other factors that might generate homogeneous attitudes toward obesity.

APPROACHES FOR MORE EFFECTIVE PREVENTION AND TREATMENT OF OBESITY

Left alone, obese children and adolescents do not outgrow their condition; they become obese adults. Since the cure of obesity is rare once it is well established, with few exceptions they remain obese adults. Other persons, nonobese until adulthood, are afflicted with obesity at maturity and are never cured. Therefore, prevention or early treatment is vital if prevalence rates of obesity are to be substantially decreased.

Moderately successful methods of weight reduction already exist, but no appreciable inroads have yet been made into the high prevalence of obesity. Weight reduction efforts by persons acting by themselves or under the direction of their physicians have been widespread in this country for many years. These measures alone do not seem to reach enough people, are often expensive, and consume a great deal of the time of health professionals who are involved in treatment, although they should certainly not be abandoned.

Group rather than individually organized efforts might have more hope of success in reaching the millions of persons who require some kind of expert support and guidance, yet whose obesity does not require highly-specialized medical supervision because it is uncomplicated by other medical problems. Such group efforts have the added attraction of being less expensive to the patient in terms of medical manpower and cost. The more successful group programs mentioned below deal with persons who are obese or at high risk of becoming so. They might be organized on a broader scale in order to test their adaptability as weight-control programs on a public health basis.

Many health agencies have begun anticoronary clubs for middle-aged persons, particularly men, which combine calorie restriction with low-cholesterol, highly unsaturated fat diets. These are designed to decrease weight as well as serum cholesterol and consequently, to reduce the risk of coronary heart disease. Most of these groups encourage their members to exercise, and some provide sports facilities and organized classes as well. Others also try to attack the smoking problem, another risk factor involved not only in heart disease but in various lung conditions. Such clubs have been quite popular in many cities, and their methods do indeed seem to substantially decrease risks of heart attacks.

The past few years have also marked the epidemic spread of "Weight Watchers" and similar clubs for reducing among women. Most of these groups are private, profit-making organizations. The reducing diets prescribed by such clubs are usually a standardized low-calorie diet of roughly 1200 calories. Strict adherence to the rather limited choice of foods and weighing of portions is required. Many people are losing weight through such clubs, whose techniques contain many useful elements of group support and group therapy that might be adopted more widely by health professionals. Members are usually friends or acquaintances. This lends a social nature to meetings, and the fact that the members know each other apparently generates social pressure to succeed in dieting by developing a spirit of camaradie and good-natured competition among the members of the group. Meetings are held in a neighborhood church or school at times convenient to members. The format is partly social, partly business; the members are weighed, exhorted to follow the club's particular diet, and given helpful hints and low-calorie recipes.

From the large membership lists of such clubs and the substantial, if temporary, weight-loss records of members, it appears that many American women are amenable to this type of weight reduction program. However, the clubs have two failings. First, in some states they are outside the realm of supervision by knowledgable physicians or health agencies so that they are difficult to monitor. Second, the major qualifications for the instructors is that they have themselves reduced successfully and are good leaders, but they are given no training in the science of nutrition or the other health sciences. Consequently, they have often given fallacious information on nutrition and weight control to members who regard it as authoritative knowledge. Unfortunately, the instructors' well-intentioned effort to explain why their diet works are usually derived from the pseudoscientific theories presented in the mass of books and articles written by prolific quacks who find the topic of weight control so profitable.

There is an urgent need to educate these instructors in the rudiments of scientific nutrition, with particular emphasis on energy balance, energy metabolism, and weight control, so that such misconceptions will not be disseminated further. However, the deficits in these programs with respect to nutrition education should not discourage nutritionists and other health professionals from adopting the more positive aspects for designing weight-control programs tailored to fit the needs of the community.

Unfortunately, the implementation of weight-control programs on a wide-scale basis at present seems far off. One shortcoming of such efforts, in any case, is that many of them possess the inherent disadvantage of being curative rather than truly preventive programs. Attempts to organize weight-control programs among adults run into the problem that adults are difficult to assemble on a regular, frequent basis, even if motivation is high. Children are more accessible. Schools have captive populations of youngsters who are easy to reach. Moreover, working with persons early in life often makes it possible to prevent obesity, or to arrest its progress. Therefore, school-based group approaches to preventing obesity in children in order to decrease the potential reservoir of obese adults offer great promise.

The first objective of such school programs should be the improvement of nutrition education with regard to obesity. Strong in-service courses in nutrition for teachers, with special emphasis on weight control in the context of adolescent development, as well as more coordination between different teachers whose subjects touch nutrition, are desperately needed to improve the quality and presentation of weight-control-related topics in the classroom.

A second objective should be to increase the efforts of school health personnel in combating overweight. Periodic screening procedures should be instituted to enable early diagnosis of weight problems. Because they lack the time, only a few school health nurses and physicians can give students direct assistance in initiating weight-control measures and supervising their dieting efforts. This service gap could be filled by augmenting the staff with a part-time nutritionist who could prescribe therapeutic diets and assist students. At the least, there should be an adequate referral system to alert parents and family physicians to the problem. Although direct intervention in altering food habits is beyond the scope of the school, the school cafeteria manager could cooperate by serving special low-calorie lunches to those who wished them, to demonstrate and encourage sensible dieting.

The third objective should be to improve physical education programs. Schools can intervene directly in matters relating to the activity component of overweight, since most of them have compulsory physical education classes, as well as a variety of extracurricular athletic programs. Presently most school physical education programs cater to the physically fit rather than to the unfit. Obese youngsters are inactive and sensitive about their clumsiness and lack of skill. Needed here are in-service instruction of physical education teachers about the special needs of the obese and an extension or redirection of departmental programs to furnish intensive, frequently-scheduled special classes in physical education adopted to the handicaps of the obese.

Two projects have demonstrated the feasability and success of a combination nutrition education-physical fitness program for controlling adolescent obesity. Christakis et al. (1966) used nutrition lectures, individual dietary consultations, and extra biweekly programs of physical fitness in addition to regular classes to attack obesity in high school boys. A larger and more intensive program carried out among junior-high-school boys and girls by Seltzer and Mayer (1970) concentrated on special before- and after-school physical education classes several times a week. Some nutrition advice was given, but no supervised dieting was attempted.

Certainly, even if well-organized programs to control obesity were instituted in every elementary and secondary school in the land today, we would still be far from solving the obesity problem, since we still would not have reached the millions of obese adults. However, this would be a good beginning and an excellent investment in the health of the adults of tomorrow. A "spin-off" effect of such programs might be to excite interest in weight reduction in the children's parents.

Another means to make dieting as painless as possible for large groups of people would be the expanded development of low-calorie, high-nutritive-value foods that are tasty, safe, and competitively priced. Such products of modern food technology would allow dieters to lose weight while maintaining satisfactory nutritional status in other respects and eating food that both looked and tasted good, without suffering the social stigma and lack of gustatory satisfaction that often accompany the eating of many of the bland, unexciting, and expensive diet foods now on the market.

A final approach to facilitating weight control that has hardly been begun yet in this country is the impovement of opportunities and facilities for exercise and the development of physical activity programs for adults. These programs might do much for the activity component of the energy balance equation.

In summary, this review has attempted to shed light on the epidemiology of weight-loss behavior and the processes that lead to it. Hopefully it will stimulate better teaching, more sympathetic counseling, and more effective treatment of those with real or imaginary weight problems, and help to identify points at which intervention might be effective in encouraging weight control or establishing preventive programs.

REFERENCES

Adams, J. F.
    1966 "Adolescents' identification of personal and national problems." Adolescence 1 (Fall):240–250.
Alexander, W. R.
    1968 "A study of body types, self image, and environmental adjustment in freshmen college women." Dissertation Abstracts 28:8A:3048.

Behnke, A. R.
1961 "Quantitative assessment of body build." Journal of Applied Physiology 16 (November):960–968.

Bruch, Hilde.
1958 "Psychological aspects of obesity." Borden's Review of Nutrition Research 19 (July–August):57.

Bullen, B. A., L. F. Monello, H. Cohen, and J. Mayer.
1963 "Attitudes toward physical activity, food, and family in obese and nonobese adolescent girls." American Journal of Clinical Nutrition 12 (January):1–11.

Canning, H., and J. Mayer.
1966 "Obesity: its possible effect on college acceptance." New England Journal of Medicine 275 (November 24):1172–1174.
1967 "Obesity: an influence on high school performance." American Journal of Clinical Nutrition 20 (April):352–354.
1968 "Obesity: an analysis of attitudes, knowledge, and weight control in girls." Research Quarterly 39 (December):894–899.

Christakis, G., S. Sajeckie, R. W. Hillman, E. Miller, S. Blumenthal, and M. Archer.
1966 "Effect of a combined nutrition education-physical fitness program on weight status of obese high school boys." Federation Proceedings 25(1) (January–February):15–19.

Deischer, E., and D. Mills.
1963 "The adolescent looks at his health and medical care." American Journal of Public Health 53 (December):1928–1936.

Dwyer, J. T., J. J. Feldman, and J. Mayer.
1967 "Adolescent dieters: who are they? Physical characteristics, attitudes, and dieting practices of adolescent girls." American Journal of Clinical Nutrition 20 (October):1045–1056.

Dwyer, J. T., J. J. Feldman, C. C. Seltzer, and J. Mayer.
1969 "Body image in adolescents; attitudes toward weight and perception of appearance." Journal of Nutrition Education 1(2) (Fall):14–19.

Dwyer, J. T., and J. Mayer.
1967a "Variations in physical appearance during adolescence: part 1. boys." Postgraduate Medicine 41A (May):99–107.
1967b "Variations in physical appearance during adolescence: part 2. girls." Postgraduate Medicine 41A (June):91–97.
1968 "Psychological effects of variations in physical appearance during adolescence." Adolescence 3 (Winter):353–380.
1970 "Potential dieters: who are they?" Journal of the American Dietetic Association 56 (June):510–514.

Glucksman, M. L., and J. Hirsch.
1968 "The response of obese patients to weight reduction: a clinical evaluation of behavior." Psychosomatic Medicine 30 (January–February):1–11.

Goldblatt, P. B., M. C. Moore, and A. J. Stunkard.
1965 "Social factors in obesity." Journal of the American Medical Association 192 (June 21):1039–1044.

Goldman, R. F., B. A. Bullen, and C. C. Seltzer.
1963 "Changes in specific gravity and body fat in overweight female adolescents as a result of weight reduction." Annals of New York Academy of Science 110:913–917.

Hassan, I. N.
1968 "The body image and personality correlates of body type stereotypes." Dissertation Abstracts 11A:4446.

Hathaway, M. L., and E. D. Foard.
1960 Heights and Weights for Adults in the United States. Washington: Home Economics Research Report 10, Agricultural Research Service, U.S. Department of Agriculture, Government Printing Office.

Hinton, M. A., E. S. Eppright, H. Chadderdon, and C. Wolins.
1963 "Eating behavior and dietary intakes of girls 12–14 years old." Journal of the American Dietetic Association 43 (September):223–227.

Huenemann, R. L., M. C. Hampton, L. R. Shapiro, and A. Behnke.
1966a "Adolescent food practices associated with obesity." Federation Proceedings 25(1) (January–February):4–10.

Huenemann, R. L., L. R. Shapiro, M. C. Hampton, B. W. Mitchell, and A. R. Behnke.
1966b "A longitudinal study of gross body composition and body conformation and their association with food and activity in a teenage population: views of teenage subjects on body conformation, food, and activity." American Journal of Clinical Nutrition 18 (May):325–338.

Maddox, G. L., C. F. Anderson, and M. D. Bogdonoff.
1966 "Overweight as a problem of medical management in a public outpatient clinic." American Journal of Medical Science 252 (October):394–403.

Maddox, G. L., K. Back, and V. Liederman.
1968 "Overweight as social deviance and disability." Journal of Health and Social Behavior 9 (December):287–298.

Maddox, G. L., and V. Liederman.
1969 "Overweight as a social disability with medical implications." Journal of Medical Education 44 (March):214–220.

Matthews, V., and C. Westie.
1966 "A preferred method for obtaining

rankings: reactions to physical handicaps." American Sociological Review 31 (December):851–854.

Mayer, Jean.
1968   Overweight: Causes, Costs, and Control. Englewood Cliffs: Prentice-Hall.

Metropolitan Life Insurance Company of New York.
1959   "New weight standards for males and females." Statistical Bulletin 40 (November–December):2–3.

Monello, L. F., and J. Mayer.
1963   "Obese adolescent girls: an unrecognized minority group." American Journal of Clinical Nutrition 13:35–39.

Moore, M. C., A. J. Stunkard, and L. Srole.
1962   "Obesity, social class, and mental stress." Journal of the American Medical Association 181 (September 15):962–966.

National Center for Health Statistics.
1966   Weight by Age and Height of Adults: 1960–62. Washington: Vital and Health Statistics, Public Health Service Publication #1000, Series 11, #14, Government Printing Office.

Newman, James.
1957   Motivation Research and Marketing Management. Boston: Division of Research, Harvard Business School.

Seltzer, C. C.
1965   "Limitations of height-weight standards." New England Journal of Medicine 272 (May 27):1132.
1969   "Overweight and obesity: the associated cardiovascular risk." Minnesota Medicine 52 (August):1265–1270.

Seltzer, C. C., and J. Mayer.
1964   "Body build and obesity: Who are the obese?" Journal of the American Medical Association 189 (August 31):677–684.
1967   "How representative are the weights of measured men and women?" Journal of the American Medical Association 201 (July 24):221–224.
1969   "Body build (somatotype) distinctiveness in obese women." Journal of the American Dietetic Association 55 (November):454–458.
1970   "An effective weight control program in a public school system." Journal of the American Public Health Association 60 (May):679–690.

Sheldon, W. H., S. S. Stevens and W. B. Tucker.
1963   The Varieties of Human Physique. New York and London: Hafner Publishing Company.

Staffieri, J. R.
1967   "A study of social stereotypes of body image in children." Journal of Personality and Social Psychology 7 (September):101–104.

Stunkard, A. J., and V. Burt.
1967   "Obesity and body image II: age at onset of disturbances in the body image." American Journal of Psychiatry 123 (May):1443–1447.

Stunkard, A. J., and M. Mendelson.
1961   "Obesity and body image I: characteristics of disturbances in body image of some obese persons." Journal of the American Dietetic Association 38 (April):328–331.

Tarini, J. A.
1962   Do Fat People Like to Be Fat? Chicago: Weiss.

U.S. Public Health Service, Center for Chronic Disease Control.
1966   Obesity and Health. Washington: Government Printing Office.

Wyden, Peter.
1965   The Overweight Society. New York: Morrow.

Social Factors in Obesity

Phillip B. Goldblatt, MD, Mary E. Moore, PhD,
and Albert J. Stunkard, MD

The relationship between obesity and several social factors was investigated among 1,660 adults representative of a residential area in midtown Manhattan. An inverse relationship previously described between obesity and parental socioeconomic status was also found between obesity and one's own socioeconomic status. Obesity was six times more common among women of low status as compared to those of high status. Furthermore, upwardly mobile females were less obese (12%) than the downwardly mobile (22%). Finally, the longer a woman's family had been in this country, the less likely she was to be obese. Similar but less marked trends obtained for the men. Suggestive relationships between ethnic and religious factors and obesity were also found for both sexes. These findings suggest opportunities for more effective weight control measures through programs specially tailored for populations at high risk.

This report is an extension of our previous finding that social factors play an important role in human obesity.[1] Current theories as to the etiology of obesity, whether behavioral, biochemical, or physiological, have directed their attention to the individual. We were, therefore, very much interested in a finding incidental to our earlier study, which was undertaken to assess the relationship of mental health to obesity in a large, representative, urban population.[1] Parental social class, introduced as a controlling variable, showed a high correlation with the prevalence of obesity and was a more powerful predictor of overweight than a number of psychological measures. The present study, undertaken to investigate this relationship further, showed obesity to be related to each of the following additional social variables: the respondent's own socioeconomic status, social mobility, and generation in the United States.

From the Department of Psychiatry, University of Pennsylvania, Philadelphia.

Read in part before the Section on Nervous and Mental Diseases during the 114th annual convention of the American Medical Association, New York, June 24, 1965.

Reprint requests to 3400 Spruce St, Philadelphia 19104 (Dr. Stunkard).

Methods and Materials

The data reported here were collected as part of the Midtown Manhattan Study, a comprehensive survey of the epidemiology of mental illness. The details of the sample and the data collection techniques have been fully described elsewhere.[2,3] The data in the present analysis were obtained from the Midtown Home Survey of 1,660 adults, consisting of 690 males and 970 females between the ages of 20 and 59. One female in the Home Survey was omitted from our study because she was under four feet (122 cm) in height. The population was divided into three weight categories—"obese," "normal," and "thin"—based upon the self-reported heights and weights as described in our previous paper. The validity of such reports has been attested to by an independent survey.[4]

The relationships of these categories to the widely accepted standards for "desirable" weight of the Metropolitan Life Insurance Company[5] is shown in Table 1. The "desirable" weights are those for which the mortality rates are lowest, so that even the group which we have designated "normal" exceeds their "desirable" weight by about 10%. The means for our "obese" groups were 34% and 44% above the "desirable" weight, indicating a significant degree of overweight. The corresponding means for the "thin" groups were 13% and 16% below the "desirable" weight.

The respondent's own socioeconomic status (SES) at the time of the interview was rated by a simple score devised by Srole et al[2] based upon the respondent's occupation, education, weekly in-

Table 1.—Relationship of Midtown Home Survey Weight Categories to Standards of "Desirable" Weight*

Midtown Weight Category	Average % Over (+) or Under (−) Desirable Weight	
	Females	Males
Thin	−13	−16
Normal	+11	+ 9
Obese	+44	+34

*Standards of Metropolitan Life Insurance Company for desirable weight.

come, and monthly rent. Each of these four variables was subdivided into six categories. In the scoring, each variable was given equal weight. Thus, an individual in the lowest category of each variable (unskilled labor, no schooling, income less than $49 per week, and monthly rent less than $30) received a score of four. Conversely, an individual in all of the highest categories (high white collar, graduate school education, income over $300 per week, and monthly rent greater than $200) received a score of 24. (Unmarried working women were rated on the basis of their own occupation. Unmarried nonworking women were classified by their fathers' occupation. Married women, whether working or not, were rated on the basis of their husbands' occupation.) In order to obtain subgroups of sufficient size to permit control by variables which the analysis showed to be relevant, the population was divided into three socioeconomic groups as nearly equal in number as feasible. Individuals with scores of 4 to 10 were designated low status; those with scores of 11 to 16 were middle status; and those with 17 to 24 points were high status.

In our first paper we used the respondent's social class of origin as a controlling variable. This measure was employed so as to avoid any reciprocal relationship that might exist between a respondent's present SES and his obesity. Obesity may in part depend on social status but, at the same time, social status may in part depend on obesity. The SES of origin is a measure of important social influences on a respondent which are in no sense a product of his obesity. The social class of origin was based on the education and occupation of the respondent's father when the respondent was 8 years old.

The scores for SES of origin were divided into "low," "medium" and "high" socioeconomic categories in a manner analogous to that used for the respondent's own SES. These two sets of scores permitted us to study the relationship of obesity to social mobility by comparing the socioeconomic status of the respondent at the age of 8 with that at the time of the interview.

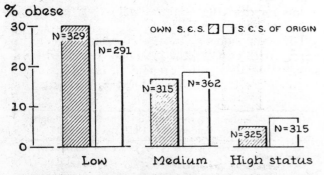

1. Decreasing prevalence of obesity with increasing socioeconomic status (SES). Data exclude one female about whom no information on the socioeconomic status of origin was available.

Results

The present analysis extended in a most dramatic way our previous finding of the importance in the understanding of human obesity of one socioeconomic variable—socioeconomic status of origin. Every one of the three additional social factors investigated was also strongly related to obesity. Furthermore, each was more strongly related to obesity among women than among men. The analysis of the data for women will be presented first.

Obesity Among Women.—Own Socioeconomic Status.—There was a marked inverse relationship between the prevalence of obesity and the respondent's own SES. Figure 1 shows that the prevalence of obesity among lower SES women was 30%, falling to 16% among the middle SES, and to only 5% in the upper SES. A chi-square test of the relationship between socioeconomic status and the three weight categories was significant at the 0.001 level ($X^2 = 120.7$).

Socioeconomic Status of Origin.—Just as the respondent's own socioeconomic status was inversely related to her obesity, so also was her socioeconomic status of origin ($X^2 = 66.5$, $P < 0.001$). This latter finding, reported in greater detail in our earlier study, is also shown in Fig 1. Note that the relationship between this factor and obesity was nearly as strong as that between the respondent's own socioeconomic status and her weight category.

Social Mobility.—The close correspondence between the results for the respondent's own SES and SES of origin suggested the possibility that these two variables were measuring the same underlying dimension. This would be the case in a society in which the vast majority of people lived out their entire lives in the same social class into which they were born. Such was not the case, however, in Midtown Manhattan which showed a high degree of social mobility. Indeed, 44% of the women belonged to a different social class from that of their parents. In other words, many people were classified differently by our two indices of social status, and these two variables did not measure the same underlying dimension. A measure of this discrepancy between the respondent's own SES and the SES of her origin is given by our index of social mobility.

Figure 2 shows the relationship of social mobility to obesity. Of women who remained in the socioeconomic status into which they were born 17% were obese, whereas among women who moved down in social status there was a higher prevalence of obesity (22%), while among those who moved upwards there was a lower prevalence (12%) ($X^2 = 20.5$, $P < 0.001$). Thus, movement *among* the social classes as well as membership *in* a social class was predictive of obesity.

Generation in the United States.—The fourth variable, generation in the United States, was also strongly linked to obesity. To assess this variable,

| | Generation | | | | | | | | | | | |
| | I | | | II | | | III | | | IV | | |
	Own SES Low	Own SES Med	Own SES High	Own SES Low	Own SES Med	Own SES High	Own SES Low	Own SES Med	Own SES High	Own SES Low	Own SES Med	Own SES High
Obese, %	30	21	7	34	19	6	22	6	2	13	4	4
N (100%)*	194	113	58	96	126	78	23	52	87	15	23	102

Table 2.—Percentage of Obese Females by Generation in United States—Controlling the Factor of Socioeconomic Status (SES)

*N = Number in sample falling into particular category, eg, 30% of 194 first generation low SES females are obese. Excludes two females about whom no information on generation is available.

respondents were divided into one of four groups on the basis of the number of generations their families had been in this country. Generation I consisted of foreign-born immigrants; generation II, of all those native-born respondents with at least one foreign-born parent; generation III, of all those who were native-born of native-born parents but had at least one foreign-born grandparent; and generation IV, of all those who had no foreign-born grandparents and who otherwise met the qualifications for generation III.

Figure 3 shows that the longer a woman's family had been in this country, the less likely she was to be obese. Of first generation respondents 24% were overweight, in contrast to only 5% in the fourth generation ($X^2 = 56.5, P < 0.001$).

It seemed probable that generation in the United States was closely related to socioeconomic status, and that the longer a family had been in this country, the higher its status was likely to be. The data in Table 2 show that this is indeed the case. Thus, in the first generation, 194 out of 365 respondents were of low SES, while in the fourth generation, 102 out of 140 were of high SES ($X^2 = 235.6, P < 0.001$).

To determine whether this phenomenon accounted for the finding that obesity was less common the longer a respondent's family had been in the country, we examined the prevalence of obesity for each SES within each generation. Table 2 clearly demonstrates that the inverse relation between obesity and generation was independent of socioeconomic status. Of the generation I respondents who were of low status 30% were obese, but only 13% of generation IV low-status females were overweight. This trend obtained in all the social classes (X^2 for low SES = 21.5, $P < 0.01$; X^2 for middle SES = 18.1, $P < 0.01$; X^2 for high SES = 21.5, $P < 0.01$).

Obesity Among Men.—The relationship between social factors and the prevalence of obesity among males paralleled that among the women, but in each instance was less marked.

OWN SOCIOECONOMIC STATUS.—There was an inverse relationship between his own SES and obesity. Figure 4, however, shows that the effect was far weaker than in the case of females ($X^2 = 17.4$, $P, < 0.01$). Whereas obesity was six times more common among women of lower socioeconomic status than among those of high status, the corresponding ratio among men was only 2:1.

SOCIOECONOMIC STATUS OF ORIGIN.—Socioeconomic status of origin had an effect upon the prevalence of overweight among men, although, as was true for women, the effect was weaker than that of the respondent's own SES. Furthermore, the influence of SES of origin was far weaker among men than among women. Whereas obesity was four times more common among women of lower socioeconomic status of origin than among those of high status, the corresponding ratio among males was less than 2:1.

SOCIAL MOBILITY.—Social mobility was even more common among the men in our sample than among the women, with 47% of the males belonging to a different social class than their parents.

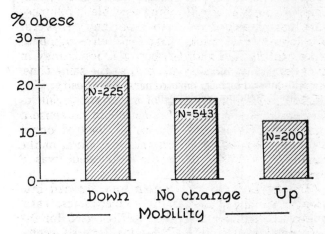

2. Decreasing prevalence of obesity with upward social mobility. Data exclude one female about whom no information on mobility was feasible.

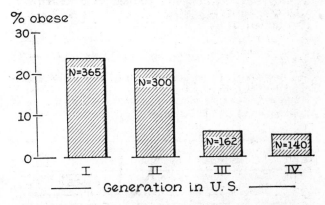

3. Decreasing prevalence of obesity with increasing length of time of respondent's family in United States. Data exclude two women about whom no information on generation in United States was available.

133

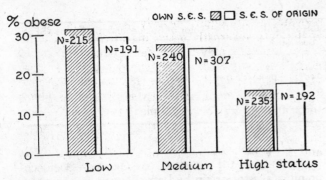

OWN S.E.S. ▨ □ S.E.S. OF ORIGIN

4. Decreased prevalence of obesity with increased socioeconomic status (SES).

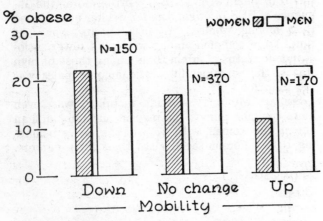

WOMEN ▨ □ MEN

5. Slight trend toward decreased prevalence of obesity with upward mobility among men as contrasted to significant trend among women.

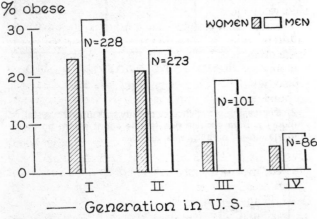

WOMEN ▨ □ MEN

6. Decreasing prevalence of obesity with increasing length of time of respondent's family in United States. Data exclude two men about whom no information on generation in United States was available.

Table 3.—Weight Categories by Respondent's Own Socioeconomic Status (SES)

Weight Categories	% of Each Weight Category in Each SES					
	Low SES		Middle SES		High SES	
	Males	Females	Males	Females	Males	Females
Thin	10%	9%	9%	19%	12%	37%
Normal	59	61	64	65	73	58
Obese	31	30	27	16	15	5
N (100%)*	215	329	240	315	235	325

*Number of individuals in sample falling into particular category.

Figure 5 shows the prevalence of obesity among those men who moved downward, stayed in the same class, or moved upward. Once again the same trend obtained as for females; in this instance, however, the chi-square did not reach a level of statistical significance.

GENERATION IN THE UNITED STATES.—Among the men as among the women the percentage of obese respondents decreased as the number of generations in the United States increased. Figure 6 reveals that obesity was three times more common among the males in the first generation as compared to those in the fourth generation ($X^2 = 18.7$, $P < 0.001$). There was, however, no sharp drop in the percentage of obese between generation II and III, as was the case among females. As among women, these findings resulted even when socioeconomic status was held constant.

The Thin Category.—At the beginning of the analysis of the weight categories, we expected that "thinness" would behave as though it were the opposite of obesity. We found, however, a striking difference in this regard between men and women. With increasing status, women moved from the "obese" to the "thin" category, whereas men moved from the "obese" to the "normal." Thus, thinness did operate as the opposite of obesity for women, but not for men. Table 3 shows that there were four times as many thin respondents among women of high status as there were among those of low status. Among men, however, about 10% were thin in all classes, and it was the percentage of normal-weight respondents that increased with increasing status.

Comment

The most important finding of this study was the remarkable consistency with which social factors correlated with body weight. Such a strong correlation, appearing in all the factors investigated, is highly significant. The only other attempt to study obesity as a social phenomenon, that by Pflanz[6] in Germany, has reported similar findings. It is now apparent that obesity can no longer be viewed as simply an abnormal characteristic of the individual. It must also be viewed as one of the possible, and not too infrequent, normal responses of persons in certain subgroups of society to the perceived expectations of their social milieu.

Although not being obese, indeed, being thin, seems culturally desirable for the women of Midtown, almost one out of three lower class females was obese. Such a high percentage implies that in this subgroup of Midtown society, overweight is common enough that it need not be viewed as abnormal.

In the Midtown society we do not have to look far to see the image of the slim, attractive female as portrayed throughout the popular culture. Motion picture stars, television personalities, women in advertisements, fashion models, and, indeed, the fashionable clothes themselves, all reflect the definition of the beautiful female as the one who is thin. How does such an ideal of beauty exert its impact on the body weight of persons in the different elements of society? At least two mechanisms seem plausible.

First, a selection process may operate so that in any status-conferring situation, such as a promotion at work or marriage to a higher status male, thinner women may be preferentially selected over their competitors.

Second, an acculturation phenomenon may be operating. For example, an individual's adult weight can be seen to be partly a product of social influences operating in his childhood. That this occurred in Midtown is demonstrated by our finding of a marked relationship between obesity and the SES of one's origin. A similar process may also be operating throughout life. Thus a female who acquires upper socioeconomic status for desirable attributes other than thinness will perceive that among her new peers more emphasis is placed upon being slim than was true in her old environment. She is likely, therefore, to make a greater effort to lose weight than she might previously have done.

The lesser importance of social factors as related to body weight among men, as contrasted to women, may arise from a lesser importance that society attaches to the physical appearance of men, as well as from a different definition of culturally desirable weight for them. In advertisements, for example, men are as likely to be exhorted to avoid being "97-lb weaklings," as to avoid being obese. It is, perhaps, not surprising that the normal weight category correlates so highly with upper socioeconomic status.

The extent to which a respondent has adopted the Midtown values about body weight apparently depends upon at least two factors: first, on the length of his family's exposure to these values (as measured by number of generations in the United States) and second, the amount of pressure to conform to these values, which is a function of his proximity to the upper classes where the values are most strongly exemplified.

Although generation and socioeconomic status are related to each other, it has been shown in this study that each makes an independent contribution to the prevalence of obesity. It is unfortunate that the size of the sample precluded more precise estimates of their relative contributions.

It is obvious that there were important differences among our respondents besides those of class and generation. The Midtown sample included nine ethnic groups (British, Russian-Polish-Lithuanian, German-Austrian, Irish, Puerto Rican, Italian, Hungarian, Czech, and fourth generation American) as well as many religions and sects. We discovered several relationships between ethnic and religious backgrounds and obesity. These were so intertwined with each other and with other social factors, such as generation and socioeconomic status, that we were unable to control all of the relevant factors simultaneously. Nevertheless, some of the data are worth describing briefly.

For example, only 9% of female respondents of British descent were obese, whereas 27% of those of Italian extraction were in this weight category. These differences diminished when social class was the control. Thus, for example, when only the upper classes of both ethnic groups were contrasted, the prevalence of obesity was 10% for the British and 20% for the Italian. Such differences can be related to what is known about the traditional diets and social implications of eating of these two ethnic groups. Joffe,[7] for example, has reported that first generation Italian mothers regard obesity in their children as protection against tuberculosis. Childs[8] found the basic diet of Italian-Americans to have a high fat content. Finally, a recent study in a small Pennsylvania town inhabited almost entirely by Italian-Americans revealed that the diet had a greater proportion of fat than that of the average American diet and that the prevalence of obesity was also significantly above average.[9]

Another example of such a phenomenon may be found among our data for Americans of eastern European extraction. Joffe notes that the Czechs love food and are less Americanized than the Poles as far as cooking habits are concerned. Among the Czechs, there is a great deal of visiting on Sundays during which time large quantities of food are consumed. Refusing a second or even a third helping of food is considered impolite. Our data reflect the results of these customs. Of the lower-class Czechs 41% were obese as compared with only 18% of the lower-class Polish-Russian-Lithuanians that were obese.

We also found differences among respondents of different religions. Lutherans, for example, were more often obese (24%) than Episcopalians (3%), but any statement made about the Lutherans and Episcopalians reflects also the difference between respondents of German and of British extraction. Unfortunately, we did not have enough cases to sift out the effects of religion per se.

What has been reported in this study about obesity in Midtown in 1954 is not necessarily applicable in toto to any other country, or any other urban area, or even to the Midtown of today. Indeed, Pflanz found an increased incidence of obesity among upwardly mobile German men and a decreased incidence among German women; in contrast, a decreased incidence among the upwardly mobile of both sexes was found in the present study. It thus appears that the same social mechanisms which discourage obesity among the socially mobile in this country may encourage it among German men. Even though Pflanz's specific findings differed from ours, his conclusion was the same: human obesity must be understood in part as a social phenomenon.

Many of the present theories about human obesity were formulated by psychiatrists on the basis of their treatment of middle and of upper class women, for whom obesity was a severe social liability. In other segments of society, however, obesity appears to be by no means such a handicap. Future researchers will have to explore the ways in which some respondents in all classes develop the attitude that a slim appearance is very important. Studies will be needed to determine the reasons why certain subgroups have a higher incidence of this belief than others, the mechanisms by which this belief is inculcated, and the ages at which it appears with differing frequencies in differing social classes. Future theories will have to take into account the differing implications of overweight for the different social classes.

It seems quite possible that the lack of success in the control and treatment of obesity stems from the fact that until now physicians have thought of obesity as always being abnormal. This is certainly not true for persons in the lower socioeconomic population. Obesity may always be unhealthy, but it is not always abnormal.

Unfortunately, our weight control programs have directed their appeals in a nonspecific way to rich and poor alike. The present study reveals an unexpected opportunity for increasing the selectivity of public health measures for the control of obesity. Would it not be more effective to initiate programs tailored specifically for subgroups of society where obesity is most common? The success of a similar approach has been demonstrated by Johnson et al,[10] who studied the epidemiology of polio vaccine acceptance in Dade County, Fla. They pointed up the importance of ethnic background and social class as an index of commonly held beliefs, shared feelings, group values and attitudes, and social participation. Utilizing such information in work with a high-risk population (lower class, Spanish-speaking residents of Dade County), they significantly increased the percentage of respondents who took polio vaccine over the percentage who had done so in previous campaigns.

The present study shows the feasibility of identifying obese populations at high risk. Such identification has generally been a prerequisite for effective public health programs. Recognition of the significance of social factors in obesity may lay the foundation for our first effective public health program for the control of obesity.

This investigation was supported by a Public Health Service research grant from the National Institute of Mental Health.

The data used in this study are from the Midtown Manhattan Study of the Department of Psychiatry, Cornell University Medical College and the New York Hospital, both in New York. Permission to use the data was granted by Alexander H. Leighton, Director of the Midtown Manhattan Study, but the contents of this paper represent independent work by the authors.

Technical assistance was rendered by several other members of the Midtown Group, especially Leo Srole, PhD, Stanley T. Michael, MD, and Thomas Langner, MD.

Financial support for the Midtown Study was provided by the National Institute of Mental Health, the Milbank Memorial Fund, the Grant Foundation, the Rockefeller Brothers Fund, and the Corporation Trust, all in New York.

References

1. Moore, M.E.; Stunkard, A.; and Srole, L.: Obesity, Social Class, and Mental Illness, *JAMA* 181:962-966 (Sept 15) 1962.

2. Srole, L., et al: *Mental Health in the Metropolis: Midtown Manhattan Study,* New York: McGraw-Hill Book Co., Inc., vol 1, 1962.

3. Langner, T.S., and Michael, S.T.: *Life Stress and Mental Health: Midtown Manhattan Study,* New York: The Free Press of Glencoe, Inc., vol 2, 1963.

4. Perry, L., and Learnard, B.: Obesity and Mental Health, *JAMA* 183:807-808 (March 2) 1963.

5. New Weight Standards for Men and Women, *Statist Bull Metrop Life Insur Co* 40:2-3 (Nov-Dec) 1959.

6. Pflanz, M.: Medizinische-soziologische Aspekte der Fettsucht, *Psyche* 16:575-591, 1962-1963.

7. Joffe, N.F.: Food Habits of Selected Subcultures in United States, *Bull Nat Res Council* 108:97-103 (Oct) 1943.

8. Childs, A.: Some Dietary Studies of Poles, Mexicans, Italians, and Negroes, *Child Health Bull* 9:84-91, 1933.

9. Stout, C., et al: Unusually Low Incidence of Death From Myocardial Infarction: Study of Italian American Community in Pennsylvania, *JAMA* 188:845-849 (June 8) 1964.

10. Johnson, A.L., et al: *Epidemiology of Polio Vaccine Acceptance — Social and Psychological Analysis,* monograph No. 3, Florida State Board of Health, 1962.

Influence of Social Class on Obesity and Thinness in Children

Albert Stunkard, MD; Eugene d'Aquili, MD; Sonja Fox; and Ross D. L. Filion, PhD

Several social factors have been closely linked to obesity and thinness in adults. This study, based on 3,344 measurements of triceps skin-fold thickness found similar relationships in white urban children. Obesity was far more prevalent in the lower-class girls than in those of the upper class—nine times as prevalent by age 6. Similar though less striking differences were found between boys of upper and lower socioeconomic status. The pattern of thinness among girls was similar to that previously reported in women, with significantly more thinness in the upper-class group. Among boys, as among men, there were no such differences. The remarkably early onset of class-linked differences in prevalence of obesity underlines the importance of attempts to prevent the disorder in childhood. These attempts should be directed particularly toward those at high risk because of their lower socioeconomic status.

This report continues our assessment of the influence of social factors on obesity in man. In earlier studies, carried out in New York City, we demonstrated a strong inverse relationship between socioeconomic status and obesity. Obesity was six times more prevalent among women of lower than among women of upper socioeconomic status.[1,2] Correlation between parental socioeconomic status and prevalence of obesity was nearly as strong, indicating that socioeconomic status was cause as well as correlate (Fig 1).

We also demonstrated significant inverse relationships between social mobility and obesity, and between number of generations in this country and obesity. In addition, several ethnic and religious variables appeared related to the prevalence of obesity.[3,4] Subsequently, we found similar results in a study in London.[5] In all these investigations, the relationship between social factors and prevalence of obesity among men paralleled that in women but in each instance was less marked.

The present study was designed to establish the age at which the influence of socioeconomic status on body weight becomes apparent. We also wanted to delineate the subsequent evolution of the relationship between socioeconomic status and obesity and thinness.

Materials and Methods

To assess the prevalence of obesity we measured the skin-fold thicknesses of 3,344 white school children in three Eastern cities. The 11 schools in the study were chosen so as to provide a population of both upper- and lower-class children. The respondent's socioeconomic status was determined on the basis of the father's occupation, according to *Intermediate Occupational Classification for Males*, a 1950 publication of the Bureau of the Census. The respondents were 5 to 18 years old.

We decided on the use of the triceps skin-fold thickness as the best index of obesity for a large field study on the basis of Seltzer and Mayer's extensive work with this measure,[6-9] as well as the view of Dugdale et al[10] that it is the best anthropometric measure of adiposity. Furthermore, Shephard et al[11] have presented evidence that the triceps skin-fold provides an especially accurate assessment of obesity in children and adolescents. To avoid interobserver error, all measurements were made by the same observer (S.F.), using the Lange skin-fold calipers. Reliability coefficient of the measurements was 0.93.

Since there is no generally accepted criterion for obesity in children, we chose two criteria that had been utilized in other studies and that seemed

From the Department of Psychiatry, University of Pennsylvania and the Philadelphia General Hospital, Philadelphia. Dr. Stunkard is now on sabbatical leave at the Center for Advanced Study in the Behavioral Sciences, Stanford, Calif.

Reprint requests to 3400 Spruce St, Philadelphia 19104 (Dr. Stunkard).

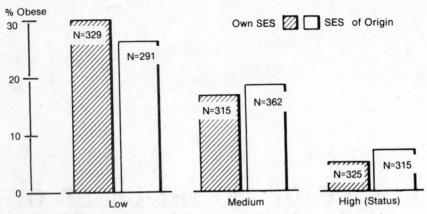

Fig 1.—Decreasing prevalence of obesity with increasing socioeconomic status (SES) among women in an Eastern city.

reasonable. The first criterion was the values for skin-fold thickness reported by Seltzer and Mayer in their study of Boston school children. They defined as obese those children whose skin-fold thickness exceeded one standard deviation from the mean for their age and sex. Table 1 shows the minimum triceps skin-fold thickness indicating obesity according to Seltzer and Mayer.[7]

Malina has criticized the Seltzer-Mayer criterion as inapplicable to other populations[12] and, indeed, the standard deviation for some age groups in our population differed from that of Seltzer and Mayer. Accordingly, we subjected our data to a second criterion of obesity. We also defined as obese the 10% of each sex in the total population that had the thickest skin-folds; and we used the minimum skin-fold thickness of this group to define obesity within each age group. Hampton et al effectively used a similar percentile criterion to define obesity and leanness.[13] In fact, according to Dr. Joseph Brozek, the percentile criterion is favored by many physical anthropologists, in part, at least, because it has the advantage of showing that obesity increases with age, a trend that is obvious in the raw data. Furthermore, by using percentiles we were able to define thinness in children, for whom no such standard is now available. We defined as thin the 10% of each sex with the thinnest skin-folds and analyzed the data as for the obese group. These empirically derived values for obesity were 23 mm for girls and 18 mm for boys. For thinness they were girls, 8 mm, and boys, 6 mm.

In the course of studying the 3,344 white children we measured also the skin-fold thicknesses of 1,903 black and Puerto Rican children. Since blacks, Puerto Ricans, and whites have different distributions of skin-fold thickness, it was not possible to analyze all 5,247 respondents as a single population. Hampton et al had also found significant differences in anthropometric measurements among teen-agers of different racial origins and cautioned against using the same standards for different races. Furthermore, the small number of upper-class blacks and Puerto Ricans made it impossible to run separate analyses of blacks and Puerto Ricans relating socioeconomic status to obesity. For these reasons the analysis reported here was confined to the 3,344 white respondents. Of these, 2,310 were classified in the upper socioeconomic status (occupational categories I and II by 1950 Bureau of Census listing); 857 were classified as of lower socioeconomic status (occupational categories III and IV); the remaining 167 could not be clearly classified. Table 2 shows the number of respondents at each age according to socioeconomic status and sex.

Results

We found marked differences in the prevalence of obesity between the upper- and lower-class children. Moreover, these differences were apparent by age 6.

Obesity in Girls.—Figure 2 shows the relationship between socioeconomic status and prevalence of obesity for girls, using the Seltzer-Mayer criterion. At age 6, 29% of the lower-class girls were obese as compared with only 3% of the upper-class girls. This class-linked difference continued through age 18, but fell to a minimum at age 12, when 13% of lower-class and 9% of upper-class girls were obese. Table 3 shows the four-fold contingency table relating high and lower social class obesity or its absence.

When we applied the percentile criterion, we also demonstrated the marked difference in the prevalence of obesity between social classes (X^2 = 70.838, $P < 0.001$). At age 6, the lower socioeconomic group contained 8% obese girls, while the upper-class group had no obese girls at either age 6 or 7. This difference was maintained until age 18, as with the Seltzer-Mayer criterion. In addition, the percentile criterion demonstrated an increase in the prevalence of obesity as a function of increasing age in both socioeconomic groups. Figure 3 shows further that the slopes for the upper and lower classes differ, with a greater yearly increment in the percentage of obese in the lower class. Obesity is not only more prevalent among poor girls, but this greater prevalence is established earlier and increases at a more rapid rate than among upper-class girls.

Obesity in Boys.—Lower-class boys showed a greater prevalence of obesity than did those of the upper class, although here the differences were not as striking as among the girls. Figure 4 shows the data for boys as analyzed by the Seltzer-Mayer criterion. At age 6, a marked difference between the two socioeconomic groups is already established, with 40% of the lower socioeconomic group classified as obese, compared with 25% of the upper-class group. Unlike the pattern among the girls, however, the difference between the boys is not continuous to age 18. Note the reversal at age 12, when the upper-class group has a greater percentage of obese. But by age 14 the lower-class group again shows a greater prevalence of obesity, and this difference is maintained until age 18. These data are summarized in Table 4.

Figure 5 shows the data for boys analyzed by the percentile criterion. Although the profile differs from that in Fig 4, where the Seltzer-Mayer criterion was utilized, the basic trend is

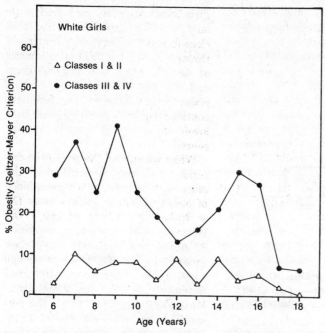

Fig 2.—Socioeconomic status and obesity by social class among girls (Seltzer-Mayer criterion). Lower class girls show far higher prevalence than upper class girls, especially during younger years.

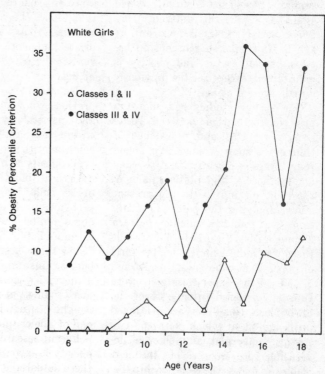

Fig 3.—Socioeconomic status and obesity by social class (percentile criterion). Apparent increase in prevalence of obesity with age probably reflects physiological facts.

Fig 4.—Socioeconomic status and obesity by social class for boys (Seltzer-Mayer criterion). Lower class boys show greater prevalence of obesity than upper class boys, but differences are less striking than among girls.

Fig 5.—Socioeconomic status and obesity by social class for boys (percentile criterion).

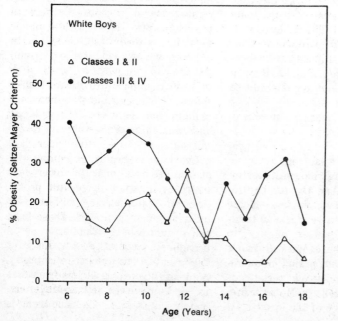

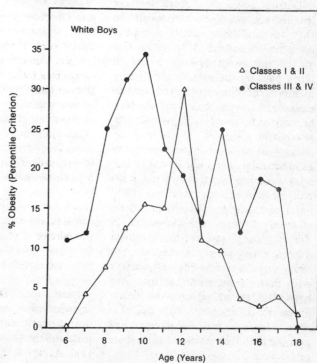

similar ($X^2 = 40.439$, $P<0.001$). Once again a significant difference between social classes is apparent by age 6. This inverse relationship between social status and obesity is maintained, except for the previously noted reversal at age 12.

Our earlier studies had shown a positive correlation between socioeconomic status and prevalence of thinness among women. We found four times as many thin women among those of high status as among those of low status. In the present study, applying the percentile criterion, we found a similar pattern among girls. Figure 6 shows that there was more leanness among girls of upper socioeconomic status. At age 6, 15% of the upper-class girls were thin as compared to only 4% of the lower-class. This difference continued until age 12, at which point the two groups converged and showed decreasing prevalences of thinness. Table 5 shows the relationship between high and low socioeconomic status and leanness or its absence.

Thinness in Boys.—Our earlier studies had shown no association between socioeconomic status and leanness among men. About 10% of each group was lean. The data on boys similarly failed to show such an association. Figure 7 demonstrates this absence of any clear trend.

Comment

During the past ten years, we have learned a great deal about obesity in the United States, and the results have been a surprise. Our conception of the nature of obesity, based in large part on the results of treating members of the upper and middle classes, has been shaken by the discovery that obesity is largely a problem of the lower classes. It now appears that socioeconomic status and related social factors have more to do with determining whether a person will be obese than does individual psychopathology.[1,14] The implications of these findings are far reaching. For one, they suggest that we need not be constrained by current psychodynamic formulations of obesity and their pessimistic outlook for treatment, when dealing with the group most afflicted with the disorder. Instead, an educational approach that recognizes the impor-

tance of social factors and is designed to influence the values and life-styles of large groups, may be more appropriate and more effective than conventional psychotherapeutic techniques.

The study reported here extends previous work and defines a discrete and particularly vulnerable group within the high-risk population—the children of the poor. Not only is childhood obesity a major problem in its own right, but the prognosis for the obese child magnifies the over-all problem for obese children become obese adults. The most authoritative estimate is that 85% of obese children follow this course.[15] Furthermore, the odds against an obese child becoming a normal-weight adult, which are more than 4:1 at age 12, rise to 28:1 if weight has not been reduced by the end of adolescence.[16]

Recent research into juvenile-onset obesity in laboratory animals adds to these actuarial cautions a possible explanation and a cause for further concern. In rats, the cellularity of adipose tissue, and consequently its lipid storage capacity, is determined very early—probably during the first three weeks of life—and primarily by the animal's level of food intake.[17] Overnutrition during this critical period leads to marked increase in the cellularity of adipose tissue, increased body size, and obesity; undernutrition has the opposite effect. Nor do changes in diet after infancy have any effect on the number of adipose cells. Caloric restriction reduces weight solely by reducing the lipid content of these cells, often to an abnormally low level. The depleted cells then remain ready to return to their initial levels of adiposity whenever sufficient lipids are available. By contrast, adult-onset obesity is produced by cellular hypertrophy, and weight loss returns the adipose tissue cells to a more normal size.

Although data of comparable precision for man are lacking, available information strongly suggests a similar pattern.[18,19] And the mechanism described offers a convincing biologic explanation for the remarkable tendency of juvenile-onset obesity to persist into adult life. We still do not know precisely what period in human development corresponds to the critical first three weeks in the rat's life.

However, the fact that such a large percentage of lower-class children is obese by age 6 suggests that hypercellular adipose tissue accounts for at least part of this increased incidence of obesity.

While we know that childhood obesity tends to persist into adulthood, we do not know what proportion of obese adults has juvenile-onset obesity. Even if the contribution is not greater than the one third that has been suggested, however, juvenile-onset obesity remains a serious problem. For all the pathologic correlates and sequelae of obesity are more prevalent and more severe in adults with juvenile-onset obesity, from diabetes and atherosclerosis to emotional disturbance. Furthermore, the juvenile-onset obese have special problems. Any psychopathology is likely to be related to obesity, and fully half of persons with juvenile-onset obesity suffer from body-image disturbances.[20] In persons with adult-onset obesity, on the other hand, psychopathology is usually coincidental and disturbance in body image rare.

One aspect of these findings deserves special note. The prevalence of thinness among the lower-class children was very low despite the poverty in which they lived. This finding surprised us, coming as it did in the midst of reports of widespread hunger among the poor, and its significance is unclear. Perhaps skin-fold calipers failed to detect evidence of undernutrition. However, they have proved adequate to the task of assessment of the undernutrition of anorexia nervosa. Perhaps the level of poverty associatied with frank undernutrition is lower than that of the children we studied. But we sought out the children with the lowest level of socioeconomic status that could be found in New York, Philadelphia, and Wilmington. It may be that white children, at least, in these cities do not suffer from undernutrition.

Conclusion.—Before we can institute effective measures to prevent or treat a disorder, it is helpful to define the population at high risk. This all-important step has now been taken for obesity. The lower socioeconomic class is the one with by far the greatest prevalence of obesity. Some of the preventive and therapeutic measures that this finding sug-

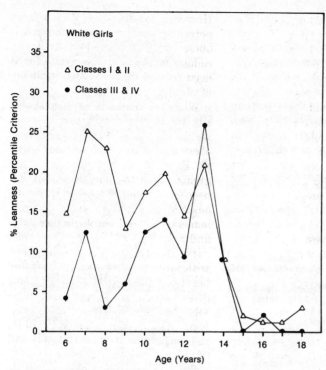

Fig 6.—Socioeconomic status and thinness by social class for girls (percentile criterion). Upper class girls show greater prevalence of leanness until age 12 when condition essentially disappears for both groups.

Fig 7.—Socioeconomic status and thinness by social class for boys (percentile criterion). Lack of association apparent.

Table 1.—Obesity Standards in White Americans According to Seltzer and Mayer		
	Minimum Triceps Skin-Fold Thickness Indicating Obesity (mm)	
Age (Yr)	Males	Females
5	12	14
6	12	15
7	13	16
8	14	17
9	15	18
10	16	20
11	17	21
12	18	22
13	18	23
14	17	23
15	16	24
16	15	25
17	14	26
18	15	27
19	15	27
20	16	28

Table 2.—Number of Respondents in Each Age Group by Socioeconomic Status (SES) and Sex				
Age (Yr)	Upper SES		Lower SES	
	Boys	Girls	Boys	Girls
5	47	5	21	25
6	67	34	27	24
7	71	40	17	16
8	79	56	24	32
9	80	54	16	17
10	90	52	26	32
11	107	56	31	21
12	74	77	33	32
13	84	76	38	31
14	103	66	44	44
15	167	84	42	53
16	216	80	48	55
17	206	80	29	43
18	114	33	19	15

gests have already been described.[1]

We have now taken a second step and pinpointed a discrete population at particularly high risk—the children of the poor. As early as age 6, the prevalence of obesity is far higher among the lower classes, particularly among girls, than it is among those of higher socioeconomic status. Furthermore, application of the percentile criterion, as illustrated in Fig 3, demonstrates that obesity is not only more prevalent in poor girls, but this prevalence is established earlier and increases at a more rapid rate than among upper-class girls.

These findings help define our task, and they should encourage us in the fight against obesity. For the remarkably early age at which obesity begins among so many of the poor bespeaks faulty nutritional practices by parents. We do not yet know to what extent these faulty nutritional prac-

Table 3.—Distribution of Obesity by Socioeconomic Status (SES) (Girls)*		
	Upper SES	Lower SES
Obese	41	93
Nonobese	747	332

*$X^2 = 81.367$, $P < 0.001$.

Table 4.—Distribution of Obesity by Socioeconomic Status (SES) (Boys)*		
	Upper SES	Lower SES
Obese	187	100
Nonobese	1,269	294

*$X^2 = 37.210$, $P < 0.001$.

Table 5.—Distribution of Thinness by Socioeconomic (SES) Status*		
	Upper SES	Lower SES
Thin	88	28
Nonthin	700	387

*$X^2 = 6.078$, $P < 0.02$.

tices result from lack of information or from lack of appropriate food. An effective program of obesity control among poor children requires that we distinguish between these two causes. Research that will enable us to determine more precisely what causes poor nutrition among the poor—nutritional misinformation or economic deprivation—is sorely needed. We have recently embarked upon such a project. One final note—Despite the poverty in which our lower-class children lived, they were no more likely to be thin than were the upper-class children.

This investigation was supported in part by a research grant MH-15383-03 from the National Institute of Mental Health.

References

1. Goldblatt PB, Moore ME, Stunkard AJ: Social factors in obesity. *JAMA* 192:1039-1044, 1965.
2. Moore ME, Stunkard A, Srole L: Obesity, social class, and mental illness. *JAMA* 181:962-966, 1962.
3. Stunkard AJ: Environment and obesity: Recent advances in our understanding of regulation of food intake in man. *Fed Proc* 27:1367-1373, 1968.
4. Stunkard AJ: Obesity, in Freedman AM, Kaplan HI (eds), *Comprehensive Textbook of Psychiatry*. Baltimore, Williams & Wilkins Co, 1967, pp 1059-1062.
5. Silverstone JT, Gordon RP, Stunkard AJ: Social factors in obesity in London. *Practitioner* 202:682-688, 1969.
6. Seltzer CC, Goldman RF, Mayer J: The triceps skinfold as a predictive measure of body density and body fat in obese adolescent girls. *Pediatrics* 136:212-218, 1965.
7. Seltzer CC, Mayer J: A simple criterion of obesity. *Postgrad Med* 38:A101-107, 1965
8. Mayer J: Some aspects of the problem of regulation of food intake and obesity. *New Eng J Med* 274:610-616, 1966.
9. Seltzer CC, Mayer J: Greater reliability of the triceps skinfold over the subscapular skinfold as an index of obesity. *Amer J Clin Nutr* 20:950-953, 1967.
10. Dugdale AE, Chen ST, Hewitt G: Patterns of growth and nutrition in childhood. *Amer J Clin Nutr* 23:1280-1287, 1970.
11. Shephard RJ, Jones G, Ishii, et al: Factors affecting body density and thickness of subcutaneous fat. *Amer J Clin Nutr* 22:1175-1189, 1969.
12. Malina RM: Patterns of development of skinfolds of negro and white Philadelphia children. *Human Biology* 38:89-103, 1966.
13. Hampton MC, Hueneman RL, Shapiro LR, et al: A longitudinal study of gross body composition and body conformation and their association with food and activity in a teen-age population. *Amer J Clin Nutr* 19:422-435, 1966.
14. Holland J, Masling J, Copley D: Mental illness in lower class normal, obese and hyperobese women. *Psychosom Med* 32:351-357, 1970.
15. Abraham S, Nordsieck M: Relationship of excess weight in children and adults. *Public Health Rep* 75:263-273, 1970.
16. Stunkard AJ, Burt V: Obesity and the body image: II. Age at onset of disturbances in the body image. *Amer J Psychiat* 123:1443-1447, 1967.
17. Knittle JL, Hirsch J: Effect of early nutrition on the development of rat epididymal fat pads: Cellularity and metabolism. *J Clin Invest* 47:2091-2098, 1968.
18. Salans LB, Knittle JL, Hirsch J: Role of adipose cell size and adipose tissue insulin sensitivity in the carbohydrate intolerance of human obesity. *J Clin Invest* 47:153-165, 1968.
19. Hirsch J, Knittle JL: Cellularity of obese and nonobese human adipose tissue. *Fed Proc* 29:1516-1521, 1970.
20. Stunkard AJ, Mendelson M: Obesity and body image: I. Characteristics and disturbances in the body image of some obese persons. *Amer J Psychiat* 123:1296-1300, 1967.

An Anthropological Approach to the Problem of Obesity

Hortense Powdermaker

M Y role as an anthropologist is to attempt to set the problem of obesity in the context of the culture. In this day of specialists we cultural anthropologists are the specialists in a holistic approach. In our studies of primitive or preliterate tribal societies, we have asked questions concerning relationships between different elements of culture. How are the functioning of the family, the economic and class organization, the political system, the religious and magical beliefs, the values that men live by, related to each other and integrated in that abstraction we call culture? In this chapter I shall give a cultural approach to the problem of obesity, raise questions, and, quite tentatively, offer some hypotheses. These will provide some understanding of the complexities of the problem and a basis for future research.

In setting the problem of obesity in the frame of the culture of contemporary society, my focus will be on the roles of food and of physical activity in our value systems. Incidentally, I wonder why so much of the education designed to reduce the incidence of obesity is centered on food rather than on activity. Is it assumed that food habits may be modified more easily than those of physical activity?

My basic questions are concerned with the symbolism of fatness and thinness in our society and the relationship of each to other symbols and to our values. I would be interested in differences in the symbols and in the relative strength of the same symbols in class, ethnic, religious, sex, and age groups, and among individuals. I would assume that there might be conflicting values concerning fatness and thinness, about eating and physical activity, as there are in many other areas of our life, and that some of this conflict might stem from the fact that we live in a rapidly changing society, where traditional values linger beside new ones. I would also be interested in the cultural study of people who are not obese as well as those who are, i.e. some kind of control group in which variables are limited. As an anthropologist, I am naturally interested in a comparative approach, i.e. the symbolism of obesity and thinness in other cultures and the many-sided role of food and eating in them, assuming that this comparative knowledge would illuminate the problem in our society.

Beginning with the last point, let me summarize briefly some relevant facts from pre-literate, tribal societies. In a large number of these societies the economy was a subsistence one, whether characterized by food gathering, hunting, fishing, agriculture, raising cattle, or some combination of these activities. A major part of all activity was concerned with the production of food. Tools were crude—a wooden hoe and a stone axe. The only means of transportation was by foot or canoe. Food-growing plots were often several miles from the village; the clearing of the dense bush in tropical and semi-tropical parts of the world by the men was a strenuous job, as was also the planting and weeding by the women. Strenuous physical activity was the norm for men and for women, whatever the type of economy. But although everyone worked hard and long in the production of food, hunger was a common experience. Famines and periods of scarcity were not unusual. Seasonal changes, plagues, pests, and many other natural causes tended to produce alternate periods of shortage and relative plenty. It is, therefore, not difficult to understand that gluttony, one of the original sins in our society, was an accepted and valued practice for these tribal peoples whenever it was possible. In anticipating a feast a Trobriand Islander in the Southwest Pacific says, "We shall be glad, we shall eat until we vomit."[1] A South African tribal expression is, "We shall eat until our bellies swell out and we can no longer stand."[2]

The function of food and eating was, and still is, not restricted to the biological aspects. Food is the center of a complex value system and an elaborate ideology centers about it. Religious beliefs, rituals, prestige systems, etiquette, social organization, and group unity are related to food. Throughout the Pacific, in Africa, and in most other parts of the tribal world, kinship groups work together in the production of food. Distribution of food is part of traditional obligations between people related biologically and through marriage ties, between clans, and between chiefs and their subjects. The accumulation of food, particularly for ritual occasions, is a major way of obtaining prestige. At all significant events in the individual's life history—birth, puberty, marriage, death—there must be a feast, and the amount of food reflects the prestige of those giving it. Less formal but of equal significance, is the relationship of food-giving to hospitality, valued even more among tribal peoples than among ourselves.

The importance of food is not limited to relations among the living. It plays a significant role in relationships with dead ancestors and gods. Offerings of food are made to them, so that they will grant the requests of the living and protect them from sickness and other misfortunes. The spirits of the dead and the ancestral gods presumably have to eat and, among some tribes, observe the same eating etiquette as do the living. In Haiti the gods are very demanding, and providing their food becomes a means of controlling and manipulating them, for the gods depend on men for their strength. In the same country death is symbolized in many instances as being "eaten" by evil gods and, in a modern context of a railroad accident, the locomotive is said to be a machine that eats people. This oral aggression of evil gods (and, presumably, the locomotive, too) is regarded as being motivated by the desire to acquire strength through being fed.[3] The function of food in magical and religious practices throughout the world is well known, and food taboos are part of many religious rituals in both tribal and modern societies. We could go on almost indefinitely describing the social role of food.[4, 5]

But we turn now to the more personal role of food for the individual. The infant's first relationship with his mother is a nutritive one. In primitive societies it is fairly common for a child to be nursed at his mother's breast for several years. For the infant in all societies, suckling and eating appear to be among the earliest sensory experiences and pleasures. The psychoanalysts call it the oral stage. We tend to agree with them that early infantile experiences have lasting effects. In some tribal societies such as the one I studied in the Southwest Pacific, the stomach is the seat of the emotions. "Bel belong me hot" is the pidgin English way of expressing deep feeling, whether occasioned by anger, sexual desire, or eating well.[6] The same concept appears in Africa and other parts of the world.

Given the scarcity of food and the ever-present fear of famine in many tribal societies, the significant social role of food, and the lasting impact of the infant's first sensory satisfactions, it is not surprising to find that stoutness or some degree of obesity is often regarded with favor. This is particularly true for the concept of female attractiveness. Among the Banyankole, a pastoral people in East Africa, when a girl began to prepare for marriage at the age of eight, she was not permitted to play and run about, but kept in the house and made to drink large quantities of milk daily so that she would grow fat. By the end of a year she could only waddle. "The fatter she grew the more beautiful she was considered and her condition was a marked contrast to that of the men, who were athletic and well-developed." The royal women, the king's mother and his wives, vied with each other as to who should be the stoutest. They took no exercise, but were carried in litters when going from place to place.[7]

Among the Bushmen of South Africa, the new moon is spoken of as a man because of its slenderness, and the full moon is a woman because of its roundness. Masculine and feminine endings are given to the same roots to denote sex: male endings for strong, tall, slender things and female for weak, small, round ones.[8] Today in a mining community on the Copperbelt of Northern Rhodesia where I have done fieldwork, in one popular song a young man sings,

> Hullo, Mama,* the beautiful one, let us go to town;
> You will be very fat, you girl, if you stay with me.

---

* "Mamma" is a term of address for a woman.

The standard of beauty for a woman here was not the fatness which we mentioned earlier, but rather a moderate plumpness.

Summarizing briefly for tribal pre-literate societies, we note that hunger was common and that a high proportion of men's and women's energy was spent in producing enough food to stay alive; that food was not only a biological necessity, but that its social and psychological functions were also very significant. The giving of food was a prominent part of all relationships: between kindred, between clans, with dead ancestors, and with gods. Food played a role in ritual, magic and witchcraft, and in hospitality. The accumulation of food was a mark of great prestige. Fatness was a mark of beauty and desirability in women.

We turn now to our contemporary society. It is characterized by an economy of plenty as compared to the economy of scarcity in tribal societies. We eat too much. We have too much of many things. According to the population experts, there are too many people in the world, due to the decline in mortality rates. A key theme in this age of plenty—people, food, things—is consumption. We are urged to buy more and more things and new things such as food, cars, refrigerators, television sets, and clothes. We are constantly advised that prosperity can be maintained only by ever-increasing consumption. This is in sharp contrast to our own not too distant past, when saving and thrift were among the prized virtues and emphasis was on production rather than consumption.

Another important change in our modern industrial society is that physical activity is almost nonexistent in most occupations, particularly those in the middle and upper classes. We think of the ever-increasing white-collar jobs, the managerial and professional groups, and even the unskilled and skilled laborers in machine and factory production. For some people there are active games in leisure time, probably more for males than females. But, in general, leisure time activities tend to become increasingly passive. We travel in automobiles, we sit in movies, we stay at home and watch television. Most people live too far away to walk to their place of work. Walking for pleasure is very rare. Former President Truman's daily walk is regarded as one of his peculiarities. The trend for those who are advised to take exercise and who also have the necessary wealth is a passive form—massage, the electric table which vibrates the body, and other electrical devices.

But while people may exercise less and live in an economy of plenty, they are becoming increasingly aware of the problem of obesity. There is a continuing enlargement of our knowledge of nutrition, of the relationship between obesity and certain diseases, and to health and longevity in general, and a wide popularization of this knowledge. This past month we had a "Nutrition Week," and every day our mass media—newspapers, radio and television—carried information about food and its relationship to health, disease, and physical attractiveness.

Our standards of beauty, particularly for the female, have undergone a great change from tribal societies and from our own past. The slender, youthful-looking figure is now desired by women of all ages. The term "matronly," with its connotation of plumpness, is decidedly not flattering. Although the female body is predisposed to proportionately more fat and the male to more muscle,[9] the plump or stout woman's body is considered neither beautiful nor sexually attractive. Our guess is that a hundred years ago the term "matronly" was not unflattering. The role of a wife today as an active sex mate, as compared to her role in our more Puritanical past with its emphasis on motherhood rather than on the pleasures of sexual experiences, may be significant in this context. For this and for other reasons the contemporary cult of youthfulness appears to be stronger among women than among men. At almost any middle and upper class gathering of middle-aged men and women, a large proportion of the latter will have dyed their hair, while most of the men will have the symbolic grey hair of aging. It is generally assumed that physical attractiveness is more important for the female than for the male in their respective search for a mate. Success, wealth, and vigor are significant eligibility criteria for potential husbands and fathers. Of course, sex appeal is important for men, too, but it seems not to be so much associated with seeming youthfulness as it is for women.

However, the cult of youthfulness is not confined to women. As science enables us all to live longer and longer, men and women want to remain young longer and longer. This is not a new desire. The quest for the fountain of youth is one of the well-known themes in mythology. The desire to remain healthy and "fit" as long as possible seems quite normal to us. Yet our excessive need to *look* young may also be related to other trends in our culture. Middle-aged people often find it difficult to get jobs, and they are faced with enforced, and sometimes unwanted, retirement at a fixed age. The cult of youthfulness may also have some connection with our apparent concern about sexual potency and sexual pleasure. Many books and articles discuss these as a difficult problem, and their large sale presumably indicates considerable anxiety about sexuality in our culture. Do people with this kind of anxiety have more, or less, difficulty in dieting and keeping their bodies young-looking?

We have indicated a number of strong trends in our culture which run counter to obesity. The desire for health, for longevity, for youthfulness, for sexual attractiveness is indeed a powerful motivation. Yet obesity is a problem. We ask, then, what cultural and psychological factors might be counteracting the effective work of nutritionists, physicians, beauty specialists, and advertisements in the mass media? We have a number of hypotheses. We think there may be considerable ambivalence for many people in regard to being fat or thin, to overeating or to dieting. This ambivalence could, in turn, come from conflicting patterns in our culture.

I have a hypothesis that, consciously or unconsciously, our symbolism for a maternal woman is on the plump or obese side. There is the figure of a pregnant woman and, as already indicated, the infantile satisfactions gained from food given by a mother or mother-surrogate. The image for mother and for mate may be in conflict.

Then, too, food is a very significant symbol in our prestige system. The kind of food, the quantity, and the manner in which it is served are among the important criteria of social class. In most tribal societies, even those with a highly stratified social system, everyone—royalty and commoners—ate the same kind of food, and if there was famine everyone was hungry. In our society there are sharp distinctions. Although there are probably relatively few people today who know sustained hunger because of poverty, poor people eat differently from rich people. Fattening, starchy foods are common among the former, and in certain ethnic groups, particularly those from southern Europe, women tend to be fat. Obesity for women is therefore somewhat symbolic for lower class. In our socially mobile society this is a powerful deterrent. The symbolism of obesity in men has been different. The image of a successful middle-aged man in the middle and upper classes has been with a "pouch," or "bay-window," as it was called a generation ago. We are all familiar with pictures of this type, resplendent with gold watch chain across the large stomach. Today this particular male class-symbolism is changing, probably because of the increased knowledge of the relationship of obesity to heart-malfunctioning and to other diseases.

Although slenderness becomes increasingly a symbol of social status, the food of the wealthy is still rich and plentiful, and their dinner parties are often, quite literally, a sign of conspicuous consumption. With the ever-increasing diversity of foods, food has become not only a matter of social status, but also a mark of one's personality and taste. More and more people are becoming gourmets, and with the declining number of servants, the hostess—and often the host, too—display their individual style and taste in cooking.[10] We become more personally interested in food as we become more aware of the problems connected with overeating.

The giving of food to people who are in trouble is a still widely prevailing folk custom and is reflected in our radio "soap operas." When someone is having marital or financial problems, or when there is illness in the family, a good neighbor brings in food and says, "You must eat to keep up your strength." The same correlation of eating with strength runs through many food advertisements, particularly those designed to reach young, growing children in the television audience. It would be interesting to do an analysis of the mass media advertisements of food which are directed toward children. It would be equally desirable to analyze the advertisements concerning reducing foods, pills, and other products, directed toward adults.

Our symbols for fatness or thinness are not clear-cut, as old and new patterns mingle. We have the beliefs that fat people are good-natured, contented, likable, funny, and also that they are foolish, "greasy," and greedy. There is the well-known image from Shakespeare's *Julius Caesar*, in which Caesar prefers his followers to be fat, and fears those who are lean and hungry.* A study of heroes and heroines and villains in our mass media, in terms of their fatness and thinness, might be revealing. I cannot offhand remember any fat movie villains, male or female. But this would be interesting to check.

While the family in our society is no longer an economic unit for the production of food, as it was in primitive society, the family meal remains one of the few times when the family is united and drawn together. Parents still are the givers of food, and most of us are aware of the intense interest with which young siblings watch mother cut a pie and their anxiety over whether the slices are even. This is true in homes where food is plentiful, and obviously food is a symbol for the mother's favoring or not favoring one child more than another.

Eating well, a full stomach, is still one of our main ways of achieving a state of euphoria. A really good dinner sets all of us up. This is probably connected with the fact that one of the earliest forms of security and of sensory pleasure is connected with the intake of food, and that about it are centered the first human relations. The eating of food and the giving of it thus remains a symbol of love, affection, and friendliness, as well as a source of pleasure in itself.

It is often stated and rather commonly believed that indulgence in overeating is a conscious or unconscious compensation for frustration or neurotic problems. We ask a further question: why do some people seek this form of compensation rather than another form? Is there, for instance, one type of person who tends to be alcoholic and another to overeat? A number of studies have indicated a comparatively low rate of alcoholism among Jews.[11, 12] They show that sobriety is a strong moral virtue among orthodox and pious Jews, and that drunkenness is associated with the outgroup, the Gentiles. The Jewish norms of moderate drinking and sobriety are

---

* "Let me have men about me that are fat,
  Sleek-headed men, and such as sleep o'nights:
  Yond Cassius has a lean and hungry look;
  He thinks too much; such men are dangerous."
   Shakespeare, William. *Julius Caesar*, Act I, Scene 2.

149

bound up with the ceremonial and ritual observances, with their religious beliefs, and with the value of remaining separate from Christians. It is assumed that Jews have the same proportion of neurotic and other problems that could lead to alcoholism as do Christians. The norms favored by any group for meeting problems are part of its culture and are internalized in childhood. It would be interesting to find out whether overeating and obesity are more common among orthodox Jews than among reformed Jews and Christians of the same class. We think, too, that there could be regional as well as religious differences in attitudes toward obesity. One suspects that there would be considerable difference between the South and New England.

We have a number of other questions concerning possible correlations of cultural and psychological factors with obesity. Is the ability to diet, and to diet consistently, related to belief in a measure of control over one's fate? Is it related to the strength of the belief in science? Is obesity correlated with orientations toward asceticism versus sensory pleasures? Has there been any study of obesity among monks and nuns? Do people who value sensory pleasures in general, such as those derived from perfumes, from physical contacts, from sexual experience, demonstrate an ability to diet more, or less, successfully than others? The degree of emphasis on sensory pleasure may be culturally determined, may vary from one historical period to another in the same culture, and from one class and ethnic group. And within each group there can be variations due to genetic idiosyncratic factors in the life history of individuals.

There are time limits to the number of questions we can raise. We have tried to indicate some of the cultural factors underlying the problem of obesity. Our society, with its economy of plenty and lack of physical activity, as compared to the economy of scarcity and the hard physical work in tribal societies, provides increasing opportunities for people to eat more food and to become obese. At the same time, other cultural factors, such as the knowledge of nutrition and of the relationship of obesity to disease and longevity and the popularization of the knowledge, our cult of youthfulness and the emphasis on the beauty of the slender body, particularly for the female, our class stereotypes, all tend to keep people from taking advantage of the opportunities to gorge on food. Yet there are many who overeat. We have hypotheses that this may be related to our deeply imbedded desire for the euphoria which comes from a full stomach, with other sensory indulgences or a lack of them, with conflicting imagery about a motherly woman versus a sex mate, with the use of food as a status symbol and as an expression of personality tastes, and with cultural norms about food and standards of beauty in different religious, class, ethnic, and regional groups. We have asked a number of questions relating to possible cultural correlations, for which there is no data. Mainly we have tried to show some of the intricate and complex ramifications of eating and of obesity in the tribal societies of the past characterized by too little food, and in our contemporary culture characterized by too much food.

REFERENCES

1. Malinowski, B.: *Argonauts of the Western Pacific*. New York, E. P. Dutton and Co., 1922, p. 171.
2. Kropf, A.: *Das Volk der Xosa-Kaffern*. Berlin, 1889, p. 88.
3. Bourguignon, E.: Persistence of folk belief: Some notes on cannibalism and zombis in Haiti. *J Am Folklore*, 72:42, 1959.
4. Richards, A. I.: *Hunger and Work in a Savage Tribe*. Glencoe, Ill., The Free Press, 1948.
5. Radcliffe-Brown, A. B.: *The Andaman Islanders*. Cambridge Univ. Pr., 1922.
6. Powdermaker, H.: *Life in Lesu. The Study of a Melanesian Society in New Ireland*. New York, W. W. Norton and Co., 1933, pp. 232-34.
7. Roscoe, J.: *The Northern Bantu*. Cambridge Univ. Pr., 1915, p. 38. Ibid., *The Banyankole*, 1923, pp. 116-17, 120.
8. Schapera, I.: *The Khoisan Peoples of South Africa; Bushmen and Hottentots*. London, Routledge and Keegan Paul, 1930, p. 427.
9. Scheinfeld, A.: *Women and Men*. New York, Harcourt, Brace and Co., 1943, p. 147.
10. Riesman, D., Glazer, N. and Denney, R.: *The Lonely Crowd*. New York, Doubleday and Co., 1953, pp. 168-69.
11. Bales, R. F.: The "Fixation Factor" in Alcohol Addiction: An Hypothesis Derived from a Comparative Study of Irish and Jewish Social Norms. Doctoral dissertation. *Arch Widener Libr*, Harvard Univ., 1944.
12. Snyder, C. R.: Culture and Jewish Sobriety: The Ingroup-Outgroup Factor. In *The Jews, Social Patterns of an American Group*, M. Sklare, ed. Glencoe, Ill., The Free Press, 1958.

Culture, History and Adiposity,
Or Should Santa Clause Reduce?

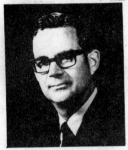

Kelly M. West, M.D.

"..a man hath no better thing under the sun than to eat, and to drink, and to be merry..."
Ecclesiastes 8:15

Prince Hal pretending to be King Henry IV denounces the corpulent Falstaff: "...that trunk of humors, that bolting hutch of beastliness, that swollen parcel of dropsies, that huge bombard of sack, that stuffed cloak bag of guts, that roasted...ox with pudding in his belly..."
Shakespeare
Henry IV: II, iv.

During the past several years I have had the good fortune to compare the fatness of thirteen populations in widely diverse parts of the world.[1-3] In several of these populations, I also had an opportunity to compare subpopulations of differing races, religions, and cultures. Results of these studies supported the view that the risk, extent, and prevalence of obesity are related to numerous and complex variables which include both genetic and environmental factors. One of the more impressive findings was the *degree* to which environmental factors may influence adiposity in populations with similar genetic makeup. For example, the

Address requests for reprints to: Univ. of Oklahoma School of Medicine, 800 N.E. 13th St., P.O. Box 26901, Oklahoma City, Okla. 73190.

the author . . .

about

Kelly M. West, M.D., Professor of Medicine and Continuing Education, University of Oklahoma School of Medicine, received his medical degree from the same institution. He is a past director of the Oklahoma Regional Medical Program.

middle-aged black women of Oklahoma have, on the average, about eight times as much body fat as their black counterparts in Panama! Under certain circumstances economic factors seem to play a predominant role. For instance, obesity was extremely rare in all the economically deprived subcultures of Pakistan and Malaya, and in the rural areas of El Salvador, Panama, and Guatemala despite widely varying cultural, environmental and genetic circumstances of these Chinese, Pakistani Indians. Malays, Hindus, Moslems, blacks, whites, and Central American Indians. After a certain critical level of economic attainment has been reached, the potential importance of other factors is often seen. In Uruguay, for example, we found that the urban people were much fatter than their rural counterparts even though income levels and racial origins were similar. But it is not my purpose to report here the results of these epidemiologic studies or to discuss the many factors which influence fatness. I will only be commenting upon what people in various societies of this and other ages have thought about how fat they and their peers ought to be, and upon the influence that these notions may have in determining the girth of the group.

"I am resolved to grow fat and look young till forty, then slip out of the world with the first wrinkle and the reputation of five-and-twenty."

John Dryden (1631-1700)
The Maiden Queen; III, i.

"O fat white woman whom nobody loves..."
Frances Cornford (1886-1960)
To A Fat Lady Seen From A Train

There is need for systematic research to define better the character and extent of the influences of peer group attitudes upon the adiposity of populations. Yet certain crude and unsystematic observations already strongly suggest that such influences are sometimes quite important. I am currently studying a group of Plains Indians who are exceedingly fat. Middle-aged women from this group believe they should weigh roughly 50 pounds more than what would be considered ideal by women from the upper-class white cultures of Oklahoma and the United States. In more systematic studies in girls five to 18 years of age from urban environments of the eastern United States, Stunkard and his associates found that obesity was nine times more prevalent in those from lower social classes than in those from upper classes.[4] Investigators have also found interesting links between obesity and other social and cultural factors such as religion, and inverse relationships with social mobility and period of time since immigration of the family to America.[5] When poor and more affluent children were compared in a sample representing the entire nation, there was not much class-related difference in adiposity in either boys or girls from six to eleven years of age.[6] In modern London, fatness of adult women is inversely related to social and economic status, but the men of the lower classes are leaner than men of the middle classes.[7]

"I don't want her, you can have her, she's too fat for me."

Ross MacLean and Arthur Richardson
Too Fat Polka, American popular song of 1947

"W'at good eesa wife eef she don'ta be fat?"

Thomas Augustine Daily (1871-1948)
Da Stylish Wife

The explorer Speke was the first white man to encounter the East African kingdom of Karagwe. He gave a fascinating account of the extraordinary corpulence of the young girls in the King's harem. Apparently certain elements of this culture had assigned a close relationship between sex appeal and adiposity. The harem girls "were so fat they could not stand upright, and instead grovelled like seals about the floor of their huts. The diet was an uninterrupted flow of milk that was sucked from a gourd through a straw, and if the young girls resisted this treatment they were force-fed like the *pate de foie gras* ducks of Strasbourg: a man stood over them with a whip."[8] By comparison, the nudes painted by Peter Paul Rubens in 17th century Holland were slender. Even so, I have estimated that these well-padded young women of Rubens would have had triceps skinfolds of about 30 millimeters and weights exceeding our present "ideal" by about 35%. Since these bountiful maidens were probably idealized conceptions of the same general culture from which ours and that of modern Western Europe is derived (the *Playboy* centerfolds of their time), it is interesting how much these ideals may change over time in the same culture. The present "Miss Holland" or "Miss New York" (Miss New Amsterdam) is likely to have a triceps skinfold of about 16 millimeters, a height without shoes of 67 inches and a weight (in her bikini) of approximately 120 pounds.

It is also interesting that the dimensions of modern Western sex appeal are well *under* the medians for "desirable" or "ideal" weights suggested by the weight-for-height charts that are so widely employed in the same culture. These height-weight standards have some appropriate uses, but they are sometimes given an official and definitive status that is hardly justified by the circumstances of their derivation. The need for caution in using these charts is well exemplified by noting that Miss America in recent years has a weight that is typically 10% to 15% below standard, while All-American football players are on the average about 25% "overweight."

"He was a lord ful fat and in good point (shape)."

Chaucer
Prologue to *Canterbury Tales*

Concepts of ideal weight within both previous and present societies have often been multifaceted, with optimum fatness being assigned on the basis of role, function, age, sex, and so forth. In most Polynesian societies, before the white man arrived, the natural and appropriate state for men and women was leanness; yet even then people of royal blood were often quite corpulent. In many cultures women are expected to be substantially fatter than men. Comanche Indians (men and women) now expect women to gain considerable weight between ages 20 and 40, while men are not expected to gain so much. This view is also held in certain Italian subcultures, while leanness is considered the natural state in both middle-aged men and women by Indians of rural Guatemala. Before this century, the Comanche Indians of both sexes and of all ages were almost uniformly lean, but occasionally those of special prominence and affluence were fat. For example, the richest Comanche of the buffalo era was a chief who owned 1500 horses. He was so fat, however, that he could not mount or be lifted upon any of these horses. (His name was Chief Big Fall By Tripping.) This phenomenon has also been observed in Caucasian societies. The Englishmen ruled by Henry VIII were quite lean, but he became so fat that special machinery was sometimes required to transport him from one part of his castle to another. Another slim society was ruled by Louis the Fat. This 11th century French monarch was Louis VI. His precise dimensions are unknown, but he was also known as "the bruiser." He was a popular and respected king, and circumstances suggest that in his case the term "fat" was descriptive but not pejorative. Apparently people regarded fatness as unusual even in kings—but not necessarily undesirable. Even in certain modern societies adiposity is prestigious. This is true, for example, in Fiji and in certain Polynesian cultures.

Very little specific data are available prior to the 20th century on the frequency distribution of adiposity in populations, even on the most famous citizens of these societies. Although Leonardo da Vinci had designed a self-indicating scale in the early 16th century, such devices were little used to weigh people until very recent times. Because of the paucity of specific scientific data concerning the adiposity of previous societies, we must look to the work of their writers and artists to gain insight on how fat people were and how fat they wanted to be. The examples given here from literature and the arts are not offered as scientifically representative samples. But even though the selection process was arbitrary, I do believe the examples will serve to illustrate the main point that, to a strong degree, cultural notions shape, and are shaped by, the fatness of a society. Using these parameters of art and literature, I have been unable to identify in history a general population where the prevalence of obesity approached that now seen in some of our modern subcultures such as the Pima and Comanche Indians, certain Polynesian communities, and the middle-aged black women of several societies. Obesity is common enough in American white women, but the data of a recent National Health Survey showed that the mean weight of American black women (of equal height) was eleven pounds greater.[9] In contrast, black men were four pounds lighter than their white counterparts.

"Other men live to eat, while I eat to live."
Socrates

"Reason should direct and appetite obey."
Cicero

"A well-governed appetite is a great part of liberty."
Seneca

Apparently ancient societies, both civilized and barbaric, were thin. Sages of ancient Greece and Rome usually idealized continence of appetite and silhouette. The prevalence of these admonitions suggests, however, that obesity was not unknown even though it was probably uncommon in the privileged classes and quite rare in the masses. Venus de Milo is not at all skinny, but she is decidedly more slender than the aforementioned young ladies of Rubens. The adiposity of Venus is roughly equivalent to that of Lillian Russell who served as a "pin-up" girl for our soldiers in the Spanish-American war. Venus de Milo is somewhat better endowed with fat than most other products of the ancient artists. For example, in the National Museum of Naples a drawing created in 400 B.C. shows five Greek women playing at knucklebones. All are considerably more slender than Venus de Milo. Perhaps to some extent the recent fame of Venus de Milo may be attributed to the tastes of the more modern European societies who came to prefer women whose fat depots were relatively well-developed.

An extraordinary Egyptian wall painting decorates the tomb of Huy, or Amenhotep, viceroy in Nubia during the reign of Tutankhamen (1361-1352 B.C.). The several princes and a single princess who are shown are all exceedingly slender. I would estimate their body weights at 80 percent of our present standard, and their triceps skinfolds at about three millimeters. Wall paintings in Turkish Anatolia created about 8,000 years ago show a series of slender men.

"Eat with moderation...What can procure digestion?—Exercise."
Voltaire (1694-1778)

Generally speaking, the invention of agriculture made it possible for some royal personages to become fat, while the industrial revolution brought this prospect within reach of the common man. The industrial revolution greatly increased food supply by making food production more efficient. But quite possibly its effect on human energy expenditure was even more important in increasing the risk of obesity. Even in very privileged circumstances obesity seemed to be rather uncommon before physical exercise was made virtually unnecessary in much of the western world by the technologic acumen of recent generations.

"A fat paunch never breeds fine thoughts."
St. Jerome
Letter to Nepotian

For the Dark Ages not many models are available, but for the most part depictions were of slender people. A 12th century manuscript is decorated with a picture showing a group of monks paying their respects to the King of France and his party as they depart on a crusade. All of the twelve persons shown are slender, including the King. The main portal at the Chartres Cathedral has upon it a large number of carved figures. Even the kings and queens are slender, suggesting that Europeans of the Gothic period probably regarded leanness as the natural state of man. The Gothic statues now at St. Denis show a very slender Solomon and Queen of Sheba.

"Mothers soften their children with kisses and imperfect noises, with the pap and breast milk of soft endearments; they rescue them from tutors, and snatch them from discipline, they desire to keep them fat and warm and their feet dry, and their bellies full, and then the children govern, and cry, and prove fools and troublesome."
Jeremy Taylor (1613-67)
Holy Dying; III

"He was one of lean body and visage, as if his eager soul, biting for anger at the clay of his body desired to fret a passage through it."
Thomas Fuller
Life of Monica (1642)

The creations of the artists of the Renaissance were somewhat variable in build but usually ranged from slender to medium. In general, girth increased from early to late

Renaissance. The women of the artist Sasseta (born about 1392) were decidedly slender, while those of Raphael, Leonardo, and Michaelangelo were a bit fatter. We would now regard most of them as having average adiposity. Indeed, from the time of the Renaissance until the present, there has been within each era considerable evidence of a spectrum of opinion about the optimum degree of adiposity. Thus, as noted above, Jeremy Taylor was concerned in the 17th century about flabby children, while his contemporary, Fuller, reflected on the unwholesomeness of leanness. It is an indication of Shakespeare's genius that he recognized and expressed so well the divergent notions men have held about leanness and fatness. The quotation above from Jeremy Taylor illustrates the divergence of opinion that has often prevailed among and within past and present cultures about whether it is good for babies to be fat. It would also be interesting to study the attitudes of various cultures concerning the optimum adiposity of pregnant women. The possible importance of these notions concerning maternal and infant adiposity is indicated by recent work which suggests that the number of fat cells may be determined very early in life.

Although there seems to have been a crude association between the fatness of a society and the adiposity of the depictions of its artists, this relationship is of course imperfect. It would seem, for instance, that most young women of the time of Rubens were more slender than his creations. The 19th century French illustrator-artist Doré was fond of drawing fat men, perhaps because he was good at it. Even though obesity was not rare in his age, its prevalence in his excellent work might mislead one. Thus, considerable caution is warranted in such judgments. But one is impressed, for example, with the substantial difference in the average fatness of the representations of 12th century artists as compared with those of the 17th and 18th century artists.

"In general, mankind, since the improvement of cooking, eat twice as much as nature requires."

Benjamin Franklin

"Why shud a woman want to be thin unless she is thin? Th' idee iv female beauty that all great men, fr'm Julius Caesar to mesilf, has held is much more like a bar'l thin a clothespole."

Dissertations by Mr. Dooley
Royal Doings (1906)

The beautiful statue of "The Bather" by Houdon (1741-1828) suggests a weight of about 90% of our present standard and a triceps skinfold of about 12 millimeters. In contrast, nude creations of other artists of that era exhibit a more abundant adiposity. We see, of course, the same diversity of taste within our own society, some elements of which prefer Audrey Hepburn and Mia Farrow while others prefer the more abundant Sophia Loren. In the 1930s we had both Greta Garbo and Mae West.

There seems to have been less variation through the ages in the adiposity of the idealized young man. The degree of muscularity preferred seems to have been more variable than fatness. The Davids of Bernini, Donatello, and Michaelangelo are all lean, but the muscularity of these three figures varies markedly. Men of Britain and the United States have been growing heavier in recent generations, while women in these two countries are a bit more slender.[10] It seems quite likely that cultural standards have had something to do with this recent trend in women toward slimming in certain affluent cultures. Although almost all societies have idealized the lean young man, there is divergence and ambiguity concerning the extent to which weight gain with age is natural and desirable. Even *within* past and present cultures there is some remaining disagreement on this point. Nor have modern scientists reached a consensus concerning whether adults are entitled to a modest weight gain as the years go by.

"For the sake of health, medicines are taken by weight and measure, so ought food to be, or by some similar rule."

Philip Skelton (1707-1787)

"They have digged their grave with their teeth."

Thomas Adams' Works (1630)

"They are as sick that surfeit with too much as they that starve with nothing."

Shakespeare
The Merchant of Venice; I, ii.

This discussion has concerned mainly the esthetic aspects of cultural attitudes, but of course this is only one of several culture-related factors that may affect adiposity. These include prevailing opinions about what and how much should be eaten by whom how often under what conditions; and views on exercise. Another factor is the attitude of the society concerning the optimum adiposity for good health.

Most ancient and modern sages have related health and longevity to leanness. It is well known that in many past and present cultures, corpulence has been considered a sign of good health. Apparently the peers of Chaucer held such a view (see above). Most of my older Oklahoma Indian women patients worry a little when my diets cause them to fall below 170 pounds. And many say they don't feel as well when they are so peculiarly "thin." They tell me of concerns of friends and family to whom they may appear dangerously frail at weights under 200.

"Let me have men about me that are fat."
(line of Julius Caesar)
Shakespeare
Julius Caesar, I, ii.

"... If to be fat be to be hated, then Pharoah's lean kine are to be loved."
Shakespeare
Henry IV, I, ii.

The modern Japanese ideal is still a relatively lean model, but the highly corpulent Sumo wrestlers are great heroes for whom weights of 400 pounds are deemed quite natural. Even though most oriental populations are and have been quite lean, it is interesting that many depictions of Buddha are decidedly fat. But it is also noteworthy that the adiposity of the figures of Buddha is quite variable among various oriental subcultures, and has changed with time in some of these cultures. It is said that Buddha was reared in luxury and was the son of a king.

That wonderful and generous personage, Santa Claus, had "...a little round belly, that shook when he laughed, like a bowlful of jelly."
Clement Clarke Moore (1779-1863)
A Visit from St. Nicholas

"Leave gourmandizing: Know the grave doth gape for thee thrice wider than for other men."
Shakespeare
Henry IV; V, v.

From a recent informal and unscientific poll I learned that most Americans still believe that Santa Claus ought to be fat. A majority told me they would make him at least a little fat even if they had an opportunity to reinvent him. None of my interviewees had given much thought to the possibility that Santa might be sustaining an increased risk of diabetes, arthritis, and hypertension. Apparently it was the popular view that, if he could fly a well-stocked and very heavy sled without the assistance of wings or jets, he could be expected to attend successfully to the trivial problems of operating his metabolism. It is, however, noteworthy that the degree of corpulence of Santa Claus, Kriss Kringle, Saint Nicholas, and Father Christmas has varied among cultures, and over time in the same culture.

"Lean, hungry, savage, antieverythings."
Oliver Wendell Holmes
A Modest Request: the Speech

"Who ever hears of a fat man heading a riot, or herding together in turbulent mobs."
Washington Irving
Knickerbocker's History of New York

I did not gather enough data to determine definitely why America expects Santa to be fat. But it would appear to be mainly attributable to the still prevalent feeling that the various degrees of adiposity have associations with certain characteristics of personality, mood, and behavior. Santa is fat; villains are usually lean; the devil is usually very lean; and witches are always skinny to the extreme. Even those who believe it is unhealthy to be fat usually "feel" a certain

association between generosity of adiposity and generosity of spirit; while leanness and meanness are still linked to some degree by most cultures.

Many important cultural effects on adiposity are indirect. Cultural attitudes may, for example, affect economic and social conditions with indirect but important effects on adiposity.

A Conclusion

The purpose of this essay has been more to entertain than to instruct or enlighten, but it is my hope that this discussion will dramatize the very considerable importance of culture and attitude on susceptibility to obesity. It is probably fair to say that our past and present efforts to prevent and mitigate obesity have been largely a failure. We need to "re-think" our approaches to what has become a very serious problem in many societies. Of course we do need more fundamental research on the genetic, metabolic, and biochemical phenomena that are relevant in the pathogenesis of obesity. At the same time we need to keep in mind the profound effects of environmental factors in this blubber epidemic.

The opinions, feelings, and attitudes that people have about adiposity are only one element of the spectrum of these environmental factors. Moreover, our knowledge of the extent and character of these "cultural" effects is still rather limited. There is now, however, enough evidence available from the experiences of history and through recent scientific observations to suggest the crucial role of these attitudes in determining the risk of obesity. Finally, an urgent need is evident for further systematic studies of interactions between cultural factors and the adiposity of various elements of society.

REFERENCES

1. West KM and Kalbfleisch JM: Influence of nutrition on prevalence of diabetes. *Diabetes* 20:99, 1971.

2. West KM: Epidemiologic evidence linking nutritional factors to the prevalence and manifestations of diabetes, in Froesch ER and Yudkin J, eds, *Nutrition and Diabetes Mellitus, VI Capri Conference*, Italy, Il Ponte, 1972, pp 405-28.

3. West, KM: Epidemiology of adiposity, in *Proc Internatl Conf on Adipose Tissue Mass*, Marseilles, 1973. *Excerpta Medica*, 1974. In press.

4. Stunkard A et al: Influence of social class on obesity and thinness in children. *JAMA* 221:579, 1972.

5. Goldblatt PB, Moore ME, Stunkard AJ: Social factors in obesity. *JAMA* 192:97, 1965.

6. Hamill PVV, Johnston FE and Lemeshow S: Height and weight of children: socioeconomic status. *U.S. Data from the National Health Survey, National Center for Health Statistics. Series 11, No 119*, DHEW Publication (HSM) 73-1601, 1972.

7. Silverstone JT, Gordon RP and Stunkard AJ: Social factors in obesity in London. *Practitioner* 202:682, 1969.

8. Speke J: in Moorehead A, *The White Nile*, New York, Harper and Row, 1960.

9. Roberts J: Personal communication in 1973 of unpublished data of the National Center for Health Statistics obtained in 1960-62 by the National Health Survey.

10. Montegriffo VME: Height and weight of United Kingdom adult population with a review of anthropometric literature. *Ann Hum Genet* 31:389, 1968.

Part III: Weight Control Fads and Fallacies

Many overweight people are so anxious to lose weight that they can be sold any program which promises to help them take it off easily. Various dietary and weight reducing regimens, ranging from bizarre faddish diets to mechanical devices that will melt the pounds away have been explored in quest of a way to achieve that "ideal" figure.

According to the Food and Drug Administration, 10 million Americans spend at least half a billion dollars annually on diet books, programs, and cures for real or imagined nutritional ills. Trick reducing diets, mystery foods, weight control pills, candy, and other contrivances for losing pounds painlessly are bought and paid for by persons of both sexes and all ages. They either fool themselves or are uninformed to the degree that they can be convinced that fad diets and other devices may be a substitute for their inability to maintain a satisfactory level of weight. Fatality or actual physical harm, or both, may be involved in the use of many quick weight reducing schemes.

Scientific journals and reliable mazagines try continually to combat unwarranted enthusiasms for fad diets, whether they are the "Hollywood" or the "holiday" diet, or the frivolous or fabulous formulas. But there are still "miracle diets," "revolutionary discoveries," and "reducing formulas" that are worded to appeal to the overweight college professor as well as to the buxom socialite. Advertisements offer tablets that will "flush fat right out of your body," "tranquilize away your reducing problems," encourage you to "drink your fat away with a reducing cocktail," or "lose ugly fat without dieting or hunger—no calorie counting! no diets! no exercise!" Testimonials such as "I thank you for my new body" or "My husband asked me for a date"

play upon emotions rather than appeal to intelligence.[1] These exaggerated claims and similar ones have aroused concern in government circles as well as among health personnel and educators.

This section is a discussion of some of the common weight control fads and fallacies as presented by some of the leading authorities in the field.

It should be obvious that one important way of dealing with such myths and encouraging proper diet and weight control lies with a longitudinal program of nutrition education, particularly with the young.

It seems that workers and educators have the right and, indeed, the obligation to present to the public information that will make for rational decisions. It is highly desirable to communicate knowledge about the association between overeating and longevity and between overeating and disease. It further seems appropriate to communicate information on the availability of effective control methods, assuming such technology is developed. Information does not necessarily create motivation to behave adaptively, but neither can there be motivated, adaptive behavior in the absence of information. Those most unlikely to behave adaptively are people who do not believe that they are overweight, or that being overweight has negative effects on health and longevity, or those people who have no confidence that there are effective means to change their habits or who are using ineffective "fad" methods. People who have been properly informed may choose *not* to behave adaptively—and the choice is theirs—but the probability of adaptive behavior will be increased.

[1]Mitchell, Helen S. "Don't Be Fooled by Fads," *Food — The Yearbook of Agriculture.* 86th Congress, 1st Session, House Document No. 29.

DIET MADNESS

What hazards lie in many well-publicized schemes for quick weight loss?

Walk into any bookstore today and you'll find a section marked "Diet Books" right next to "Cookbooks." Open any newspaper, tune in the TV, and you'll be confronted with ads urging you to "reshape your figure through our program of exercise and nutritional guidance." Attend a cocktail party and your opinion of the latest diet fad will be eagerly sought. Listen in on any conversation and you're sure to hear something like this: "I simply *have* to lose some weight!"

Weight control has become a national obsession—and it's not surprising. Fully one-third of the American population is overweight. According to weight-mortality statistics gathered by insurance firms, half the men between the ages of 30 and 39, and almost as many women, are 10 per cent overweight and one-fourth are at least 20 per cent too heavy. Between the ages of 50 and 59, almost two-thirds of the population in that age bracket is 10 per cent overweight and one-third is 20 per cent over ideal weight.

Data on children are not as readily available. But based on his observations, Dr. Jean Mayer of Harvard University's School of Public Health estimates that 10 per cent of schoolchildren weigh too much.

No one is unaware of the dangers of being fat. Conditions associated with obesity—diabetes, diseases of the digestive system, cerebral hemorrhage and heart disease—contribute to a mortality rate nearly one-half greater than that among those at ideal weight. The cost of being fat, in terms of comfort, appearance, and social ease, is also considerable.

Diet fads

Americans rightly want to lose weight, say the country's nutrition experts. But they're going about it in the wrong way. Diet experts are concerned that overweight Americans are risking their health and that of their children, including the unborn, on fad diets advanced by dieticians, physicians, do-gooders, and quacks. Most overweight people, if asked what they expect from a diet, will reply: "A method of losing weight that's quick and easy," and, only as an afterthought will they add, "One that's safe."

Over the years Americans have been urged to try the ice cream diet, the lollipop diet, the champagne diet, the sweet tooth diet, the grape diet, the whipped cream diet, the cottage cheese diet, the coffee and cigarette diet, the Zen macrobiotic diet, the water diet, the grapefruit diet, the egg diet, the raw food diet, the working man's diet (eat sensibly Monday through Friday, eat anything weekends), the Roman orgy diet (gorge and vomit), the total fasting diet (eat nothing) . . .and so on.

Deluge of books

The public has been deluged by books ever since William Banting, a London undertaker, published a pamphlet in 1863 entitled *A Letter on Corpulence Addressed to the Public*, in which he revealed how at the age of 66, he lost 46 pounds in a few months by following a meal plan that Dr. William Harvey had given him to treat his deafness—avoid bread, butter, milk, sugar, beer, soup, potatoes, and beans; instead eat only flesh, fish, and dry toast.

The years that followed have brought *Eat and Grow Thin: the Mahdah Menus; Why Die?; Faith, Love and Seaweed; How I Lost 36,000 Pounds;* the *Amazing Hypno-Diet; Pray Your Weight Away; Edgar Cayce on Diet & Health; The Official Eight and a Half-Ounce Mashed Potato Diet Book;* the *Boston Police Diet & Weight Control Program; The No Willpower Diet; Calories Don't Count; How Sex Can Keep You Slim; The Thin Book by a Formerly Fat Psychiatrist; Strong Medicine; Eat Fat and Grow Slim, Diet Dynamics, The Doctor's Quick Weight Loss Diet;* the *Low Carbohydrate Diet;* the *Drinking Man's Diet;* the *Air Force Diet; Dr. Atkins' Diet Revolution;* and *The Psychologist's Eat-Anything Diet,* to name just a few publications.

Seventy-two books on reducing were published in one year alone. Dr. Frederick J. Stare, Chairman of Harvard University's Department of Nutrition, attributes the commercial success of these books to the American belief in "diet magic. Every couple of years a book comes out that tells us we can eat all we want and, presto, our weight problem will disappear. We believe it."

Nutrition and dieting

Nutrition experts do not doubt that fad or crash diets can result in pounds lost. "By definition," says Dr. Morton B. Glenn, past president of the American Nutrition Association, "a crash diet is an overwhelmingly quick way to lose weight." What does worry nutritionists, however, is that such diets are potentially dangerous. "Losing weight alone is not a criterion of a successful diet," claims Dr. Lawrence E. Lamb, former chief of the Clinical Science Division of the United States Air Force School of Aerospace Medicine, and author of *What You Need to Know About Food & Cooking for Health*. "The goal is proper nutrition, proper weight and maintenance of health."

Fad diets are not nutritionally adequate. According to Dr. Neil Solo-

> "The macrobiotic diet, consisting of cereals and few liquids, has resulted in at least one death. And cases of scurvy, anemia, and loss of kidney function have been reported."

mon, Maryland's chief health officer and author of *The Truth About Weight Control*, "Fad or crash dieting is like trying to run an expensive engine on French perfume. It will run at first because of the alcohol, but the oils and aromatics will soon make it run raggedly, and eventually it will stall, its exquisitely machined parts a mess beyond repair. So also with fad diets and reckless dieters."

The macrobiotic diet, consisting of cereals and few liquids, has resulted in the death of at least one adherent. Cases of scurvy, anemia, hypoproteinemia, hypocacemia, emaciation, and loss of kidney function have been reported. Total fasting has culminated in heart failure, renal failure, lactic acidosis in diabetics, and acute volvulus of the small bowel.

Sensible dieting

The only sensible diet, most experts agree, is the traditional one—one that restricts caloric intake while supplying proteins, carbohydrates and fats. Dr. Mayer believes that "the basics of a good diet have not changed over the years. The secret ingredients are: eat a varied diet; eat enough; don't eat too much."

Dr. Glenn says that "ideally, a reducing diet should simply be an exaggeration of proper eating habits," which means balanced meals. The "high-protein, moderate-carbohydrate, low-fat diet has withstood the test of time." None of the elements vital to continued good health is missing, and the reinforcement of proper eating habits helps to *keep* the weight off once it is lost.

Crash diets, on the other hand, do not aid in maintaining long-term weight loss. Once the weight is off, "there are no well-balanced dietary guidelines by which to revise eating habits," says Dr. Solomon. "Without these it is almost impossible to maintain healthy low weight." As it is, surveys indicate that less than 15 per cent of all dieters, including those under physician care, succeed in maintaining their weight loss beyond two years.

In addition, the fad diet, with its concentration on one or two nutrients, can throw the body's metabolic system out of balance with unpleasant results.

The trouble with the sensible, balanced eating regimen, according to most dieters, is that weight loss is slow—an average of two pounds a week. So, the majority of dieters try any one or all of the diets promising faster weight reduction. These diets invariably involve a drastic alteration in the proportion of protein, carbohydrates, and fats ingested.

High-protein diet

The high-protein diet contains a high proportion of protein to carbohydrates, but is not devoid of any nutritional essentials. Meat, cheese, eggs and fish form the diet's backbone. The danger in this diet is that a kidney infection or malfunction may result in urea retention, coma and death.

High-fat diet

Too much fat in the diet can cause constant diarrhea, resulting in the loss of essential vitamins, minerals and cofactors. Dehydration and electrolyte imbalance (loss of magnesium, potassium, and sodium) can lead to coma and death.

High-carbohydrate diet

For the patient with hypoglycemia, an overabundance of carbohydrate can trigger increased insulin production and a lowering of blood sugar to dangerous levels. For the normal dieter, too many carbohydrates can lead to elevated cholesterol and triglycerides, as well as high blood pressure and weight levels.

Low-fat diet

The body is unable to manufacture certain essential fats. These must be part of the daily diet. A diet too low in fats will result in dry skin and scalp and decreased joint mobility due to decreased lubrication. Fats are a concentrated form of energy and combine with phosphorus as part of every cell. A layer of fat under the skin cushions

the nerves and muscles and insulates the body against sudden temperature changes. Studies demonstrate that rats fed fat-free diets become emaciated and develop skin rashes and kidney disorders.

Low-carbohydrate diet

The low-carbohydrate diet has been around since William Banting's publication. Periodically, the diet has been revived in slightly different forms. In 1953, it appeared as the Pennington diet, again in 1959 as *Eat Fat and Grow Slim*, followed in quick succession by the *Air Force Diet* (1960), *Calories Don't Count* (1961), the *Drinking Man's Diet* (1964), the *Low-Carbohydrate Diet* (1965), *The Doctor's Quick Weight Loss Diet* (1967), and the current bestseller, *Dr. Atkins' Diet Revolution*.

Low-carbohydrate, low-calorie diet

Opinion is divided on the merits of a low-carbohydrate, low-calorie diet. There is some evidence (notably the work of Dr. John Yudkin, emeritus professor of nutrition, University of London) to indicate that restricted carbohydrate intake can lead to weight loss. As reported in the *Am. J. Clin. Nutr.* (24:190), researchers found that subjects consuming 30 gm. of carbohydrates daily lost an average of 16.8 kg. after nine weeks, compared to a loss of 12.78 kg. in subjects ingesting 60 gm. carbohydrates, and 11.85 kg. in those consuming 104 gm. All subjects were on a low-calorie (1,200) diet. Physical activity was not followed. Some diet experts (Dr. George A. Bray of the University of California School of Medicine, for one) favor a reducing regimen of 1,000 calories and between 30 and 50 gm. of carbohydrates daily.

Other diet authorities, however, are concerned about the effect low-carbohydrate intake might have on body cell function. Dr. Lamb notes that "a small amount of carbohydrate is necessary to protect the cells in the liver, kidney, spleen, heart and skeletal muscles, as well as all the other vital structures of the body. No carbohydrates can result in the failure of the body to build protein in the vital cell repair and replacement process necessary to maintaining youthful health." Dr. Mayer reinforces this: "We need carbohydrates—which come from cereals, fruits and vegetables and milk, as well as sugar—for two main reasons: our muscles work most efficiently when burning carbohydrates, and our brains burn nothing but a carbohydrate, glucose."

Low-carbohydrate, high-calorie diet

Whatever the merits of a low-carbohydrate, low-calorie diet may be, the medical establishment is appalled by the low-carbohydrate, high-calorie diet outlined in *Diet Revolution*. Dr. Atkins claims that by eliminating carbohydrates altogether for one week and thus becoming ketotic, dieters can consume all the proteins and fats they want and still lose weight. After the first week, dieters can increase their carbohydrate intake gradually up to 50 gm. daily. In the first month, the average weight loss for a man is 15 to 20 pounds, for a woman, 10 to 15. Dr. Atkins has yet to produce any data on patients following his diet, although he claims to have files on 11,000 dieters.

Medical reaction

Criticism of the Atkins' diet has been widespread. The American Medical Association's Council on Foods and Nutrition has labeled the book "unscientific and potentially dangerous to health," and issued a 16-page condemnation which concludes by saying: "The rationale advanced to justify the diet is, for the most part, without scientific merit . . . There is no evidence advanced that controlled studies were ever carried out to validate the observation that weight can be lost by sedentary subjects who consume a carbohydrate-poor diet providing 5,000 calories per day."

The Medical Society of the County of New York has warned that ketogenic diets may result in "weakness, apathy, dehydration, calcium depletion, lack of stamina for prolonged exertion, nausea, hyperlipidemia and hyperuricemia, kidney failure, tendency to fainting, possible cardiac irregularity,

and potential danger to the unborn child."

"If I were a fetus, I would forbid my mother to go on such a diet," says Dr. Karlis Adamsons, an obstetrician at Mount Sinai Hospital in New York.

Some physicians are particularly upset that the Atkins diet has achieved such popularity at a time when the relationship between diet and the incidence of heart disease is getting clearer. Says Dr. Stare: "Coronary heart disease is the principal cause of death in the United States, and any diet which tends to be high in saturated fats and cholesterol tends to elevate the chance that the individual will get heart disease. Any book that recommends unlimited amounts of meat, butter and eggs, as this one does, is, in my opinion, dangerous."

Senate committee meetings

Nutritionists are not the only ones concerned about the American diet. The Senate Select Committee on Nutrition and Human Needs has begun hearings devoted to "overnutrition." Committee chairman Senator George McGovern of South Dakota said that it would seek means to protect overweight Americans from reducing schemes, including fad diets, that might be "worthless, fraudulent" and dangerous. "The overweight consumer," said Senator McGovern, "is certainly the most unprotected consumer of all."

Witnesses before the committee, however, have indicated that perhaps what the consumer needs is not protection, but education. Americans are "nutritional illiterates," say the experts. According to Dr. Mayer, "The public has no idea about how many calories go in from food and how many go out from exercise." Dr. George M. Briggs and Helen D. Ullrich, two California experts, estimate that our nutritional ignorance is costing $30 billion a year in medical bills.

Legislative action, say nutritionists, "is urgently needed to develop and disseminate nutrition information." Dr. Mayer believes that $100 million per year will be needed to change American eating habits.

One of the measures being considered by the committee is a mandatory warning to be printed on the cover of all diet books, urging the buyer to consult his doctor before embarking on the diet.

Research on obesity

Ironically, while overweight American adults are busily trying every new diet that promises a "new you," researchers are looking into the possibility that fat people may be, to a certain extent, "born" and not "made."

One of the more important studies in recent years was conducted by Dr. Jules Hirsch and colleagues at Rockefeller University, who have devised a method of counting the actual number of fat cells in the human body. After making fat-cell counts at various points in individual growth, Dr. Hirsch concluded that the actual number of fat cells in the human body is determined within the first few months after birth. Following Dr. Hirsch's work, Dr. Jerome L. Knittle has shown that the obese "have a higher number of fat cells than the non-obese, and the fat cells are generally bigger than in non-obese persons . . ."

This research indicates that, popular belief to the contrary, one does not develop new fat cells as one gains weight. Drs. Ethan A. H. Sims and Edward S. Horton of the University of Vermont Medical School have determined, using the Hirsch cell-counting technique, that the fat cells of overfed men expand, rather like sponges, to accommodate the excess weight, while the actual number of fat cells remains the same. When the subjects in their experiment returned to their normal weights, the fat-cell counts again remained the same while the cell size decreased.

The implications of this research are enormous. While the influence of hereditary and environmental factors on weight control is yet to be determined, it has been suggested that by controlling infant nutrition, we might one day be able to fix the number of fat cells an individual forms at a non-obese level.

This is still way off in the future. And until that time, overweight Americans will continue to search for that magic cure.
—Anastasia Toufexis

The Realities Of Obesity and Fad Diets

Cigarette smoking, drunken driving, and flirting with other men's wives are widely indulged in. The remedy for each is self-discipline. The same may be said for obesity. Nobody has to be fat if he possesses the will power to starve himself and is not lured onto the easy road of popular magic-formula diets.

by SEYMOUR K. FINEBERG, M.D.

The foundation of the treatment of obesity must be the physician's unremitting effort to teach his patients the necessity of adhering religiously to a diet that is restricted in calories but balanced in terms of nutrient content.

"Calories" and "balance"—these are the key words. There is no other way to treat—or, more accurately put, to control—obesity. The patient must be made to understand that if he is to reduce his weight, keep it down, and not harm himself in the process, he must practice the self-discipline that is needed to adhere to a balanced diet of reduced caloric content. This requires strong motivation on his part. He must not waver in his determination to change his style of life and eating habits. Once he has made the change, he must abide by the new regimen no matter how great the temptation to stray from this straight, narrow path.

These are the harsh, plain realities. And perhaps because they are so stark and simple, obesity is for the physician one of the thorniest problems he has to tackle in his daily practice.

Although there are many fine points

Dr. Fineberg is Chief of the Diabetes and Obesity-Diabetes Clinics at the Metropolitan Hospital in New York, Assistant Clinical Professor of Medicine at the New York Medical College and Flower and Fifth Avenue Hospitals, and Chief of the Department of Medicine, Prospect Hospital, Bronx, N.Y.

involved in the effective application of the simple rules of caloric restriction and nutritional balance, they are all that medical science has to offer for the management of obesity at this time. No wonder so many patients seek a way out of this harsh and difficult-to-accept reality and turn to some "magic" diet formula instead, which offers a welcome escape. That the balanced, calorically restricted regimen has a high rate of failure is not surprising because it demands so much of patient and physician alike. The extent and duration of success seem to be directly related to the degree of personal effort applied by the physician. But sometimes the best that an enlightened and conscientious physician can do will fail in cases of very pronounced obesity because the patient sooner or later concludes that the treatment is worse than the disease or his fear of the consequences. This is true especially in massive obesity, a state in which the unfortunate individual's weight is two, three or four times the desirable level. It is extremely rare for such a person to achieve and maintain satisfactory control of his affliction.

INVISIBLE FACTOR

Before considering the fallacies and inadequacies of fad and crash diets, the composition and requirements of a nutritionally sound, balanced diet which will produce a significant rate of weight loss in the vast majority of cases should be reviewed in more detail. A sensible reducing diet should accomplish its

purpose, the loss of fat from the body stores, with a minimum of risk to the individual and the least variance from a diet of commonly used foods. Caloric restriction is the essential prerequisite if the patient is to lose weight. The daily caloric deficit should be great enough to cause a loss of at least 2 to 3 lbs. per week during the early weeks of dieting. Most experienced therapists in the field are convinced that a majority of severely obese people, owing to an error or errors in their metabolism, have a daily caloric requirement for maintenance of ideal weight that is far below the levels set forth in the 1968 revision of the Recommended Dietary Allowances of the National Research Council's Food and Nutrition Board: 2800 calories for men and 2000 for women. This inherently lower caloric requirement, combined of course in most instances with ingestion of calories in excess of the average requirement, is the root cause of severe obesity. Without such errors in body chemistry these severely obese individuals would still have grown fat but probably to a lesser degree. Far too frequently, this totally invisible underlying factor is disbelieved or ignored by the physician, and all the blame for massive obesity is placed on an unmeasured and perhaps only moderately excessive caloric intake.

The traditionally prescribed 1000-calorie diet was most likely chosen originally by trial and error since its long-term application does produce satisfactory weight loss in practically all individuals. The actual degree of restriction may be varied according to individual response between 800 and 1400 calories daily.

However, such a calorically restricted diet should be a balanced diet, including a maximum of the required nutrients. It should comprise one or more servings a day from the Four Basic Food Groups, the milk, meat, vegetable-fruit and bread-cereal groups, and include a small amount of fat. These, in fine, are the bare elements of a balanced diet, often mentioned but seldom described. This simple regimen will provide a mixed nutrient intake of carbohydrates, proteins, fats, vitamins and minerals; the only drastic change is in the amount of calories. Much of the caloric reduction is in fat and some in carbohydrate, while protein intake is reduced least and remains entirely adequate. Proportionately, of course, this means a higher intake of protein. Even this sensible diet should very soon be supplemented, as an added precaution, by a multiple vitamin-mineral preparation to guard against the possible development of subclinical or borderline deficiencies.

This weight-reducing diet is the only suitable one for the treatment of obesity because all that is needed to make it a proper balanced diet for maintenance—as opposed to reduction—of weight is an increase in the size of portions. In this manner it prepares the patient for continued dietary control of his obesity for the rest of his life.

Anyone who has ever become seriously obese will always be a prime candidate—even after successful weight reduction—for rapid reversion to his previous overweight state. Even after attainment of the ideal or desirable weight, therefore, obesity should be considered to be controlled but never cured. The obese individual should be a permanent diet watcher! Like the diabetic or the hypertensive patient, he should remain under treatment at all times. The sensible diet I have described teaches him how to eat and what to eat for the rest of what may possibly be closer to a normal life span. The physician's major contribution to the program is his success in persuading the patient to accept and adhere to this new way of life.

The greatest obstacle to the proper medical management of obesity is posed by reducing diets that have been concocted by a combination of faulty reasoning and wishful thinking. Adherence to such ill-advised diets may upset the obese individual's nutritional equilibrium and produce a state of malnutrition. This condition can develop in a number of ways.

WISHFUL THINKING

All diets, balanced or unbalanced, "fad" or "crash," will produce weight loss if the total calories they provide in twenty-four hours amount to less than the individual's caloric requirement for weight maintenance at the start of dieting. At an equal—or slightly greater—intake of calories, weight loss will appear to be somewhat faster on some diets than on others. But no diet will result in loss of fat if it ignores the principle of the conservation of energy and the first law of thermodynamics by not providing for significant caloric restriction.

Probably the most misleading type of fad diet is derived from the school of thought that permits unlimited consumption of certain high-protein foods. Examples of such "Eat-All-You-Want" diets that are being widely promoted are the "Calories-Don't-Count" diet, which adds safflower oil to unlimited proteins and fats with very little carbohydrate; the "All-the-Meat-You-Want" diet; and "The Doctor's Quick Weight Loss Diet" allowing unlimited amounts of certain meats, fish, eggs and cheeses and requiring ingestion of at least 8 glasses of water daily. The life span of each of these diets is brief because it takes at most a few days or weeks for the people misled into following them to discover that they cannot continue to follow them. In desperation, these individuals then turn from one fad diet to another, unable to find a way out of their adipose predicament. The reason for the failure of these diets is simple enough: they run counter to the basic principles of balance, minimal change, and the teaching of good dietary habits for permanent control.

After a short time on one of these diets the patient is only able to choke down a limited amount of calories. He usually becomes repelled or satiated and winds up with an unplanned reduction in calories which does cause loss of weight. If he tolerates the diet better than most, he will not lose weight and may even gain. These diets may spring from an unconscious delusion but as a rule they are a deliberate ploy on the part of the "expert" prescribing them. Belief in them is self-delusion on the part of the victim. The dieter neither finds the diet satisfactory nor does he achieve anything approaching a lasting loss of weight.

Another type of fad diet may requir some caloric restriction but deman either a sharp reduction of carbohydrate intake or no carbohydrate at all. An example is "The Drinking Man's Diet," which substitutes alcohol for carbohydrates. As Dr. Frank L. Iber of Tufts University pointed out in NUTRITION TODAY (January/February 1971), alcohol calories are not only nutritionally empty but are devoid of the type of energy that muscle tissue can utilize. Other diets of this type have been cloaked in a mantle of respectability by such names as "Mayo Clinic Diet"—a name that has been applied over the years to more than a dozen diets, none of which of course had the frailest connection with this renowned institution—or "Air Force Diet." This last, needless to say, has been emphatically disowned by the Air Force. In these diets, carbohydrate intake is reduced to 60 grams or much less, while fat and protein are usually unlimited. The "scientific" explanation being offered for the alleged effectiveness of low-carbohydrate diets is that in the fat person carbohydrate is rapidly converted to adipose tissue rather than being used for energy, whereas calories from fat and protein are burned up in the metabolic processes and are not stored as body fat. This is simply not true. What does appear to be true to some extent is that excess calories from whatever source, carbohydrate, protein, or fat, are less readily utilized and more readily stored in the fat person, in whom the process of lipogenesis is enhanced. *The initially greater weight loss resulting from a low-carbohydrate diet providing the same number of calories as a balanced, mixed-nutrient diet is actually due to an additional loss of body water, not fat.* Ignorance of this scientifically proven fact has probably led to more confusion in the dietary treatment of obesity than any other single factor. To understand this, a strong differentiation must be made between fat loss and scale-weight loss. The scale measures total weight only—and cannot distinguish fat loss from water loss or loss of vital lean tissue. It can never indicate what portion of a weight increase or decrease is due to change in fat content and what portion to a change in water content. A diet that contains carbohydrates but is well below the individual's caloric require-

740-CALORIE "NORMAL PROTEIN DIET"

BREAKFAST	Calories
4 oz. orange or grapefruit juice **or**	
5 oz. tomato juice	50
Portion of cooked cereal	100
Coffee with artificial sweetener	
	150
10:00 A.M.	
4 oz. buttermilk or fat-free milk	50
LUNCH	
4 tablespoons cottage cheese	60
Lettuce and tomato salad	40
Canned fruit—unsweetened, or gelatin	50
Tea or coffee	
	150
3:00 P.M.	
4 oz. buttermilk or fat-free milk	50
DINNER	
4 oz. chopped lean steak **or**	
3 oz. hamburger meat **or**	
6 oz. chicken or fish	260
1 leafy vegetable	30
	290
10:00 P.M.	
4 oz. buttermilk or fat-free milk	50
Total Calories	**740**

ment in total caloric content will produce a reduction in scale weight which will parallel fat loss for only a few weeks in most individuals. Then, although the body fat of these persons continues to decrease, retention of water will set in and mask or counterbalance the fat loss. The patient's weight as measured on the scale may show little or no change. This metabolic abnormality of water balance, the cause of which remains unknown, has been conclusively demonstrated to be due to the carbohydrate portion of the diet. It is not uncommon to see extreme examples of this in which patients will actually begin to gain weight on the scale while in negative caloric balance. If the diet contains little or no carbohydrate, this apparently disturbing and obstructive phenomenon does not occur, hence the greater effectiveness of such diets. It is of extreme practical importance to recognize that uncorrected salt and water retention is often responsible for the failure of obese patients to lose weight on a low-calorie diet of mixed nutrients to which they actually adhere. Failure to recognize and correct this retention by the judicious use of diuretics is probably the most important single reason for lack of response to the treatment of obesity in patients who are properly motivated and cooperative. This can be a very frustrating experience for them.

ENERGY FOR THE BRAIN

Yet carbohydrate must be furnished in the diet, despite this disadvantage, for a number of compelling reasons.

First of all, if lifetime calorie control is to be acceptable to the patient, the diet must have some palatability and appeal. Much of the variety and taste in foods is furnished by carbohydrates. In addition, carbohydrate is an essential nutrient although not quite as indispensable as certain of the amino acid constituents of protein. The body has a specific need for carbohydrate as a source of energy for the brain and for other specialized functions. The Food and Nutrition Board of the National Research Council has suggested that the normal adult requires approximately 500 carbohydrate calories daily. If these are not provided in the diet, they will be derived from the breakdown of protein and fat, by the process of gluconeogenesis. Glucose is synthesized from protein only in certain body tissues and at a rate insufficient to meet specific demands. Carbohydrate is required so that fat, either endogenous or exogenous, may be completely oxidized in the body. In the absence of a sufficient amount of carbohydrate, an intermediary product of fat metabolism, acetylcoenzyme A, is formed, which condenses to form ketones. When the ability of the kidneys to excrete ketone bodies is exceeded, they accumulate in the blood, producing ketosis. This is an abnormal and undesirable metabolic state which occurs in starvation and in individuals on unbalanced, carbohydrate-deficient diets.

Another category of fad diets are those which are low or inadequate in protein. An example is the greatest crash "diet" of all time, "total fasting"! This is a recent fad of medical origin. The victim is given non-caloric liquids only and of course no protein. Other examples are the experimental low-protein "Rockefeller Diet," the Grapefruit Diet, the Watermelon Diet, the Skimmed Milk and Banana Diet, and the "Doctor's Quick Inches-Off Diet." An adequate protein intake is a basic requirement for health. A reducing diet, just like a normal diet, must contain sufficient protein to maintain the body structure. The recommended daily minimum is almost a gram of protein per kilogram of desirable body weight. If this amount is not furnished in the reducing diet, the vital need has to be filled by the breakdown of the individual's own lean, non-fat, protein tissue. Most of this will come from muscle and some of it from organ tissue. Instead of mobilizing and reducing only the excessive and harmful stores

of body fat, there is actual catabolism of healthy, vital body structure. Metabolic studies of nitrogen balance performed in obese individuals undergoing total fasting revealed that 65% of their weight loss was due to loss of lean body tissue and only 35% was due to loss of adipose tissue. These studies have shown that fasting and diets with insufficient protein cause rapid weight reduction, but at the expense of lean tissue. To put it mildly, this is physiologically undesirable! A low-calorie weight-reducing diet must provide for a sufficient intake of essential amino acids to prevent any breakdown of body protein and insure that the weight loss produced is entirely due to the mobilization and utilization of fat.

ILLUSIONARY LOSS

Because of the constant metabolic need of the body for protein replacement, the total eventual weight lost on a diet of no calories, or total starvation, will not be greater—paradoxical as this may seem—than that resulting from adherence to a 700 to 900-calorie diet providing adequate protein! It has been observed repeatedly that the weight lost owing to catabolism of lean tissue is rapidly regained upon resumption of even a very low-caloric intake which includes protein. This is due to the rapid replenishment of the stores depleted during the period of negative protein balance. For every pound of protein replaced, there will be an increase of four pounds of body weight; apparently, three pounds of water are incorporated into the intracellular portion of each pound of actual protein mass. Even though the individual is still in negative caloric balance on the refeeding diet, he will thus continue to gain weight until the protein has been completely restored. In the long run, therefore, only the weight lost from fat depots can be prevented from returning. A reducing diet which contains no protein or insufficient protein not only causes weight to be lost from the wrong storehouse but much of the total weight loss is an illusion created by loss of water. Worst of all, this type of weight loss is completely futile because even with careful refeeding recovery of the lost weight cannot be prevented! This can have a serious, traumatic psychological effect on the actively cooperating fat person who has starved or half-starved himself for a prolonged period of time. He cannot understand why his weight should rapidly increase again with very little increase in calories. Many such victims of crash or unbalanced dieting or "dieting with malnutrition" have only slightly less understanding of this phenomenon than their physicians. At this point they may even conclude that they are hopeless "glandular" or metabolic freaks whom no doctor understands or can help and become totally discouraged from further efforts to control their obesity.

In order to realize fully the fallacies, pitfalls and dangers of all fad diets, past, present and future, we should keep in mind the basic principles of the sensible approach to long-term dieting and good nutrition. Some of these are axiomatic in the light of our medical knowledge of nutrition and may be summarized as follows:

1. A diet must produce a negative caloric balance if any weight loss is to occur.

2. No weight will be lost through any conceivable change in proportion, combination, or omission of certain nutrients unless the caloric intake falls below the caloric requirement.

3. An estimated average daily allowance of calories derived from a diet of mixed nutrients is the fundamental basis for lifetime control of obesity.

4. Obesity of the common type should be considered to be controllable but not curable.

5. Any individual who has ever developed a serious or massive degree of obesity must watch his diet for the rest of his life.

6. Even reaching a "normal" or "desirable" weight is futile and possibly harmful if this weight is maintained for a relatively short time only.

7. The loss of fat weight must be accomplished by a method whose major tool is a diet which, once weight reduction has been achieved, can be easily adapted for permanent control and is not detrimental to health.

8. Diets very low in carbohydrate or protein may seem more efficient in that they produce some added weight loss for a given amount of caloric deficit, but this is a transient illusion attributable to water loss or changes in water balance. Actually, no added loss of fat is produced.

9. A diet based on such an unbalanced "magic formula" is plainly injurious to health if the patient adheres to it for any length of time because he is then, in reality, "dieting with malnutrition."

There seems little doubt that the penalty of obesity is fewer years of life. Not only is life shortened by undue overweight, but death is usually preceded by a host of acute and chronic illnesses.

1000-CALORIE BALANCED DIET
(Balance of carbohydrate, protein, fat plus vitamins and minerals)

BREAKFAST (160 calories)
1 serving of fruit juice
1 egg or substitute
½ slice of bread
Coffee or tea

Egg Substitutions:
A. 4 tablespoons cottage cheese
B. 1-inch cube American cheese
C. 3 crisp bacon strips
D. 1½ oz. meat
E. ½ cup oatmeal without cream or sugar **or** cornflakes with 4 oz. skim milk.

LUNCH (260 calories)
A. 1 cup vegetable soup (can)
1 hard-boiled egg
½ slice of bread
1 cup (6 oz.) fat-free milk
or
B. 1 cup vegetable soup (can)
4 tablespoons cottage cheese
½ slice of bread
1 medium tomato and ¼ head lettuce
1 serving of fruit
Coffee or tea (no cream or sugar)
or
C. 3 oz. lean hamburger
½ slice of bread
1 serving of fruit
Coffee or tea (no cream or sugar)

3:00 P.M. (50 calories)
½ glass fortified, fat-free milk (4 oz.)

DINNER (500 calories)
2 cubes bouillon
1 serving of meat, 4 oz.
2 servings of vegetables (with a pat of butter or margarine)
1 slice of bread
1 serving of fruit
Coffee or tea (no cream or sugar)

EVENING OR BEDTIME (50 calories)
½ glass fortified, fat-free milk (4 oz.)

It is, therefore, all the more distressing that there are a great many people and not a few physicians and dietitians who continue to believe that the demand for people to do everything possible to keep from becoming or remaining obese is based entirely on some sort of vain pursuit of the "slim look." If many people continue to look upon slimness of figure as a fad, then, to the degree that they do so, our efforts to get at the root of the malady are vitiated.

At present, medical science is not trying as hard as it should to come to grips with the causes of obesity, and there seems little doubt that the failure to accept obesity as a disease or at least as the prodromal condition for other diseases is abetted by the frustrations most physicians experience when they try to do something about it.

FACTS OF OBESITY

The advice to slim down is based on sound medical thinking, and it may well be accepted even more widely in the future. Medical advice about eating habits and food selection in all states of health, including obesity, is in fact taken more and more seriously. Physicians should therefore not allow themselves to be discouraged when an obese patient says he cannot or will not follow his advice.

Regrettably, scientific half-truths, unproven and unsubstantiated conclusions, and just plain bunk about obesity and its treatment are still being welcomed by many as the ultimate truth and are often enthusiastically espoused. Inasmuch as medical knowledge in the entire field of nutrition is still hazy and incomplete, the patient is faced with the impossible chore of trying to separate fact from fiction. The trouble with most popular books about obesity and reducing diets is that only half of what they say is accurate but the reader does not know which half! This is not surprising since there are as yet few ironclad and immutable facts in any branch of medicine. Medicine is a "practice" and appropriately so called. It is based on valid conclusions drawn from an accumulation of data and experience, and these conclusions are continually being subjected to review and amendment as additional experience is gained. Nutrition is a relatively new science, and only in the last few decades have we assembled sufficient data to incriminate obesity as the forerunner of many diseases. No wonder, therefore, that the doctor often finds himself in a dilemma where obesity is concerned.

These, to this physician, are the facts of obesity. It seems inescapable to conclude that if the obese patient will abjure fads, ignore gossip, and be deaf to rumor and all the other cajolements that prey upon our natural human weakness in seeking shortcuts to health, he will realize that he cannot escape the torturous path leading to weight reduction, and he will finally be motivated to face up to the reality that weight can be lost only through serious, hard work. Not many are able to work so hard on themselves. But many more could if they would only learn from the repeated disappointments they have suffered by swallowing nutritional half-truths and trying fad diets.

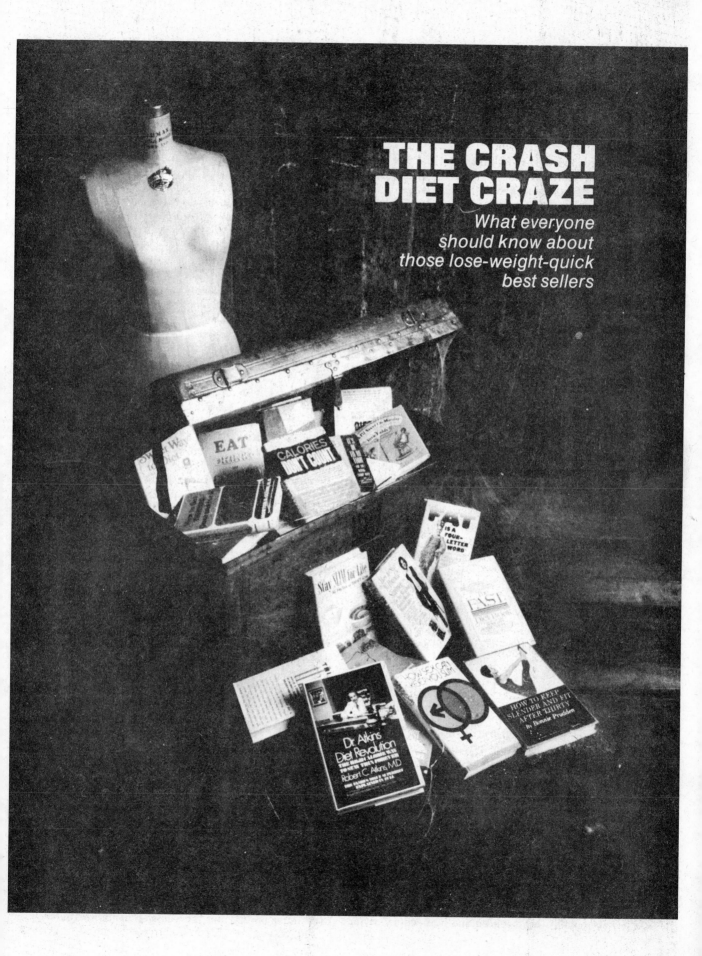

THE CRASH DIET CRAZE

What everyone should know about those lose-weight-quick best sellers

Crash diets, according to Peg Bracken, author of the *I Hate to Cook Book*, do have their merits. "There is one for everybody, regardless of race, creed, or color," she observes, "and it's something to get up in the morning for, just to see what today's is going to be: booze it up, eat it up, live high on the fat, low on the sugar, or heavy on the egg noodles."

In other words, whatever else crash diets may be good for, they are certainly good for a laugh. Among the fascinating diets that Peg Bracken describes are the vanilla ice cream and poundcake diet (one woman who tried it reports, "It was delightful for breakfast, mildly interesting for lunch, and an abomination for dinner—visions of raw carrots kept dancing through my head"); the mainly watercress and skim milk every January and February diet; the eat everything you want three times a day for just two minutes diet (she suggests that those who try it "charge admission at feeding time").

Magazines in recent years have heralded such curious regimens as the sweet-tooth diet, the lollipop diet, the whipped-cream diet, the champagne diet, the grape diet, the operant-conditioning diet, the Stone Age meat diet, and the working man's diet (eat sensibly Monday through Friday, eat dumbly Saturdays and Sundays). Book publishers have regaled us with the *Amazing Hypno-Diet* ("Get a clear picture of yourself refusing second helpings"); *Pray Your Weight Away* ("Three years and 100 pounds ago, I dropped to my knees and prayed, 'Dear God, I've tried for 15 years to whip this problem of obesity . . .'"); the *Boston Police Diet & Weight Control Program* (it sounds like an anticlimactic sequel to the U.S. Air Force Academy diet); *Edgar Cayce* (the "sleeping prophet") *on Diet & Health*; *The Official Eight and a Half-Ounce Mashed Potato Diet Book*; *A Sensuous Approach to Losing Weight & Looking Younger*; and *The No Willpower Diet* (the Chicago Nutrition Association's review: "It seems questionable that the dieter will have much success with this program that advises him to make up his own diet as he goes along, to eat the foods he likes best, and to cut out only those foods he can resist"). The only gimmicky reducing-diet book that has not yet been published, it would seem, is one waggishly announced some 20 years ago: *Lincoln's Doctor's Dog's Diet*.

The continuing cornucopia of new diet regimens testifies to both the ingenuity of the human mind and the inefficacy of human perseverance. But the situation also has its grim side, as even Peg Bracken admits. She tells of a young woman who dieted on cottage cheese and pears for ten months and succeeded in losing 40 pounds, inclusive of her gallbladder. In no time at all, she grew back the 40 pounds but not, unfortunately, her gallbladder.

Indeed, for a number of reasons many nutritionists consider crash diets a public health problem. For physicians, crash diets present an additional problem, because in recent years some of the most criticized crash-diet books have been written by doctors, and some of the books carry the name of the doctor or the word doctor in the title (*The Doctor's Quick Weight Loss Diet* and, most recently, *Dr. Atkins' Diet Revolution: The High Calorie Way to Stay Thin Forever*, which has been on the best-seller list for

five months). "It's fairly easy to cope with food faddism," says Jean Mayer, Ph.D., professor of nutrition at the Harvard University School of Public Health, "except when it's under the sponsorship of a man who has an M.D."

The trouble with crash diets is not, of course, that it's undesirable for the overweight to reduce. Nor is it that crash diets fail. Nutritionists agree that virtually every reducing diet, if followed carefully, will cause the dieter to shed poundage, because most crash diets are crashing bores and will lead to a decline in calorie consumption. Moreover, as Dr. Walter Modell of Cornell University has pointed out, many overweight people lose weight "on entering any new treatment or even an association with a new physician." In fact, there is evidence that the obese will reduce if they are simply told to eat just what they always eat.

For a one-week control period in a diet experiment conducted by Dr. John Yudkin, professor emeritus of nutrition at the University of London, ten moderately overweight subjects were taken to a posh hotel and "constantly reminded that, so far as possible, they should eat as they would at home." Despite the instructions, Dr. Yudkin expected "that in the pleasant holiday atmosphere in the hotel, with no housework, and with the very attractive food that was served, they would tend to overeat." One subject remained at the same weight. The nine other subjects, to Dr. Yudkin's amazement, lost weight—an average of 4.2 pounds, with a range up to 7 pounds. Dr. Yudkin's explanation is that "obese subjects under close supervision are likely to restrict their diets even when specifically asked not to do so."

The real trouble with crash diets, according to the experts, is that they are potentially dangerous. Certainly some current reducing diets mentioned by Dr. Philip L. White, director of the department of foods and nutrition of the AMA, fit this category—the all the coffee you can drink and all the cigarettes you can smoke diet (used mainly by college students) and what might be dubbed the classic Roman regurgitation diet (everything you can eat, followed by a finger down the throat). Other extreme examples include the macrobiotic diet, which has caused cases of scurvy, and the total-fasting diet (alias the zero-calorie diet), which has led to deaths from heart failure, acute volvulus of the small bowel, renal failure in a patient with glomerulonephritis, and lactic acidosis in a diabetic patient, but whose most common complication, according to two English physicians, is "surreptitious eating."

In the view of Dr. Morton B. Glenn of New York City, an internist who is a past president of the American Nutrition Association, all crash diets are dangerous because all crash diets are unnutritious. "A crash diet, by definition, is an overwhelmingly quick way to lose weight," he says. "And the only way to lose weight overwhelmingly quickly is an unhealthy way. Giving someone a crash diet is the equivalent of telling your daughter, 'If you're late for an appointment, don't bother looking at the traffic lights.' A sensible diet, for most people, results in the loss of approximately two pounds a week. The heavier one is, the taller one is, and the younger one is (because of the faster metabolic rate), the more one may safely lose, and a man tends to lose more quickly than a woman because of his greater activity."

A second trouble with crash diets is that, like color TV sets, they rarely if ever come with a two-year guarantee. Surveys have shown that 85% of all dieters, including those under professional care, do not reduce and stay reduced for over two years. Besides, "there's some evidence that obese individuals who lose weight and gain it back have a gradual increase in their blood cholesterol and blood lipid levels," says Dr. White, "and the next time they lose weight and gain it back, these levels are even higher. It must be tough on the psyche," he adds, "for anyone to go on a crash-diet program, then see all the weight come right back again. I think that the discouragement that could ensue might be enough to make a person lose all interest in physical fitness and just balloon away."

If a physician discovers that his patient is on a crash diet, or plans to go on one, says Dr. Glenn, what the physi-

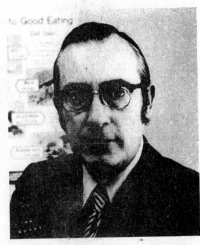

Dr. White: 'It does no good to hand a person a sheet of recommendations that are alien to his way of eating. That's why there's no such thing as an AMA diet.'

cian must do is educate the patient to the dangers and drawbacks of such diets—and outline a sensible diet. "The important thing in weight control," he goes on, "is to get the patient to *keep* his weight off. The only way I know to keep weight off is to have good eating habits, and the best place to learn such habits is during the dieting regimen. Ideally, a reducing diet should simply be an exaggeration of proper eating habits. When you drop the exaggeration, you're left with the good eating habits. Never having cake or pie on the diet is the exaggeration; after the diet is over, the patient has cake or pie in moderation, or has fruit instead.

"The reducing diet that has withstood the test of time best, I think, is the high-protein, moderate-carbohydrate, low-fat diet," notes Dr. Glenn. "But any diet, to be successful, has to face three basic facts: one's nutritional needs, one's cultural needs (people eat differently at home, at play, at a business lunch), and one's psychological needs—food, after all, is the world's most acceptable and available tranquilizer."

Similarly, Dr. White emphasizes that a diet must be tailored to the individual. "What works for one person may not work for another," he says. "It does no good to hand a

person a sheet of dietary recommendations that are alien to his way of eating. That's why there's no such thing as an 'AMA Diet.' "

Before putting someone on a diet, Dr. White says, a physician should determine whether the patient really should reduce. "There is a definite school of thought that it isn't until a person gets 30% or 40% above his desirable weight that you begin to see enough of a difference in the mortality and morbidity rates to be worrisome, and that people who are only 5%, 10%, or 15% overweight may be left alone." If physicians want to recommend a particular diet for someone who has been weighed and not found wanting, Dr. White continues, they might make sure that the patient receives a reasonable variety of foods, and that he also exercises "portion control." One diet that Dr. White recommends is the American Diabetic Association's Food Exchange System. But to achieve any success in treating obese people, he stresses, the physician must have "magnificent rapport with his patient"—if only to make sure that the patient is following the diet without cheating.

Unfortunately, many physicians working with obese people have a lot of dead weight to carry. The first handicap we shall pass over very quickly: "A significant number of doctors are overweight," says Dr. Glenn. "Patients look at them and think, 'If *they* can't lose weight, how are they going to help *me*?' "

Second: Many physicians do not seem to recognize the gravity of the subject. "They aren't willing to spend the considerable amount of time that may be necessary to instruct the patient," says Dr. Mayer. "A physician will certainly spend whatever time is required on an acute condition, even if it is not very serious, but he does not feel he has the time to instruct a patient on a chronic condition that may take 20 years off the patient's life expectancy." Dr. Glenn adds that "obesity has been a very unrewarding area of practice, in terms of success. Physicians generally don't like to treat conditions that don't remit—senility, osteoarthritis, and so forth. And with the obese, it's not the doctor who is doing the work. It's up to the patient. If you get enough patients who do not follow your advice, you get upset with them and with the whole thing."

Third: Many physicians are just not very knowledgeable about nutrition and dieting. "It's a subject hardly taught at all in medical school," says Dr. Glenn. "That is why, I am convinced, the medical profession has lost the lead in nutrition to nonmedical people—to nonmedical experts like Jean Mayer, as well as to quacks. I think that academia is at fault."

Dr. Mayer himself says: "Nutrition and preventive medicine in general are very poorly taught subjects in medical school. In surveys of what people know about nutrition, we found that junior and senior physicians in a Boston hospital had a very fragmentary knowledge of nutrition. This knowledge tended to be very highly theoretical—they had no knowledge of food composition and therefore were unable to translate their theoretical knowledge into practical advice."

Hard evidence that physicians have not been strikingly successful with the overweight comes from Dr. Albert J.

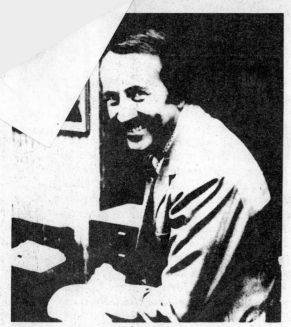

Dr. Atkins isn't sorry he wrote his book even though it has drawn unprecedented attacks.

Stunkard, a psychiatrist at the University of Pennsylvania, who found that a lay organization, TOPS (Take Off Pounds Sensibly), was quite as effective in getting the obese to lose weight as were physicians specializing in the problem—and more effective than "a distinguished teaching hospital" (*Postgrad Med*, 51:143 May '72).

The solutions to all these problems are, of course, obvious. Overweight physicians should reduce. Medical schools should beef up their nutrition departments. Physicians uninterested in obesity should refer patients to doctors who are interested, as well as knowledgeable; or, Dr. Glenn suggests, refer patients to a hospital's therapeutic dietician. The physician who is interested, but does not have sufficient time, "should hire a dietician for perhaps just a few hours a week," Dr. Glenn says, "and get all his obese patients together for proper instruction. I have a dietician in my office, and I can't work without her."

(Among her jobs is explaining to patients the difference between 99% fat-free milk and what Dr. Glenn calls "Dr. Glenn's miraculous 96.4% fat-free milk," which tastes quite as good as regular whole milk because it is regular whole milk. Each percentage point of fat carries 23.5 calories in an 8-oz glass, however, so Dr. Glenn advises his patients to consume skimmed milk.)

An alternate proposal comes from Dr. Stunkard, who suggests that family physicians and internists turn over to TOPS "the jobs of weight monitoring and psychologic support for obese patients," so that the physician's role can be "confined to periodic assessments of their diets and weight goals. We believe that such a plan is feasible and that it would result in larger weight losses for obese patients and in conservation of the physician's time and energy."

One final obstacle to the physician's success in treating overweight patients seems to be the crash diet—the fat man's fata morgana, the illusory safe, quick, and easy way to lose weight.

The reducing diet rage is not so new as people tend to think. Before we had TOPS and Weight Watchers, we had the Defensive Diet League of America; before Dr. Atkins' current best seller, we had *Eat and Grow Thin: the Mahdah Menus*, which by 1914 had gone through 112 printings; before the low-carbohydrate diet, we had the uric-acid-free diet of 1914, and the contemporaneous Rankin farm diet, which spoilsports at the U.S. Public Health Service promptly dubbed the pellagra-producing diet; before books with catchy titles, like *Calories Don't Count*, *How I Lost 36,000 Pounds*, and *Faith, Love and Seaweed*, we had what was unquestionably the catchiest book title of all time, Eugene Christian's forgotten 1928 dietary classic, *Why Die?*

Physicians have never been slouches at coming up with reducing diets. There was Dr. Philippe Karrell's 1866 diet: three or four glasses of creamy milk. There was Dr. William Howard Hay's diet of the 1930s, which proved re-

GENESIS OF THE LATEST BEST SELLER

"I don't expect to receive a red cent from my book," says Dr. Robert C. Atkins, the physician whose best seller everyone is talking, if not shouting, about. "There will probably be litigation pending forever, suits that will be forever postponed, tying up the money." Already, one suit—for $7.5 million—has been brought against him, his colleague, and his book's publisher by a former patient who claims the diet led to his angina pectoris and heart attack.

"But I didn't write the book for money," Dr. Atkins goes on. "I didn't imagine for a moment that more than a couple of thousand dollars would derive to me." In fact, he accepted an unusually low percentage (40%) of the advance and royalties from the publisher, which should have already given him paper earnings of up to $300,000. Dr. Atkins says that he felt that his editorial assistants—those helping with the book's recipes, with the rewriting—needed the money more than he did.

The 42-year-old physician, who graduated from Cornell

University Medical College, started practice in 1959 as a cardiologist and gradually shifted his specialty to metabolism and obesity. He says he wrote his book "because there was a need for it—and because publishers were asking me to write such a book. I felt that the counting-calories diet is very rarely followed, and people should be shown an alternate and better way of dieting." To lose weight, he himself became the first patient on the diet, nine years ago, and lost 28 pounds after six weeks. (The idea for the diet came partly from a similar regimen suggested by Dr. Alfred W. Pennington.) In the nine years since, he has put 11,000 patients on the diet. He charges $125 for the first visit, $20 for later visits.

As of April 6, his book had sold 953,000 copies, though Dr. Atkins says that sales have now been hurt by attacks coming from organized medicine. He is not sorry he wrote the book, though. And he is buoyed by reports he has heard "over the grapevine" that three medical centers are conducting controlled studies of his diet.

markably popular despite the common misconception that the Hay diet called for the ingestion of dried grass. (What it actually recommended was at least a week of fasting followed by the avoidance of so-called incompatible foods, such as proteins and carbohydrates.) But, for a long time, doctor-written diet books just did not go anywhere. In 1959, a *Life* magazine writer lamented that "the books written on this subject by physicians have been consistently outsold by a book written by a diet faddist named Gaylord Hauser." Two years later, the writer's prayer was answered when a doctor's ghost-written book left Gaylord Hauser's books light-years behind—Dr. Herman Taller's *Calories Don't Count.*

Today, it almost seems that every other reducing-diet book has been written by a doctor. The Boston police diet comes to us via Dr. Samuel S. Berman. Dr. Peter G. Lindner has brought us *Doctor Lindner's Point System Food Program.* Dr. Bernard A. Bellew's contribution is *Diet Dynamics.* Dr. Abraham I. Friedman has titillated us with

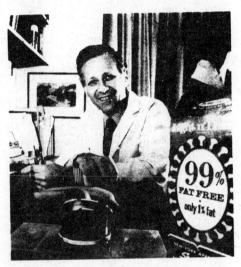

Dr. Glenn: 'All crash diets are dangerous because all crash diets are unnutritious. A sensible diet results in the loss of approximately two pounds a week.'

How Sex Can Keep You Slim ("In my opinion, based on 25 years of medical practice and experience in treating obesity, the most frequent cause of emotional overeating stems from sexual problems and frustrations"). And Dr. Theodore Isaac Rubin has weighed in with a thin book called *The Thin Book by a Formerly Fat Psychiatrist.*

According to Dr. White, good dieting books by doctors outnumber bad dieting books by doctors, and among the former he mentions Dr. Glenn's *How to Get Thinner Once and For All,* Dr. Norman Jolliffe's *How to Reduce and Stay Reduced,* and Dr. Ancel Keys and Margaret Keys' *Eat Well to Stay Well.* Still, it would seem that a slight edge in the won-and-lost record is nothing for the medical profession to brag about. And some doctor diet books have really taken a roasting. Dr. Morris Fishbein said of Dr. Blake F. Donaldson's regimen, outlined in *Strong Medicine* as mainly walks and meat with fat, that "his book is hardly scientific, so presumably what the physician was taught in his youth he has forgotten in his later years." Dr. Keys (who developed World War II's K-rations) said of Dr. Richard Mackarness' *Eat Fat and Grow Slim* that it "offered no scientific evidence, but he wrote well and his car-

toons of imaginary biochemical processes are amusing, though they have nothing to do with scientific reality."

Dr. Fredrick J. Stare, chairman of Harvard University's department of nutrition, said of Dr. Taller's *Calories Don't Count* that "there is hardly a word of sense in the whole book"; the *American Journal of Clinical Nutrition* called it "nutritional nonsense"; and Dr. White said that "this book is a grave injustice to the intelligent public and can only result in considerable damage to the prestige of the medical profession." By comparison, Dr. Bellew's *Diet Dynamics* has escaped relatively unscathed: The Chicago Nutrition Association said only that it is "another of the many sources of misinformation available to the already misinformed public. In addition to misinterpretation of data and research information, there are many instances of either confused thinking or factual errors."

Yet the doctor's dieting book that has probably drawn more immediate flak from organized medicine than any other is Dr. Atkins' current best seller. Dr. Atkins' "revolutionary" diet is a low-carbohydrate diet, and as such it echoes Dr. Stillman's *The Doctor's Quick Weight Loss Diet* (1967), which is the kissing cousin of the *Low Carbohydrate Diet* (1965), which resembles the *Drinking Man's Diet* (1964), which is not dissimilar to *Calories Don't Count* (1961), which harks back to the *Air Force Diet* (1960), which summons up remembrances of *Eat Fat and Grow Slim* (1959), which is akin to the Pennington diet (1953), and whose common progenitor is the Dr. William Harvey diet of 1863.

Dr. Mayer says, with undisguised rancor, "One of the things that irritates the hell out of me is that this same diet is sold, and I use the term advisedly, by physicians year after year under different guises, each time claiming that it is something new. Each time, only a wrinkle is different. With Stillman, it was drinking six glasses of water; with the *Drinking Man's Diet,* it was, I presume, drinking six martinis. With Dr. Atkins, it is just about as extreme as you can make a ketogenic diet. And whatever the merits of the low-carbohydrate diet, it's obvious that if it worked for the long pull, it wouldn't have to be reinvented every year." Dr. Atkins says, "Look at how long these diets have been popular. They may not be the *doctor's* diet, but they are the *dieter's* diet."

Dr. Atkins admits that his diet is not all that revolutionary, and that Dr. Stillman's low-carbohydrate diet was also ketogenic (though Dr. Atkins criticizes its prescription of six glasses of water a day). The newness in his own book, Dr. Atkins says, lies in his enlistment of the reader to monitor his own metabolic response to the ketogenic diet by means of ketone testing paper, and in terms of progressive weight loss, his feeling of well-being, etc.

What really makes Dr. Atkins' diet unique is that it has been violently attacked in a 16-page monograph by the AMA Council on Foods and Nutrition and publicly bombed by the Medical Society of the County of New York.

The AMA monograph's first criticism of Dr. Atkins' book is that it is not new and not revolutionary. Dr. Atkins asks why, then, it has occasioned the stir that it has.

Dr. Mayer suggests some possible answers. Perhaps Dr. Atkins' book was the "last straw." Perhaps organized

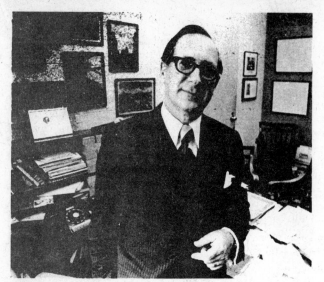

Dr. Mayer: 'Doctors aren't willing to spend necessary time instructing diet patients.'

medicine was still nursing its wounds from criticism that it acted too slowly against Dr. Taller's book. Dr. Mayer adds, "Here, every conscientious internist in the country has been trying to reduce cholesterol in patients, and I think that they are very alarmed by Dr. Atkins' book."

Dr. Atkins urges his diet's followers to embrace ketosis with all the abandon of a 13th-century mendicant embracing scrofula. The typical dieter starts off for a week consuming no carbohydrates, so that he becomes ketotic. So long as he remains ketotic, he increases his carbohydrate intake, up to a limit of 50 gm per day. He remains ketotic until he has achieved his desired weight loss. Meanwhile, he is permitted to consume all the proteins and fats he wants, as long as he is losing weight. According to Dr. Atkins, the average obese man loses 15 to 20 pounds the first month; the average woman, ten to 15 pounds.

There is evidence that people on low-carbohydrate diets lose weight, and the reason may be that these diets are also low-calorie diets. "All research," says Dr. White, "shows that people consume fewer calories and less total food when carbohydrates are restricted." The likely explanation is that proteins and fats tend to be more satiating than carbohydrates. Perhaps it is just that "fat takes longer to digest and absorb than proteins and carbohydrates and rumbles around in the stomach longer," as Dr. White says. "That may be why, after an Oriental dinner, people seem to be hungry in an hour or two. Generally, Oriental dinners are low-fat."

Some diet experts consequently recommend a low-carbohydrate regimen for their patients. Thus, Dr. George A. Bray, associate professor of medicine at the University of California School of Medicine, Los Angeles, says that, for obese adults, "It is my current feeling . . . that a 1,000-cal diet with restriction of carbohydrate to 30 gm to 50 gm is preferred."

But if the low-carbohydrate, low-calorie diet has its supporters among nutrition authorities, the low-carbohydrate, *high*-calorie diet does not. And this is what the critics of Dr. Atkins' diet say his diet is.

In defending his diet, Dr. Atkins maintains that no one—except himself—has any good data showing what happens when patients follow his exact diet. His own data consist of studies on 11,000 patients. He has not published the data, although he has urged his critics to check them

and says that he does intend to publish them. His critics argue that his data must be wrong, because they fly in the face of accepted scientific knowledge. Thus, the AMA suggests that Dr. Atkins is claiming to have "found a way of circumventing the first law of thermodynamics." Judged by existing nutritional knowledge, says the AMA monograph, "the notion that sedentary individuals, without malabsorption or hyperthyroidism, can lose weight on a diet containing 5,000 cal/day is incredible." Dr. Atkins says it may be incredible, and he does not know why it happens, but he sees it time and again.

The AMA's major indictments of the Atkins diet are: First, that "the rationale advanced to justify the diet is, for the most part, without scientific merit." Dr. Atkins had proposed, for example, that people lose weight because of the loss of ketones, but there is evidence that the most a person can lose a day is 100 cal worth of ketones. Second," the council is deeply concerned about any diet that advocates an 'unlimited' intake of saturated fats and cholesterol-rich foods. In individuals who respond to such a diet with an elevation of plasma lipids and an exaggerated alimentary hyperlipemia, the risk of coronary artery disease and other clinical manifestations of atherosclerosis may well be increased—particularly if the diet is maintained over a prolonged period." (A low-carbohydrate diet, in the opinion of various authorities like Dr. Mayer, is a high-fat diet—because, as Dr. White explains, "Protein is pretty yucky stuff, and usually high-protein foods come with a fair amount of fat.") Third, the Atkins diet allegedly does not lead to a "lifetime change in eating habits" that a practical diet would lead to.

The Medical Society of the County of New York has also stated that the adverse effects of a ketogenic diet reportedly include "weakness, apathy, dehydration, calcium depletion, lack of stamina for prolonged exertion, nausea, hyperlipidemia and hyperuricemia, kidney failure in individuals with kidney disease, tendency to fainting, possible cardiac irregularity, and potential danger to the unborn child." According to Dr. Mayer, no one really knows what the long-term effects of ketosis are, but the short-term effects include damage to the gallbladder in borderline patients.

Dr. Atkins makes a spirited defense. First, he says his diet is not necessarily a high-calorie diet: "If a person is given instructions to eat all he wants, and if his objective is to lose weight, and if he does not lose weight, he will not continue to consume high calories." He adds: "We do have a significant number of patients who were able to follow the diet on a high-calorie basis—not eating less but still losing weight. There's a large body of these patients."

Next, he denies that his dietary regimen will frequently lead to increased cholesterol levels. "Although it is clear and obvious that a high-fat diet raises cholesterol, this is *not* true when carbohydrates are cut down to the ketogenic level, though I do not know why. In the majority of my cases, the mean cholesterol level drops. And triglycerides drop dramatically. I know for a fact that there are no conflicting data in the entire medical literature. I'm not saying there aren't cases where cholesterol does go up on my diet. But the protocol of the diet very

boxyl cellulose, also commonly found in over-the-counter preparations, are "bulk producing products." Bulk producers swell up when they absorb water. When they are taken before meals they are supposed to swell up in the stomach and diminish hunger contractions.

However, bulk producers generally pass quickly into the small intestine, particularly when taken on an empty stomach. And even if they remained in the stomach, there has been no conclusive scientific proof that the jelly-like mass would in fact serve to reduce hunger contractions. Finally, even if hunger contractions were somehow reduced, there is no proof that this would have any bearing on the appetite of an overweight person. People who overeat often do so even when their hunger pains are satisfied. A person's appetite is based on complicated physical and psychological causes. Bulk producers have not been proved to have much, if any, effect on those causes. Modell found that methyl cellulose had no weight-reducing effect at all, and that the given dosage of sodium methyl cellulose also had none.

Thiamine mononitrate, Modell said, would not depress the appetite at all in any dose. Thiamine is more commonly referred to as Vitamin B1. Riboflavin, more familiarly known as Vitamin B2, in the dose contained in the Anapax tablets, also would not depress the appetite. The presence of B-vitamins in most of the over-the-counter weight-reducing preparations, including the ones which are not advertised fraudulently, stem from the fact that these preparations are often, if not always, accompanied by a high protein or low carbohydrate diet to be followed in conjunction with the pills (or gum, or wafers).

But the ad for Anapax, you will recall, seemed to dispense with the need for a diet. Nevertheless, included along with the pills, was a modified high protein diet. The fact that the diet was included, despite the implication of the ad, was one of the reasons the District Attorney's Office began its investigation in the first place.

More often than not, the diets which are mailed along with such pills are of dubious value in themselves. According to Neil Solomon, M.D., Secretary of Health and Mental Hygiene of the State of Maryland, author of The

Truth About Weight Control, "If you examine most physicians' diets, you will note that, providing you are a healthy individual, they contain a high proportion of protein to carbohydrate; however, they are not diets devoid of carbohydrates, nor are they lacking in any other nutritional essentials . . . If you embark on the 'high protein' diet and, unhappily, are unaware of a kidney infection or malfunction, it is conceivable that you might retain urea, lapse into a coma, and die. This is, of course, the most extreme possibility, but in any case, this diet, without the proper supplements, is eventually only going to compound the problem."

This year, says the Better Business Bureau, the public will be bilked out of $2-10 billion by "medical quackery," including reducing machines, belts and creams.

The *Anapax* plan is typical of a number of frauds in that it contained the diet even though the ad stated that it was unnecessary, and that the pills contained a more or less standard mix of benzocaine, bulk producers and vitamins. Given the included doses, the pill was harmless. This is not always the case, however. A common ingredient in many of the recorded frauds is a class of chemical which can produce drowsiness, and thereby "help" the person to refrain from eating. Bel-Doxin, a pill taken off the market in 1969, contained such a drug; *scopolamine aminoxide*. In a letter to the District Attorney, Herbert D. Bank, Executive Secretary of the Pharmacological Society of the State of New York, wrote: "One of the ingredients which ingested even in small doses by a person allergic to this drug, may cause serious complications."

What is clear from all of this is that these common magazine, TV, radio or newspaper mail order ads should be regarded with suspicion. If you have any doubts about these ads, or insist upon embarking upon these plans without first consulting a doctor, you can write to:

The Federal Trade Commission, Bureau of Investigation, Washington, D.C. 20580;

The United States Postal Service, 1200 Pensylvania Avenue, N.W., Washington, D.C. 20260—for mail order products—such as Anapax;

The U.S. Food and Drug Administration's District Offices listed in local telephone books of their branch cities, or the national office, Washington, D.C. 20201;

The American Medical Association, Department of Investigation, 535 North Dearborn Street, Chicago, Illinois 60610;

Council of Better Business Bureaus, Inc., 845 Third Avenue, New York, N.Y. 10022;

Your state or local health department, medical society, food and drug enforcement agency, or consumer affairs or consumer frauds agency.

But, first of all, you might ask yourself this question: Is the advertisement promising me that, if I send my money in, I'll receive something that will enable me to lose weight without undue effort on my part in a marvelously short time?

If so, beware!

Some diet misrepresentations, however, may be made in good faith, and with scientific backing—and yet may still be considered misrepresentations by conservative nutritionists.

Here, for example, is a program which is based on the findings of a man with impressive medical and scientific credentials, which has had proven results published in respectable professional journals, which involved regular consultation with physicians, which states explicitly the necessity of a regulated diet, which is characterized by the principle that in order to lose weight, new eating patterns must be established and maintained. What do you do? You read. And above all, you think.

In the 1950's, a British endocrinologist, A. T. Simeons published a number of papers which established that remarkable weight losses resulted when patients were put on a 500 calorie per day diet, and regular injections of a hormone called human chorionic gonadotropin, taken from the urine of pregnant women, were given on the average of six days a week for between six and seven weeks. Simeons established a clinic in Rome, Italy, and physicians in this country began to use the program and swear by it. Research was conducted in the United States, and Simeons' findings were confirmed. By this year, a number of clinics have been established, some of which charge from between $450 and $700 for the program. Articles have been written about the program for magazines: *Mademoiselle, Harper's Bazaar* and *Cosmopolitan*.

While it is true that some attention has been paid to the miraculous nature of the hormone, it is also true that many of the physicians who use the treatment, and Simeons himself, have emphasized the necessity of the cooperative efforts of the patients and the physicians, the discipline required to stick to the diet and the encouragement towards the ultimate goal of proper eating habits.

But there seem to be a number of problems with the regimen. One concerns the scientific basis of the program itself. What is the precise relation of the hormone to the admittedly confirmed loss of weight? While Simeons and his supporters refrain from making the explicit claim that human chorionic gonadotropin is the cause of the weight losses, they do claim that it is involved with the breaking up of deposits of certain types of fat. However, there has been no conclusive proof of this.

So that brings you back to the question: can you achieve the same kind of weight loss keeping all of Simeons' conditions except the use of the hormone? This kind of experiment has not been performed by Simeons and his followers, but a number of doctors writing in the *Lancet* and the *American Journal of Clinical Nutrition* did conduct one.

This is how they did it:

They put one group of patients on a rigid diet, and gave them regular injections of the hormone. Simultaneously, they put another group of patients on the same diet. But instead of the hormone they injected a placebo (a predetermined substance which would have no physical effect). But neither the patients nor those giving the injections knew whether a given shot contains the hormone or the placebo (thus "double-blind"). In each group, the weight losses were similar. In each group, the changes in body measurements were similar, and in each group other changes, or lack of them, in physical appearance and appetite were similar.

Last March, Charles Cargille, M.D., of the National Institute of Child Health and Human Development, wrote in the *Journal of the American Medical Association:*

"In my opinion, a 500-calorie diet without chorionic gonadotropin, if combined with daily interviews and encouragement, would be an equally effective, short-term management for obesity, while less costly and painful than if chorionic gonadotropin were used additionally. However, it is indeed possible that deep intragluteal daily needle-sticks *per se* are an indispensible component of the Sim-

---

There is no medical evidence that any topical applicant, such as a cream or an emollient, can have the effect of reducing weight.

---

eons' regimen. This painful experience may enhance patient acceptance of the stringent dietry restrictions imposed."

The "stringent dietary restrictions," present another problem. William J. McGanity, M.D., in an article in the *Journal of the American Medical Association*, wrote: "We agree that with such starvation, loss should be observed. The important aspect is, however, that continued adherence to such a drastic regimen is potentially more hazardous to the patient's health than continued obesity."

There are very few, if any, people who are likely to be able to spend the rest of their lives on diets of 500 calories a day. The most important factor in long-term weight reduction is the formation of new and stable eating habits. Those habits are not formed in the chorionic gonadotropin program. More likely than not, after the completion of the program, most if not all of the patients will revert back to their previous eating habits and will find themselves as heavy as they were before they began the regimen.

The Simeons method is not an outright fraud, but many medical authorities and nutritionists question whether it is based on incomplete research and faulty nutritional premises.

And it should come as no surprise to an overweight person that the responsibilities he incurs when he commits himself to the decision to lose weight are very great indeed. In the first place, he must take care that he isn't being swindled, and in the second place he must be careful to ask himself and others the right questions about the methods he chooses. How sure is he that he knows what he should about the causes of his problem? How much are they related to his need to overeat? How much are they related to his genetic and glandular make-up? Does the patient have the self-discipline to change his habits to get his weight down and, even more difficult, keep his weight loss permanent?

Those are hard questions to ask oneself, let alone one's physician. In the meantime, many of us continue to respond to come-on advertisements about reducing panaceas, such as creams, emollients or bath oils. For instance, David Ruff, executive director of the Better Business Bureau of Greater Newark (New Jersey), cites a substance called XR-6 which promises the purchaser that he will lose 61 pounds if he puts two capfuls of the substance in his bath and does so for five successive baths.

"The nation is being swept with gadgets and pills and body wraps that claim to take inches off a person's body without the difficult regimen of diet and exercise," says Woodrow Wirsig.

"But since the claims for these products and techniques have never been proved, the Better Business Bureau considers them deceptive and their advertising misleading to the public." There is no medical evidence that any topical applicant, such as a cream or an emollient, can have the effect of reducing weight.

What about the recurrently popular grapefruit diets? Most advertisements for them focus on an extensive use of grapefruit in combination with a low-carbohydrate, high-protein diet, such as the *Super-C Grapefruit Diet Reducing Plan*. The Post Office Department, in refusing this plan the right to the mails, had this to say: "The grapefruit itself has no special properties as a metabolizer of fat. Depending on how much you eat, if followed for a long term without medical supervision, it could be harmful to persons with certain kinds of heart or kidney problems."

Well, if not grapefruit, how about the sex-instead-of-supper regimen? Sounds attractive, but does it work? According to Neil Solomon, M.D., sex is good exercise, as is any phsical exercise. And it can't hurt. But there is no substitute for a combination of diet and exercise, under the control of a physician.

Amphetamines? Jean Mayer, M.D., of Harvard University, one of the world's most respected nutritionists, stresses that the weight loss resulting from courses of amphetamines are often short-term. In the long-term only psychological dependency and deleterious side effects may result.

Again and again, scientists, researchers, nutritionists report—as the result of controlled experiments—that whatever the panacea for weight loss, people tend to regain the weight they think they have lost forever.

Maybe it shouldn't come as a surprise, but it almost invariably does. In 1968, Dr. Jean Mayer wrote about a study conducted in Boston:

"Four similar groups were constituted, each of a hundred patients recognized as overweight. The first group was left untreated; the second group was referred to a dietary clinic at a university hospital; the third group was treated by group psychotherapy; and the fourth by individual psychotherapy. Three years later the individuals involved in the experiment were again examined. Although the various treatments had yielded some measure of temporary success, the long-term result was about equally dismal for all four groups. At the conclusion of the three-year period, a small minority in each group had lost weight, a somewhat larger number—again in each group—had gained weight, and the majority of patients were in about the same position they had occupied before the experiment commenced. Their weight had bobbed up and down . . . None of the therapeutic groups led to an effective improvement over the untreated group."

This past August, Abraham Weinberg, M.D., a New York psychiatrist and Alvan Feinstein, M.D., of the Yale Medical School, both were quoted as saying that out of any given 100 patients on weight control programs, only two can be expected not to regain the weight within a year after losing it.

They are victims of their own situations. Is it any wonder that they are so prone to becoming victims of others?

Here are some basic guidelines anyone who is overweight and wants to lose weight can follow to assure a sound, healthy life of reducing':

● Diet alone, without exercise, is seldom sufficient. Beware especially of diets that have special "gimmicks."

● Exercise alone, if directed at particularly portions of the body, such as the hips, the abdomen, is not effective if you don't work at it. Exercise and diet, under a physician's direction are best.

● If you go to a clinic or gym, and are told you are receiving a special program, make sure everyone isn't also receiving the same "special" program. And, before you sign a contract, have your lawyer examine it to make sure you can get out of it, if necessary.

Above all, to thine own self be demanding. Leaving out people who have medical or hormonal difficulties, the way to lose weight is by eating less but more soundly, and exercising more.

You have to expend more energy than you take in.

Any other claim you can suspect to be a fraud.

BEFORE YOU BELIEVE THOSE EXERCISE AND DIET ADS read the following report

by Robert Sherrill

THE PATH to instant happiness for the average adult American can be capsuled in two words: *inches off.*

To the medical doctor, excess fat may signal heart disease, but to nearly everyone else it means something much more grim. Fat is what wallflowers are made of; fattys look bad in minis or bikinis and never know true love. And fattys must lose weight fast, fast, fast.

The most indifferent television viewer or magazine reader has only to bring his eyes to rest to absorb this siren-like pitch from the omnipresent advertiser. A frenetic national campaign urges that we *take inches off* . . . inches off the waist, hips, thighs and, as the diet ads persist in calling it, the tummy.

With this heightened, albeit manufactured desire for *inches* off comes impatience. Otherwise mature adults, who have dedicated a lifetime to putting on fat, now expect to shed it in a matter of hours. How? By heeding advertisers who promise anything, and then deliver to the fat-fighters only inefficient, if not worthless pills and, more recently, the questionable gadgets that squeeze, shake, rattle, juggle and electrically roll-away excess *avoirdupois.*

The results? Just short of chaotic. A new and often dangerous huckster preys upon the gullible American public, bilking us of more than $250,-000,000 each year. Some experts believe the bill for this consumer fraud is even higher, placing the total at one billion dollars.

Moreover, with his special blend of hucksterism, this predator brings a share of heartache as well as other, more permanent injury.

A bona-fide physician can keep his anti-fat speech to five words: "eat less and exercise more." But, in the rococo world of the advertiser, exemplified in the pages of the popular women's magazines, no element of life can be restricted to five words—particularly when the subject is diet!

For example, between March 1969 and February 1970, 26 diet articles appeared in *Harper's Bazaar, Mademoiselle, Good Housekeeping, Ladies' Home Journal, Vogue, Seventeen* and *Redbook.*

And that, apparently, was only a warmup. Over the next 12 months, 38 more diet articles were featured in these same magazines, including sage and relevant advice on "Dieting by Computer", "Chewing Your Way to Health, Sexual Vitality, Peace", "Hot Dog Diet the Three Star Way" and, under a joint byline, "We Lost 409 Pounds."

Despite the occasional news story about deaths from diet pills—despite congressional investigations of "fat doctor" rackets—despite continued warnings from the American Medical Association and other counselors in the health field, this con game continues.

It can be argued, of course, that the public has no one to blame but itself, if it believes that magic tonics are able to transform Kate Smith into Twiggie.

One might also argue that the public would not be so gullible had it not been led to believe that federal agencies are keeping a sharp eye out for untested advertising claims, and that these agencies employ investigators who come down hard on predators, exposing their fallacious and often harmful advertising claims.

Let's look at the record. When I called recently at the Federal Trade Commission in Washington to ask agency officials what they had been doing to keep the *inches-off* industry honest, I was referred to the case against Tone-O-Matic. I was given a press release which, in a few terse paragraphs, explained that the commission had commanded this manufacturer of weighted belts to cease and desist from false advertising.

Tone-O-Matic had boasted that simply by wearing their weighted belt an individual could "whittle inches off your waist (firm up your thighs and hips, too) ."

True? False, said the FTC, adding that by wearing the weighted belt some individuals could "physically injure" themselves.

Beyond this press release, however, the agency spokesmen were reticent, almost uncommunicative, to the point of being unwilling to explain how a belt-wearer injured himself. I decided to telephone Tone-O-Matic in St. Petersburg, Florida, where, according to the FTC release, the belt manufacturers had their headquarters.

I was frustrated, however, for the Florida operator had no number for the company. I learned why from the St. Petersburg Chamber of Commerce.

"Tone-O-Matic?" said my inform-

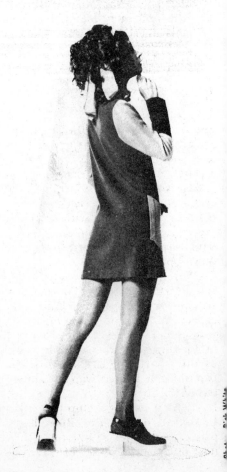

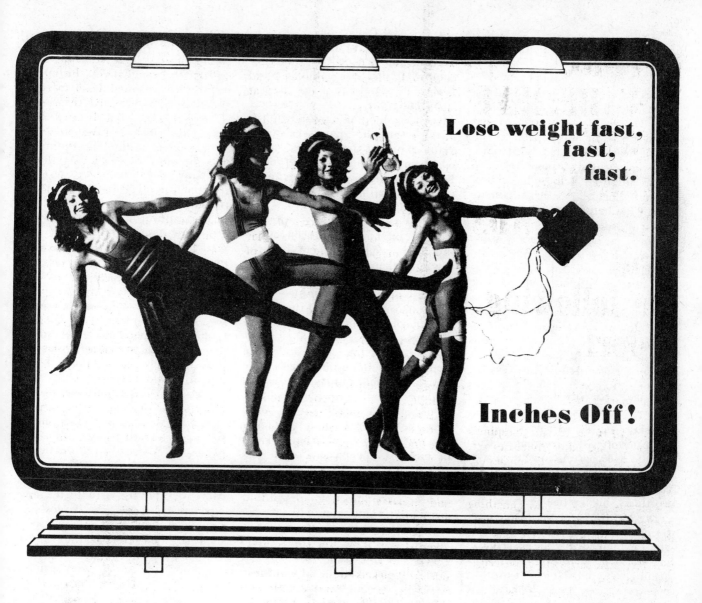

Lose weight fast, fast, fast.

Inches Off!

ant. "They're out of business. Our records show they went out of business on December 1, 1970."

The date on the government press release was April 8, 1971. The Federal watchdog had issued its stern order to the company, with press fanfare, exactly four months and eight days after Tone-O-Matic had shut down operations.

Of even more significance perhaps, is the FTC duty roster. To keep tabs on all false advertising claims, the agency employs one young man four years out of law school. He is assisted in making preliminary evaluations by three part-time law students and two full-time lawyers who have other responsibilities.

These six men make up the entire Consumer Protection Bureau—six pair of eyes to review the multi-million dollar outpouring of advertis-

ing from Madison Avenue, U.S.A.

Naturally — understandably – this cadre is overwhelmed. They cannot humanly keep pace, so they don't try. Their monitoring of television advertising consists of one "sample day" each month. What happens on the three major networks the other 29 or 30 days is lost to the FTC.

Harder times may be ahead for advertisers, though, because on June 9 the commission announced that hereafter it would require advertisers to prove their claims ahead of time. (Many believed this was in response to pressure exerted by consumer champion Ralph Nader.) The FTC has had the power to demand this kind of performance since 1914, the year the agency was established. Clearly, if it does intend to enforce the new regulation, it will have to add to both the size and the enthusi-

asm of its small investigatory staff.

Another government agency with a spotty record for policing the inches-off peddlers is the Food and Drug Administration. The FDA's most notable success against the fat-quack fraternity came last year, when it forbade any but prescription sales of the Relaxacizor.

The Relaxacizor is an electrical device that transmits current to the muscles via contact pads strapped on the body. The electrical current then forces the muscles to contract. This was alleged to "firm up" the body and reduce girth.

When assembled and turned on, the Relaxacizor made the user look like a character out of television's *Chiller Theatre.* Making a fool out of the buyer wasn't the end of it, however. In the hands of some 400,000 amateur and unsuspecting owners, the Relaxacizor could, literally, be a death trap.

Acting upon evidence provided by the FDA, a federal judge issued a court order halting the future sale of the machine. He then declared that the Relaxacizor was capable of inducing heart failure. He also attributed to the machine the power to add to "gastrointestinal, orthopedic, muscular, neurological, vascular, dermatological, kidney, gynecological and pelvic disorders."

Moreover, he said it very possibly aggravated "epilepsy, hernia, multiple sclerosis, spinal fusion, tubo-ovarian abscess, ulcers, and varicose veins."

Historically, federal agencies have been slow to move against businessmen, and the sales of Relaxacizors and similar devices have proved that the *inches off* machines are very big business. Relaxacizor first appeared on the market in 1949, and was sold for 21 years before the government "crackdown." Estimates are that the Relaxacizor, with prices ranging from $100 to $400 per instrument, grossed $40,000,000—for a machine that the courts ultimately ruled not only worthless, but extremely dangerous.

Dr. Joe Davis, of the FDA's office for evaluation of medical-clinical devices, explained why the government moved so ponderously. He was disarmingly candid: "It wasn't until we got worried about the electrical dangers of the machine, frankly, that we found out much about it.

"They had started out saying the device would reduce weight, and we eventually got them to stop that advertising.

"Then they claimed it would reduce girth, and we got them to stop making that claim. They also said it would tone up muscles, and we disagreed with that. I guess we fussed with them four or five years before we took them to court, and after that we were in court for five or six more years.

"After we went to court, we made them give us copies of all the complaints they had received, including people who were injured. There were around 1,000 complaints, and of these about 500 said they had been injured by the device. Our men investigated 150 complaints and selected the 50 best cases for witnesses. They represented every kind of injury. One woman was so shocked by the machine that she fell off the sofa and broke her arm."

Dr. Davis says that 10 years experience in Washington have taught him to respect people's right to be stupid. "How much of the taxpayer's money," he asks, "should be spent protecting the gullible? The government says, 'Protect the fools, but not the damn fools.'"

In his time, Dr. Davis estimates, the FDA has forced about 500 companies to change labels where the error was more than minor, but only a few of these cases involved firms offering diet pills or devices promising weight-loss. The inference is that the agency did not consider diet quacks as public enemies.

"And many times," he adds, "we were only spinning our wheels. The companies could just change the misleading statement on the label and go on selling a worthless item. Moreover, the law is written in such a way that even if we forced a company out of business, the owners could just sell to a nephew and start up again.

"It's a very lucrative market," he added, "because people are gullible. Naturally businessmen will take advantage of people who think that by wearing a piece of innertube around their waist, and doing a few exercises, they can take off all the fat they want. Why, any woman who has ever worn a girdle should know what that sort of thing can do for you."

A third government agency involved in the "sometime war" against diet and device quacks is the Post Office Department. Here I found a little more action and spirit in the enforcers. Perhaps this is because they feel personally involved; after all, the hucksters depend on letter carriers to do most of their work. But, like the FTC and FDA, postal authorities rarely seek a criminal penalty. The Post Office only presses for a "civil agreement" from the cheaters, who they hope will then stop cheating people in that particular way.

To support this observation, I asked one of the Post Office lawyers if, as a result of their investigations and civil prosecutions, hucksters ever had to pay fines.

"No," he said, "and let's not use the word punishment. Our goal is not punishment but protecting the public."

Regrettably, their efforts haven't always been successful. This fact is manifest in the agency's running battle with mail-order peddlers of diet pills. Earlier this year Post Office authorities closed down Anapax Products Inc., of Brooklyn, N.Y. The company had been doing a brisk trade with sandy-colored pills whose principal ingredients were those old pharmaceutical familiars *benzocaine* (for quieting the taste buds) and *methylcellulose* (for supplying bulk to the stomach and intestine and thereby, supposedly, giving a feeling of "fullness").

During the postal hearing against the Anapax manufacturers, the government's expert witness testified that the tablets were worthless as diet pills. Dr. Lawrence E. Putnam said the pills could neither cause a weight reduction or help a person maintain a disciplined diet.

Anapax was out of business, but in similar cases when diet pill companies have been shut down by the government, they have simply begun anew under a different brand name. Moreover, they use virtually the same advertisements ("Yes, I lost 83 pounds of ugly fat in only two short months"), the same mailing house, and continue to ship the inevitably worthless pills along with printed diets that could, in fact, produce weight-loss. However, the skimpy diet plan is hardly worth the price of pills —usually around $5.95 for a 30-day supply.

Another factor favoring diet quacks is time. It takes time for the Post Office to investigate and test a product, and it requires additional time to draw up and file a complaint and bring the case to a hearing. As one Post Office lawyer said, "Time is what these people trade on. As long as they can keep operating, with mail returns of anywhere from 100 to 1,000 pieces a day, they couldn't want any more. Every day means big money to them."

According to this lawyer, a diet quack generally is in operation at least three months before the Post Office hears about him. Then he's free to market his product for another nine months before he must answer charges at a hearing. Meanwhile, he can average 500 daily orders, at $5.95 each. Total gross income: $1 million.

Millions of overweight Americans, conditioned by advertising to join the *inches-off* crusade, offer an irresistible market for profit-bent manufacturers of "effortless" reducing devices.

One of the most successful of these new products is called the Sauna Belt; it is a phenomenon worth examining.

Several years ago, an articulate Californian named Jack Feather who, with his wife, runs a chain of health spas, sprained his knee. He wrapped an elastic Ace bandage around the knee and left it on for several weeks. When he removed the bandage he noticed the knee was, he says, about an inch thinner than the uninjured knee. He deduced that the bandage had produced a weight loss.

"I thought perhaps the combination of constrictive bandage and activity made the difference.

"Anyway, it was worth trying. So we got a number of Ace bandages and had our women customers wrap their upper arms before they exercised. We found it helped to tighten and firm the arm and diminish girth much more rapidly than exercising without the bandages."

It may not have been the greatest discovery since the wheel, but for Mr. and Mrs. Jack Feather it meant money—lots of it.

After the initial success with Ace bandages, the Feathers began wrapping the waists of their lady exercisers with gauze. Then, around 1962, Jack Feather started using a rubber belt. Six years later, in October 1968, the plastic Sauna Belt was announced. It proved to be the mother lode. More than 600,000 have been sold, at about $10 per belt.

The belt differs from its predecessors. It is inflated before exercising and left on for a time after the exercise to let your midsection "steam".

The manufacturers guarantee its performance, promising: "If you do not lose one to three inches from your waistline in just three days of use, you may return the belt and receive an immediate refund of your money."

The Post Office investigators, however, don't believe in the belt. They maintain it won't do anything that plain exercising of the vigorous type

Sauna Belt dealers recommend won't accomplish. Their view is shared by some 14,000 dissatisfied customers who have asked for refunds. The federal examiners have also said that the belt can prove harmful for some, and that it is hardly a "new" device.

(The department's files tell of a device described as an elastic abdominal belt which was ruled off the market 21 years ago. The charge: fraudulent advertising.)

But postal authorities, and the doctors they hired to do their research, were especially offended by the idea, promulgated by the manufacturers, that the belt could reduce dimensions *without reducing body weight.*

In other words, if Sauna Belt's claims are accurate, the device causes the fatty deposits at the waist to move—to some other body area.

This contention was a focal point at an administrative hearing brought by the Post Office department. Lawyers, doctors and other witnesses argued for and against the claim.

Both advocate and adversary ran tests. Sauna Belt's test subjects, who included company employees, all were said to have lost from one to 3.87 inches at the waistline after using the belt three days. The government's testers all said they showed no loss.

The lay witnesses were followed by medical experts. Here is a sampling of their contradictory testimony:

Dr. Sedgwick Mead, a 1938 Harvard University graduate now at Kaiser Foundation Rehabilitation Center and Hospital in Vallejo, Calif., testified for the government:

"There is no really successful way of reducing the waistline without reducing body weight as a whole. . . . (The) inert fatty substance cannot be in any way increased or decreased in volume by massage, compression or exercise."

This was considered standard medical opinion concerning the possibility, or impossibility, of so-called "spot" reduction.

Challenging this view, and generally defending the Sauna Belt claims, was Dr. H. J. Ralston, professor of physiology at the University of the Pacific. Professor Ralston insisted spot reduction had taken place, explaining it was a "redistribution of the fat layer. There is no other reasonable

explanation. There is some kind of distribution of fat which is not dependent on weight changes . . . I am going to investigate this further. . ."

Dr. Ralston also testified that there "are rather peculiar things happening under the belt. The temperature seems to go up during the exercises, and although the subject sits for over an hour, the temperature keeps going up, instead of rising for a couple of minutes and then dropping . . ."

Postal officials aren't certain why, but they lost their case against Sauna Belt. Searching for an explanation, one investigator lamented that "we were up against thousands of those so-called satisfied customers."

Undaunted, the agency built a case against sauna shorts. They chose 30 prison inmates and ran well-controlled tests. Those who wore the "girth-reducing" shorts, now so widely advertised under a variety of trade names, lost no more than other inmates who followed the same exercises without shorts.

In this case, the government was testing for a complaint against Sauna Shorts Inc., of San Fernando, Calif., which had placed ads in most of the popular women's magazines. The ads guaranteed to take inches off, or the money would be refunded ($9.95 for regular size, $14.95 for longees).

When the Post Office investigators approached the manufacturer, setting forth their evidence, the company president promised to have his ads rewritten, giving more credit where credit was due, namely, to exercise.

In summary, government regulators win a few skirmishes, lose others, and are able, because of manpower and resources, to hector only a handful of the diet and exercise hucksters. And things aren't likely to improve until we have tighter laws and the will to press criminal prosecutions where warranted, more investigators and lawyers, and, above all, the technique for filing class actions—firing a legal suit at all the cheaters, not just one or two.

The protectors of consumer rights can't hope to nibble an entire industry into shape. That's no way to reduce; any number of boys in the *inches-off* business will swear to that. ▦

diet books THAT POISON YOUR MIND... and HARM YOUR body

A concerned look at popular weight-loss programs

By Don A. Schanche

A few months ago two fit-looking men appeared on a television panel show in Houston. The subject was dieting and nutrition.

One of the panelists was a physician who was deeply concerned about the millions of gullible, overweight Americans who swallow spurious diet books almost as readily as they gulp down food.

The other was a self-proclaimed "successful" dieter who boasted that he owed his strikingly lean shape to the best-selling book *Dr. Atkins' Diet Revolution: The High Calorie Way to Stay Thin Forever*, by Robert C. Atkins, M.D.

Visually the show was a standoff, but verbally it turned into a real contest. If one could judge from the reactions of the panel's moderator and the small studio audience, the glib dieter won, hands-down. The physician's sober warnings against the potential hazards of Atkins's discredited high-protein, low-carbohydrate diet were no match for the sparkling wit and evident success of the high-calorie advocate.

But viewers missed the show's ironic sequel. The very next day the seemingly healthy dieter called his fellow panelist and urgently asked for a professional appointment. Sheepishly, he explained that while rising from his morning bath he

had blacked out, struck his head on the tub, and very nearly drowned.

As it turned out, he had suffered a spell of what doctors call "postural hypotension"—a dramatic drop in blood pressure when one shifts from a supine to a standing position—when he stood up in the bathtub.

Most low-carbohydrate dieters—and there are many millions in the United States—know the feeling: a slight dizziness when rising from a chair or getting out of bed. In this man's case it was more severe. His brain momentarily lacked sufficient blood flow to sustain consciousness. He was lucky to survive with only a bad headache.

The cause, according to the physician, was *Dr. Atkins' Diet Revolution*, a book that has been condemned by the Council on Foods and Nutrition, of the American Medical Association, as being not only "without scientific merit," but fraught with hazards.

Reduced blood pressure is but one of a number of ill effects directly traced to Atkins's and other immensely popular diets which promise that you can lose weight and inches while consuming all the calories you want. All you must do, the diet books say, is stick to copious servings of protein and fats—such as

eggs, meat, and cheese; and stay away from carbohydrates—such as bread, potatoes, and sweets.

One of the worst problems (and, paradoxically, the greatest lure) of such diets, according to Philip L. White, Sc.D., Secretary of the AMA Council, is that they "create a situation that is not dissimilar to the metabolic pattern of diabetes." The high-fat, low-carbohydrate diets trigger an abnormal body response called ketosis, the increased production of compounds called ketones—usually associated with conditions of impaired metabolism, such as diabetes. In normal quantities, ketones play a routine part in the body's metabolic process. But when they flood the system in excessive quantity, they suppress appetite.

Presto! Diet magic. Since the dieter no longer is stuffing down all the calories he *thought* he wanted to eat, he loses weight.

But, like the rueful TV panelist who toppled in the tub, he or she may end up paying a very high price in general health for this seemingly magical ketogenic effect. Even if he succeeds in maintaining the weight loss (less than 10 percent of dieters achieve that goal), he still may be in trouble.

Physicians have reported hundreds of

cases of men and women hospitalized from the side effects of such dieting programs. One example, that of an old-fashioned case of scurvy, in a young women dieter, was recently mentioned to me by Theodore B. Van Itallie, M.D., the internationally known nutrition expert and professor of medicine at New York's Columbia University.

Among other health problems directly linked to low-carbohydrate diets are fatigue, apathy, dehydration, calcium depletion, kidney trouble, and threatening elevations of blood lipids (cholesterol and triglycerides) which are associated with heart disease. Therefore, according to C.E. Butterworth, Jr., M.D., the AMA Council's chairman, "the full impact . . . may not become apparent to an individual's health until many years later."

As a druggist once said to an unsteady but pleasure-bent young sailor who anxiously ordered a bottle of Dramamine and a box of contraceptives, "If it makes you sick, why do you do it?"

Because, says Dr. Van Itallie, this is the "Age of Caloric Anxiety." The anxiety stems from the inherent conflict between our thin standards of beauty and desirability, to which Americans are conditioned from childhood, and our fat standard of living. Not just plump: Fat!

Between 25 and 45 percent of us are officially obese (that is, more than 20 percent overweight) according to Richard F. Spark, M.D., of Harvard Medical School. Our diets, even among the non-obese, are tilted out of balance—too many of the wrong kinds of calories.

Fat, for example, constitutes 43 percent of the average American's daily calories (50 percent among college students and businessmen surveyed by the U.S. Department of Agriculture). Nutrition experts say it should be 30-35 percent, at most.

One out of five of us skips breakfast; and many of us snack around-the-clock, mainly on foods which are high in calories and low in nutritional value. Per capita consumption of such "empty" foods as potato chips and sugared soft drinks has doubled during the last two decades.

At the same time, the energy crisis notwithstanding, we're more sedentary than ever. For every jogger, hiker, and tennis player you see working off his excess calories, there are 20 soft bodies parked behind a table or a TV set.

"We have inherited a body made to hunt—to run after deer and club them—

not to sit at a desk," says Jean Mayer, Ph.D., of the Harvard School of Public Health.

It is no wonder that we are anxious about our weight and that in our anxiety we have spawned a $10 billion industry that caters, often irresponsibly, to our wishful hope of getting off that fat.

The industry that has sprung up promotes everything from "hot pants" (worthless rubber sweat-suits whose overuse can drain vital body minerals such as sodium and potassium and cause congestive heart failure) to luxurious fat farms (where pampered dieters often lose more money than weight). The most conspicuous and widely used products, for which Americans apparently have an insatiable appetite, are diet books and pamphlets.

No one knows just how many diets there are, because so many circulate in mimeographed and handwritten private editions. But there are literally hundreds of diet books on the open market, and they sell by the millions, annually. Except for Bibles and dictionaries, nothing in the history of world literature has surpassed them in volume.

A few of the more recent offerings, such as How Sex Can Keep You Slim, by Abraham Friedman, M.D. ("reach for your mate instead of your plate"), probably won't hurt you, which is more than can be said for the vast majority of weight-loss regimens. The idea behind the book is that sex, not overeating, is the better substitute for the unsatisfied emotional needs of many overweight people. Psychiatrists say that emotional food-stuffing is a lot more complicated than that, but at least sex is less fattening than a bedtime snack.

"It sounds like a real fun way to reduce," says Dr. White, who can manage, simultaneously, to place his tongue in cheek and lift his eyebrows over Dr. Friedman's assertion that the average sex act consumes more than 200 calories of energy (roughly equivalent to jogging a mile). More seriously, Dr. White adds that "there's no real harm in a book like this, except the economic loss to the person who buys it and fully believes what he reads—and the unwanted pregnancies that may result."

Two others of the emotional genre, minus the joys of sex, are Think and Grow Thin, by Morton Walker, M.D., and Joan Walker, and The Psychologist's Eat Anything Diet, by Leonard Pearson, M.D., and Lillian R. Pearson. These

books joined The Thin Book by a Formerly Fat Psychiatrist, by Theodore Isaac Rubin, M.D., on the self-help shelf. Any one, or all three of them, may actually benefit dieters who have the strength and emotional maturity to recondition themselves psychologically as well as physically. All, in different ways, try to help the reader establish his own internal signals to tell him when enough is enough. But the fact that 90 percent of American dieters fail to maintain their weight loss after any diet, even a medically prescribed one, indicates that few can manage such a psychological flip-flop without professional help.

But those are tough, demanding books, as is The Truth About Weight Control: How To Lose Excess Pounds Permanently, by Neil Solomon, M.D., with Sally Sheppard. Dr. Solomon, of Johns Hopkins University Medical School, in Baltimore, Maryland, offers no magic and no gimmicks—just sound, nutritional advice for people who are willing to work at sensible, healthy weight control.

Unhappily for our national state of health, the public, by its overwhelming dollar-vote in the diet-book marketplace, still opts for fads and gimmicks that do little good and can do much harm. Last year, for example, Senator George Mc-Govern's Select Committee on Nutrition and Human Needs turned up 51 new "egg and grapefruit" diets, all of which were at least figuratively fruitless and distressingly alike.

The diets were variations of an old perennial that usually surfaces under the name "Mayo Diet," even though no identifiable Mayo, including the prestigious medical center of that name, has ever had anything to do with it.

The bogus "magic" of the diet is the false implication that grapefruit, because of its tart, acid quality, has the extraordinary property of "dissolving" body fat. No food can do that. A grapefruit merely adds 110-120 calories, plus some healthy nutrients such as vitamin C, to the dieter's plate. Eggs, as every dieter knows, have high protein content and are one of nature's richest producers of cholesterol—one of the chief villains of cardiovascular disease.

Fortunately, most people who try such high-protein fad diets (or their opposite numbers: low-protein/high-carbohydrate) do not stick with them very long, so they probably do little immediate harm. But persistent dieters who go off-again on-again in a never-ending cycle of fat chasing can suffer from what Dr. White and Dr. Solomon call a "yo-yo" or "roller-coaster" effect. Its process was demonstrated in a recent experiment at the Harvard University School of Public Health. The results of blood tests on student volunteers revealed a surprising organic response to dieting. The cholesterol levels would rise a little higher with each dieting experience—almost as if the body were taking two steps down the weight ladder for each three steps up the blood-fat ladder. The experiment was curtailed to avoid doing permanent harm to the subjects, because such incremental increases in blood lipids can be dangerous.

That danger is one of many reasons why medical experts and nutritionists are virtually unanimous in singling out diets that are high in fat and protein and low in carbohydrates for special condemnation. These are the ketogenic diets, such as *Dr. Atkins' Diet Revolution.*

Careful scientific analyses of the diets and their hazards have received such widespread publicity that almost everyone, by now, must know of their dubious qualities. Yet ketogenic diets remain at the top of the list of best-sellers and promise to stay there until all of us drop in our bathtubs.

Actually, none of these popular diets is "revolutionary," nor do they differ much from one another. All stem, in fact, from the same source, a slender pamphlet published in 1863.

That was the year that William Banting, a portly Londoner, slimmed down on an experimental diet prescribed for him by a surgeon named William Harvey (not to be confused with the revered physician, William Harvey, who first described the mechanism of blood circulation two centuries earlier). Harvey drastically restricted Banting's carbohydrates but let him eat all the meat and dairy products that he craved. In tribute to his doctor, Banting wrote "A Letter on Corpulence Addressed to the Public."

Almost a century later, Banting's diet became the foundation of an immensely profitable, quasi-literary trade in ketogenic weight-loss plans, most of them written by men who, like Banting, knew little or nothing about the hazards of their course of eating.

The best known among the early entrées were the so-called "Air Force Diet" (variously and falsely attributed to both the Canadian and U.S. Air Forces); *Calories Don't Count* (which earned its author, Herman Taller, M.D., a mail-fraud conviction); and *The Drinking Man's Diet* (which merely added the numerous "empty" calories of booze to its adherents' low-carbohydrate meals).

Sales of these books, while brisk, were relatively small potatoes by today's standards. In a way, they were to diet-book publishing what an advance man is to politics: merely paving the way for the two biggest and most profitable ketogenic diet acts of all time.

The first came in 1967, when Irving Stillman, M.D., a Coney Island physician, and his highly visible ghost-writer, Samm Sinclair Baker, brought out *The Doctor's Quick Weight Loss Diet.* It was soon followed on the doctor's profitable quick-publishing schedule by four warmed-over spin-offs: *The Doctor's Inches Off Diet; The Doctor's Teen-Age Diet; The Doctor's Quick Weight Loss Diet Cookbook;* and a 25¢ abbreviated version in pamphlet form.

The books and pamphlet have so far sold 20 million copies and are still going strong, according to Baker. And he adds that the indomitable ketogenic collaborators are readying another number, *Dr. Stillman's 14-Day Shape-Up Program,* which promises to puff its way onto the best-seller lists by midyear. The book's "new" quality is that it adds exercise to the old diet, along with the astute observation that if you do your 15-minute daily workout in front of a television set, it won't turn out to be so boring.

Stillman and Baker may stand alone in terms of sheer productivity and sales, but they will never top Atkins in record-setting impact. Within a year after his revolutionary version of the same old diet was published, he had sold more than a million hardcover copies, at $6.95 apiece. Industry sources say that's an all-time record for *any* hardcover book of *any* kind.

Curiously, when the AMA's Council on Foods and Nutrition took the unprecedented step of issuing a warning against the book (as well as some of the others mentioned above), *Diet Revolution* experienced only a "brief and spotty lag in sales," according to the publisher, David McKay Company. Then it took off again.

When the paperback version hit the stands last fall, it moved even faster. Bantam Books reports that Dr. Atkins is now in his fourth paperback edition, with 2.45 million copies in print—all of which suggests that there are vast numbers of us who will swallow anything in our quest for fashion-model figures. For reasons which no one has satisfactorily explained, there seems to be a mystique to the psychology of overweight and dieting that even trips up usually skeptical scientists.

A few years ago, for example, many professional readers of the normally somber *Journal of the New York Academy of Sciences* pondered a weighty psychological monograph that purported to shed new light on "the relationship between eating habits and personality traits." The article disclosed several startling psychonutritional findings, one of which was attributed to an exhaustive psychoanalytic study of a group of asparagus eaters.

Its author reported that people "who spontaneously attack and eat the *tip* of the asparagus first are likely to be immature, fearful, dependent, and unable to defer gratification—even briefly.

"Those individuals who proceeded from stem to tip," on the other hand, "rated high in such personality parameters as frustration-tolerance, self security, and confidence. . . . In the American psychosocial tradition, (they) showed faith in the future, confidence in the Judeo-Christian ethic, and a conviction that delayed gratification is morally correct."

The title of the paper was "Freud Eggs." It was an obvious spoof. Yet the journal's chagrined editor reported that many of his scientist readers took its findings seriously.

While that may say something about the humorlessness of some scientists, it probably says more about the general public's apparent eagerness to believe anything in print that links food with emotional hang-ups. There is plenty of evidence to support the link in at least some obese people, although most overweight Americans can blame their lifestyles, not the hang-ups, for excess pounds and inches.

Unless we have deep-seated problems or extreme obesity, most of us ought to be able to shape up on our own, without expensive psychiatric attention or diet books that play Russian roulette with our metabolism. All one really requires, say experts such as Dr. White, Dr. Van Italie, and Professor Mayer, is a balanced, nutritious, low-calorie diet. Eat normal foods but less of them. On such a meal regimen of 1,000 to 1,200 calories a day, the average chubby American will lose between two and two-and-a-half pounds a week and learn something about healthful eating in the process.

You've heard that before, right?

Well, if it's not for you, try eating your asparagus from stem to tip, then reach for your mate. It can't hurt. **TH**

Two authorities suggest that recent best-selling books on weight control and nutrition recommend programs that may be ineffective at best, and hazardous to health at worst.

the dangers in diet advice

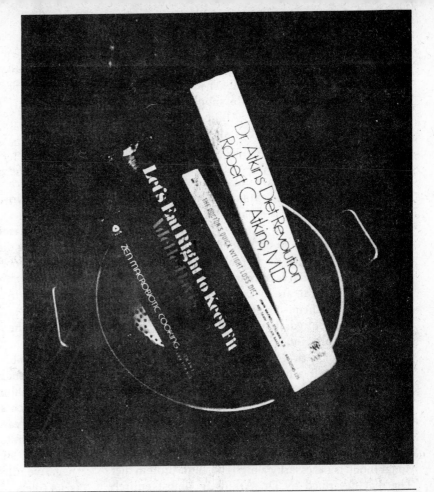

DR. ATKINS' DIET REVOLUTION: COMMENTARY BY PHILIP L. WHITE, Sc.D.

Dr. Atkins' Diet Revolution[1] is neither unique nor revolutionary, but it has nevertheless become one of the most popular of all diet books. In the process, states the AMA Council on Foods and Nutrition, it has exposed the dieter to definite health hazards.[2] The diet consists of the intake of no carbohydrates whatsoever the first week, followed by a low-carbohydrate regimen of such nature as to create intentionally deep ketosis. The author instructs readers to test for ketosis with a dip stick and to reduce carbohydrates until the test is positive.

Dr. Atkins developed some rather fanciful biochemical pathways and an unverified hormone in his attempt to introduce originality and credibility into his book. He failed in both instances, but the public doesn't seem to mind. To set the stage for his essentially total condemnation of carbohydrates, he dismisses dietary carbohydrates as having anti-nutrient properties. ". . . carbohydrates—not fat—are the principal elements in food that fatten fat people. They do this by preventing you from burning up your own fat and by stimulating your body to make more fat. Protein and fat combinations alone do not do this."[1,p.7]

Now the unverified hormone appears. According to Dr. Atkins, the diet promotes the production of "fat mobilizing hormone" (FMH), which is claimed to be the whole purpose of the diet and the reason it works when all others fail. "FMH releases energy into your bloodstream by causing the stored fat to convert to carbohydrate. Thus, the fatigue clears without having to call upon the defective insulin mechanism."[1,p.73] This fanciful biochemistry comprises "the diet revolution; the new chemical situation in which ketones are being thrown off—and so are those unwanted pounds, all without hunger."[1,p.13]

The Council on Foods and Nutrition, in its review, points out that no such hormone as a "fat mobilizing hormone" has been unequivocally identified in man.

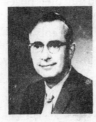

Dr. White is secretary of the Council on Foods and Nutrition of the American Medical Association; he served as a panel chairman of the White House Conference on Food Nutrition, and Health in 1969.

"... the existence and physiological role of a putative FMH in man remain to be established."[2] Atkins presents no evidence of his own to support its existence in man. Fat, according to Dr. Atkins, is converted to carbohydrate, presumably thus supplying the body's needs. In point of fact, other than the glycerol moiety of the triglyceride, fatty acids composed of an even number of carbon atoms are not converted to carbohydrates to any appreciable extent. Essentially all of the stored fat in man is composed of even-numbered carbon acids.

A considerable point is made that calories "flow out of the body" with the ketones and that this extra calorie loss is a special feature of the regimen. Actually only about 100 kcal. are lost via ketone excretion.

Incredible biochemistry appears to be the hallmark of the low-carbohydrate diet books, since Atkins' predecessors Taller[3] and Stillman[4] were just as free and easy with physiological pathways. Fanciful biochemistry is not of itself a hazard to the dieter, although it misleads him into believing that the discourse is authoritative and new. Other hazards await the unwary dieter, and it is precisely these hazards that prompted the Council to speak out.

A low-carbohydrate diet designed around conventional foods is necessarily a high-fat, high-protein diet. The diet described by Dr. Atkins is almost entirely composed of animal products very high in fat and

The risks do not justify using the ketogenic diet

protein. Unlimited food intake is encouraged, so that large amounts of uric acid and fat are circulating in the blood stream. These two features of the regimen, plus ketosis, set the stage for problems.

The high-cholesterol, high-saturated-fat diet poses a threat to the obese individual already in jeopardy of coronary artery disease. "The Council is deeply concerned about any diet that advocates an 'unlimited' intake of saturated fats and cholesterol-rich foods. In individuals who respond to such a diet with an elevation of plasma lipids and an exaggerated alimentary hyperlipemia, the risk of coronary artery disease and other clinical manifestations of atherosclerosis may well be increased—particularly if the diet is maintained

over a prolonged period."[2] The following listing of potential problems related to a mineral-depleting, dehydrating, high-fat, high-protein, low-carbohydrate diet has grown out of discussions of the Atkins book: weakness, nausea, apathy, dehydration, calcium and other mineral depletion, kidney stones, renal failure, cardiovascular disease (vascular thrombosis, atherosclerosis, cardiac arrhythmias, and possible congestive heart failure), gout, fetal damage, and last but not least anorexia.

It is reasonably well accepted now that a ketosis-producing diet does induce anorexia, and the resultant reduced food intake, along with attendant dehydration, probably causes the weight loss. The Council does not state that a ketogenic diet wouldn't work, but it does feel that the risks do not justify using this diet without the safeguard of careful medical supervision. In addition, "it is unlikely that such a diet can provide a practicable basis for long-term weight reduction or maintenance, i.e. a life-time change in eating and exercise habits."[2]

Research should continue on the ketosis associated with starvation and that induced by high-fat, low-carbohydrate diets. Blackburn, for instance, recently described studies of a starvation-like ketosis without negative nitrogen balance.[5] His experimental diet consists solely of lean meat to provide 0.6 to 1.0 g. of protein/kg. of body weight/day. He reports that hunger was not a problem and that weight loss was consistent. This regimen, however, differs significantly from one permitting unlimited intake of fat and protein. Until more research is accomplished, physicians are urged to observe the admonition of the Council: "Physicians should counsel their patients as to the potentially harmful results that might occur because of adherence to the 'ketogenic diet.' Observations of patients who suffer adverse effects from this regimen should be reported in the medical literature or elsewhere, just as in the case of an adverse drug reaction."[2]

But it seems reasonable to assume that a rash of similar books will follow, each with exaggerated advertising claims and promotion by the authors. After all, this has been going on without interruption for over 10 years, progressing from *Calories Don't Count*[3] (1961) through *The Doctor's Quick Weight Loss Diet*[4] (1967) to *Dr. Atkins' Diet Revolution*[1] (1972). Many science writers have asked whether the Council on Foods and Nutrition will continue to speak out against fad diets and reducing diets promoted to the public. Clearly, there are so many self-serving books and schemes that it would require inordinate amounts of time to respond to each one individually. An advisory panel to the Council has advised it to respond with critiques of fads when there is known or suspected biological harm attendant upon their use. Thus the Council in 1971 advised the profession of the inherent dangers of the "Zen Macrobiotic Diet." The Council's critique of low-carbohydrate diets[2] indicates the extent of its concern that physicians and others be advised of the hazards of such regimens promoted to the public. □

1. Atkins, R. C. *Dr. Atkins' Diet Revolution: The High Calorie Way to Stay Thin Forever.* New York: David McKay, 1972.
2. Council on Foods and Nutrition. A critique of low-carbohydrate ketogenic weight reduction regimens: a review of Dr. Atkins' Diet Revolution. *JAMA 224* (1973), 1415-1419.
3. Taller, H. *Calories Don't Count.* New York: Simon and Schuster, 1961.
4. Stillmen, I. M. and Baker, S. S. *The Doctor's Quick Weight Loss Diet.* Englewood Cliffs, N.J.: Prentice-Hall, Inc., 1967.
5. Blackburn, G. L. and Flatt, J. P. Preservation of lean body mass during acute weight reduction. *Fed. Proc. Abstracts 32* (1973), 916.
6. Council on Foods and Nutrition. Zen macrobiotic diets. *JAMA 218* (1971).

ADELLE DAVIS' BOOKS ON NUTRITION: COMMENTARY BY EDWARD H. RYNEARSON, M.D.

Unquestionably Adelle Davis is the best-known "nutritionist" in the United States; the reason for putting quotations around nutritionist is that she is not so regarded by the members of any of the scientific organizations in the specialties of dietetics and nutrition. This in no way implies that she has not had adequate training. By training she is eminently qualified. She is excluded from professional societies because of what she has done with this excellent training.

The 1927 University of California Yearbook records her transfer from Purdue University and her graduation from the Department of Letters and Science, where she was elected to the honor society and received the Bachelor of Arts degree with a major in household science. Her classmates and members of the faculty remember her as a pleasant, active and intelligent student whom they enjoyed and respected. For further training in dietetics she went to Bellevue Hospital and Columbia University, and received her M.S. degree in biochemistry from the University of Southern California Medical School in 1938. She has worked as a consulting nutritionist with physicians in various New York and California clinics.

Each classmate or teacher with whom I have corresponded expressed regret that a woman of her attributes and with her training should use them to disseminate half-truths and untruths. As one of her teachers said, "What bothers me about Miss Davis is that she has found it financially profitable to make a good story for food faddist preparations to the extent that she pays little attention to the accuracy of her subject matter. . . . She does have the capacity to interest people in nutrition—coupled with very few inhibitions about the accuracy of her statements—provided she can make a good story." Another associate writes, "She has long since forgotten the principles she learned and her books show an abysmal lack of knowledge of physiology." Still another states, "From the beginning of her professional life she has had an urge to explore and expound—sometimes beyond the field of her training."

Perhaps the most popular of the books she has written for the public is *Let's Eat Right to Keep Fit* (Harcourt, Brace & Jovanovich). It was written in 1954 and revised in 1970. Early in this work she squares off against physicians by saying, "We often forget that the study of medicine is *a study of medicine.* From the first day of medical school throughout the years of a physician's practice this study is primarily one of disease rather than health. . . . The tragic result is that nutrition is tremendously underemphasized, misinformation is given patients, much suffering continues needlessly, and drugs are expected to do what good food could accomplish." (p. 18) This is simply not true, and a great many other statements throughout the 272 pages are similarly inaccurate.

George V. Mann, M.D. of the Department of Biochemistry of Vanderbilt University School of Medicine, who took the time to read every page and to mark the mistakes (as defined by nutritionists and physicians), discovered an average of about one mistake per page!

The Journal of Nutrition Education referred this book to Dr. Ruth Okey, Emeritus Professor of Education at the University of California at Berkeley, who was one of Miss Davis' teachers. Dr. Okey says, "We wish we could believe that inositol would prevent blindness, that vitamin E would prevent or cure muscular fatigue or even muscular dystrophy, or that niacin would do away with blue Mondays. Most of us would hesitate to take 100,000 units of vitamin A per day for four weeks. . . . There are limits to the philosophy that if a little of a necessary nutrient is good, more is always better. The danger in a book like this lies in its use by the zealot."

Let's Get Well (Harcourt, Brace and World), written for the more serious students of nutrition, appears to be what is commonly referred to as a "cut and paste job." Almost certainly Miss Davis and her assistants compiled this book by reviewing a large amount of medical and scientific literature relating particularly to medicine, dietetics and nutrition. When she decided to make a statement of prejudice, she simply listed these references by number as support for the statement. These references were accepted by her publishers without verification.

A check of the references reveals a great discrepancy between them and the author's statements. For example, she says on page 406, "Because cancer has been produced in animals by feeding petroleum products (p. 373), fruits and vegetables sprayed with paraffin waxes should be avoided, and the use of these sprays prohibited by law." The references cited do not support this statement. In certain instances strong chemicals had been incorporated into a paraffin base and applied externally to mice; this caused some ill-defined skin cancers, but the interpretation of the authors was that these changes were related to the chemicals and not to the paraffin.

On the next page, 374, Adelle says, "Autopsies reveal that 90 per cent of persons dying of kwashiorkor have cancer [25]" and gives reference to an article written by Dr. J. F. Brock from Capetown, South Africa. There was no such support in Dr. Brock's article and in response to our query he replied, "Thank you very much indeed for drawing my attention to the misquotation in Miss Davis' book. I have never met her nor have I seen her book. This statement is, of course, nonsense."

Other misleading references abound. On page 154, Miss Davis says, "It has also been shown that the changes in aging skin are practically identical to those in the skin of young people overexposed to sun," and documents this as reference 57. But the article cited as reference 57 deals with the effects of vitamin E on the reproductive cycles and sexual development in rats. In Chapter 22 there are 50 references in less than eight pages, again showing a high incidence of carelessness and misrepresentation. Miss Davis discusses vitamins "so readily discarded during refining" when the article she quotes makes no mention of the refining process.

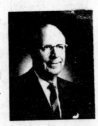

Dr. Rynearson is emeritus professor of medicine, Mayo Graduate School of Medicine, and emeritus consultant, sections on metabolic diseases, Mayo Clinic, Rochester, Minn.

She claims that "magnesium is particularly involved with the normal function of the brain, spinal cord and all nerves," and the references omit any mention of this mineral. She refers to a baby formula administered to 300 infants; the article deals with 54. On page 157 in a discussion of "Sore lips, whistle marks, and cracks at the angles of the mouth. . . ." she gives reference 18. This certainly is incorrect since the article is a summary regarding influenza, apoplexy and aviation safety.

Any physician or dietician will find the book larded with inaccuracies, misquotations, and unsubstantiated

---

«The danger in a book like this lies in its use by the zealot»

---

statements. For example, on page 374 "I have yet to know of a single adult to develop cancer who has habitually drunk a quart of milk daily." When I addressed a very large group of senior citizens in Sun City, Arizona I asked how many people in the audience ever had known of anyone who had "habitually drunk a quart of milk daily." Only two hands were raised.

Rona Karney, a graduate student in the School of Public Health of the University of California at Los Angeles and her professor, Roslyn B. Alfin-Slater, Ph.D., the Professor and Division Head of Environmental and Nutritional Science, plan to publish at least two chapters from Miss Davis' book where they have checked the references and found that approximately half of the references had no data leading to the conclusions drawn by the author.

Miss Davis is graciously received on television talk shows and guest appearances, usually in company with other "authorities" on food faddism from the entertainment field. They may have great talents as entertainers, but very few have had any training to qualify them as experts in nutrition.

One typical appearance was on *The Merv Griffin Show* on the evening of June 28, 1971. Other guests included Carlton Fredericks, who was introduced as "the leading nutritional consultant to industry, government and the professions"—a lofty title for a man with no scientific credentials. He and the three television personalities applauded the entrance of their star, Adelle Davis, who very quickly dismissed physicians as men and women who have never studied nutrition. She then commenced extolling the wonders of vitamin E. At this point Merv pointed to a member of the stage crew who had received a facial scar. Merv's wife followed Adelle's advice and prescribed Vitamin E for the man; to cut the capsules in half and rub them on the scar. "And as you can see the scar disappeared." Miss Davis' comment was, "Just think. You cheated a poor plastic surgeon out of his fee." Millions of Americans watch this nonsense, and there is no opportunity for orthopedic and plastic surgeons to report that this simply is not true.

When Miss Davis is confronted by experts, however, she does not fare so well. *Glamour* magazine, for its July, 1971 issue, arranged to have her meet with three other persons for a panel discussion; one of them was Dr. Leo Lutwak, then Professor of Clinical Nutrition at Cornell, now Professor of Medicine at UCLA. In this taped interview her supposedly scientific statements received rough handling. For example, when she

Physicians must deal with patients mislead by self-appointed experts

said, "The organic eggs are supposed to have more vitamin B12 and to have quite a different hormonal makeup," Dr. Lutwak replied, "Chicken hormones! What kind of hormones do chickens produce that the mammal requires? Chicken hormones are probably treated as foreign toxic substances by the human body." When Dr. Lutwak mentioned that high doses of vitamin C sometimes produce diarrhea, Miss Davis contradicted him, saying that this had never been her experience—a statement that conflicts with that in *Let's Get Well*, "Extremely large amounts of vitamin C will sometimes cause diarrhea." (p. 149).

Occasionally Miss Davis does admit errors. At a meeting in Washington which was called by the Division of Nutrition of the Food and Drug Administration, she was asked by Dr. Allen Forbes, Deputy Director of this agency, why she advocated large doses of vitamins A and D when it is known that these are harmful to some people. He gave as an example a case of a child undergoing brain surgery for a suspected tumor when the problem was really an excessive intake of vitamin A. Miss Davis' reply was, "I will accept your criticism and will watch carefully and take it seriously." Robert Choate asked, "You've written that calcium is a good

pain killer. What is the source for this?" Miss Davis said that many people feel that calcium kills pain: "The idea has been around awhile. I may be wrong." Dr. Eleanor Williams of Columbia University took issue with Miss Davis' claim that pregnant women should not drink skim milk "because it might cause cataracts in their babies." Again Miss Davis concluded her discussion by saying, "I could be wrong."

Dr. Russell E. Randall, Jr., M.D., Professor of Medicine and Chief of the Division of Renal Disease is very disturbed by her misquotation of his work and by her whole chapter relating to the kidney. "It is fraught with errors and inaccurate statements that are extremely dangerous and even potentially lethal, (such as the suggestion that patients with nephrosis take potassium chloride)."

She states in her introduction to *Let's Get Well*, "The hundreds of studies used as the source material for this book have been conducted almost entirely by doctors, perhaps 95 per cent of whom are professors in medical schools." (p. 9) This simply is not true; my guess would be that not 10 per cent are professors, and I feel quite certain that not five per cent of these were ever approached by Miss Davis or her publishers to ask for permission to quote from their articles or books. Although such permission is not a requirement for writing a book, it is a courtesy. I wrote to many of the professors and emeritus professors asking whether Miss Davis had corresponded with them concerning her use of their names and findings; of the 35 replies I received, not one had any record of correspondence with her, and not one endorsed her books.

I am not particularly concerned with Miss Davis' emphasis on "organic foods;" I believe that if people wish to pay two or three times as much for "organic honey" or fertilized eggs, it's their business and their money. What does concern me is that Miss Davis and so many others are opposing the pasteurization of milk and other foods. All of the studies performed by state, national and independent laboratories report that pasteurization and homogenization have almost no measurable effect on the nutritional character of the food. A great many of us can remember the ravages of many diseases before pasteurization became a standard procedure.

It is my hope that this article has not been a simple exercise in futility. Miss Davis' books have sold over 10 million copies, and she writes so authoritatively that her readers believe she writes the truth. A recent survey by National Analysts, Inc., indicates that a majority of citizens prefer information obtained from faddists and quacks; physicians must deal with the resistances they will encounter in patients who have been misled by these self-appointed experts. It is my sincere wish that what I have written here may counteract some of the erroneous and dangerous propaganda of Adelle Davis. ☐

Dr. Philip L. White tells
WHICH DIETS WORK—WHICH DON'T

*In a no-punches-pulled interview, one of America's top nutrition experts evaluates
the full range of popular diets and recommends the most sensible approaches to losing weight.*

JUST LOOK into the possibility of taking off a few pounds and you'll discover the merchants of America coming at you. They'll tempt you with such painless fad regimens as the "Drinking Man's Diet," the "Calories Don't Count Diet," the "Doctor's Quick Weight-Loss Diet," the "Inches-Off Diet" and others—all the while recommending that you consume everything from rice and bananas to alcohol and steak.

America responds by paying out $100 million a year to the weight reduction industry. But the question is: Do these diets really work? Are they helping or hurting your general health? In the following interview, noted nutritionist Dr. Philip L. White, director of the American Medical Association's Department of Food and Nutrition, answers the question by examining the above-mentioned popular diets (and others) and offers his recommendations on how to diet intelligently.

Dr. White, do fad diets have any value at all?

Commercially, I'm sure they are of enormous value to their promoters. Nutritionally, I'm not so sure. Some of them are useless and a few are even dangerous.

But a lot of people claim to have successfully lost weight with some of the more popular diets.

Sure, you can lose weight with a commercial diet, I can't deny that. But there is more to proper dieting than just losing weight. Once you've lost the weight, you must change your eating habits so you won't gain it all back again. And the diet should be nutritionally sound or it could endanger your health.

All reducing plans—both good and bad—work on the principle that any time there is a serious deficit of energy or an important nutritional imbalance, the result is weight loss. We need certain quantities of protein, fat, carbohydrates, vitamins and minerals every day for health and normal weight maintenance.

In a sound reducing plan, the nutritional element you want to reduce is the number of calories in the food. You do that by simply reducing the quantity of food, without taking away any of the nutrients you need.

How do the fad diets work, then?

The gimmick common to most of the commercial diets is high-protein, high-fat, low-carbohydrate intake. The theory is that protein is "less fattening" than carbohydrates. But that's not true—*any* food can be fattening, depending on how much you eat and what you eat with it.

You mean commercial diets are all about the same?

More or less. Those that aren't high-protein, low-carbohydrate are probably just the opposite—low-protein, high-carbohydrate. They work on the same spurious principle.

But the most popular diets seem to be the high-protein ones. Some of them are simply variations on the old "Calories Don't Count" diet of Dr. Herman Taller, which was a version of something earlier called the Pennington Diet. It had to do with the all-meat diet that explorer Vilhjalmur Stefansson followed on one of his extended explorations in Alaska. Some authorities trace that high-protein diet clear back to a regimen concocted for an English dignitary in the 18th Century. In other words, it's nothing new.

Let's talk about some of the more popular diets. The biggest seller in recent years seems to be the "Doctor's Quick Weight-Loss Diet," by Dr. Irwin Stillman. What is that like?

That's a high-protein, "no-carbohydrate" diet. It can be very satisfying to the dieter because it offers meat, cheese and eggs. In addition, Dr. Stillman urges the dieter to drink at least eight glasses of water a day.

I suspect the reason he put that in was because a number of people had criticized the high-protein diets for tending to cause dehydration (excessive loss of body water), and that can be quite unhealthy. It seems Dr. Stillman has capitalized on the water part of it. To some of the people who try his diet, it seems a mystery that you can drink all the water you want and still lose weight. Of course, most people excrete exactly as much water as they take in, so it's no mystery, but the "Quick Weight-Loss Diet" implies that it is the water that makes the diet successful.

Is that an unhealthy diet?

It can be. Most of these diets tell you to eat very little carbohydrate, and with some diets you consume less than 60 grams of it a day. The National Research Council suggests that persons accustomed to normal diets need at least 100 grams per day to avoid ketosis—excessive protein breakdown—and other undesirable metabolic responses. Carbohydrates—sugars of all kinds and starches—are important for many different functions in our bodies, brain and nerve cell maintenance, for example.

What about the second Stillman diet, the "Doctor's Quick Inches-Off Diet"?

In my judgment, this diet can be extremely hazardous, because it is very low in protein. So low that it can in fact cause the dieter to lose protein from his own body, to use up muscle and organ tissue and generally weaken the body. Anyone who is already unhealthy because of organ damage—liver problems, kidney damage, heart disease, anemia—can be put in a very hazardous situation by further tissue depletion.

The "Inches-Off Diet" says you can lose weight in selected spots, wherever you want to. That's a complete fallacy. Even if it were true, this kind of diet would cause loss of muscle tissue as well as fat.

What about the "Calories Don't Count" diet you mentioned earlier? Is that still popular?

I think it has outlived its usefulness. Like most of the fad diets, it was a high-protein, high-fat, low-carbohydrate regimen. Its originator, Dr. Herman Taller, was convicted in 1967 of mail fraud and violation of the Food, Drug and Cosmetic Act. What ultimately got Dr. Taller and his publishers in trouble was a commercial promotion for safflower oil capsules tied into the book. Safflower oil containing polyunsaturated fatty acids was supposed to flush body fat out of the system. That, of course, is a complete hoax.

What about the Air Force Diet?

Again, the same thing. It is sometimes called the "Low Carbohydrate Diet." You were supposed to be able to eat lots of meat and poultry with few vegetables, cheese or eggs. The amount of carbohydrates in this diet was dangerously low, far below the National Research Council's suggested levels. The diet, by the way, has no connection with the U.S. Air Force.

The "Drinking Man's Diet" was popular in certain circles a while back. Was there a gimmick to that diet, too?

That was just a variation of the "Calories Don't Count" plan. The gimmick was that, according to the promoters, the calories in alcohol "don't count." Its popularity was built on the contention you could drink all the booze you wanted and it wouldn't cause weight gain. That's nonsense. Actually, alcohol is quite high in calories, though it has little nutritive value.

There is something called the "Mayo Clinic Diet" that seems quite popular. Is that just another commercial enterprise?

I'm not sure of its origin, but it has nothing at all to do with the Mayo Clinic in Rochester, Minnesota. The clinic disavows any relationship with it at all.

The diet seems to vary according to who mimeographed it last, but generally it promotes grapefruit and eggs as the basic regimen. Grapefruit was supposed to chew up and dissolve body fat, which is an asinine supposition. No food has such properties.

Most fad diets seem to be based on the same concept, that certain foods or combinations are less fattening than others. But you say that concept is erroneous. Why is the idea so popular, then?

People who commercialize these diets like to be able to say, "You can eat all you want and still lose weight." And the foods they tell you to eat sound very attractive: lean meat, eggs, cheese—these are all fine foods.

But the notion that you can eat all you want and lose weight is a fallacy. Some people say they've been successful with these diets, but I suspect it's because over a period of time the diet becomes so monotonous and boring that they eat less. They may not notice the difference in quantity, yet in the tenth week of a high-protein diet they may be eating a great deal less than they did in the first week. Because they are eating less—not because of what they are eating—they lose weight. Unfortunately, that may

not be the best or safest way to do it.

Why not?

First of all, that kind of diet is likely to provide insufficient nutrition. We do need certain amounts of all nutrients every day for proper health maintenance. Take away one of those nutrients and you're putting yourself in a hazardous situation, even if you are losing weight.

Second, these concocted commercial diets teach the dieter nothing that can lead to a new way of eating for the rest of his life. It's fine to lose weight, but once you've lost it you've got to keep it off. And for most people who are overweight that means new eating habits. I think it is important for the dieter to learn good eating habits during the dieting experience so he can adopt a healthy weight-maintenance regimen once he's down to his desired weight.

But if a person started gaining weight after a successful diet, couldn't he simply go back on that diet and

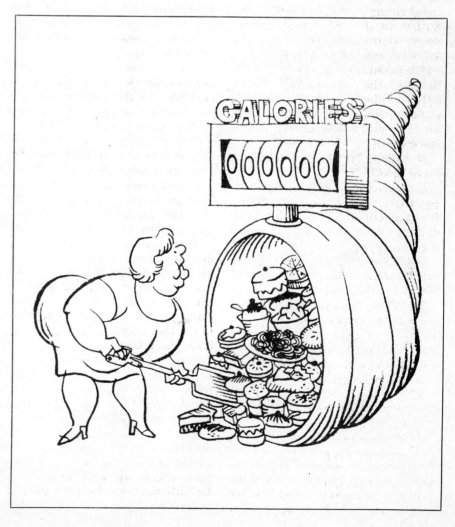

easily take the extra weight off again?

He could, but it would be better to maintain a steady weight. Losing and gaining weight periodically like that is what's called the "roller coaster effect;" it might be rather exhausting and possibly quite unhealthy. A number of authorities have stated that when this happens the level of blood cholesterol keeps creeping up. The level goes down each time you lose weight, but when you regain the weight the cholesterol level goes up higher than it was before, and the net result is that your health may be placed in serious jeopardy. That theory hasn't been well established yet, but it is certainly something to be concerned about. I'm not talking of weight fluctuations of just a couple of pounds or so—that's normal, and nothing to be alarmed about.

Is there a guaranteed "sure-fire" way to lose weight?

To hear the diet salesmen talk, there is, but that is nothing but pure commercialism and phony advertising come-ons. Actually, human nature is such that a simple answer to your question is impossible. Theoretically, if one simply adopts a regimen of calorie restriction without reducing the normal amount of exercise and activity he will lose weight. But there is more to it than that. People eat for a lot of different reasons, both

physical and psychological—we call those reasons the internal and external "clues" to eating—and different individuals react to different cues. A diet plan that does not take into consideration the psychological reasons a person eats is almost certainly doomed to failure. So I can't really say there is a "sure-fire" way to lose weight. First of all, of course, an individual must want to lose weight badly enough to change his eating habits.

Assuming a person does want to lose weight and is willing to stick with it, how should he plan a diet?

First, before he starts his diet, he should check up on what he normally eats for its nutritional value. He should make sure he's getting enough meats, vegetables, fruits, dairy products and other foods to get the right amounts of all nutrients. Then, he should simply reduce the portions he takes of all those foods—assuming he is choosing his foods carefully for good nutrition—until he begins to lose weight. Once he is down to his best weight, he should continue to eat the same foods, but in moderate weight-maintenance quantities. I think it is absolutely essential that a dieter's meals mimic a conventional, nutritionally sound maintenance regimen.

But how is the dieter supposed to know how much food he can eat and

still lose weight?

Well, you have to experiment with it. Each individual has slightly different nutritional needs. What the dieter must find out is how much food his body needs for normal day-to-day operation—that is, how many calories of energy his body uses. If he is overweight, then he is probably eating food in quantities that contain more calories than his body needs and the excess is being turned into fat. To lose weight, he must take in fewer calories than his body needs so that fat will be burned up to meet energy requirements. The dieter will simply have to try different quantities of foods. For instance, he might start out by simply cutting his portions by one-fourth. If after a few weeks or so he hasn't lost any weight, then he should cut down the portions even more, until he begins to lose weight gradually.

Isn't there any easier way to do it?

No, I'm afraid not, even though that's what 50 million Americans spend $100 million trying to find.

But I think people will find that once they get started on a regimen of eating less and exercising more it won't be so hard to take. You get used to it, and the benefits are worth the effort: You look better, feel better and stand a good chance of living longer than you might otherwise. **⊞**

—Edited by Roy Petty

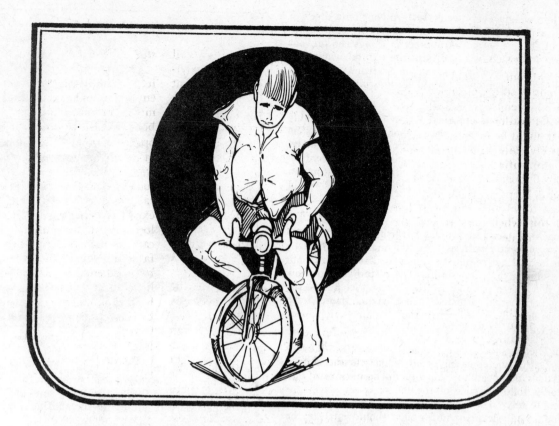

The truth about the 25 most common weight control myths

- Eating grapefruit burns excess fat.
- Dieters should take supplementary vitamins every day.
- Steam baths and massages help you to reduce.
- To gain weight, a thin person should stop exercising.

Belief in myths such as these has prevented many overweight and underweight persons from solving their problem. In some cases, belief in weight control myths even has led to physical damage. To get the scientific facts about 25 of the most common of these myths, *The Better Way* consulted the Good Housekeeping Institute, which has long been concerned with effective and healthful diets and weight control, as well as leading nutritionists and medical authorities.

DIETS

Myth: It is best to lose excess weight as quickly as possible. **Fact:** Most physicians recommend a weight loss of one to two pounds a week, unless there is a specific reason for which the physician wants a patient to lose more rapidly. Fast loss usually means a person resorts to a "crash" or fad diet. These can be hazardous to health if they do not provide a proper balance of nutrients.

The ideal weight-reduction program is one that provides all of the nutrients needed for good health but is restricted in calories. The diet should be within the framework of normal eating habits. The greatest advantage of this diet is that the dieter learns good nutritional habits for the rest of his life that will permit continuous weight maintenance. A proper exercise program also is important.

Myth: If you stay on a diet all the time, you *continued on next page* will lose weight every week. **Fact:** Anyone on a diet can reach a plateau where he will temporarily stop losing weight. This is normal. A number of things can prevent weight loss, such as changes in the natural water balance of the body. Physicians say that when a dieter does reach a plateau he will eventually lose more pounds if he continues to follow the diet.

Myth: Certain diets are good for spot reducing (taking inches off certain parts of the body). **Fact:** A person on a diet tends to lose weight uniformly over the body. Spot reducing can best be accomplished by concentrating on exercises that will strengthen muscle tone in problem areas and make you appear firmer once weight is lost through dieting.

Myth: After being on a diet for several weeks, the stomach shrinks. **Fact:** Studies have shown that if a person *permanently* reduces the total quantity of food he eats, he will not require as much food to feel full, but the stomach does not shrink. These studies also show that if a dieter stays away from sweet, rich foods, the body becomes accustomed to not having them. Some dieters actually feel ill when they eat these rich foods once again.

Myth: Dieters should take supplementary vitamins every day. **Fact:** A dieter eating a nutritionally well-balanced diet does not need to take vitamin preparations. If a dieter is following one of the fad or crash diets, it is wrong to rely on vitamin preparations for adequate nutrition. A physician or nutritionist should analyze the nutritional adequacy of your diet and decide if additional vitamins are needed. An iron supplement also may be needed since it is difficult for women to meet their full iron needs while on a low-calorie diet.

INDIVIDUALS AND WEIGHT PROBLEMS

Myth: A fat baby is a healthy baby. **Fact:** No medical evidence supports this. A high correlation has been shown between obese children and obese parents, and if one or both parents are obese or tend toward obesity, special attention should be directed to the diet and activity pattern of an infant from his birth.

Myth: A child will lose his baby fat as he becomes older. **Fact:** The earlier a child becomes obese, the less likely he is to lose weight. Research shows that gross overfeeding of infants and children is producing adults who have a larger number than normal of fat storage cells, says Dr. Philip L. White, director of the department of foods and nutrition of the American Medical Association. Once these cells are formed, they do not seem to break down. Throughout life these persons are much more likely to be overweight.

In general, parents should consult a physician to determine if a child is overweight and to prescribe the proper food program for the child. Parents should not put children on a weight control diet without consulting a physician. Improper nutrition can interfere with a child's growth and development.

Myth: The less weight gained during pregnancy the better. **Fact:** Obstetricians now agree that maternal weight gains are necessary because of the nutritional requirements of the fetus. Dr. Allan B. Weingold, professor of obstetrics and gynecology at New York Medical College in New York City, says that "if we analyze statistically the outcome of pregnancy compared with weight gain, the best outcome is associated with a

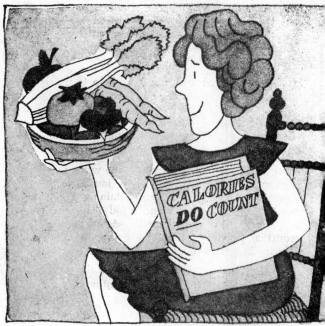

Illustrations: Lee Albertson

maternal weight gain of 25 to 27 pounds based, of course, on a sound nutritional program that is best suited to pregnancy." Dr. Weingold says the weight gain is necessary regardless of the starting weight.

Myth: As long as a fat person feels well, it is not necessary to lose weight. **Fact:** An excessive amount of weight always creates an extra hazard for an otherwise healthy person and can affect normal body functions. A fat person may have respiratory difficulties or less tolerance for exercise. Certain diseases are associated to a significant degree with excessively fat people, such as gallbladder disease, gout, diabetes, hypertension and cardiovascular diseases. Furthermore, excess weight aggravates certain conditions, such as arthritis. An overweight patient faces more risks in surgery, and mortality rates are higher among overweight persons compared with normal weight individuals.

Myth: Thin people naturally eat less. **Fact:** Many lean people are hearty eaters, but their bodies may utilize food less efficiently than an overweight person whose body stores unused calories as fat. However, being underweight, like overweight, depends on many factors—genetic, environmental, cultural, economic and familial influences and the amount of physical activity the person undertakes.

Myth: It is easier to gain than to lose weight. **Fact:** For the underweight person, gaining pounds can be as difficult as reducing is for the overweight. To gain a pound a week, a person must eat an additional 500 calories worth of food a day and, often, a constitutionally lean person has a difficult time eating this additional food.

WEIGHT CONTROL AIDS

Myth: Appetite suppressant pills or shots are all that is needed to lose weight. **Fact:** Any weight reduction procedure that does not include a restriction of calorie intake will not result in a permanent weight loss. Drugs only help curb appetite. Any drugs used should be taken under the supervision of a physician in the exact dosage he prescribes. The main disadvantage of drugs is that the patient often relies solely on the drug and learns little about adjusting his diet pattern to a lower caloric level so that he can permanently maintain a lower weight.

Myth: Steam baths and massages help a person lose weight. **Fact:** No scientific evidence shows that steam baths and massages are of value in a reducing program. A steam bath does cause a quick loss of water through sweating, but when the person drinks water, the loss is replaced.

Myth: If a person is underweight, one way to gain is to stop exercising. **Fact:** Exercise is important whether a person is gaining, losing or maintaining weight. Exercise gives added muscle mass and helps the gained weight to be distributed evenly. As part of a weight reduction program, exercise will expend calories and help the body develop good muscle tone.

Myth: Mechanical vibrating devices melt away fat or break up fat deposits. **Fact:** No scientific evidence supports this claim.

FOODS

Myth: Alcoholic beverages stimulate the appetite. **Fact:** When some people are tense, their appetite can temporarily disappear. Alcohol has a relaxing effect and, in this way, can help the appetite's return. However, any factors that help relax a person would have the same effect.

Myth: Toast has fewer calories than bread. **Fact:** The toasting process does not change calorie content.

Myth: Margarine has fewer calories than butter. **Fact:** Margarine and butter have the same amount of calories (100) per tablespoon. Diet margarine has approximately half the amount of calories of regular margarine and butter.

Myth: Washing rice and spaghetti after cooking reduces their calorie content. **Fact:** Washing does not reduce the amount of calories to any important degree, but it does rinse away some vitamins.

Myth: Milk should not be included in a weight-reduction diet. **Fact:** Milk is an excellent source of protein, calcium and the B vitamins. Sixteen ounces or more of milk each day is recommended for an adult. Skim milks (fluid and nonfat dry) have fewer calories than whole milk.

Myth: If a person eats large amounts of fish, he will lose weight. **Fact:** No single food will cause a weight loss. It is the total amount of calories you eat in a single day that is important in a weight control program. Most forms of fish contain less fat and therefore are lower in calories compared to meats.

Myth: Grapefruit burns up fat in the body. **Fact:** No foods will dissolve body-fat tissue.

Myth: Snacking makes you gain weight. **Fact:** You can eat snacks, so long as the total calories you eat in a day do not go over the amount of calories allowed.

Myth: Drinking vinegar has a slimming effect. **Fact:** There is no truth to the belief that body fat melts by drinking vinegar.

Myth: Different salad oils have different calorie values. **Fact:** All oils, including safflower, corn, peanut and olive, have the same amount of calories, approximately 125 per tablespoon. ◄

Ten common misconceptions about overweight and dieting

A third of the people in this country are overweight. Another third are struggling to keep their weight stable. Dieting has become a national American preoccupation, generating as much folklore as fact.

This article debunks ten of the most popular myths about dieting and being overweight. Each statement in bold type is a myth.

1 **Overweight people have something wrong with their glands.** Hardly ever true. Some people *are* overweight because of glandular diseases—such as an underactive thyroid, a malfunctioning pituitary or adrenal gland, or perhaps a diseased pancreas.

But blaming glands is a cop-out for most overweight people.

2 **Dieting is the best way to lose weight.** Wrong. Dieting usually means going on a crash program of eating at a near-starvation level. Crash diets are always doomed to failure because of their short-term, crisis nature—and because they don't provide adequate nutrition. They wear you down physically—and emotionally.

Experts agree that the best way to lose weight is to change your way of eating and living. You must eat less (particularly carbohydrates) and exercise more. If you have a sedentary job, you need only about 2,500 calories a day; but make sure you get them in a nutritionally balanced way.

Do some mild form of exercise regularly, including walking and calisthenics. Never take an elevator when you can take the stairs; never drive your car on an errand when you can walk or bicycle instead. And push rich desserts away.

3 **Fat people eat the wrong kinds of food.** Not necessarily. Fat people

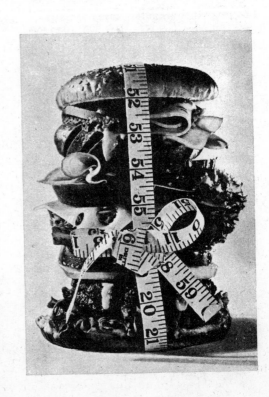

simply eat too much food, and are too inactive physically. They continually consume many more calories than they spend, day in and day out.

Think of it this way. You have a daily caloric budget, but it isn't constant. In the winter, especially if you spend time outdoors, you use up calories just to keep warm. You also automatically use up so many calories every day to stay alive, so many more calories to energize your muscles so you can move around (unfortunately, sitting, thinking, or talking doesn't burn many calories). You really need only as many calories as you use each day; what's left is "banked" as fat.

Naturally, some of the foods fat people love to eat are those more likely to be converted to fat by the body, such as rich desserts. Because of the complicated chemistry of your metabolism, carbohydrates—sugars and starches—are converted to fat more readily than are protein and fat. But that only means *some* of the foods fat people eat are wrong. Their problem really is that they eat far more food than they need day after day.

4 **Fat people are simply gluttons.** Nothing is simple about gluttony. There are many reasons people eat too much and get fat. Obese people often have some nervous or emotional problem that compels them to want more food than their bodies need. To some, food represents love. Many fat people have been that way since childhood, raised by fathers who showed their love by loading up the refrigerator, and by mothers who stressed second helpings and rich desserts as tokens of their love. As a result, these people grew up relying on their stomachs to give them comfort and security. When they feel blue, frustrated, or lonely, they often eat more to relieve their anxiety.

Another surprising fact is that many fat people act like gluttons only at night. They may have only coffee for breakfast, then skip lunch, and eat a modest dinner. Before going to bed, however, they stuff themselves with 3,000 or 4,000 or 5,000 calories. This compulsive gluttony is so common that doctors call it the Night-Eating Syndrome.

5 **Heredity has nothing to do with obesity.** Actually, heredity may have a great deal to do with an expanded waistline. Of course, if you're overweight, you put on that fat yourself; nobody bequeathed it to you. But it's quite possible you inherited a susceptibility to gain excess weight.

This genetic fact at least partially explains why some individuals can eat enormous amounts of food and stay thin —while others may eat only meager portions and get fat. Much of this difference relates to what a person's body does with food. Those lean people who are hearty eaters have bodies which are less efficient in using the calories in food. If you're overweight, there is a chance your body is a more efficient food-burner, which certainly is a mixed blessing. You've then inherited your body's ability to use food efficiently and store the excess, unused calories as fat.

Many studies have shown that overweight parents tend to have children who become overweight. Also, certain diseases associated with obesity, such as diabetes, are inherited.

Even so, this doesn't mean you're doomed to be fat. Recent studies of identical twins separated at birth showed that the twin reared by overweight parents who pushed food on him usually was overweight, while the identical brother or sister reared by normal-weight parents was of normal weight. The implication is that you can counteract your genetic tendency to fatness. But you'll have to be even more careful about eating than are people your own age born of normal-weight parents.

6 **You can eat as much as you want of some foods.** It's not true, despite all the diets around that are based on the idea of eating exclusively noncaloric or very-low caloric foods. The claim is that such diets provide a full feeling and curb your appetite for all other foods. One diet uses water, for example, and another fresh green or yellow vegetables such as celery or carrots.

Of course, you're a lot better off to reach for a stick of celery or a carrot than a piece of candy when   *Continued*

195

the urge to snack comes over you. But if you eat enough carrots to turn you yellow, or enough water to keep you running to the toilet 20 times a day, you're liable to do yourself harm. To stay healthy, you must eat a well-balanced diet that contains all of the necessary food nutrients. By eating *only* fresh green vegetables, for instance, you'll get plenty of vitamins and iron, but you'll no doubt lack proteins, fats, and carbohydrates.

There also are fad diets that let you drink as many martinis or other alcoholic beverages as you want, as long as you watch your carbohydrates; or eat as much fat as you want as long as you eat lots of grapefruit; or the latest craze with the young, a diet which calls for only rice—and brown rice at that.

The main ingredient of these diets is baloney, and not the kind you eat. In the long run, fad diets are dangerous because they don't give you a well-balanced menu. You really need to eat every kind of food; the trick is to eat only what you need of any kind.

7 Height-weight charts are your surest guide to ideal weight. They may be your fastest guide, but they definitely are *not* your surest guide. First, the charts most commonly used are based on data from thousands of Metropolitan Life Insurance Company customers. These policyholders do *not* necessarily represent the American population and its composition of people from diverse ethnic and racial backgrounds, living at all levels of economic conditions.

Yet even if their data were perfect, the tables still don't give you enough information to figure your ideal weight accurately. The tables are categorized by Small Frame, Medium Frame, and Large Frame. How do you judge your frame? Besides, the categories don't take into account normal variations such as a short trunk and long legs, or vice versa.

Fortunately, there are better guides to ideal weight. One is the pinch test: with your finger and thumb, gently pull on the loose skin at the back of your upper arm or at your waist and measure the thickness. It should be between a half-inch and an inch thick. If it's thicker, you're too fat.

An even better test is your mirror. Look critically at your nude body and decide if *you* think you're too fat. If you see more of yourself than you would like to see, you're not at your ideal weight. Or ask your mate, but brace yourself for the brutal truth.

8 You can actually exercise fat away. This is a half truth. On the positive side, exercise is one of the most important things you can do to keep your weight under control. It is the expenditure part of your daily caloric budget. If you eat the same number of calories you did when inactive, and then start exercising, you'll soon lose weight. Think of it this way: 34 minutes of swimming burns up a hunk of apple pie, which otherwise could be converted to fat; or 49 minutes of walking uses the same number of calories in an ice cream soda; 49 minutes of bicycle riding uses as many calories as are in a serving of strawberry shortcake. These are, admittedly, examples of lots of exercise for relatively little weight loss, but they can add up to a substantial amount. To lose even more weight, you could stop eating these desserts completely and begin exercising; then you'll double your loss. For every 3,500 calories you burn up, you'll lose a pound.

But there is a negative side to the weight-loss-by-exercise idea. Too many people forget the diet part of their calorie account. They feel that by exercising regularly, they don't have to worry about what they eat, that the fat will merely "melt away." This is no more true than the claim that belts and other kinds of "exercising at rest" vibrating devices will rid you of fat. These contrivances only reduce your bankroll.

9 Certain pills make weight loss easy. No. They actually make it much more difficult. The first thing you should remember is that any diet pills you buy in a drug store or supermarket without a prescription contain little medicine and have very limited effectiveness. And the potent pills a physician can pre-scribe are almost always only chemical crutches for desperate dieters to lean on. Here's why.

A person on a strict diet usually loses weight very quickly at first, and then levels off to a slow weight loss over a period of weeks or months. Along the way the dieter often gets discouraged and is ready to give up. What's happened is that the body is retaining water. During this discouraging period, the dieter's doctor may prescribe a drug called a diuretic to trigger water weight loss. It gives his patient inspiration to stay on the diet, and there's no great harm in that. Less justified is the use of amphetamine drugs, which stimulate a person physically while curbing his appetite. These pep pills can be habit forming, and once hooked on them an individual may have to resort to still other pills to relax. This is the road to drug dependency—and there's a greater danger in that than in being overweight.

Equally hazardous are the "miracle drugs" pushed by some diet doctors. These can be, for example, pep pills with thyroid extract to boost metabolic rate and some digitalis thrown in to spur your heart. You seriously risk weakening your heart if you try to lose weight this "easy way."

10 You should eat only three meals a day. Apparently not. Many experts feel we'd all be better off if we ate five or six small meals a day instead of three big ones. Such a nibbling diet can reduce fat and even lower weight. The idea is to feed the body machinery with an even stream of calories during the day, rather than with two fair-sized portions at breakfast and lunch and a huge input at dinner. By consuming small amounts throughout the day, the body uses calories as they come.

This doesn't mean, however, that you can forget about total daily calories. Even with the nibbling diet, you still have to watch the crucial balance of calories eaten and calories burned. ■

(Written in cooperation with Theodore Berland, a noted science writer, Chicago.)

Part IV: Overweight and Obesity in Childhood and Adolescence *

Apart from the fact that the untreated overweight child or adolescent invariably becomes the obese adult, childhood and adolescent obesity must be treated for its own sake. The fat child is at a grave disadvantage physically, socially, and psychologically.

Children in many parts of the United States are overweight. Obese children and adolescents are a major reservoir for obesity in adult life. They are more likely to remain obese as adults and to have more difficulty in losing fat and maintaining fat loss than the people who become obese as adults.

One excellent reason for the prevention of obesity, particularly during childhood and early adolescence, is the apparent persistence of early obesity.

It appears that obesity which develops before age 10 or after age 16 has a somber prognosis for eventual weight reduction. Obesity developing just before or with the onset of puberty may be an exaggeration of a normal physiological process and is often benign and self-corrects in the next few years. It is evident that early diagnosis and rapid initiation of preventive measures are essential if the obesity of early childhood and adolescence are to be avoided. While prevention of middle-age obesity is also of importance, it will be seen that obesities occurring in younger years are particularly damaging from a psychological viewpoint.

The psychological aspects of obesity may be a most compelling reason for prevention rather than waiting until obesity occurs and treating it. This is particularly true for children and adolescents.

Physicians and others who have studied and treated obesity in children have long believed that obesity exposes youngsters to difficult situations and damaging pressures.

These may be as important or even more important than the underlying psychological factors that could have etiologic significance.

The impact of uncomfortable pressures on the psyche of obese children has been illustrated in studies comparing obese girls in weight reduction camps with control subjects in a typical summer camp. Projective tests such as word association, sentence completion, and picture description revealed that the obese girls had personality characteristics strikingly similar to the traits sociologists have shown to be typical of youngsters in oppressed minority groups who were victims of intense prejudice.

One such trait is "obsessive concern" or heightened sensitivity and preoccupation with one's status. This was clearly illustrated in word association tests. Passivity and withdrawal were also characteristic. Passivity was illustrated in particular by picture description, which also revealed the obese group's feeling of isolation and rejection by their peers. The obese girls considered obesity and hence their own bodies as undesirable and as cause for shame.

The lack of an "in group" and particularly the lack of family support actually seemed to expose the obese youngsters to even greater tensions than experienced in minority groups. In relation to their own family, the obese youngsters appeared to be in both a situation of greater dependence and at the same time greater tension than the girls who were not obese.

The foregoing findings may be related to observations about obese subjects with "distorted body images" who exhibited attitudes remarkably similar, once again, to the "obsessive concern" and "identification with the dominant group" noted in ethnic and racial minorities. They had an exaggerated preoccupation with weight; they judged people in terms of weight, feeling contempt for fat people and admiration for thin people, and they felt that their obesity was a handicap responsible for all disappointment.

The individuals who displayed these attitudes had all been obese since childhood or since adolescence. The others had all become obese as adults. The crucial difference may be the extent to which punitive social pressures affected their personalities. Children and adolescents are sensitive to such pressures and would be expected to respond more strongly than adults.

Enough has been said to make it obvious that prevention of obesity, and the possible resulting psychological traumas, is an infinitely more desirable goal than mere treatment of an already obese person.

It appears likely that the psychological results of obesity, such as passivity and withdrawal, tend to accentuate the physical inactivity of obese youngsters and thus make the obesity self-accelerating or at least self-continuing.

Recent studies have demonstrated the extreme inactivity of the majority of obese children.

While the effects of obesity are particularly traumatic in children and adolescents, similar effects can be observed in middle-aged women and even in men who have lost confidence in their appearance and fitness. By "giving up" and "letting themselves go," the middle-aged obese epitomize the difficulty of restoring and maintaining pride in one's body once this pride has been lost.

Many youngsters are trying to maintain their body weight at a level lower than desirable for optimum health and fitness. A great deal of the malnutrition observed is self-inflicted, with the youngsters putting themselves on fad diets that are severely deficient in calories.

This section presents a comprehensive review of the criteria, classification, prevalence and etiology of childhood and adolescent obesity. There is also a thorough presentation of proposed treatment programs as well as suggestions for prevention.

*Excerpts from: *Obesity and Health*, U.S. Public Health Service Publication No. 1485.

Fat Babies Grow Into Fat People

That cute, chubby baby—isn't she the picture of health? Mother may think so, but sadly, that overfed infant is embarking on a lifelong weight problem

By Dr. Jean Mayer
Professor of Nutrition
Harvard University

Whenever our press, weary of reporting on bombings, crime rates, and unemployment statistics, looks for something more cheerful to convey to the American public, we are told that our children are getting bigger. And indeed they are: in Boston, the average 14-year-old is six inches taller than his counterpart of 100 years ago. Over 25 percent of our young men are more than six feet tall, as compared with only 4 percent in 1900.

But, alas, there is another altered physical characteristic—one which is rarely commented upon: Americans are getting fatter even faster than they are getting taller. Our Boston 14-year-old is not only taller, he is also over 30 pounds heavier than his 1870 model.

From 1940 to 1960, the average weight of American men went up 10 pounds. And the increase is accelerating, with recent statistics of the U.S. Public Health Service indicating that over half of adult men are overweight! Forty percent of adult American women also weigh more than is conducive to greatest longevity. In suburban Boston schools, the proportion of "obese" children has grown in 20 years from 12 to 20 percent.

One reason for this increased prevalence of overweight is obviously the growing physical inactivity of our population and, in particular, of our children. A number of years ago, I showed first in experimental animals, then in people of various ages, that while appetite is a fair-

ly good guide to the amount of food needed by active people, it is not a reliable measure for inactive subjects. While daily exercise is minimal, most children and adults eat more than they need. In other words, if you walk 10 miles during the day you will automatically be hungrier than if you walk two miles, but it does not follow that if you don't walk at all you will want to eat less than if you walk two miles. You will probably eat as much—and you will get fatter.

We also found that individuals who are endowed with a large bone and muscle mass (the type physical anthropologists call "mesomorphs") need to exercise more than ectomorphs (elongated types with narrow hands and feet) to reach the point at which their appetite automatically dictates the right amount of food for them to eat.

In a number of studies, stretching over 20 years, we showed that the big difference between most overweight children and adolescents and their thin contemporaries was not that the overweight youngsters eat more, but that they exercise far less than other children who are of normal weight.

Unfortunately, a number of school systems have dropped the requirement for even the sketchy physical-exercise program once offered to all students. With the growing affluence of the middle class, more and more American families own a second—and a third—car. This means that if by some chance children

don't ride a school bus, Mother drives them to school. And if the youngsters are old enough, they will drive themselves to school. In a number of urban schools, with land at a high premium, school committees have converted playground areas into student parking lots!

The effect of the elimination of walking is compounded by the hours spent daily in front of the television set. While every educator in America worries about the results of exposing our children's impressionable minds to hours of mediocre television fare, I worry also about the effect on their bodies. A recent foundation study discloses that preschool children watch TV an average of five hours a day (and, incidentally, see an average of 5000 food commercials a year—most of them for foods of high-sugar and low-nutrition content). Our studies of children's schedules show that a great deal of this "viewing" (and sitting) time has replaced playing time—active games in the back yard or neighborhood playground. This drastic curtailment of physical activity has been both so gradual and so nearly universal that most parents seem unaware of it. But it shows up in the lack of fitness and the overweight of too many children.

There is worse to come. A number of nutritionists and pediatricians are beginning to show deep concern over the possibility that we are overfeeding babies in a way that will produce an enormous

199

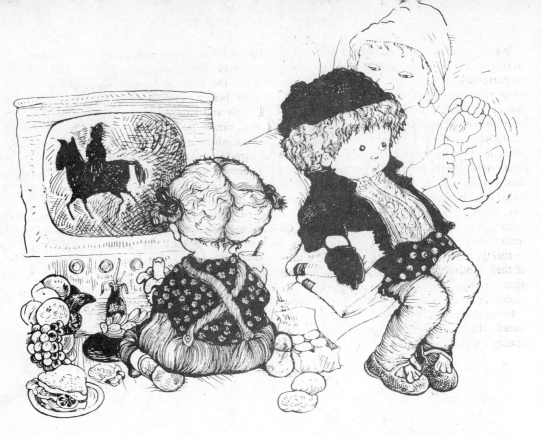

proportion of fat babies, and also actually modify their anatomy so that they will be prone to obesity for the rest of their lives! Specifically, we feel that the recent practice of giving babies not only high-calorie formulas, but baby foods that contain many more calories than mother's milk, may lead them to eat more than they need for harmonious growth. This practice also may induce the formation of additional fat cells which *all their lives* will greedily sop up nutrients from their blood, leading them to overeat and become excessively fat.

To appreciate these two risks, you need to understand a little basic physiology. First, the mechanism of appetite is probably different in newborn infants than in older children and adults. Humans have an automatic "calorie counter" in the hypothalamus, the part of the brain that regulates a number of basic body functions such as temperature control. The "satiety" centers of the hypothalamus send special messages to other parts of the brain to turn off your desire to eat when you have had enough calories. The volume of food seems far less important than the calorie content. Laboratory experiments show that most adults can adjust almost instantaneously to changes in calorie content. You'll stop after eating a small piece of a calorie-rich cheesecake, whereas you might consume a larger portion of food with fewer calories. Actual "fullness" of the stomach has little lasting effect and is

not the reason why you stop eating. In fact, studies show that even removal of part of the stomach (in cancer or ulcer operations) has slight bearing on the amount of food consumed in the course of a day—it just leads to consumption of a larger number of smaller meals.

By contrast, our studies at Harvard and those of Gordon Kennedy of Cambridge University in England show that this hypothalamic system is not yet fully operating in very young animals, and that babies probably stop eating because they are literally full. Most babies cannot be overfed by parents who try to make them consume a larger *volume* of milk or formula than they want. A baby will turn his head away and close his mouth or, if forced to ingest extra milk, will regurgitate it immediately. (An old pediatric adage is that it's impossible to overfeed a breast-fed baby.) However, babies may have very little defense against being fed an over-concentrated diet. For aeons, young infants have consumed mostly breast milk—with 65 calories per 100 milliliters. Solid and semi-solid foods fed young infants may contain up to 200 calories per 100 milliliters. Prepared baby foods, such as egg yolk, meats, cereals, desserts, some meat dinners, and most fruits (which often have considerable added sugar), contain more calories per unit than breast milk, in many cases two to three times as much!

Young infants may not be able to handle such high concentrations—and the younger they are, the less they're able to adjust. Premature infants seem to be the least capable of adjusting to great variations in calorie content.

We also must remember that in the young infant, the fat cells are still multiplying. In older children and adults, the number of fat cells seems fixed, like that of the brain and nerve cells. Getting fat simply means that you are filling up these specialized "reservoir" cells with fat. But these cells are still dividing in young infants. A number of experiments, conducted at Cambridge University by Dr. R. A. McCance and Dr. Elsie Widdowson, and at Rockefeller University by Dr. Jules Hirsch, have demonstrated that overfeeding very young animals leads to the development of extra fat cells, which presumably persist throughout life. And studies have repeatedly shown that obesity is most stubborn when it has occurred early in life. Too many mothers "jump the gun" with solid foods. While well-informed pediatricians nowadays usually do not prescribe solid foods before the age of three months, we find that a great many young mothers believe that the use of such foods is some sort of status symbol—something like taking that first step or getting a first tooth. As a result, they start babies on solid foods at two months or sometimes even as early as six weeks.

Many new mothers, obsessed by weight as the only measure of growth (unfortunately, they don't routinely measure the length of their babies), often rejoice at what is, in fact, evidence of overfattening. Yet they should be particularly wary if (a) a number of their own or their husband's relatives are overweight; (b) the baby looks fat, or at least is a "broad" rather than a "long" baby; or (c) the baby is unusually inactive. All too often, mothers forget that babies, too, need exercise. They may seem to be little bundles of activity, but in reality, too many babies spend most of their waking hours confined in playpens, strollers, or car seats, rather than exploring their worlds.

In our studies, all these traits are associated with an above-average risk of obesity—which may be lifelong. For such high-risk infants, your pediatrician may well suggest the following:

• Wait until the baby is four to six months old before introducing solid foods. Cereals and strained foods such as egg yolk, meats, desserts, and high-meat dinners, which are high in calories, may be introduced late and used sparingly. Preference may be given to relatively low-calorie foods, such as canned breakfasts, dinners, and vegetables (with no starch or sugar added).

• Give unsweetened juices (and water!) as an alternative to milk for slaking thirst, especially during hot weather when children drink more.

• Recheck the baby's formula after a few weeks to insure that it is not too rich. If your baby is gaining too much weight, your doctor may dilute the formula or switch to skim milk.

Remember, your children have individual differences in their eating behavior and physical development. The last thing your pediatrician wants to do is to thwart the harmonious growth of your baby. But there is no point in pushing a susceptible baby into the health risks and unhappiness of being too fat.

To summarize, don't start your infants earlier on solid foods than your pediatrician recommends; also, check with him before pushing more high-calorie baby foods into your baby. Play with your small children and keep them active. At the risk of being thought an ogre, ration TV time. You'll be giving your offspring a great physical (and mental) head start over their peers. ∎

The Portly, Corpulent or Obese American

Margaret A. Flynn, Ph.D.

Poor feeding habits on the part of mothers, reinforced by the inattention or lack of information on the part of the physician, can create physiological changes in the infant which are difficult, if not impossible, to reverse in the adult. Particular emphasis is placed upon allowing the appetite of the infant to serve as a guide to total consumption. Unnecessarily complicated feeding programs tend to be expensive and to increase the chance of overeating.

continued

Family practitioners and pediatricians, along with "Mom," must assume some of the blame for the large number of fat children in our country. Obese infants have a higher probability of becoming fat adults. One third of all Americans are by definition overweight when compared to accepted height-weight ratios. Many of them are in this condition because of food habits established in infancy and early childhood which persist throughout life *(Figure 1)*. Obesity is a chronic condition. It is resistant to treatment, prone to relapse, and it has no cure.

Because the infant is a favored health consumer, physicians, including pediatricians, who administer family medical care, can serve as pivotal influences in the prevention of juvenile-onset obesity. In spite of this, there appears to be an increasing "laissez-faire" attitude on the part of physicians who care for healthy babies. This may in part be due to the fact that the art of feeding infants has been relinquished to the scientists who formulate commercially sold infant foods. Since the physician is no longer required to calculate formulas and periodically modify them, he tends to be less concerned about height-weight relationships.

Relatively few infants in the United States are breast-fed. Breast-feeding may be one excellent answer to the prevention of obesity in the first year of life. Besides having the nutritional advantage of species-related biologic formulation, breast milk is packaged in a vehicle that does not permit visible estimation of quantity. This is advantageous because most lactating women assume that when the baby ceases

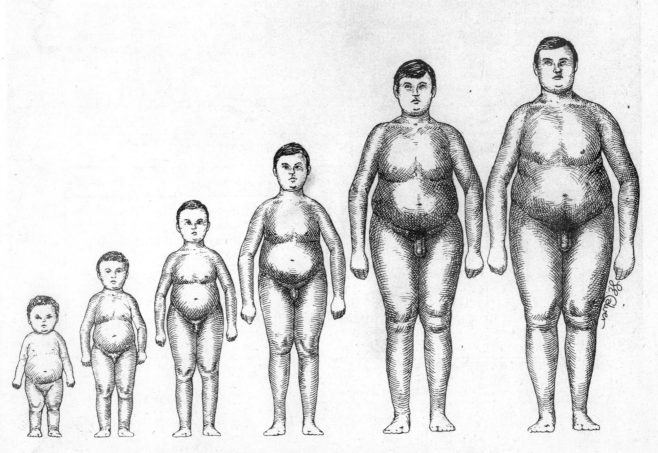

Figure 1. Obese infants have a higher probability of becoming fat adults.

to suck and swallow, he has had enough food. In contrast, a woman who uses bottle feeding as a mode of sustenance may frequently encourage the infant to drain the contents of the bottle because the doctor recommended a specific amount of the formula at a specific age rather than allowing appetite influenced by growth demand to set the pace. From this point of view, bottle feeding may become a subtle form of force-feeding fostered by the physician and mother.

Juvenile-Onset Obesity

Obesity beginning in childhood differs from that which starts after maturity in its effect upon the *number* of fat cells used for storage. Evidence in both animal and human experimental studies suggests that the number of fat cells is determined early in infancy, during prepubescence when the growth spurts of children occur.[1] Overeating of foods high in calories during these critical periods stimulates the creation of a greater number of fat cells. In contrast, the numbers of fat cells in adult-onset obesity do not multiply; rather, the fat content of the existing cells increases. Further, when weight reduction is attempted by caloric restriction in either

age group, a decrease in size, but not numbers, of fat cells occurs.

Weight reduction in humans who have been obese since childhood is under any circumstances a difficult task, whether the physician attempts to manage it alone or with the aid of a health care team, a qualified nurse practitioner or a nutritionist. The juvenile-onset obese individual, if he is to reach a normal height-weight-status, must empty his greater number of fat cells to disproportionately low levels of fat. This is quite difficult since weight reduction requires loss of lean body mass as well as fat.[1]

Weight *reduction* programs for children are discouraged by some physicians and nutritionists because of the possible poor intake of nutrients associated with decreased caloric ingestion. Some place great confidence in juvenile summer camps for weight reduction. Some endorse drastic diets which unfortunately tend to induce ketosis through the accompanying depressant effect upon the appetite. Interestingly, only a few physicians prefer increased exercise as a method for weight reduction. A substantial number of health professionals attempt to avoid the issue by responding, *"He'll outgrow the baby fat."* No one of these responses by itself consti-

continued

TABLE 1				
SCHEDULE FOR ADDITION OF SOLID FOODS TO INFANT DIET				
3 months	4 months	5 months	6 months	7 & 8 months
CEREAL—1 srvg. 3 T. Rice Cereal	CEREAL—1 srvg. (3 T. Rice Cereal)	CEREAL—1 srvg. (3 T. Rice Cereal)	CEREAL—1 srvg. 3 T. Rice Cereal	CEREAL—1 srvg. 3 T. Rice Cereal
	FRUIT—1 srvg. (4½ T.)	FRUIT—1 srvg. (4½ T.)	FRUIT—2 srvg. (9 T.)	FRUIT—2 srvg. (9 T.)
	VEGETABLE— ½ srvg. (2 T.)	VEGETABLE— 1 srvg. (4½ T.)	VEGETABLE— 2 srvg. (9 T.)	VEGETABLE— 2 srvg. (9 T.)
		MEAT—½ srvg. (2 T.)	MEAT—1 srvg. (3½ T.)	MEAT—2 srvg. (7 T.)
ALL MEASUREMENTS ARE LEVEL T. = tablespoon 1 jar fruits & veg. = 9 T. (134 gm) srvg. = serving 1 jar meat = 7 T. (100 gm)				

tutes adequate treatment for juvenile-onset obesity. The condition is usually based upon a way of life that often includes parental belief that, *"a fat child is a healthy child."* It may include a distorted self image of proper body appearance, or bizarre eating habits related to emotional problems.

Prevention of Obesity

Physicians responsible for the health maintenance of children must focus upon the *prevention* of obesity for maximum success. How many physicians regularly and emphatically say to the obese child's mother, *"We need to review Carol's diet. She is putting on more weight than her height needs to carry. We don't want her to grow wider than she is tall."*? What percentage of family physicians on the first visit for health maintenance make the verbal observation that, *"Because there is an increasing number of fat babies, we'll have to periodically check Carol's height and weight whenever dietary changes are contemplated."*? Either approach, although quite direct, would be an improvement in the majority of practices.

Where obesity exists or potentially exists, a standard set of procedures for change in diet should include communication with the physician before foods are arbitrarily added to the infant's diet. For all children, more involvement of physicians, nurse practitioners and nutritionists is needed to offset the persuasiveness of "sales pitches" for food supplements, particularly where the control of calories is critical. Industries which supply baby foods have placed hundreds of well advertised baby foods in the supermarkets. The caloric content of many of these foods is inflated by the overuse of sugar.[2] Sub-

stantial emphasis has also been placed on the early addition of solid foods to the infant diet to the point that some pediatricians have advised adding baby cereal at 2 weeks of age.

Objective studies have shown that the modern infant formulas contain all the known required nutrients for babies up to 3 months of age. Solid foods simply are not needed until that time. (See *Table 1* for schedule for addition of solid foods to infant diet.) Cereal in the first month does *not* make the baby sleep through the night. It does take a great deal of the mother's time to administer.[3] Foreign protein may sensitize an infant whose genetic background predisposes him to allergies if too much is introduced too early in the infant's diet. In addition, many of the baby food mixtures, particularly in jars, contain large amounts of water making them a poor economic investment.[2] Curbing the use of unneeded early solid food additions is one way the physician can intervene in some of the common present day practices of infant feeding that often add unnecessary calories. Mothers should be cautioned against "across the fence" dietary advice. They should understand that feeding practices used for a previous child may lead in the current circumstance to the undesirable production of a fat baby. If he is to practice preventive medicine, the physician must have more knowledge about nutrient needs of infants than that provided with most commercial formulas.

For instance, if the formula contains iron, the cereal added to the diet at 3 months of age does not have to be iron-enriched. Infant food additions should be plain vegetables and plain fruits prepared to facilitate chewing and swallowing, given at 4 months, with meats given at 6 months. This procedure has proved completely effective in assuring proper weight for height growth. Commercially bottled "dinners," "breakfasts," "desserts," or other infant mixtures are unnecessary and should be avoided when they contain large amounts of sugar, water, or thickening agents. The physician has a direct responsibility for the proper instruction of

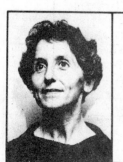
Margaret A. Flynn, Ph.D.
Associate Professor
Community Health and Medical Practice
Nutrition/Dietetics
University of Missouri
School of Medicine
Columbia, Missouri 65201

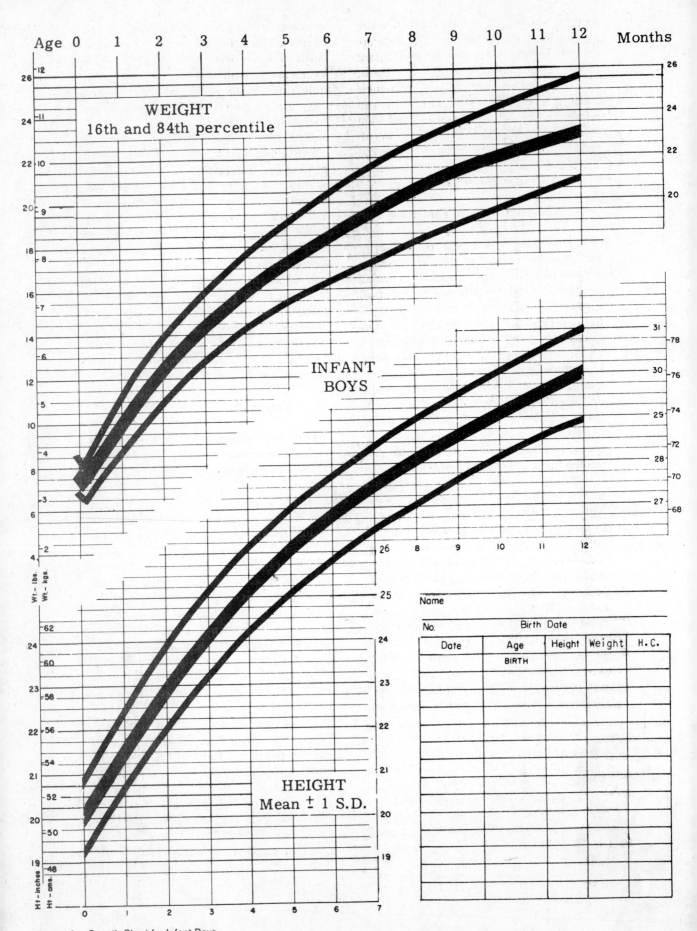

Figure 2. Growth Chart for Infant Boys.

206

mothers about appropriate diets. If more physicians spoke against the inappropriate use of high caloric commercial infant foods, fewer mothers would buy them, and the food industry would stop their manufacture. The infant with teeth can satisfactorily eat mashed, non-spiced food from the family table. This transition can be made without the use of commercial "junior" foods so long as sanitation in food preparation is not an issue.

Discontinuation of Formulas

The American Academy of Pediatrics has recently recommended the use of iron-fortified commercial formulas through the first year in order to curtail iron deficiency anemia.[4] This has changed the previous practice of direct conversion to milk after a few months of commercial formula. For those physicians who believe this is necessary, the discontinuation of commercial formulas can be staged in several ways: (a) by prescribing 2 per cent cow's milk by the fourth month in order to keep the intake of saturated fatty acids low; (b) by advising the use of whole pasteurized cow's milk at 4 months; or (c) by using diluted whole cow's evaporated milk at 4 months. Evaporated milk has the advantage that it is sufficiently heat treated to change cow's milk protein to a less allergenic form (some physicians have continued to recommend the use of evaporated milk for making formula in the home because it is less expensive and because it is allowed in the maternal and child supplemental foods). The record is clear that children have grown equally well in weight and height with commercial formulas, evaporated milk formulas, human milk, or soy bean milk formulations when their weights have been within the normal range for height.[5]

The measurement of weight-for-height ratio is usually recorded on growth charts in the physician's office such as the one reproduced here (Figure 2). As long as the height and weight measurements for a child correspond in distance from the mean or median value of the chart, growth in size is likely to contain proportionate amounts of lean mass. If an infant's weight begins to climb above his height, 2 per cent cow's milk and less use of other fats and sweets are recommended rather than skim milk since whole milk contains essential fatty acids and fat soluble vitamins not found in skim milk.

With the increased physical activity of crawling and walking, the child's need for protein can also be met by increased use of meat, fish, cheese and legumes so that his milk intake may be kept within reasonable limits. Snacks such as fruit, fruit juices, 2 per cent milk and cheese are recommended at mid-morning, mid-afternoon and bed time after the child is 1 year of age. Such snacks should be part of the plan for a total day's nutrient. Sugared cereal, cookies, candy, carbonated beverages, pastries, donuts, potato chips, etc., should be used sparingly if at all since they have a high caloric content of carbohydrates but few other nutrients.

Necessary Amount of Food

The development of sound judgment on the part of parents and children concerning total amount of food necessary is important in the prevention of childhood obesity. Too often the family which claims a child is a "good eater" is acknowledging a member who cleans his plate quickly and pleasurably and then asks for more food. A truly "good" eater is the one who knows when his body needs have been met and stops eating at that point.

Besides watching *how much* and *what* is eaten, it is important to add definite patterns of physical activity to the daily regimen. An attempt should be made to emphasize those recreational activities which will continue for a lifetime. Television watching time should not be allowed to substitute for needed physical exertion. This holds for the child, parents, teachers and the physician. Swimming, volleyball, tennis, handball and hiking are more likely to be enjoyed by adults if they program their minds and bodies to accept them as sports and good health measures in childhood. Not every child should engage in competitive sports, but every child should be allowed, and if necessary, encouraged to exercise vigorously—if only to run, climb, jump and walk during the day. The family physician can assist by emphasizing the importance of acquiring the physical skills when physical exams are given for health maintenance during childhood years. In obese children, it is particularly appropriate with the review of dietary habits.

Whether children under the care of the family physician become portly—connoting dignity, corpulent—connoting bulk, or obese—connoting an unpleasant excess of fat, he must accept at least part of the blame for future obese adults and their resulting health problems.   ☐

References

1. Knittle, J.: When to start dieting? At birth. *Medical World News.* Sept. 7, 1973.
2. Anderson, T. and Fomon, S.: Commercially Prepared Strained and Junior Foods for Infants. *J. Am. Diet. Assn.* 58:520, 1971.
3. Gutherie, H.: Effect of Early Feeding of Solid Foods on Nutritive Intake of Infants. *Pediatrics* 38:879, 1966.
4. Committee on Nutrition. Amer. Acad. Ped. *Pediatrics* 47:786, 1971.
5. Jackson, R.L., Westerfeld, R., Flynn, M.A., Kimball, E.R., Lewis, R.: Growth of "Well-born" American Infants Fed Human and Cow's Milk. *Pediatrics* 33:642, 1964.

Childhood Obesity

If obesity at any age is undesirable, that occurring
in the early years of life would seem to be the most unwanted.
New ideas are emerging that may explain why it occurs.
They may indicate ways to treat the condition.

by MYRON WINICK, M.D.
Reprinted with permission of
Nutrition Today, Copyright ©1974
by Nutrition Today, Inc.

In November 15 and 16, 1973, a Conference on Childhood Obesity was held in New York City. This meeting, the first of its kind, was the second annual symposium on nutrition held by the Institute of Human Nutrition of Columbia University, College of Physicians and Surgeons. Its purpose was to bring together a group of physicians and biochemists to discuss what we are beginning to believe may be a very dangerous form of obesity, childhood obesity.

The first day of the conference began with a discussion of certain cellular and tissue changes which may be unique to "early onset" obesity; progressed to observations on the clinical picture of obesity in infants, children, and adolescents; and closed with a discussion of some of the major long term consequences of obesity in early life. On the second day, treatment was discussed from the standpoint of dietary management, hormones and behavioral modification.

FAT CELLS

The first investigator to be heard was Jules Hirsch, Professor of Experimental Medicine at Rockefeller University. Dr. Hirsch spoke at length about his work on the newest concept of obesity, namely the relation of the condition to the number and size of adipose cells in both experimental and clinical obesity. According to this point of view, the fat in the adipose tissue may be packaged in a large number of small cells or in a smaller number of larger cells. Dr. Hirsch has pioneered methods to determine cell number and cell size in adipose tissue.

Dr. Winick is Professor of Pediatrics and Director of the Institute of Human Nutrition at Columbia University, College of Physicians & Surgeons in New York.

The problems in methodology that still exist, are related primarily to determination of total body fat, the representativeness of any one biopsy site, and the fact that an "adipocyte" can be recognized only after fat has begun to accumulate. Nevertheless, classification according to relative number and size of fat cells is regarded by many as a major breakthrough in our understanding of the fundamental tissue changes that take place in obesity. Early in his studies, Dr. Hirsch noted that the adipocytes of non-obese individuals averaged 0.6–0.7 mg of fat per cell, whereas those of obese individuals averaged about twenty percent more. Further, the non-obese individual had approximately three hundred billion fat cells, and the obese individual usually had about twice that number. Thus in very obese adults, the really mammoth cellular difference was in the number of fat cells. When such adults lost weight, the effect at the cell level was almost entirely on cell size. Cell number changed very little, if at all.

Further studies, conducted on a larger number of subjects, suggested that there are actually two types of obesity: one, wherein the patient has too many fat cells and would be said to be suffering from "hyperplastic obesity;" the other, wherein the patient has fat cells that are too large, a condition called "hypertrophic obesity." It appears that early onset (childhood) obesity is primarily hyperplastic, whereas late onset (adult) obesity is hypertrophic. Although these findings appear to be "statistically" valid, there is always "overlap" in both directions; some adult onset obesity was hyperplastic and some early onset was hypertrophic, according to the report given by Dr. Hirsch.

In order better to characterize these types of obesity, animal studies were undertaken. During normal growth, the number of epididymal fat pad cells of a rat reached a maximum at around 12 weeks of age, according to the Rockefeller investigator. Nothing done to the animal after this time changed cell number. From then on, the rest of growth of the fat pad was hypertrophic. He also reported that when a lesion was made in the ventro-medial portion of the hypothalamus at 7 weeks age, marked hyperphagia and obesity ensued but, again, cell number was not affected; cell size, however, increased enormously. Thus even though new fat cells were still appearing at that time, cell number reaches the same plateau as in the non-lesioned.

On the other hand, dietary manipulation during the first three weeks of life alters the number of fat cells. Recent experiments by Marci Greenwood, a post-doctoral fellow at the Institute of Human Nutrition at Columbia University, College of Physicians and Surgeons, have shown that cell division, as measured by thymidine incorporation into DNA, in cells destined to become adipocytes, stops at about 2 to 3 weeks of age. Thus even though cell number increases by the histometric osmium method beyond 7 weeks of age, the division of fat cells actually stops long before this. These data raise important questions about human obesity, because the methods presently employed to discover when the number of fat cells is determined are histometric.

Cell division may actually cease much earlier than we have thought. The realization that adipocytes stop dividing early in life has led to an examination of cellularity in genetic obesity. The cells

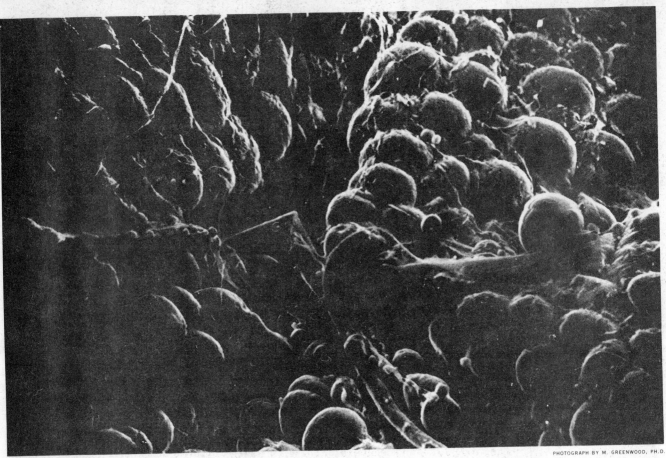

White adipose tissues magnified 280 times (above) and 1400 times (below).

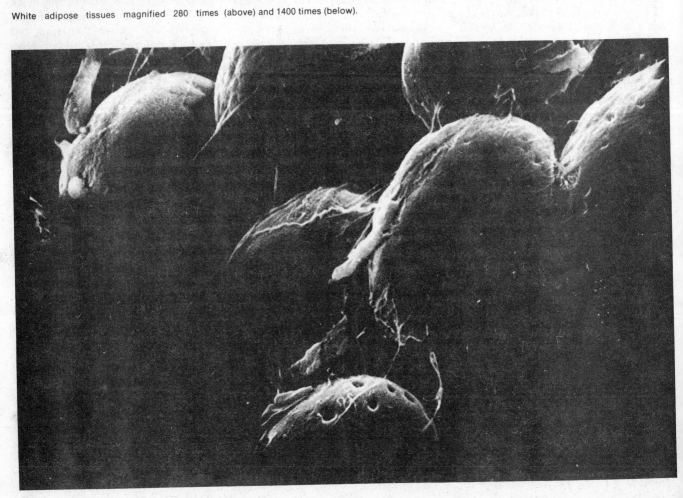

of most genetically obese animals are too large, and obesity begins in the adult life of these animals. By contrast, the "Zucker" rat, named after its discoverer, Marjorie B. Zucker, a genetically obese strain with too many fat cells, becomes obese early in life. Also, manipulation of these rats' diet early in life alters the expression of their genetic obesity. Subsequent *ad libitum* feeding allows the gene to be expressed, but prevents the animals from being as obese as they would have been had their diet not been restricted early in life. Even genetic types of obesity, therefore, may be amenable to nutritional manipulations at critical times during development.

What are the critical periods in man? These are not yet known but, in Dr. Hirsch's opinion, the last trimester of pregnancy, the first three years of life, and adolescence are crucial in determining whether a person will be obese. Stanley Garn, from the Center for Human Growth and Development at the University of Michigan, Ann Arbor, examined childhood obesity in epidemiologic terms. He defined an obese person as one who is above the 85th percentile for triceps fat fold for age and sex, and a lean person as one below the 15th percentile in the same measurement.

Dr. Garn called attention to several physical changes that are characteristic of the obese child but are not usually appreciated by physicians. He said, for example, that obese boys and girls are taller than their lean peers. In addition, skeletal development is advanced in the obese youngster, giving him a body of greater skeletal mass than his peers. Whether the increase in skeletal frame results from the stimulus of having to carry more weight or whether it is a concomitant phenomenon of obesity is not known. Also, obese children show higher-than-normal levels of hemoglobin and certain vitamins in their blood. Surprisingly, they have an increase not only in fat tissue but in fat free weight (F F W).

FAT PEOPLE

Obesity is influenced by socioeconomic status. The children of the poor are leaner than those of more affluent parents, and this is not due entirely to differences in food intake. Differences also occur in various populations. Black infants are, as a rule, fatter than white infants, but the reverse is the case in later childhood. This is true even when income levels are kept constant. Puerto Ricans are fatter than either blacks or whites at the same economic level.

Dr. Garn next spoke on the relationship between childhood and adult obesity. He pointed out that, in males, poverty results in thin children who grow to become thin adults. By contrast, in females poverty appears to lead to thin children who become fat women, whereas affluence results in heavy children who become slim women. From these data, Dr. Garn attacked the theory that obesity in childhood leads to obesity in the adult. Going one step further, he took the position that since there seems to be little relation between childhood and adult obesity, the entire theory of hyperplastic and hypertrophic obesity espoused by Dr. Hirsch only minutes before was open to serious question.

It must be noted that data Garn presented was cross-sectional. The lean children studied were not the same individuals grown to obese adults. We don't know whether these adults were lean twenty, thirty, forty, or fifty years ago. Only longitudinal data, which are not available, can answer this question. Moreover, Dr. Garn pointed out that the poor, adult female who is obese has a low F F W. This is in contrast to the poor female children who have high F F W Based on body composition, obesity in poor, adult females would appear to be of a different type than that which occurs in childhood. Could obese women have hypertrophic obesity, whereas obese children have hyperplastic obesity?

Dr. Garn elegantly described the characteristics of childhood obesity, as evidenced by his extensive cross-sectional studies. The criteria he set forth for the obese child are extremely useful, both from a research and a clinical standpoint. In using his cross-sectional data to argue that *all* fat children do not become fat adults, he is on good ground. But when he argues that this raises serious problems with the theory of hyperplastic and hypertrophic obesity, as enunciated by both Dr. Hirsch and Jerome Knittle, of Mount Sinai Medical School, in this symposium, his ground is much less firm. In fact, what suggestion there is from Garn's data is perfectly consistent with the Hirsch-Knittle hypothesis.

While Dr. Garn concerned himself with the total amount of fat and its percentage when compared to other tissues, and Dr. Hirsch was concerned with the manner in which this fat is packaged, Sami Hashim, Associate Professor of Medicine and Director of the Metabolic Unit of the Institute of Human Nutrition at Columbia, concerned himself with the quality of the fat being deposited in the

obese person. He noted that, although unsaturated fat will cross the placenta, little of it gets into the fetal adipose tissue, and the newborn infant has almost one hundred percent saturated fat in his adipose depot. Within three months of birth, however, the infant's fat tissue will change reflecting the fat in the diet. Since most dietary fat is long, even chained, this is what is found in the fat cells of most people. These long-chain fatty acids are transported, via the thoracic duct to the systemic circulation and then deposited in the fat. Medium chain triglycerides (MCT), on the other hand, are transported from the intestine, through the portal circulation, to the liver, where they are metabolized and, therefore, do not reach the fat depots. Thus, Dr. Hashim hypothesizes, feeding

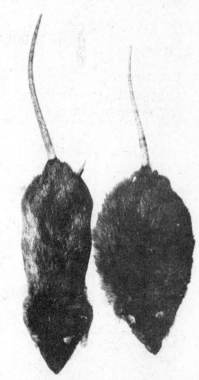

PHOTOGRAPH BY P. R. JOHNSON, M.D.
Of the two litter mates, the Zucker rat (right) born with the obese gene. The other rat was normal.

MCT might be one way to treat obesity and, perhaps even more important, would modify the rate of adipocyte cell division in childhood. The composition of the fat can be altered not only by feeding naturally occurring polyunsaturates, but by feeding synthetically made, odd-chained fatty acids. The resultant adipose cells will then contain odd-chained fatty acids in their fat globules, and will release them when necessary (*i.e.*, during starvation). In contrast to the even numbered carbon molecules, odd-chained fatty acids can be partly broken down to glucose, sparing both glycogen and body protein. This could have important effects, especially during the growing period, when preservation of body protein is essential. Dr. Hashim's work, while not yet at the "practical stages," is a new and exciting approach to the problem of childhood obesity.

The meeting then moved from fat tissue to fat people: infants, children, and adolescents. William B. Weil, Jr., Professor and Chairman of the Department of Human Development at Michigan State University, led off with comments on the general problems of obesity in infancy. Defining obesity in terms of weight for length and of weight gain, Dr. Weil noted that although very fat infants

mobility might play a role. By this he meant that a slim girl from poor circumstances who remained slim might have been able to move upward, and would, therefore, appear in the affluent adult group. By contrast, an obese girl might have moved downward and would appear in the less advantaged adult group.

Dr. Weil then turned from this topic and called attention to some of the factors involved in the etiology of infant obesity. These include: maternal weight gain during pregnancy, brain damage, over-zealous bottle feeding, early introduction of certain high caloric solid foods, and such less tangible factors as the mother's and the family physician's attitude towards weight gain. Finally, the Michigan physician cautioned that when an infant begins to show evidence of too

chance of the child being obese. If one parent is obese, the chance is forty percent whereas, if both parents are obese, the chances jump to eighty percent. Environmental factors are also important, but as society de-emphasizes physical activity, the genetic potential has more and more chance of being expressed. According to Mayer, physical activity is by far the most important environmental variable affecting obesity. Obese children and adults often eat the same amount, he said, and usually the same nutrient proportions as their lean counterparts, but they exercise much less. Studies, accompanied by motion pictures, were said to show that fat girls exercised one third less than lean girls. Other studies have shown that there is no correlation between weight gain in babies and the amount of food ingested. However, fat babies were placid and thin babies active. Having made these observations, Dr. Mayer then discussed some of the consequences of being a fat child. He noted that such children are rejected, citing as evidence a study demonstrating that fat girls have only one third the chance of being accepted into college that lean girls have. These societal pressures are reflected in the child's personality. Psychologic testing reveals a profile similar to other types of children who have experienced prejudice and discrimination. Therapy in childhood obesity must be instituted in a number of directions simultaneously. Not only must the diet be controlled, but exercise must be increased and the child must be supported psychologically. This regimen of increased activity must be long-term or the obesity will recur.

OBESITY HALLMARK

Felix P. Heald, Professor of Pediatrics at the University of Maryland School of Medicine, reported on his studies of the obese adolescent. The hallmark of adolescence is rapid change, he said. Boys increase their height by around twenty percent; they almost double their body mass during this period. There is also a normal deposition of fat, especially in adolescent girls. Two historical patterns may be noted in obesity, which begins when the young girl enters adolescence. The first is a distinct family history of obesity that begins in infancy. The second is no family history of obesity, but the child commences to grow fat at about the time of some specific stressful event in his or her life.

There are three peak periods for the development of obesity in children: late

Cell Number Development

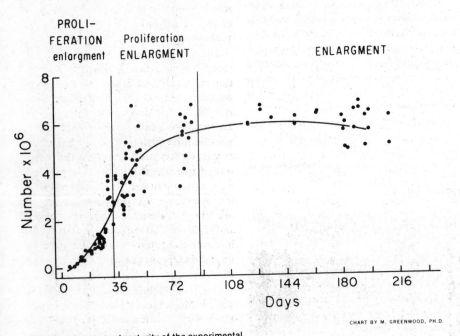

CHART BY M. GREENWOOD, PH.D.

From birth to sexual maturity of the experimental rat, adipose cell number increases greatly. However, after sexual maturity, the body makes no additional adipose cells.

do not appear to die in greater numbers than do their counterparts of normal weight, obese infants are more prone to respiratory infections and other illnesses. However, like so many others who have studied the subject, he felt the most important problem to be that fat infants might become fat children who, in turn, would become fat adults. He was not persuaded by Dr. Garn's data that this was not so, pointing out its cross-sectional nature. He also noted that class

rapid weight gain, dietary therapy to prevent obesity should be instituted.

Jean Mayer, Professor of Nutrition at the Harvard School of Public Health, moved the discussion to obesity in childhood. He noted that certain body types are associated with obesity and that, since these body types are, according to him, inherited, there is a genetic component to obesity that must be considered. For example, he asserted if neither parent is obese, there is only a seven percent infancy; early childhood, around age 6; and adolescence. As was previously noted by Dr. Mayer, Dr. Heald agreed that literature on the subject suggests that obese children do not appear to eat more than lean children. However, he pointed out that the dietary intake data upon which the Mayer statement was based were developed from 3 to 4 hour recall interviews and are of questionable reliability, because obese children and adolescents minimize food intake as a defense mechanism. Moreover, in one study, in which young patients were hospitalized and fed what they indicated was their normal intake, they lost weight. These data, however, are in contrast to the one observational study done on teenagers. That study indicated that the obese eat no more than the lean. It would seem, then, that even the most basic question about childhood obesity—Does the obese child eat more than the lean child?—is not yet answered.

One interesting observation on obese teenagers, however, is that they do not eat when they are hungry, but rather when they are bored. Examination of obese adolescents reveals that, while they are taller than their peers, and their skeletal age is somewhat beyond their body age, they grow up to be less tall adults. Puberty comes earlier. We do not know what psychological effect this one-year shortening of childhood has on these children. Obese children are rarely hypertensive but errors will occur if the arms are very fat.

Since adolescence is an anabolic period and weight reduction is a catabolic process, the teenager is particularly sensitive to weight reduction, Heald continued. Thus weight loss must occur very slowly, in order to preserve growth. This makes treatment of the obese adolescent particularly difficult. Not only must weight reduction be gradual, but therapy is difficult because the poor body image of most persons whose obesity began in adolescence, that is to say, one's perception of his own body as unattractive, is shown to have begun during adolescence. This is associated with other behavioral problems that can complicate therapy. Although some improvement can be made during adolescence, Dr. Heald thinks that therapy should be aimed at prevention.

By this time in the proceedings, it became evident that one of the major concerns with childhood obesity is the fact that these juvenile-onset obese individuals we had heard discussed are destined to have the most severe and the most-difficult-to-treat type of obesity when they grow up.

Another concern, which was discussed, was the relation between the fat content of the child's diet and the hyperlipidemias so commonly seen in our adult populations. Each of the next three speakers addressed this problem from a different perspective.

A. K. Khachadurian, Professor of Medicine at Rutgers Medical School, New Brunswick, discussed the diagnosis and management of hyperlipidemia in children. After describing the manner in which the different types of hyperlipidemias are currently classified, he focused his attention on the type of primary or genetic hyperlipidemia most commonly found in the pediatric age group, namely, familial hypercholesterolemia. Homozygotes with this disease show plasma cholesterol values approximately four times normal ($728 \pm$ S.D. 140 mg/100 ml). Clinically, these children show tendon xanthomas, corneal arcus, xanthelasma, and arthritis. Both E.S.R. and plasma fibrinogen are elevated. Atherosclerosis, once it begins, takes a galloping course; the mean age at death being 21 years (range 13–37).

The heterozygote is much more difficult to identify. Serum cholesterol elevation in cord blood above 100 mg is suggestive. In older children and adults there is a significant overlap between heterozygotes and so called normal individuals who consume high-fat diets. In the heterozygote, dietary management is the mainstay of treatment. Placing these patients on the "prudent diet" recommended by the American Heart Association will often keep cholesterol levels between 200 and 250 mg/100 ml. As age advances, however, cholesterol levels begin to creep up and dietary management becomes less effective.

Charles J. Glueck, Associate Professor of Medicine and Pediatrics at the University of Cincinnati College of Medicine, carried the discussion of hyperlipidemia further. He first pointed out that there is mounting concern that the apparent progression from fatty streak to fibrous plaques, and then to full-fledged atheromatous plaques is an indication that "coronary heart disease" may begin in childhood. He noted also that a great number of children and young adults have elevated levels of serum cholesterol.

HUMAN ADIPOSE TISSUE

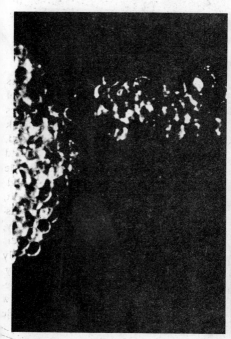

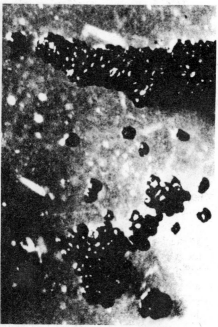

UNFIXED   OSMIUM-FIXED

Unfixed human adipose cells obtained by needle aspiration and washed free of adherent oil (left), and cells fixed with osmium tetroxide in collidine buffer to prevent breakage while being electronically counted (right) are shown magnified 40 times.

For example, in one study 6 to 7 percent of the schoolchildren had levels above 220 mg percent. In another study, 14 percent of children between the ages of 12 and 15 had cholesterol levels greater than 260 mg percent. Dr. Glueck feels, therefore, that one approach to the primary prevention of cardiovascular disease might be to identify children with elevated levels of cholesterol and triglyceride, or both, and to do whatever one can to treat them. The two most common hyperlipidemias in children are hypercholesterolemia, with a primary elevation of cholesterol and beta lipoprotein cholesterol (LDL), and hypertriglyceridemia, with a primary elevation of triglycerides and very low density lipoprotein cholesterol (VLDL). In a small number of children, cholesterol, triglycerides LDL and VLDL are all elevated.

Dr. Glueck's studies based on screening 1,800 newborns suggests a frequency for familial hypercholesterolemia of about 0.9 percent. Those 0.9 percent also have elevated levels of cholesterol at age one year. Screening later in childhood makes it difficult to separate children with familial hypercholesterolemia from those with the diet-induced form. Hypertriglyceridemia in childhood cannot be diagnosed from cord blood. If there is a family history of this condition, repeated serum levels should be taken. Since these diseases are transmitted as autosomal dominants, it is important to carry out a complete family screening, if an adult member of the family has any form of hyperlipidemia. A second approach, which has identified a high percentage of affected children, has been to screen all members of a family in which either parent had a coronary before age fifty. Finally, if resources will allow, all newborns and schoolchildren might be screened.

Experience indicates that, among school-age children, there are from two to three hypercholesterolemics whose families have no evidence of hypercholesterolemia for every one whose family does. In the former cases, dietary history often demonstrates a cholesterol intake of 600–1200 mg a day and an average polyunsaturated/saturated ratio of about 0.3–0.4. This is in contrast to an average intake of 400–600 mg a day and an average ratio of 0.2 to 0.5 among American children. A prudent, low-cholesterol diet, containing approximately 200 mg of cholesterol and a polyunsaturate/saturate ratio of 1.5 to 1, will almost always normalize the cholesterol levels of affected children. Dietary therapy for children with familial hypercholesterolemia is begun at one year, using a modification of the National Institute of Health "type 2" diet. On this diet, which contains less than 200 mg of cholesterol and a P/S ratio of 1.5 to 1, the cholesterol level in from 60 to 80 percent of children will drop to normal. As the children get older, however, fewer and fewer will respond to this type of dietary management. Hypertriglyceridemia in children is relatively easy to treat. First and foremost is weight reduction in those who are obese. This treatment will usually reduce serum triglycerides levels to normal. If, however, they remain elevated, a National Heart Institute "type 4" diet (a balanced proportion of calories, 20 percent as protein, 40 percent as fat, and 40 percent as carbohydrate and moderately rich in polyunsaturates) is effective in maintaining normal triglyceride levels. Extrapolating from primate studies, Dr. Glueck expressed the hope that keeping plasma cholesterol or triglycerides normal in children, whether their disease is familial or acquired, may limit the formation of irreversible atherosclerotic plaques.

MAJOR THEME

Prevention of coronary artery disease in adults by tackling obesity in childhood was the major theme of the paper delivered by Glenn Friedman, a practicing pediatrician on the faculty of the University of Arizona. He reminded the audience that there are five major factors that predispose to coronary heart disease: hypercholesteremia, hypertension, cigarette smoking, obesity, and sedentary living. Dr. Friedman reasoned that "since the above five risk factors probably are harmful and since they each have been related to our cardiovascular epidemic as well as to other disease processes, it would seem reasonable to reduce or prevent these factors from developing in the child and his parents without either producing anxiety or decreasing the joy of living." He argued that the time to begin prevention is in childhood because that is when patterns of living that lead to risk patterns begin. Atherosclerosis does develop in the pediatric age group and may be "reversible" in this age group. Finally by reducing developing risk factors in the

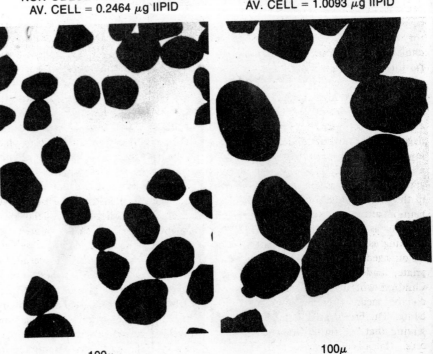

PHOTOGRAPH BY JULES HIRSCH, M.D.

ADIPOSE CELL SIZE OF HYPERGLYCEMIC–OBESE MICE

NON-OBESE MATE WT. = 25g
AV. CELL = 0.2464 μg IIPID

OBESE LITTER MATE WT. = 48g
AV. CELL = 1.0093 μg IIPID

100μ

100μ

The average cell size of a hyperglycemic-obese mouse is nearly double that of its non-obese litter mate.

child, parents' risk factors may also be reduced.

Putting this philosophy into practice, Dr. Friedman has helped to organize two screening intervention programs in the state of Arizona. In his office, some 3,400 middle-class children have been screened for serum cholesterol, blood pressure, subcutaneous fat, and maximal endurance tests on the bicycle ergometer; their histories which include details of milk consumption and exercise, have been recorded. Parents too were measured for total cholesterol, blood pressure, and subcutaneous fat. Their family histories of cardiovascular disease were taken, and notations were made on their use of tobacco and indulgence in exercise. The tests on the children were begun at the age of one month and continued at regular intervals, even on healthy children. A similar program, sponsored by the state health department, is under way in certain rural areas of Arizona.

When Dr. Friedman spots a child he considers to be at risk, he takes the following steps in the following manner: By reporting to the parents all test results in relation to "desirable levels," he motivates them to promote changes; he reinforces various segments of the program with pamphlets and visual aids; one evening a month he holds a slide presentation which is open to the community; lastly, he has the services of a nutritionist in his office.

Dr. Friedman has developed an alternative to the low-fat, low-cholesterol diet because, he said, he has found it difficult to persuade his patients to adhere to it for very long. He controls the intake of cholesterol by limiting the protein intake to the Recommended Dietary Allowances. Since protein-rich animal products are also usually high in cholesterol and saturated fat, he creates what is, in effect, a cholesterol quantity exchange diet pegged to the recommended protein allowance. If the protein recommendations are not exceeded, it is difficult for the patient to get too much fat or cholesterol in the diet. In addition to these dietary manipulations, a parent with hypertension is referred for medical help, smoking is discouraged, and parents are encouraged to lose weight, when appropriate, and to increase their exercise. Children who are obese are managed by dietary means through parental counciling. Dr. Friedman concluded by observing that "we are dealing with an iceberg. The disease process and the risk factors have their inception in the pediatric age group, where there is presently no significant screening or intervention. It is only when the problem emerges from the sea with the onset of a coronary or a stroke that we seem to get concerned. By then it is too late. We must start earlier."

FINAL PHASE

At the conclusion of these three contributions on obesity and hyperlipidemia in the young, the symposium moved into its final phase: therapy for childhood obesity. This aspect has drawn more and more interest as the diet craze has slowly filtered down from our weight-conscious adult society to the children in our midst. Three specific approaches to therapy were discussed. These were dietary management, the use of hormones in obesity, and psychological management of the fat child.

Jerome Knittle, Professor of Pediatrics at Mount Sinai Medical School in New York City, led off with his observations about various aspects of the dietary management of childhood obesity. Animal studies had shown, he said, that only when dietary management began early in life could the number of fat cells be altered. His statement was based on his studies of both normal and obese children. He showed that some obese children had acquired the adult number of fat cells by the time they were three years old. Prognosis in such cases is quite dark. Children who have too many adipocytes for their age, but still have fewer than the normal adult number, have a better chance to avoid adult obesity. However, the aim is to slow down the rate of adipocyte division while maintaining normal or, at least, near normal growth. Weight reduction is not advocated for such patients. Dr. Knittle took the position that the aim of restricting the diet is to have the child maintain his weight but "grow out of his obesity."

Hormones have very little, if any, place in the treatment of childhood obesity, according to Richard Rivlin, Associate Professor from the Department of Medicine and the Institute of Human Nutrition of the College of Physicians and Surgeons. He noted that although certain workers have claimed success with chorionic gonadotropin, the results of controlled studies are, at best, inconclusive. Thyroid hormone produces weight loss, but only while it is being taken. It depletes nitrogen and calcium stores, but causes relatively little loss of body fat. The cardiovascular effects of thyroid hormone may constitute a risk, and its known effect on skeletal growth is an even greater hazard in childhood. Thus the indiscriminate use of thyroid hormone is to be discouraged. Although its use is not practical, human-growth hormone has certain attractive features for the treatment of obesity. It mobilizes body fat and promotes nitrogen retention. However, it is only recommended for growth-hormone-deficient children. At present, then, there is no hormonal agent that can be used safely and effectively to treat childhood obesity.

Henry Jordan from the Department of Psychiatry of the University of Pennsylvania School of Medicine, Philadelphia, approaches childhood obesity as a matter requiring behavioral modification. The initial phase of treatment focuses on analyzing behavior and keeping accurate records of it to determine what behavior is maladaptive. Once that has been done, emphasis is placed on gradual changes in behavior, rather than on weight loss *per se*. This approach was tried on overweight children, and an average weight loss of 6.2 pounds in ten weeks was achieved. Follow-up was incomplete but that fact alone served to emphasize the need for physicians to develop techniques that would gradually shift the responsibility for treatment from the therapist to the parents and children. Thus, although much more research in this area is needed, the behavioral-modification approach seems to offer promise as being a useful therapeutic tool in the treatment of childhood obesity.

The conference ended with a discussion of "special diets" by a panel consisting of George Blackburn of Harvard, Francisco Grande of the University of Minnesota, and David Coursin of St. Joseph's Hospital in Lancaster, Pennsylvania. They seemed to be of the opinion that "fad" or "crash" diets are of little use to adults and are actually dangerous to the growing child.

During these two days a great deal of information was presented. New approaches were examined, current research evaluated. Some answers were forthcoming but many questions remain unanswered. Perhaps more important than any of this, however, was the fact that childhood obesity was identified as a significant health hazard. Only this realization can mobilize the medical community, the nutrition community, and concerned parents into instituting the necessary programs to study and eradicate what is perhaps the greatest "nutritional danger" in our country today.

Obesity in childhood: A problem in adipose tissue cellular development

Jerome L. Knittle, M.D., *New York, N. Y.*

From the Division of Nutrition and Metabolism, Department of Pediatrics, Mount Sinai School of Medicine of The City University of New York.

Reprint address: Department of Pediatrics, Mount Sinai School of Medicine of The City University of New York, Fifth Ave. and 100th St., New York, N. Y. 10029.

OBESITY is one of the common medical problems currently confronting the physician. This problem has received increased attention from the pediatrician, partly because of recognition that the prognosis of obesity in adults is extremely poor and that a high proportion of obese children become obese adults. Inasmuch as results of long-term treatment of overtly obese children are no better than those observed in adults, prevention of the obese state is desirable if one wishes to avoid a lifetime of dietary restriction.

The purpose of the present discussion is to focus attention upon the developmental aspects of the obese state in order to provide a rational means for its prevention.

Knowledge of morphology and function of adipose tissue in subjects of varying ages could provide bases for an understanding of the complex pathogenesis of obesity, including the mechanisms involved in the growth and development of the enlarged fat depots characteristic of most obese patients. There is need for classification of the obese state, which would be useful in assessing the prognosis of childhood obesity. Indeed, much of the confusion in the current literature regarding the outcome of childhood obesity is due to lack of agreement concerning the definition of the obese state and to variations in the methods used in determining body composition. It is hoped that the studies described herein will provide a background for a better understanding of the factors which contribute to the development of enlarged fat depots.

CRITERIA, CLASSIFICATION, AND PREVALENCE

Total body weight is made up of a number of components, each of which can contribute to differences in weight in relation to a given age, sex, or height. Thus an individual can be overweight relative to some arbitrary standard by virtue of increases in bony structure, musculature, or adipose tissue. Strictly speaking, however, the term obesity should be limited to an excessive deposition and storage of fat and is to be distinguishes from "overweight," which does not have any direct implication of fatness. It is essential, therefore, that a study of the obese state include some estimate of total body fat. Although total body fat can be determined directly by the use of inert gases or indirectly by the measurement of body density, total body water, or total body potassium, these techniques are not readily available to the clinician in practice.[1-4] He must rely on less exact methods such as skin fold thickness, body weight for height and sex, or weight charts in which obese subjects are defined as those who exceed mean values by more than two standard deviations.[5-9] In general, clinical studies assessing the incidence of obesity have utilized one or more of these height and weight relationships and have reported widely varying figures, ranging from 3 to 20 per cent of the population.[7, 10, 11] Thus while most investigators agree that obesity is a major nutritional problem, accurate figures as to its prevalence, especially in children less than five years of age, are not available.

The problem is further complicated by the fact that obese subjects represent a heterogenous population. Forbes[4] has demonstrated that at least two subgroups exist among obese children: those with increases in both lean body mass and fat and those with increases in body fat alone. Furthermore, studies of adipose tissue indicate that the enlargement of the fat depot in obese adults is due primarily to an increase in the number of adipose cells with varying increases in cell lipid content (cell size). Thus an obese subject may have an increased adipose organ by virtue of increases in adipose cell number alone or due to a combination of increased cell number and cell size.[12, 13] Further studies related to variations in body composition and adipose tissue cellularity are necessary before a meaningful classification of obesity can be achieved.

At present, any definition or classification of the obese state in childhood or adolescence is purely arbitrary and can provide only a rough guide for the clinician. Accurate estimates of the prevalence of juvenile obesity and its prognosis will not be available until one can ascertain at what time the size of the adipose depot is abnormal and to what extent it will persist into adult life and become associated with pathophysiologic processes.

NATURAL HISTORY

Studies of the long-term consequences of childhood obesity suffer from the same handicaps described above. However, the impor-tance of childhood obesity as a forerunner of obesity in adult life has been documented by a number of prospective and retrospective studies. Thus it has been shown that approximately 80 per cent of all overweight children remain so as adults, and those with the most marked obesity are most likely to become obese adults. Retrospective studies of obese adults also indicate that 30 per cent of overweight adults were heavy as children.[11, 14-16] Robertson and Lowry[18] found that 45 of 100 obese children had been overweight before the age of 6, and Asher[17] has demonstrated that children who are overweight at 6 months of age are, on the average, 4.2 Kg. heavier at 5 years of age than children whose weights are average at 6 months. However, others have shown that birth weights do not correlate with subsequent obesity in adult life; significant correlations between weight in childhood and weight as adults do not occur until about the age of 5.[6]

It would appear then that a critical period of development, with major consequences for one's adult weight, occurs somewhere between birth and 5 years of age. Mossberg[19] has suggested two peaks for the onset of juvenile obesity, one between birth and 4 years and another at 7 to 11 years.[19] Recent studies of adipose tissue cellularity, described below, tend to support his hypothesis.

Despite the evidence that the obese child becomes the obese adult, we still must rely on statistical analyses based on vague and varied criteria. Two critical questions remain: (1) Which child will be obese as an adult, and (2) how can the physician identify him or her so that proper therapy can be instituted at the most propitious time?

Unfortunately, the prognosis of childhood obesity remains poor, since many obese children are brought to the attention of the physician when the factors that promote the obese state appear to be well established. There is no correlation between the success of therapy (long-term maintenance of weight reduction) and rate of weight loss or amount lost.[16] Indeed, most of our knowledge of the treatment of this condition is based on studies performed in adults. Only within recent years has the pediatrician questioned the dictum that "a fat baby is a healthy baby." Future studies of the prognosis and pathogenesis of the obese state must, therefore, be devoted toward the earliest detection of the obese state if meaningful therapeutic measures are to be achieved.

PATHOGENESIS

A multitude of mechanisms have been invoked in studies of the development of the obese state. These include genetic defects, imbalances in caloric intake, derangements of glucose and fat metabolism, endocrine disorders, and psychological processes.[20-32] It is probable that all of these factors play a significant role and that obesity is truly a multifactorial syndrome in which the physician must weigh the relative contribution of each factor if he is to deal effectively with an individual patient. A review of all the medical literature related to the pathogenesis of the obese state is not practical in the present discussion; emphasis will therefore be placed on more recent cellular studies, which indicate the importance of early nutritional and hormonal factors and the developmental nature of this disorder.

Development of adipose tissue. The earliest studies of the development of the fat depot in man have shown that fat increases steadily for the first nine months of life. At this time a plateau is reached and thereafter a slight increment occurs until approximately age 7 years, when fat once again increases. A final spurt of deposition of adipose tissue occurs during adolescence. In females the early fat loss is less, as is the development of lean body mass; hence the average female finishes as an adult with a greater amount of body fat.[33] The growth of the fat depot is not linear, and the relative contribution of cell number and size to the growth of this organ remains unclear.

The development of a technique for obtaining multiple subcutaneous specimens of fat from the same individual by means of needle aspiration has provided a new approach for the study of human adipose tissue cellularity, metabolism, and development. The method is simple and safe and can be readily performed in an outpatient setting. The tissue obtained can then be utilized for the determination of cell size (lipid content) or for a variety of in vitro metabolic studies.[34, 35] estimate the total number of adipose cells in the body by dividing total body fat by the Once cell size is determined, it is possible to cell size previously determined.

Initial studies using this technique were performed in obese adults 21 years of age and older, who had a childhood history of obesity and in whom body fat comprised 40 per cent or more of body weight. Studies were performed before and after weight reduction and compared to the values found in a group of nonobese adults.[12] The results indicated that the expansion of the fat depot in the obese subjects was due primarily to an increase in cell number (2- to 3-fold). While some obese subjects also had increases in adipose cell size, others had normal values. Weight reduction was associated with a decrease in adipose cell size but no significant alteration in cell number was observed.

It appears that once adulthood is achieved the number of adipose cells is unchanged by dietary manipulation and the hypercellular state persists even after marked degrees of weight loss. Studies of overfeeding in adults also indicate the permanent nature of adult adipose tissue cellularity.[36] Alterations in the fat depot in adults are mediated solely by changes in cell lipid content.

A similar constancy of adipose cell number is encountered in the study of the epididymal fat pads of Sprague-Dawley rats.[37] Whereas cell size continues to increase slowly with time in these animals, cell number develops rapidly early in life and a plateau is reached at approximately 10 to 15 weeks of age. The results of caloric deprivation after this plateau is reached are similar to those seen in human adults; loss of weight is achieved exclusively by a decrease in the size of the cells without any change in number. Furthermore, procedures such as overfeeding and production of hypothalamic lesions, which

218

increase the size of adipose depots in the adult rat, result in a further increase in cell size without altering cell number. As in man, once adult number is attained it apparently cannot be altered by nutritional factors.

However, it has been shown that early nutritional influences can affect the number of the adult adipose cells in the epididymal fat pad of the rat. Caloric intake during suckling can be controlled, using the experimental design suggested by the works of Widdowson and McCance,[38, 39] in which litter sizes are altered. In addition, maternal protein-calorie restriction during lactation has been associated with changes in adipose cell number in the young.[41] Thus it has been possible to show that infantile nutritional experiences can effect a permanent change in the number of cells in the epididymal fat pad of the rat.

To date, early nutritional studies are the only experimental situations encountered in which changes in the size of the adipose depot are accompanied by significant differences in the number of adipose cells. These findings, and the fact that human obesity is accompanied by similar alteration in the number of the adipose cells, strongly suggest that early nutritional experiences, by virtue of their effect on cellularity, may be of prime importance in the development and treatment of the obese state.

The immediate questions that arise from these results are: (1) At what age in man is adult adipose cell number and size achieved? (2) At what age do obese subjects begin to deviate from normal cellular development? (3) At what age do obese subjects exceed normal adult values for size and number? (4) At what age, if any, can cell number be altered by dietary means? The questions are of more than academic interest, since the answers could provide a rational basis for the dietary control of obesity during critical periods of development.

In order to explore this problem further, subcutaneous samples of adipose tissue were obtained from obese and nonobese subjects, ages 2 to 26 years of age, and adipose cell number and size were determined.[42]

The weights for obese subjects ranged from 28 to 175 Kg. The youngest obese child studied was a 2-year-old girl who weighed 38 Kg. Indeed, all obese subjects were above the ninety-seventh percentile for weight and height when plotted on Stuart's charts, and all exceeded ideal weights by 130 per cent or more. Nonobese young adults over the age of 20 ranged in weight from 56 to 62 Kg., whereas obese subjects of similar age weighed 97 to 170 Kg.

At all age levels studied, obese children had, on the average, larger cells than nonobese children, although some degree of overlap was observed. However, it is significant that all nonobese children had cell sizes below adult values (i.e., below 0.5 to 0.8 μg of lipid/cell), whereas the fat cells of three obese children had attained adult size by age six. Indeed, by the age of 11 years, the fat cells of all obese children had attained but had not exceeded adult values.

At all ages, obese children had a greater number of adipose cells. In one subject, age 6 years, the adult range was exceeded, and all teen-age subjects either attained or surpassed normal adult values. None of the nonobese children attained adult values prior to the age of 12. It would appear that in some obese children a rapid increase in cellularity begins between the ages of 5 and 7 years or earlier, whereas in nonobese children a similar occurrence is observed between the ages of 9 and 12, with little change in number between the ages of 2 and 10.

These results indicate that cellular development proceeds at a more rapid rate in obese subjects; indeed, deviations from "normal development" were observed as early as age 2 years. The data also suggest that by age 6, one can distinguish at least two subgroups within the obese population, based on cell number: those individuals with marked hypercellularity exceeding normal adult values and those with modest increases in cell number relative to nonobese subjects of the same age but who have not exceeded the normal adult range. These subgroups can be further refined if one includes differences in cell size. Thus one has individuals with marked hypercellularity with either increased cell size or normal cell size. Two similar groups can be identified within the obese groups with only modest elevations in number. The significance of these findings cannot be assessed at present, but they could prove to be an important basis for prognosis of childhood obesity. It is reasonable to assume that subjects who have exceeded normal adult values for cellularity will most likely retain their obesity, whereas those within the normal range or below may outgrow their "baby fat." Longitudinal studies are currently in progress to test this hypothesis.

Studies of weight reduction in teen-age subjects have indicated that the hypercellular state found in this age group, as in the adult, is unaffected by dietary manipulation.[43] In addition, preliminary longitudinal studies (1 and 2 year follow-ups) have also demonstrated that hypercellularity persists.[42] It is clear then that early detection is imperative if one is to avoid a life-long history of obesity.

Metabolic and endocrine studies.

Glucose and insulin. The cellular changes found in obese adults have important metabolic consequences.[44] Many obese individuals have evidence of disordered carbohydrate metabolism and hyperinsulinemia, in either the fasting or postprandial state.[26-28, 45-50] These abnormalities of glucose and insulin metabolism often occur in the absence of other clinical manifestations of diabetes mellitus. In such patients it is not clear whether the metabolic abnormalities precede or follow the development of obesity. The absence of other signs or symptoms does not, of course, mean that diabetes does not exist, but its diagnosis on the basis of intolerance to oral glucose alone must be made with care. This is emphasized by the high percentage of "diabetic" oral glucose tolerance tests in the older population.[51] Furthermore, intolerance to oral glucose in obese individuals may be dependent upon the load administered.

In looking for clues to the relationship between obesity and diabetes, one characteristic of the obese individual stands out: the excessive size of his adipose depot. In the obese state, when carbohydrate metabolic abnor-malities are present, the adipose depot is enlarged. When there is weight loss and reduction in the size of this depot and in cell size, carbohydrate metabolism is improved.[12, 44]

In vitro studies of adipose tissue indicate that glucose metabolism, and in particular lipogenesis from glucose, proceed at a normal rate in the adipose cells of obese individuals. However, total adipose cell number is increased in these obese subjects, and total lipogenesis from glucose is increased in their adipose depots. However, lipogenesis from glucose is relatively small in adipose tissue; the major pathway of triglyceride synthesis is esterification of plasma free fatty acids. Thus far, measurement of this pathway has failed to reveal differences in the rate of lipogenesis.[34, 52]

It has also been reported that obese individuals are relatively resistant to the effects of insulin.[53, 54] This is based upon the observation that the hypoglycemic response to intravenously administered insulin is less marked in obese subjects, and the finding of insulin resistance during studies of glucose metabolism in which arteriovenous differences are measured by placing catheters into the arteries and veins that perfuse the forearm.[54] The insulin sensitivity of human adipose tissue is therefore of interest, particularly when examined in terms of its cellular characteristics.

In vitro insulin sensitivity of adipose tissue, as measured by the effect upon glucose oxidation, is dependent upon the size of the adipose cells. The larger the cell, the less responsive it is to insulin. Thus children whose cells are smaller than adult size are the most sensitive to the hormone, showing a 250 to 300 per cent increase in CO_2 production, compared with nonobese adults who show a 100 to 150 per cent rise in glucose oxidation. The enlarged fat-filled cells of obese subjects are the least insulin sensitive, showing only a 50 per cent increase in CO_2 production from glucose. This tissue abnormality could be a major factor in the insulin resistance of obesity. However, the adipose tissue of the reduced obese subject, with smaller sized cells, is normally sensitive to the action of insulin. Glucose oxidation in adipose tissue of reduced obese subjects is increased 150 per cent in the presence of insulin. The relationship between the size of the adipose cell and its insulin sensitivity is further emphasized by the observation that cells from reduced obese individuals who maintained normal body weight for 6 to 24 months remained sensitive to insulin in vitro. In vivo studies also reveal that glucose tolerance, plasma insulin, and free fatty acid levels are changed by weight reduction.[43, 55, 56] Thus abnormalities of glucose metabolism and the hyperinsulinemia found in the obese adult may be secondary to rather than the cause of the obese state.

Little is known about the causal relationships in children and adolescents since the finding of similar abnormalities at these ages have only been demonstrated in overtly obese subjects.[57, 58] Prospective studies will be needed before one can state definitely that a hyperinsulinemic state and/or abnormal glucose tolerance precedes the obese state. However, recent studies in our laboratory of newly diagnosed diabetic children, before and after therapy, indicate that treatment with insulin affects adipose cell lipid content without significantly altering cell number.[59] Thus one might predict that if the hyperinsulinemic state precedes obesity, it will lead to an increased lipid content of cells rather than to hypercellularity.

Growth hormone. Studies of the effect of growth hormone on the cellular development of a variety of organs other than fat have shown that this hormone increases cellular proliferation.[60-62] In vitro studies of adipose tissue in animals suggest that the main metabolic action of growth hormone is to increase the rate of lipolysis.[63] However, little is known about the effect of human growth hormone on human adipose tissue. In vivo studies indicate that the administration of human growth hormone increases free fatty acid release, presumably due to its effect on adipose tissue lipolysis.[64] Preliminary studies in our laboratory indicate that the treatment of growth hormone–deficient children produces significant increases in total body potassium and adipose cell number 6 to 8 months after onset of therapy.[65] These findings plus the fact that obese subjects have abnormalities in serum growth hormone levels suggest that growth hormone may also play a role in the development of the hypercellular state of obesity by virtue of its effect on cell division.[66]

Furthermore, we have found that infants of diabetic mothers studied at 6 months of age or less are relatively hypercellular in regard to adipocytes.[67] Indeed, three of the five subjects studied developed clinically evident obesity one year after the initial studies. It is tempting to postulate that frequent fluctuations of blood sugar with periods of hypoglycemia in diabetic mothers may serve as the stimulus for increased secretion of growth hormone in the fetus. This in turn could lead to an increase in cellularity of adipose tissue.

At present the role of growth hormone in the development of the obese state remains conjectural, but its importance in cellular division indicates that further studies of its action on the development of adipose tissue are warranted.

Adrenal function. Increased adrenal cortical function has been found in 30 to 60 per cent of obese subjects, but it is not clear how this may relate to the development or maintenance of the obese state.[68, 69] Weight reduction is accompanied by a decrease in 17-hydroxycorticosteroids, but little is known about the effect of corticosteroids on human adipose tissue metabolism other than its effect on lipolysis.

Studies of in vivo responses to exogenous epinephrine are conflicting; some authors suggest that obese subjects fail to increase free fatty acids after an epinephrine load, while others maintain that the response is normal.[70, 71] These differences may be due to the heterogeneity of obese persons, and no data related to adipose cell number or size are available.

In vitro studies of epinephrine-stimulated glycerol release indicate that the increase over basal values is diminished in larger adipocytes.[52, 72] As with insulin, it is not clear whether this phenomenon precedes or follows the development of obesity. However, it has been shown that weight reduction does not alter the in vitro epinephrine response in obese adults or adolescents.[43] No data relative to weight reduction are presently available in obese children who have diminished epinephrine response.[73]

One could speculate that the lack of epinephrine response serves as a stimulus for the development of new adipose cells. Thus a decrease in fatty acid release secondary to epinephrine stimulation could be overcome by providing a greater number of less responsive cells to meet energy needs. Since epinephrine acts via adenyl cyclase, one could also postulate a defect in this system. Studies of the levels of 3'5' cyclic adenosine monophosphate and adenyl cyclase in human and rat adipose tissue are currently in progress in our laboratory to explore this hypothesis.

Thyroid. At present there are few data to support any role for thyroid malfunction in the pathogenesis of obesity. Serum levels of protein-bound iodine or thyroxine all appear to be normal in obese subjects.[74] Bray[75] has recently identified a small group of obese women with exceptionally large cells that respond to T3 therapy. However, one should not use this drug routinely in the treatment of simple exogenous obesity. Furthermore, there is no evidence that similar subjects exist in the pediatric or adolescent age group.

It can be seen from the above that our understanding of the metabolic and endocrine abnormalities found in the obese state is far from complete. The extent to which any of these hormones play a role in the pathogenesis of the obese state is not clear. Indeed, the fact that weight reduction results in a more normal metabolic and endocrine profile suggests that these phenomena are secondary to the obese state rather than causal. Nonetheless, it does appear that hormonal actions can markedly affect adipose cell size by virtue of their effect on metabolism and cellular proliferation. Further studies of the complex interaction of hormonal control and early nutritional factors could provide important clues about the development and mainte-

nance of the ultimate size of the fat depot in man.

Genetic factors. The existence of genetic factors in the development of obesity has been clearly established only in animals. Most of these models are unsuitable for the study of human obesity, since the fat depots are increased solely by increments in cell size.[37] Recently, however, Johnson and Hirsch[76] have identified one strain of obese rat that does have hypercellularity of the fat depot. Early feeding studies utilizing this model will hopefully shed important light on the relative importance of nutritional intake and genetic cellular endowment.

In man, the problem is more complex; genetic obesity (i.e., individuals with specific enzymatic defects) has not been definitely detected. Family studies indicate that if one parent is obese, 40 to 50 per cent of the children will develop obesity, and the proportion rises to 70 to 80 per cent if both are obese.[21, 22] Twin studies also show that identical twins reared in the same environment have less differences in weight than do fraternal twins.[23] When the former are reared in different homes, the weight differences increase but are still less than those found in nonidentical twins. Furthermore, the weights of natural children correlate well with those of their parents, but no correlation can be found between the weights of adopted children and those of their adopting parents.[24] Thus a real genetic contribution to the control of body weight appears to be present. However, the facts that cellularity can be affected by early nutrition and that birth weight does not correlate with adult weight indicate that evironmental factors also play a role. Like all questions of genetic versus environmental factors, the answer may be found in a combination of the two. An individual is probably endowed with a certain range of adipose tissue cellularity which can be modified by a variety of environmental influences. The final depot size will in all likelihood depend upon the interaction of a genetic template with all the environmental and hormonal factors that influence number and size. However, one cannot hope for the elucidation of genetic obesity until one demonstrates a familial biochemical error that will provide a basis for the many abnormalities found in obese subjects. Indeed, a universal basic defect may not exist; there may be many different genetic types.

Psychological factors. The data presented above clearly indicate that multiple etiologic factors may act either alone or in unison to produce a variable size in the adipose depot. Although the present discussion has stressed some of the newer metabolic and cellular aspects of the pathogenesis of obesity, the reader should also be aware of the voluminous literature relative to the role of psychological factors and of disturbed eating patterns in the obese subject. Here, too, one finds a multitude of theories, all of which cannot be detailed in the present discussion. One can only state that no one psychological problem or feeding pattern can be found. Psychological factors appear to form a continuum ranging from patients in whom they play little or no role to those in whom eating has become a predominant mechanism for psychological adjustment. The same is true of eating patterns, which can range from the so-called "binge eaters' syndrome" to continuous eating without satiety.[3] As with the metabolic studies, little is known about the developmental aspects of these phenomena.

The study of subjects with juvenile onset obesity and adult onset obesity indicates that those subjects with early onset had severely disturbed concepts of body image and other psychological problems, whereas the other group did not.[30] One is still left with the question of whether the psychological problems encountered in these obese subjects precede or follow the obese state. Do psychologic factors develop primarily in response to a distorted body image in childhood, or do they antedate it? Much more information is necessary in this area, with particular emphasis on interactions between mother and child during the earliest feeding periods.

TREATMENT

In discussing the treatment of obesity it is necessary to re-emphasize that one is dealing with a syndrome rather than a disease.

The physician must be acquainted with the metabolic and psychological complexities of human obesity in order to better deal with this perplexing and frustrating problem. The concept of the obese subject as one who merely over indulges, due to a lack of self-discipline can no longer be accepted.

The treatment of obesity is at once the simplest and yet most complex of all disorders: simple in that, in the adult, all that is required is caloric restriction, and complex in that cellular, metabolic, socioeconomic, cultural, and psychological factors all militate against the maintenance of the reduced state. Unfortunately, in our society only the weight reduction period is emphasized and the obese subject is exposed to an endless variety of weight reduction programs, which include diets, drugs, hormones, hypnosis, psychotherapy, and surgical intervention.

Although drastic crash programs may be necessary in life-threatening situations, such as the Pickwickian syndrome, diabetes, hypertension, or coronary artery disease, they are usually not necessary in uncomplicated cases. Furthermore, they do not prepare either the patient or the physician for a life of continuous dietary control. This preoccupation of both the lay and medical community with weight loss alone has fostered the neglect of the postreduction period, which is in fact the more difficult problem. Thus most obese subjects live in a vicious cycle of weight loss followed by weight gain, ad infinitum, going from one "cure" to another in search of a magic formula.

The fact is that success with any weight reduction program will always be short lived if it is not followed with supportive therapy that includes nutritional information suited to the tastes and life style of the individual. One must make the subject aware of the fact that once his or her desired weight is achieved, some degree of caloric restriction must be maintained if the reaccumulation of fat is to be avoided.

Obesity is a complex disorder, and merely lecturing the patient or instilling guilt feelings by the use of such phrases as "weak willed" or "cheating" will only be counter productive. Rather one must be sympathetic and understanding of the enormity of the problem confronting the obese subject after weight loss is achieved. No one dietary program can be used for all patients, and it is up to the physician to work closely with his patient to find a program that is suitable. Any caloric restriction program that provides sufficient protein and minerals without promoting excessive ketosis or undue hunger will suffice.

Preparations for the weight loss and maintenance period should be made well in advance. The patient must be made to understand that a decrease in weight is not a cure-all. Most of the psychological and social problems that he has attributed to obesity will remain, and indeed some degree of depression and anxiety will occur as the subject realizes this fact.[77] At this time the physician must be prepared to emphasize the positive aspects of the weight loss, such as changes in body image and other medical and social benefits.

The use of drugs such as amphetamines is of little value in the long-range treatment of obesity and should be assiduously avoided. This is especially true in children and adolescents who are exposed to a drug-oriented society. The introduction of yet another medically approved drug creates the risk of subsequent harm from misuse. The short-term gain provided by these drugs is far outweighed by the long-term losses. Indeed, the reliance upon initial easy weight loss therapies may interfere with the initiation of effective weight maintenance programs by misleading the patient in regard to the nature and extent of effective long-term treatment.

The problem of dietary control is even more complicated in children. In the adult most organ systems have reached their ultimate size and cellular division is complete. Weight reduction can be achieved almost exclusively by a decrease in body fat with little or no decrease in lean body mass.[12] However, in the child one must provide sufficient calories and protein to allow for the growth and development of lean body mass, while achieving a decrease in the fat depot. The extent to which any dietary regimen will be responsible for these changes will depend upon the age at which it is instituted and the individual's level of cellular development. Unfortunately, at present our knowledge of the interrelationship of cellular growth and development of the various organ systems in the body is still incomplete. No one diet can be devised that will deny calories and protein to the fat depot while providing the necessary nutrients to other tissues. Thus one must be extremely cautious and ever alert in restricting calories in the earliest age groups, and normal linear growth rates must be maintained.

As a rule, in children under age 12 years we have used 60 calories per kilogram of ideal body weight and provide 20 per cent of calories as protein with the remaining 80 per cent evenly distributed between carbohydrate and fat. Supplements of minerals and vitamins are provided as needed, as well as iron in menstruating girls.

As in the adult one must be aware of the psychological and social problems, especially with younger children who are more dependent upon their mothers. Indeed, one cannot alter dietary patterns of obese children without an understanding of their social milieu; the full cooperation of the family and school is necessary.

Once dietary restriction is instituted, weight loss and linear growth must be carefully monitored. Calories can then be readily increased or decreased depending upon the individual's response. Weight loss should be monitored in terms of body composition rather than total body weight. Indeed, the maintenance of a constant weight with an increasing ratio of lean body mass to body fat with normal linear growth is a desirable result. Ideally, of course, one would like to provide a diet at a critical period in the cellular development of the fat depot, so that adipose cell number would be held constant or decreased with minimal effect on the cellularity of nonfat organs. Unfortunately, at the present time this cannot be done because we lack sufficient information.

However, it is hoped that studies of adipose tissue cellularity and metabolism described above, coupled with frequent longitudinal examinations of the same subject, will provide the necessary data to accomplish this end.

The development of techniques for the earliest identification of abnormal development of the fat depot and the institution of therapeutic measures to alter the development of this tissue before immutable hypercellularity occurs offer the best hope for the treatment of obesity in both children and adults.

The contribution of Dr. Fredda Ginsberg-Fellner in compiling the adipose cellular data in children is gratefully acknowledged.

REFERENCES

1. Lesser, G. T., and Zak, G.: Measurement of total body fat in man by simultaneous adsorption of two inert gases, Ann. N. Y. Acad. Sci. **110:** 40, 1963.
2. Brozek, J., Grande, F., Anderson, J. T., and Keys, A.: Densitometric analysis of body composition, Ann. N. Y. Acad. Sci. **110:** 113, 1963.
3. Owen, G. M., Jensen, R. L., and Fomon, S. J.: Sex-related difference in total body water and exchangeable chloride during infancy, J. PEDIATR. **60:** 858, 1962.
4. Forbes, G. B.: Lean body mass and fat in obese children, Pediatrics **34:** 308, 1964.
5. Heald, F. P., Hunt, E. E., Schwartz, R., Cook, C. D., Elliott, O., and Vajda, B.: Measures of body fat and hydration in adolescent boys, Pediatrics **31:** 226, 1963.
6. Wolff, O. H.: Obesity in childhood, Q. J. Med. **24:** 109, 1955.
7. Quaade, F.: Prevention of overnutrition, *in* Blix, G., editor: Symposia of the Swedish nutrition foundation, Uppsala, 1964, Almqvist and Wiksells, p. 25.
8. Jackson, R. L., and Kelly, H. G.: Growth charts for use in pediatric practice, J. PEDIATR. **27:** 215, 1945.
9. Stuart, H. C., and Meredith, H. V.: Use of body measurements in the school health program, Am. J. Public Health **36:** 1365, 1946.
10. Johnson, M. L., Burke, B. S., and Mayer, J.: The prevalence and incidence of obesity in cross section of elementary and secondary school children, Am. J. Clin. Nutr. **4:** 231, 1956.
11. Rose, H. E., and Mayer, J.: Activity calorie intake and the energy balance of infants, Pediatrics **41:** 18, 1968.
12. Hirsch, J., and Knittle, J. L.: Cellularity of obese and nonobese human adipose tissue, Fed. Proc. Symp. **29:** 1516, 1970.
13. Bjorntorp, P., Berchtold, P., and Tibblin, G.: Insulin secretion in relation to adipose tissue in men, Diabetes **20:** 65, 1971.
14. Mullins, A. G.: The prognosis in juvenile obesity, Arch. Dis. Child. **33:** 307, 1958.
15. Abraham, A., and Nordsieck, M.: Relationship of excess weight in children and adults, Public Health Rep. **75:** 263, 1960.
16. Lloyd, J. K., Wolff, O. H., and Whelen, W. S.: Childhood obesity; long term study of height and weight, Br. Med. J. **2:** 45, 1961.
17. Asher, P.: Fat babies and fat children: The prognosis of obesity in the very young, Arch. Dis. Child. **41:** 672, 1966.
18. Robertson, A. F., and Lowry, G. H.: Overweight children, Mich. Med. **63:** 629, 1964.
19. Mossberg, H. O.: Obesity in children; a clinical prognostical investigation, Acta Paediatr. **35:** Suppl. 2, 1948.
20. Mayer, J.: Obese hyperglycemic syndrome as an example of "metabolic" obesity, Am. J. Clin. Nutr. **8:** 712, 1960.
21. Rony, H.: Obesity and leanness, Philadelphia, 1940, Lea & Febiger, Publishers.
22. Angel, J. L.: Constitution in female obesity, Am. J. Phys. Anthropol. **7:** 433, 1949.
23. Von Verschuer, O.: Quoted by Mayer, Some aspects of the problem of regulation of food intake and obesity, N. Engl. J. Med. **274:** 671, 1966.
24. Withers, R. F. J.: Problems in the genetics of obesity, Eugen. Rev. **58:** 81, 1964.
25. Miller, D. S., and Payne, P. R.: Weight maintenance and food intake, J. Nutr. **78:** 255, 1962.
26. Ogilive, R. F.: Sugar tolerance in obese subjects; a review of 65 cases, Q. J. Med. **4:** 345, 1935.
27. Mostofi, A. G., Sanford, H. N., Bronstein, I. P., and Asrow, Q.: The arterial and venous glucose tolerance test in obese and nonobese children, Pediatrics **19:** 993, 1957.
28. Vajda, B., Heald, F. P., and Mayer, J.: Intravenous glucose tolerance in obese adolescents, Lancet **1:** 902, 1964.
29. Bierman, E. L., Dole, V. P., and Roberts, T. N.: An abnormality of nonesterified fatty acid metabolism in diabetes mellitus, Diabetes **6:** 475, 1957.
30. Mendelson, M.: Psychological aspects of obesity, Med. Clin. North Am. **48:** 1373, 1964.
31. Stunkard, A. J.: Eating patterns and obesity, Psychiatr. Q. **33:** 284, 1959.
32. Bruch, H.: Psychological aspects of obesity, *in* Blix, G., editor: Symposia of the Swedish nutrition foundation. II. Occurrence, causes and prevention of overnutrition, Uppsala, 1964, Almqvist and Wiksells, p. 37.
33. Falkner, F.: General considerations in human development, *in* Falkner, F., editor: Human Development, Philadelphia, 1966, W. B. Saunders Company, p. 10.
34. Hirsch, J., and Goldrick, R. B.: Serial studies of the metabolism of human adipose tissue, J. Clin. Invest. **43:** 1776, 1964.

35. Hirsch, J., and Gallian, E.: Methods for the determination of adipose cell size and cell number in man and animals, J. Lipid Res. **9:** 110, 1968.

36. Sims, E. A. H., Goldman, R. F., Gluck, C. M., Horton, E. S., Kelleher, P. C., and Rowe, D. W.: Experimental obesity in man, Trans. Assoc. Am. Phys. **81:** 153, 1968.

37. Hirsch, J., and Han, P. W.: Cellularity of rat adipose tissue, effects of growth, starvation and obesity, J. Lipid Res. **10:** 77, 1969.

38. Widdowson, E. M., and McCance, R. A.: Some effects of accelerating growth. I. General somatic development, Proc. R. Soc. Lond. Series B. **152:** 188, 1960.

39. McCance, R. A.: Food, growth and time, Lancet **2:** 621, 1962.

40. Knittle, J. L., and Hirsch, J.: Effect of early nutrition on the development of rat epididymal fat pads: Cellularity and metabolism, J. Clin. Invest. **47:** 2091, 1968.

41. Knittle, J. L.: Maternal diet as a factor in adipose tissue cellularity and metabolism in the young rat, J. Nutr. **102:** 427, 1972.

42. To be published.

43. Knittle, J. L., and Ginsberg-Fellner, F.: The effect of weight reduction on in vitro adipose tissue lipolysis and cellularity in obese adolescents and adults, Diabetes **21:** 754, 1972.

44. Salans, L. B., Knittle, J. L., and Hirsch, J.: The role of adipose cell size and adipose tissue insulin sensitivity in the carbohydrate intolerance of human obesity, J. Clin. Invest. **47:** 153, 1968.

45. Newburgh, L. H., and Conn, J. W.: A new interpretation of hyperglycemia in obese middle aged persons, J. A. M. A. **112:** 7,1939.

46. Paullin, J. H., and Sauls, H. C.: A study of the glucose tolerance test in the obese, South. Med. J. **15:** 249, 1922.

47. John, H. J.: A summary of the findings in 1100 glucose tolerance estimations, Endocrinology **13:** 388, 1929.

48. Berkowitz, D.: Metabolic changes associated with obesity before and after weight reduction, J. A. M. A. **187:** 399, 1964.

49. Forsham, P. H.: Excessive insulin response to glucose in obese subjects as measured by immunochemical assay, Diabetes **12:** 197, 1963.

50. Beck, P., Koumans, J. H. T., Winterling, C. A., Stein, M. F., Daughaday, W. H., and Kipnis, D. M.: Studies of insulin and growth hormone secretion in human obesity, J. Lab. Clin. Med. **64:** 654, 1964.

51. Streeten, D. H. P., Gerstein, M. M., Marmor, B. M.,, and Doisy R. I.: Reduced glucose tolerance in elderly human subjects, Diabetes **14:** 579, 1965.

52. Goldrick, R. B., and McLoughlin, G. M.: Lipolysis and lipogenesis from glucose in human fat cells of different sizes: Effects of insulin, epinephrine and theophylline, J. Clin. Invest. **49:** 1213, 1970.

53. Fraser, R., Joplin, G. F., Opie, L. H., and Rabinowitz, D.: The augmented insulin tolerance test for detecting insulin resistance, J. Endocrinol. **25:** 299, 1962.

54. Rabinowitz, D., and Zierler, K. L.: Forearm metabolism in obesity and its response to intra-arterial insulin; evidence for adaptive hyperinsulinism, Lancet **2:** 690, 1961.

55. Kalkhoff, R. K., Kim, H. D., Cerletty, J., and Ferrou, C. A.: Metabolic effects of weight loss in obese subjects; changes in plasma substrate levels, Diabetes **20:** 83, 1971.

56. Newburgh, L. H.: Control of the hyperglycemia of obese "diabetics" by weight reduction, Ann. Intern. Med. **17:** 935, 1952.

57. Parra, A., Schultz, R. B., Graystone, J. E., and Cheek, D. B.: Correlative studies in obese children and adolescents concerning body composition and plasma insulin and growth hormone levels, Pediat. Res. **5:** 605, 1971.

58. Paulsen, E. L., Richenderfer, F., and Ginsberg-Fellner, F.: Plasma glucose, free fatty acids and immunoreactive insulin in sixty obese children, Diabetes **17:** 261, 1968.

59. Ginsberg-Fellner, F., and Knittle, J. L.: Adipose tissue cellularity and metabolism in newly diagnosed juvenile diabetics, Soc. Pediatr. Res. **40:** 134, 1970.

60. Kenny, F. M., Drash, A., Garces, L. Y., and Susan, A.: "Catch up growth" despite hypopituitarism after craniopharyngioma removal, American Pediatric Society, May 1, 1968.

61. Cheek, D. B., Brasel, J. A., Elliott, D., and Scott, R.: Muscle cell size and number in normal children and in dwarfs (pituitary, cretins and primordial). Preliminary observations, Bull. Hopkins Hosp. **119:** 46, 1966.

62. Beach, R. F., and Kostyo, J. L.: Effect of growth hormone on the DNA content of muscles of young hypophysectomized rats, Endocrinology **32:** 882, 1968.

63. Vaughn, M., Steinberg, D.: Effect of hormones on lipolysis and esterification of free fatty acids during incubation of adipose tissue in vitro, J. Lipid Res. **4:** 193, 1963.

64. Raben, M. S., and Hollenberg, C. H.: Effect of growth hormone on plasma free fatty acids, J. Clin. Invest. **38:** 484, 1959.

65. Knittle, J. L., Sussman, L., Collipp, P. J., and Gertner, M.: The effect of treatment with growth hormone on glucose tolerance and adipose tissue cellularity in ateliotic dwarfism, Am. Diabetes Assoc., June, 1972.

66. Para, A., Schultz, R. B., Graystone, J. F., and Cheek, D. B.: Correlative studies in obese children and adolescents concerning body composition and plasma insulin and growth hormone levels, Pediatr. Res. **5:** 605, 1971.

67. Ginsberg-Fellner, F., and Knittle, J. L.: Maternal diabetes as a factor in the development of childhood obesity, Soc. Pediatr. Res. **41:** 197, 1971.

68. Migeon, C. J., Green, O. C., and Eckert, J. P.: Study of adrenocortical function in obesity, Metabolism **12:** 718, 1963.

69. Schteingart, D., and Conn, J.: Characteristics

of the increased adrenocortical function observed in many obese patients, Ann. N. Y. Acad. Sci. **131:** 388, 1965.

70. Gordon, E. S., Goldberg, E. M., Brandabur, J. J., Gee, J. B., and Rankin, J.: Abnormal energy metabolism in obesity, Trans. Assoc. Am. Physicians **75:** 118, 1962.

71. Orth, R. D., and Williams, R. H.: Response of plasma nefa levels to epinephrine infusions in normal and obese women, Proc. Soc. Exp. Biol. Med. **104:** 119, 1960.

72. Zinder, O., and Shapiro, B.: Effect of cell size on epinephrine and ACTH-induced fatty acid release from isolated fat cells, J. Lipid Res. **12:** 91, 1971.

73. Knittle, J. L., and Ginsberg-Fellner, F.: Adipose tissue cellularity and epinephrine stimulated lipolysis in obese and non-obese children, Clin. Res. **17:** 387, 1969.

74. Hung, W., Gancayo, G. P., and Heald, F. P.: Thyroxine metabolism in obese adolescent males, Pediatrics **36:** 877, 1965.

75. Bray, G. A.: Effect of diet and triiodothyronine on the activity of SN-glycerol-3-phosphate dehydrogenase and on the metabolism of glucose and pyruvate by adipose tissue of obese patients, J. Clin. Invest. **48:** 1413, 1969.

76. Johnson, P. R., and Hirsch, J.: Cellularity of adipose depots in six strains of genetically obese mice, J. Lipid Res. **13:** 2, 1972.

77. Glucksman, M. L., Hirsch, J., McCulley, R. S., Barron, B. A., and Knittle, J. L.: The response of obese patients to weight reduction. II. A quantitative evaluation of behavior, Psychosom. Med. **30:** 359, 1968.

227

When to start dieting? At birth

Obesity experts think eating and weight patterns are set in infancy

Obesity and heart disease are so widespread and so difficult to control in adulthood that many physicians favor preventive measures, particularly early childhood diet control, as the best way to tackle the problem. Authorities generally agree that it's not wise to let children grow too fat and that fresh fruits and vegetables are far better for them than the glut of snack foods and sweets modern marketing thrusts at them.

But the younger the child, the hazier the guidelines for feeding him. And the most confusion of all surrounds the question of proper diet for newborn babies.

The whole concept of preventing adult heart disease through studies of small children is itself only two or three years old, says Dr. Forrest H. Adams, professor of pediatric cardiology at the University of California at Los Angeles and past president of the American College of Cardiology. "It's very difficult, if we make a recommendation today, to tell parents—or children—with confidence that if they follow it the children won't have heart disease when they grow up," he says.

Dr. Adams heads a UCLA clinic for recognizing and treating early atherosclerosis in children. The clinic's approach is interdisciplinary, combining the services of a medical geneticist, a pediatric endocrinologist, a dietician, a cardiologist, and a pediatric cardiologist—Dr. Adams.

Children whose relatives had heart disease prematurely are screened and those at risk identified by blood-lipid tests, after which their diets are regulated. Though he is busy working with children already judged abnormal, Dr. Adams feels that the key future research project will be diet control for normal infants, with particular emphasis on prevention of childhood obesity.

Some of the blame for obesity in children can be placed on the medical profession itself, Dr. Adams feels.

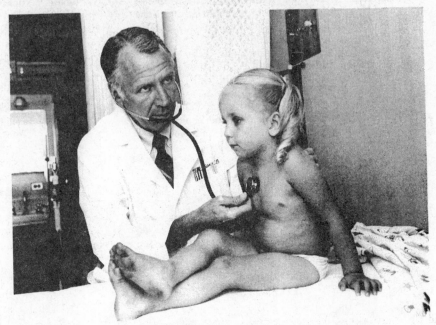

Dr. Adams says diet for normal babies should be a key research project.

"Pediatricians have possibly encouraged poor child-raising practices in that we have tended to go along with the idea that a big baby is a healthy baby," he says.

And while the effects of childhood obesity on later development are not yet fully known in humans, says Dr. Adams, "I think the evidence in animals, especially primates, is highly suggestive that if we control the diet—particularly fat intake—weight, and blood pressure, there is every indication we should be able to lengthen people's lives and make them healthier. But there is certainly nobody I know of who has the necessary information yet."

Cardiologist George E. Burch, professor of medicine at New Orleans' Tulane University, has lectured often on experimental evidence that young animals kept thin tend to live longer than their fat siblings, while adult-onset obesity seems to make no difference in animals' longevity. Dr. Burch admits this information can't be directly extrapolated to humans, but he has been known to say facetiously that free school lunches should be eliminated to keep children healthy. Nevertheless, he agrees that specific diet recommendations can't be made for infants on the basis of available knowledge.

An experimental approach to such questions was taken several years ago by Drs. Jules Hirsch and Jerome L. Knittle at Rockefeller University, who used rats to study how obesity in infancy relates to excess weight in adulthood (MWN, June 2, '67, p. 55). They found that obesity in young rats was a result of too many fat cells, while adult-onset obesity was due to an increase in the size of pre-existing fat cells.

Dr. Knittle, now professor of pediatrics at Mount Sinai School of Medicine, extended his investigations directly to obese children. He found that the two critical periods in development of fat cells are the ages from birth to two years and from eight to 12. The number of fat cells is fixed between the ages of 16 and 21; weight gain after that is accomplished by enlarging existing fat cells.

Ominously, the number of fat cells formed appears to be irreversible,

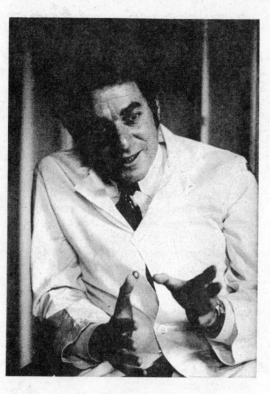

Dr. Knittle: We're not clever enough to tell a calorie: 'you go to the brain, and you go to the liver, and stay away from the adipose depot.'

and Dr. Knittle sees the significance of this in the fact that more than 80% of all obese children become obese adults. "All the people we have ever reduced in weight have done so by making cells smaller," he says. "We've never been able to reduce the *number* of cells."

But what this means in relation to adult obesity remains unclear. The New York researcher hopes obese children can be treated at a time when, even if they are hypercellular for their age, they have not yet developed more fat cells than the average adult. Says Dr. Knittle: "The question that really remains is: Given a child who has a normal adult fat-cell level at the age of six, is it possible to keep it there?"

He is following the development of over 200 children at Mount Sinai to determine whether one can feed only the lean part of a growing child without increasing the number of his fat cells. Dr. Knittle has observed hypercellularity in children as young as two, but says the weight range of infants less than a year old is so narrow it's hard to discover which babies are tending toward obesity.

But the pediatric researcher is reluctant to give specific information

about what a baby should eat to prevent the problem in the first place, because he feels not enough facts have been established about body composition. He hopes his animal studies will reveal just what does trigger development of excess fat cells. He also believes some metabolic defects might be hereditary but, cautions Dr. Knittle, "While there is a small group of children who may have genetic defects, this does not necessarily explain all kinds of obesity."

Once a physician can pick out some at-risk children at birth, the infant's diet may be controlled from the beginning. But at this point, Dr. Knittle says, "We are not clever enough to tell a calorie: 'You go to the brain and you go to the liver, and stay away from the adipose depot.' We have to learn a little more about the interdevelopment of organ systems."

The significance of his observations about fat-cell development remains controversial. Dr. Malcolm Holliday, a San Francisco pediatrician and chairman of the American Academy of Pediatrics' committee on nutrition, says: "The first year of life is not as crucial as has been believed." He adds that the fat-cell theory should not be interpreted to mean necessarily that a

fat six-month-old baby will be fat later in life, but rather that fat two-to five-year-olds run the highest risk of obesity as adults, because their eating patterns are now established.

The AAP nutrition group is preparing a paper which should be available within the next six months on infant formulas and milk as foods. While the committee has not yet reached a consensus, Dr. Holliday says his personal feeling is that mothers should breast-feed babies for six months and then start them on solid foods. But he acknowledges that mothers can't always do what is ideal. "In modern society breast-feeding is not always possible, so we need good substitutes. The old modified-milk formulas that were promoted were not ideal. The question is whether formulas more like breast milk have advantages," explains Dr. Holliday. He thinks so—he favors development of formulas that resemble breast milk as closely as possible.

Dr. Holliday doesn't feel the committee has enough information to set broad guidelines on all phases of diet for all babies. He does suggest, however, that mothers are feeding their babies solids at far too early an age—as early as two weeks after birth.

The trend toward early introduction of solids is leading to overweight in infants, and possibly to heart disease in adults, according to Dr. Sherrel L. Hammar, associate professor of pediatrics at the University of Hawaii, who says: "Particularly in families where there's a high incidence of obesity, I would try to monitor the child's weight carefully during the first year."

Infants are doubling their birth weight at a significantly earlier age than they were several decades ago, he observes. While nutrition has generally improved, weight gains are coming too rapidly, far exceeding the old formula of doubling at six months and tripling at a year. The Honolulu pediatrician also deplores the use of a bottle as a pacifier, claiming that an infant gets enough calories at mealtime and that the extra formula just provides excess calories not needed for growth. A baby is being fed enough if his weight increases by half a pound a week for the first six months, he says.

"The plump, healthy-looking infant has long been considered the hallmark of good mothering," Dr. Hammar noted in a recent paper. "The concept that maximum growth of the infant is not synonymous with optimum growth requires a reorientation in our approach to public health and nutritional education."

The controversy over neonatal feeding patterns has sociological overtones, says Dr. John Crawford, associate professor of pediatrics at Harvard and chief of the endocrine and metabolism unit of Boston's Massachusetts General Hospital. "The time of introduction of solid foods has been a matter of keeping up with the Joneses," he says, adding that what a baby is fed has been a decision by the mother, usually decided by what is tastier for her rather than for the baby. The most popular baby foods not only have too many calories but possibly a salt level that may have something to do with the high incidence of hypertension and atherosclerosis in early middle age.

But the salt question is a particularly hot one. And since not enough facts are available to make specific judgments, doctors should not restrict the salt intake of children unless there is a family history of hypertension, the American Academy of Pediatrics nutrition committee suggested in a recent bulletin.

This controversy and others point up the fact that there are more questions about how much and what a mother should feed a baby than there are answers. There is a clear need for further studies of infants whose diets are controlled from birth.

Dr. Charles Glueck at the University of Cincinnati College of Medicine has shown that infants with familial type II hyperlipoproteinemia can have normal plasma cholesterol levels in the first year of life if they are put on a special formula beginning at birth. Diet restrictions are not as effective in lowering cholesterol levels in older children.

In the study 33 hypercholesteremic newborns were selected from 3,800 consecutive live births at Cincinnati General Hospital. Fourteen of the infants were documented as having type II. Half of them were put on a normal cholesterol intake (cow's milk formulas) while the others were given cholesterol-poor polyunsaturate-rich formulas. The first group showed a mean plasma cholesterol increase at six months of age, while the second showed a decrease. Four type II children put on the low-cholesterol diet at six months were maintaining normal cholesterol levels at a year. Thirteen children with type II, over the age of six, were also put on a low-cholesterol diet. Dr. Glueck observed a 12% decrease in plasma cholesterol levels in these older children, but they still had severe hypercholesterolemia.

Studies like that of Dr. Glueck support the argument that diet can affect and possibly prevent certain children's diseases. While the children in the study were already considered abnormal, as are the children at Dr. Adams' Los Angeles clinic, there are others who have studied the effects of diet on normal infants.

One of these is Dr. Calvin W. Woodruff, professor of pediatrics at the University of Missouri at Columbia. He has done experiments comparing serum lipid levels in infants fed breast milk and those fed evaporated cow's milk. He also studied the iron deficiencies caused by feeding normal infants whole cow's milk. In his study 13 infants were fed fresh cow's milk after the age of two months and were compared with a group of 25 infants whose diet differed only in that they were fed a prepared formula without iron in the first nine months of the study. Both groups were fed iron-fortified cereal in defined amounts and strained fruits and vegetables starting at the third month of life. The milk-fed infants developed microcytosis, ferropenia, and lowered hemoglobin concentration.

"It's not hard to find parents who are willing to have their infants in nutritional experiments, as long as they're assured the baby will not be harmed," says Dr. Woodruff. He tells parents the experiments are merely trying to "find the difference between good and better methods." ∎

Treating Obesity in Growing Children

Treating obese children takes time, more time than most
physicians can spare. A competent health professional can handle
certain aspects of management. With some extra study, the
office nurse might be ideal in this role. Except in severe cases,
the goal of treatment is not dramatic weight reduction. Instead
the child should grow up to his fatness, meanwhile receiving
psychologic support and learning self-control.

JOHANNA T. DWYER, D.Sc.
CAROLINE V. BLONDE, M.D.
JEAN MAYER, Ph.D., D.Sc.
Harvard University School of
Public Health, Boston

1. GENERAL STRATEGY

Unfortunately, no new or revolutionary treatment for
obesity has emerged in recent years. However, there
have been a number of developments which the practicing physician can use to manage obesity more effectively. These will be discussed in light of our experience in
studying and treating large groups of obese pediatric and
adolescent patients.

Determination of Obesity

We strongly urge the practicing physician to invest in
a skinfold calipers and to equip himself with a set of
triceps standards.[1] The first step in determining obesity
should be the triceps skinfold measurement, since no other
method is as rapid and precise. Confirmation should come
from study of the patient's growth chart and visual inspection. These aids represent substantial improvements
over more commonly used procedures based on weight
and appearance alone.

Differential Diagnosis

History—Once the presence of excessive fatness has
been established, it is necessary to determine whether it
is simple obesity or whether it is secondary to some other
pathophysiologic condition. A thorough medical history
yields many useful clues to the origin of the obesity and
may suggest other areas which need particular attention
during the physical examination. Equally important, it
gives an opportunity to elicit from the patient (or parent)

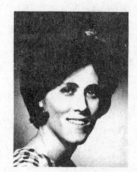

JOHANNA T. DWYER

Dr. Dwyer is assistant
professor, departments of
nutrition and of maternal and
child health, Harvard
University School of Public
Health, Boston.

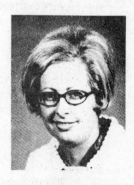

CAROLINE V. BLONDE

Dr. Blonde was formerly a
resident, department of
nutrition, Harvard University
School of Public Health, and
is now associated with the
Bureau of Nutrition, New York
State Department of Health,
Albany.

Dr. Mayer is professor of nutrition, Harvard University
School of Public Health, and consultant in nutrition,
Children's Hospital Medical Center, Boston.

attitudes toward growth in general and obesity in particular, an aspect of history taking all too often neglected. It is essential to know why medical help is being sought.

An understanding of motivation is aided by knowing the patient's social and emotional background. The sentiments of the patient and family about obesity, diet, exercise, discipline, personal appearance, and health may be crucial in determining the success or failure of a fat-reduction program. The degree of involvement of the physician and his office personnel should depend largely on what emotional support is needed and what is available in the home and school. Thus, all these questions need investigation. Time so spent pays off by enabling the physician to tailor treatment. Different approaches are indicated for an adolescent girl who seeks help on her own initiative, a prepubertal child who is brought in by her anxious mother, and an unconcerned student who is referred by a school nurse.

The discussion also often aids in identifying the few obese children with severe emotional disturbances in whom obesity treatment is usually contraindicated until the mental problems are resolved. Obviously, a patient's anxieties about obesity can be dealt with only after a careful examination. However, when a patient's presenting complaint is obesity, he needs help whether or not the physician finds him to be obese, because the patient or someone close to him is convinced that he is overfat. Often, anxious adolescents become convinced that they are obese by reading magazine articles or books on obesity. At the other extreme, a patient's parent who believes his child to be muscular or developmentally advanced may be outraged when a school physician or nurse categorizes the child as being overfat.

It is wise to inquire about the use of psychotropic drugs, particularly tranquilizers. The extremely low physical activity often associated with their use, coupled with depression or malaise and compensatory overeating or excessive sleeping, can lead to rapid weight gain. Of course, pregnancy must be ruled out in adolescent females.

Physical examination—Next a thorough physical examination should be performed, along with appropriate laboratory tests. The physician must also evaluate the patient's ability to undergo fairly vigorous exercise and dietary regulation.

Treatment

Time and responsibility for management —Few physicians can find the time to manage personally all aspects of simple obesity in a child or an adolescent. Dietary therapy and reformation of physical activity are time-consuming and not intellectually stimulating to most physicians. Moreover, such management requires a fairly high degree of sophistication and expertise in physical education and applied nutrition, particularly those areas touching on food composition, eating habits, and food preparation, subjects rarely covered in medical school.

To cope with the limitations of time, we use a system of referral for many of the aspects of treatment. The physician handles the diagnostic examination and sets overall goals for treatment. The patient is then referred to a competent health professional who is familiar with or willing to learn the management process suggested. Periodically the physician reevaluates progress and suggests modifications in the program.

Because of their special training in dealing with obesity, nutritionists or dietitians usually are the best choice for referral. When such professionals are not available, many physicians delegate to their nurses some aspects of management of obese patients. This can be a satisfactory solution *if* the nurse is willing to familiarize herself with the literature on juvenile obesity and to learn the details of managing diet and physical activity. Generally, nurses are not sufficiently trained in these matters to do a good job without further study. However, they are usually well versed in providing the psychologic support so important in treatment. The ready availability of the physician in the same office makes communication and consultation easy and is an added advantage. Several excellent sources of information are available for nurses wishing to learn more about this field.[2-8]

No matter how the responsibility is divided, the objective of treatment is essentially didactic, i.e., teaching the child to control his diet and physical activity, helping him not to forget to do so, and assuring him by frequent supportive contacts. Dialogue, by providing the necessary motivation, is just as important as advice on diet and exercise.

Anticipatory guidance—Obese children, even more than other children, need to understand the nature of growth and development and its relation to fatness. A brief presentation of this information coupled with sympathetic elicitation of and response to the child's questions on these topics is vital. The child needs to understand that the tendency to excessive fatness is a physical difference that is undesirable from the health standpoint but that is *not* a moral or physical defect about which he should feel guilty.

Self-esteem and body image are often poor in obese children. Adolescents, whether obese or nonobese, usually worry about their appearance. The physician's (or other health professional's) counsel can aid the patient to form a better, more realistic self-view. In these efforts it is useful to point out which bodily dimensions are under the patient's control and which are not. The patient needs to accept his true physical limitations and must understand how and to what extent he can control the aspects that are amenable to intervention.

Growth charts can be used to point out individual growth patterns. Full-length mirrors are useful in showing patients their good points and those that need improvement. Children approaching puberty should be apprised of the character of adolescent growth and its ramifications for fatness.[9-11] Measurement of a few bony diameters with a sliding calipers can furnish graphic evidence of relative frame size and illustrate the contribution of bones and muscles to weight. This technic is helpful in showing adolescents how people differ in body build and how these differences affect weight.

Goals and family involvement—The child needs to understand fully and agree with the goals set by the physician. Short-term goals are the basis of day-to-day motivation to continue treatment and are particularly important. They must be realistic. Except in cases of severe obesity, the long-term goal is for the child to grow up to his fatness. Dramatic immediate results are not to be expected, and this must be carefully explained to both patient and family. For many growing children a weight loss may be undesirable, and everyone concerned should understand that in a growing child, maintaining the same weight for several months or decreasing weight gain means successful fat reduction. This is a difficult point for parents to grasp, since adults measure the success of dieting by weight loss.

Height and weight should be plotted on a growth chart, and serial measurements of skinfold thickness taken. Periodically this evidence should be examined with the patient and parent and, coupled with mirror inspection, interpreted to emphasize success achieved or to point up problems still in need of solution. In addition, such a conference often uncovers anxieties and difficulties the patient might not otherwise reveal.

The ultimate goal is to inculcate habits which will bring about fat reduction and eventually maintain fatness at more normal levels. All of this must be done without compromising physical or emotional growth and development. Treatment is designed with the hope that it will allow the patient to retain (or gain) a positive as well as realistic body image and a sense of worth as a person, regardless of the outcome of therapy.

Without the understanding and support of the family, it is difficult or impossible to instill new habits in the obese child. While the mother's cooperation is vital, the father, siblings, and other family members also influence the outcome. A father may see his obese son as "husky" and fear that weight loss will mean loss of robustness, stamina and manliness. Siblings may resent the attention given to the obese child unless their support has been enlisted.

The patient also must be prepared to deal with the reactions of family and friends to his new patterns of eating and physical activity. These individuals may tempt him to abandon therapy, nag him when he forgets, chide him for making slow progress, and offer all manner of unsound advice. The adolescent particularly must be ready to cope with this "help" from peers. The opposite reaction, excessive attention given to the "brave little soldier" battling against fatness, can be equally harmful, putting so much emphasis on obesity that the more important aspects of the child's development needing praise or correction are ignored. Undue attention, negative or positive, given to the place of food and exercise in the child's life may hinder his learning to regulate these aspects *unobtrusively*.

"Quarterbacking" by patients or, more commonly, by parents who consider themselves experts on the subject complicates matters and can be exasperating. Still, it is important not to cut off honest questions about obesity in the mistaken belief that the motive is interference. Parents who do tend to intervene excessively should be told politely but firmly that this will do more harm than good, as it surely will.

Dietary advice and modification of physical activity—The plan of treatment must include explicit advice about diet and physical activity if it is to succeed. These factors will be discussed at length in part 2 of this article.

Follow-up and periodic reevaluation—Since obesity is a chronic disease and rapid cure is not to be expected, diligent follow-up observation is as important to successful treatment as a well-planned program of therapy. Initially, the office visits should be scheduled at about two week intervals. Later, when progress is good and the need for support becomes less, they may be spaced farther apart. Visits can be supplemented by telephone conferences. Adolescents especially should be encouraged to call during specific hours for answers to questions and should receive general support when necessary.

Visits, usually brief, may be conducted by the physician, nutritionist or nurse charged with handling some aspects of the case. Each visit should be regarded as a teaching session that will give the patient additional information about obesity and its control. At least every few months, the physician should personally evaluate the patient. Weight and fat changes should be explained in terms of overall growth and the effects of diet and physical activity. At various points in treatment, 24 hour records of dietary intake and physical activity are helpful for purposes of comparison in evaluating patient progress.[12]

With younger children, parental participation in interviews is useful. With a junior-high or high-school student, solo interviews may instill in the patient a greater sense of autonomy and responsibility and lessen his resistance to authority.

In conclusion, the single most important aspect of management of obesity in a child is nonjudgmental and supportive perseverance on the part of the physician. Obesity is a lifelong problem and yields only to relatively long-term corrective efforts. Thus, even if progress is not satisfactory after a month or longer, the effort should not be abandoned. Rather, patient and physician should have a frank talk about the patient's difficulties and work together to make matters better.

Part 2, to be published next month, deals with the specifics of dietary modification and regulation of physical activity.

REFERENCES

1. Seltzer CC, Mayer J: A simple criterion of obesity. Postgrad Med 38:A-101, Aug 1965
2. Mayer J: Overweight: Causes, Costs and Control. Englewood Cliffs, NJ, Prentice-Hall, 1968
3. Maddox G: The Safe and Sure Way to Reduce. New York, Random House, 1960
4. Asher P: Prevention of obesity. Dev Med Child Neurol 10:391, June 1968
5. Obesity and Health. United States Public Health Service, Department of Health, Education, and Welfare. Washington, DC, US Government Printing Office, 1965
6. Alley RA, Narduzzi JV, Robbins TJ, et al: Measuring success in reduction of obesity in childhood. Clin Pediatr 7:112, 1968
7. Wolff GH: Obesity in childhood. In Card D (Editor): Recent Advances in Pediatrics. London, J & A Churchill Ltd, 1965, p 229
8. Heald FP: Obesity. In Gardner LI (Editor): Endocrine and Genetic Diseases of Childhood. Philadelphia, WB Saunders Company, 1969
9. Dwyer J, Mayer J: Variations in physical appearance during adolescence. Postgrad Med 41:A-99, May; A-91, June 1967
10. ____: Psychological effects of variations in physical appearance during adolescence. Adolescence 3:353, Winter 1968
11. Dwyer JT, Feldman JJ, Mayer J: The social psychology of dieting. J Health Soc Behav 11:269, Dec 1970
12. Young CM: Management of the obese patient. JAMA 186:903, 1963

Most obese children actually have a calorie intake in line with or lower than that of their more active peers. Thus, exercise is the cornerstone of the regimen detailed here. Every effort must be made to increase physical activity so that the child will "spend" more calories. When dietary regulation also is needed, the calorie deficit should be only moderate, to avoid interference with growth or other harmful effects.

Treating Obesity in Growing Children

2. SPECIFIC ASPECTS: ACTIVITY AND DIET

The general strategy for treating obesity in growing children was outlined in part 1 of this article. This discussion will concentrate on the two factors in the energy balance equation which must be modified to achieve fat loss.

JOHANNA T. DWYER, D.Sc.*
CAROLINE V. BLONDE, M.D.†
JEAN MAYER, Ph.D., D.Sc.§
Harvard University School of Public Health
Boston

Modification of Physical Activity

The exercise component of clinical management is the cornerstone of our treatment of simple obesity. It can also be part of treating obesity secondary to some other condition if not clearly contraindicated. We are convinced that inactivity rather than overeating is the root of the problem in most cases.

Most patients (and many physicians) are unaware of the fact that most Americans spend more time eating than they spend in any physical activity more vigorous than strolling. If each minute spent eating or drinking were matched with a minute of vigorous physical activity, the pandemic of obesity in the United States would soon vanish. This applies in large measure to juvenile obesity as well as to obesity in adults.

In treating the obese pediatric patient, great emphasis needs to be placed on reformation of physical activity patterns. It is not necessary to make the obese child into a

sports enthusiast. Rather, the goal is to increase his physical activity to levels similar to those of nonobese children.

We have advocated special school-based physical activity programs for obese children.[1,2] If such a program is available, the child with simple obesity should be urged to join it. He should also take part in the regular gym class. Obviously, furnishing a medical ex-

*Assistant professor, departments of nutrition and of maternal and child health, Harvard University School of Public Health, Boston.

†Formerly, resident, department of nutrition, Harvard University School of Public Health; now with the Bureau of Nutrition, New York State Department of Health, Albany.

§Professor of nutrition, Harvard University School of Public Health, and consultant in nutrition, Children's Hospital Medical Center, Boston.

cuse exempting him from such classes would be counterproductive.[3] Most requests for such excuses are motivated by embarrassment with appearance and poor performance, but many stem from the child's or the parent's anxiety about overheating and fatigue after vigorous exercise. The physician can calm and re-assure child and parent if they are unduly worried. He should also try to enlist the support of the physical education teacher in

---

Many obese children are anemic; thus, foods providing vitamins and minerals such as iron should not be restricted unduly.

---

helping to develop the child's physical skills. If a special program is not available, it might be possible for the child to take extra periods of physical education.

As a general rule, obese children should be encouraged to walk as much as possible. Riding a bicycle is a good second choice. Maternal or paternal chauffeuring should be strenuously discouraged, and use of public transportation kept to a minimum. One way to encourage a child to walk rather than ride a bus is to have the parent continue to give him bus money but allow him to keep it for other things.

The physician may want to prescribe sub-stitution therapy for the obese child who watches television excessively. An approach which usually works is to tell the child that for every hour of television viewing he must log an hour of outdoor activity on his feet. The same strategy may be effective in re-ducing the time spent in another sedentary activity, telephone conversations.

With thought, it is relatively easy to in-crease physical activity during the week. Planning for weekends takes more ingenuity,

since most American families are more seden-tary at these times. The physician should suggest participation in community recrea-tional programs involving physical activity, especially those conducted on weekends. Parents should be encouraged to plan family outings which incorporate exercise. Summer vacations need especially careful planning. Camping and other activities stressing physi-cal exercise are useful. If the parents' means permit, the very obese child may benefit from attendance at one of the special camps for obese children.[4]

In general, patients know little about the energy expenditure involved in physical ac-tivity. The child or parent needs instruction in the relative benefits of various physical activities in terms of energy output and ap-propriateness. He also needs to be reminded that energy expenditure varies with the speed and duration of participation.

The obese child needs to be encouraged to "spend" calories all through the day—not to stand when he can move, not to ride when he can walk, not to take elevators when he can use the stairs—and to develop compe-tence in active pastimes such as hiking, swim-ming, tennis and skiing. Planning such a change in life-style often is easier if the pa-tient keeps an activity diary which the phy-sician can examine with him.

Counseling sessions should also touch on explanations for physical changes likely to accompany vigorous physical activities, changes which the patient may never have experienced and may consider symptomatic of illness.

Every conference or interview should in-clude assessment and discussion of the child's progress in the direction of greater physical activity. Encouragement by the physician is essential, since obese children usually do not undertake these efforts on their own volition and may not recognize how vital they are in treatment.

A step-up in physical activity amounting

to an hour of fairly vigorous exercise a day will increase calorie output by only about 150 to 200 cal. Thus, without a change in calorie intake, a dramatic drop in fatness or in weight is not to be expected. An increase in energy output of 200 cal a day achieves a loss of about a half pound of fat per week. In six months or a year this obviously can accomplish a great deal. Moreover, greater physical activity improves fitness, does not seem to increase food intake, and sometimes improves the psychologic outlook. When an adequate school program is available and obesity is only moderate, participation in the school program coupled with a regimen of increased general physical activity may be enough to control obesity.

Modification of Diet

When obesity is severe or a good school program is unavailable, adjunctive dietary modifications may be necessary. However, dieting is not an either-or proposition. It works best when combined with a program of increased physical activity.

Theory—Few of the plans and methods advanced for the dietary treatment of obesity are suitable for children.[5,6] The theoretical basis of all sound reducing diets is a restriction of calorie intake sufficient to deplete fat reserves or prevent their further accumulation. The problems inherent in applying this to obesity in a growing child are several. Growth and maturation depend in great part on energy intake, and calorie restriction must not be so severe as to retard or halt growth. Calorie restriction of a degree acceptable for mature adults may adversely affect linear growth in children.[7] Growth of nonfat tissue in the body requires adequate amounts of *all* nutrients. The lower the calorie intake, the greater is the chance that intake of protein, vitamins and minerals will be inadequate, unless food selection is carefully supervised or vitamin-mineral supplements are taken regularly.

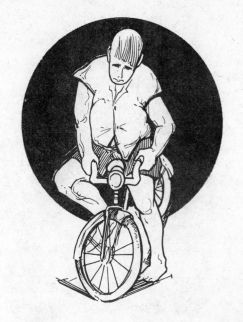

Contrary to popular opinion, most obese children have a calorie intake in line with or even lower than that of their more active peers of normal fatness status.[5,8,9] However, their intake is certainly more than is needed for the level of energy output. If intake is sharply reduced, the child will be forced to eat not only less food than his peers but in most cases different foods if he is to get adequate nutrients. This may impose a real hardship, for children tend to interpret such prescriptions as punishment rather than treatment. In particular, care must be taken not to restrict unduly the foods providing vitamins and minerals such as iron; many obese children are already anemic. In addition, diets must be planned, and periodically revised, to take into account variations in energy requirements for physical activity and growth needs during childhood and adolescence.

Adjustment of normal diet to create a moderate calorie deficit—The aforementioned factors and our clinical experience have led us to advocate relatively mild calorie restriction in treating obesity in children.

There is no workable standard low-calorie diet sheet for obese children. If the physician feels that dietary restrictions are in order, there is only one approach which will assure a fairly high probability of adherence by the patient, and that is for someone to spend the time necessary to adapt and tailor the reduced intake to the patient's existing dietary

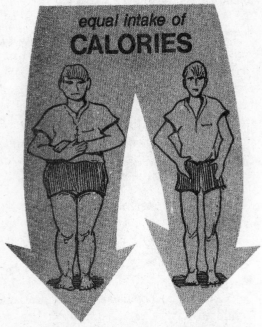

equal intake of
CALORIES

habits, making as few changes as possible.

The usual way to do this is to take a dietary history or have the patient or parent record food intake, listing the kind and amount of food eaten at each meal and snack for several days. It should be remembered that patterns on weekdays and weekends often vary considerably. This history or food diary gives the physician a quantitative estimate of calorie intake as well as of the quality of the diet with respect to nutrients and may indicate "extras" that could be eliminated to achieve a calorie deficit without compromising nutritional adequacy.

Regardless of the calorie level, if the patient can reduce his intake by 200 cal a day, he can be expected to lose the equivalent of a half pound of fat a week over the long run. The patient may be happier with a prescribed 275 cal deficit daily during the week and his previous pattern on weekends, a satisfactory alternative unless he is unable to restrain himself and eats excessively on Saturdays and Sundays.

More severe calorie deficits, e.g., 500 cal per day, should rarely be considered for children, since growth may be compromised. Even if growth is unaffected, the radical changes in eating habits are usually unacceptable and may set the obese child apart from his peers and family whenever he eats.

Even if a child follows his diet to the letter, those concerned should not expect a regular weekly loss of a half pound of weight. Accretion of bone or lean body mass may add tissue weight even as fat is lost, and shifts in water balance may mask decreases in fat content. However, within about a month, dietary modifications alone should achieve objective evidence of progress (a few pounds of weight loss). In the meantime, someone must keep in close touch with the patient, perhaps by weekly telephone conversations or even more frequent consultations in the first few weeks. These will help to clarify the inevitable questions and to motivate the patient and furnish psychologic support.

The two major strategies in paring down the regular diet are restriction and substitution. Some high-calorie foods such as candy and cookies usually have to be restricted, but they should almost never be eliminated entirely. In addition to being popular, these items have emotional significance as "reward" foods. Appealing low-calorie foods should be substituted. Substitution strategy may also be applied with benefit by using skim milk instead of whole milk. While the principles of dietary planning are relatively straightforward, it takes a high level of skill and knowledge of food composition and preparation, as well as knowledge of the individual child's personality, to produce an acceptable diet.

The rationale of the dietary recommendations should be clearly stated to the child and, if he is young, to his parents. Progress should be planned on the growth chart. Food buying practices, cooking methods, and eating habits often may need modification. Perhaps more important are any necessary changes in parental attitudes toward the child's eating. The child should not be expected to go hungry while others are eating snacks but should be given low-calorie snacks that he enjoys. Neither should he be expected to always practice moderation if the parents do not do half as well with their own dieting efforts.

When dealing with adolescent patients, we find it useful to have them start their diaries of food intake and physical activity during the first month of treatment. We provide them with food composition tables so that they can calculate their calorie intake retrospectively and see where they have deviated from the plan of treatment. We also find it useful to have them jot down in the diaries situations which give them difficulty in following their diets. These are discussed, and possible solutions suggested. All these technics are useful in that they draw the patient into the treatment, motivate him to solve his own dietary problems, and serve as an informal tutorial course on the dietary therapy of obesity.

With younger children, similar methods used with parent and child together encourage adherence to the plan. Under no circumstances do we exclude a child from discussions; we believe that this can create an unhealthy attitude of dietary dependence on the parent, when in fact it is the child who must eventually control his own diet. The child excluded from the conferences also may come to distrust the physician. Any necessary private discussions with the parent should be conducted during a separate visit or by telephone.

Summary

This discussion details a method for the clinical management of juvenile obesity using the health care team approach. The regimen emphasizes increased physical activity, carefully individualized and moderate dietary restrictions, frequent patient contacts, and patient education conducted by allied health professionals working in conjunction with the physician.

REFERENCES

1. Dwyer JT, Feldman JJ, Mayer J: The social psychology of dieting. J Health Soc Behav 11:269, Dec 1970
2. Seltzer CC, Mayer J: An effective weight control program in a public school system. Am J Public Health 60:679, 1970
3. Grossman MS: Medical aspects of the obese child in athletics. Md State Med J 18:83, Aug 1969
4. Spargo J, Heald F, Peckos PS: Adolescent obesity. Nutr Today, Dec 1966
5. Goldbloom RB: The special problem of obesity in childhood. Mod Treat 4:1146, Nov 1967
6. Crawford JD, Haessler HA: Obesity—a pediatric viewpoint. Med Times 95:1269, Dec 1967
7. Parízková J, Vamberová M: Body composition as a criterion of the suitability of reducing regimens in obese children. Dev Med Child Neurol 9:202, 1967
8. Huenemann RL: Consideration of adolescent obesity as a public health problem. Public Health Rep 83:491, 1968
9. Corbin CB, Pletcher P: Diet and physical activity patterns of obese and nonobese elementary school children. Res Q Am Assoc Health Phys Educ 39: 922, Dec 1968

Food (or energy) intake is obviously an important consideration in the causation and treatment of obesity. Its relationship to obesity is, in fact, unequivocal in view of thermodynamic principles. Recognition that it is not the only factor to consider, or necessarily the main one in individual cases, has come about through a better understanding of the complex nature of obesity and its multiple etiology, as discussed by Mayer.[1] Because food and exercise are subject to environmental control, however, they must receive prime consideration in the prevention and treatment of obesity and in attempts to explain the cause.

This report examines some of the studies of food intake of noninstitutionalized obese and nonobese adolescents and some of the implications for weight control. It also includes any findings on activity (energy expenditure) of the subjects studied.

Studies of Food Intake and Activity

Among the first of these studies was that of Johnson, Burke and Mayer,[2] who compared diets, physical maturation, and activity of 28 obese and 28 nonobese high school girls of similar height, age, and school grade. The average daily caloric intake of the obese girls was lower in most cases than that of the nonobese girls (table 1). Conversely, the control subjects spent more hours per week in active pursuits.

Stefanik, Heald and Mayer[3] in a later study compared the food intake and activity of 14 boys 13 to 15 years of

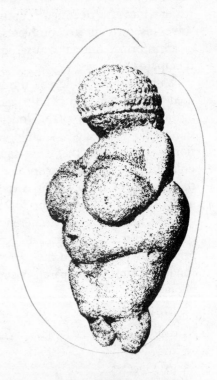

Food Habits of Obese and Nonobese Adolescents

Eating practices of adolescents, both obese and nonobese, vary highly among groups and individuals. Data representative of the United States as a whole are not yet available. Evidence indicates that the obese may eat fewer calories than the nonobese and that their nutrient intakes are likely to be lower. The overall physical activity level of adolescents appears to be low.

RUTH L. HUENEMANN, D.Sc.
University of California
School of Public Health, Berkeley

Table 1.   Average Daily Caloric Intake of Obese and Nonobese Girls*

Group	Number	Calories per Day				
		>2,500	2,500-2,000	<2,000	Mean Intake	S.D.
Obese	28	3	6	19	1,965	453
Control	28	15	10	3	2,706	633

*From Johnson, Burke and Mayer.[2]

age classified as obese on the basis of skinfold measurements and 14 nonobese controls of the same age, height and maturation. Differences in activity of these two groups were less apparent, but the authors noted that the "degree of participation in the active exercises was observed to be generally less for the obese than for the nonobese."

Bullen, Reed and Mayer[4] used motion pictures to compare the activity of obese and nonobese girls in a summer camp and found that the obese girls were far less active in three different sports.

During the four years from 1961 to 1965, my associates and I[5-9] conducted a longitudinal study of gross body composition and body conformation and their association with food and activity in about 950 high school students. Once each year we obtained anthropometric determinations of gross body composition and conformation, using the "body envelope" method of Behnke,[10] and gathered questionnaire data dealing with subjects' views on food, activity, and body size and shape. A subsample of 122 subjects kept detailed seven-day records of food intake and activity four times during the last two years of the study.

The subjects were classified according to the percentage of body fat as lean, somewhat lean, average, somewhat obese, and obese. The seven-day records showed lower mean caloric intakes for the somewhat obese and obese boys and girls than for those in the other categories (table 2). Individual intakes

varied widely, however, and standard deviations were large.

In terms of calories per kilogram of total body weight, the intakes were highest for lean and somewhat lean girls and average boys. On the basis of lean body weight, the somewhat lean girls and average boys ate the most. These same groups ate the most calories per decimeter of height.

The activity records showed clearly that the group as a whole was markedly inactive (figure 1), a finding contrary to the popular idea that the teen years are active ones. No large difference between the obese teen-agers and their nonobese peers emerged.

Each of six obese twelfth-grade girls was matched as closely as possible in terms of height and lean body weight with an average and a lean twelfth-grade girl of the same age, and their seven-day records were compared (table 3). Only in two of these groupings did there appear to be a consistent trend for the obese girls to consume more calories than their leaner peers. These findings are to be viewed as indicative of trends rather than as representative of a mean intake for the entire period. In fact, the significance of individual mean intakes based on periodic sampling may rightly be questioned. While each seven-day record appeared to be valid for the period covered, there is no assurance that it was representative of a significantly longer period.

Eppright, Coons and Jebe[11] in a study of 1200 Iowa schoolchildren found that those

Table 2. Mean Caloric and Nutrient Intakes Reported by 122 High School Students

	Mean Intake Total Group	Mean Intake by Subgroup				
		Lean	Somewhat Lean	Average	Somewhat Obese	Obese
Boys	51	9	7	19	9	7
Calories*	2,846	2,675	2,923	3,088	2,621	2,624
S.D.	116	550	1,273	566	779	817
Protein (gm)	116	107	130	126	101	107
S.D.	37.5	25.7	62.2	26.6	38.4	31.4
Calcium (mg)	1,338	1,201	1,538	1,461	1,193	1,162
S.D.	575.0	427.9	914.5	475.5	571.9	436.8
Iron (mg)	14.3	12.9	15.7	15.6	12.7	13.2
S.D.	4.86	3.28	8.91	3.62	4.02	3.66
Vitamin A (IU)	7,493	7,247	9,546	8,236	5,889	5,800
S.D.	7,007	6,671	13,774	5,139	3,394	4,583
Thiamine (mg)	1.38	1.24	1.47	1.52	1.27	1.23
S.D.	0.492	0.339	0.852	0.377	0.437	0.418
Riboflavin (mg)	2.53	2.35	2.85	2.76	2.21	2.25
S.D.	0.980	0.838	1.561	0.782	0.881	0.809
Ascorbic acid (mg)	94	78	125	107	86	62
S.D.	83.2	47.7	162.3	72.3	47.8	48.7
Girls	71	14	10	31	10	6
Calories*	1,972	2,112	2,102	1,981	1,771	1,717
S.D.	486	431	356	496	444	618
Protein (gm)	76	85	83	74	70	68
S.D.	19.9	19.2	17.5	19.1	17.7	23.6
Calcium (mg)	917	1,021	1,022	887	845	784
S.D.	400.9	415.5	305.0	388.2	406.7	492.6
Iron (mg)	9.6	10.1	10.4	9.4	9.1	9.0
S.D.	2.30	2.15	2.15	2.24	1.97	3.13
Vitamin A (IU)	5,637	4,896	6,785	5,552	5,465	6,175
S.D.	4,022	2,228	4,942	4,098	4,417	4,334
Thiamine (mg)	0.91	1.0	0.98	0.88	0.89	0.85
S.D.	0.251	0.222	0.277	0.223	0.275	0.311
Riboflavin (mg)	1.72	1.86	1.88	1.66	1.63	1.56
S.D.	0.601	0.601	0.46	0.589	0.591	0.795
Ascorbic acid (mg)	82	89	99	75	82	69
S.D.	48.2	42.9	51.6	47.3	50.7	47.6

*Calorie levels are lower than those obtained in previous studies, in part because of methodology. Intake assessments based on diet history tend to be higher than those based on diet record. These data represent seven-day records made four times during the study period.

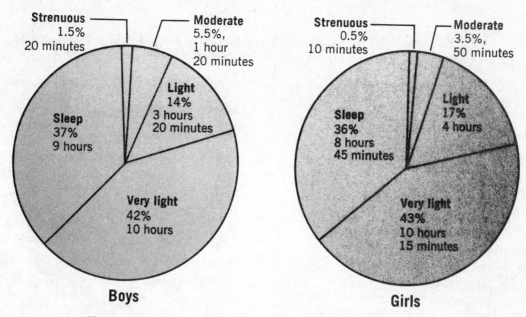

Figure 1. Time spent daily by teen-agers in different classes of activity.

Boys pie chart labels:
Strenuous 1.5% 20 minutes
Moderate 5.5%, 1 hour 20 minutes
Light 14% 3 hours 20 minutes
Sleep 37% 9 hours
Very light 42% 10 hours
Boys

Girls pie chart labels:
Strenuous 0.5% 10 minutes
Moderate 3.5%, 50 minutes
Light 17% 4 hours
Sleep 36% 8 hours 45 minutes
Very light 43% 10 hours 15 minutes
Girls

rated in channel A_3 or higher on the Wetzel grid tended to consume fewer calories than their leaner peers, according to seven-day dietary records.

Hodges and Krehl[12] in a preliminary report on the nutritional status of Iowa teen-agers noted what appears to be a conflicting finding, stating that "body weight . . . corresponded with higher caloric intake." They did not discuss obesity as such, nor did they specify the method used to obtain dietary data.

It is evident from these and other studies that most obese teen-agers tend to eat like "normal" teen-agers and that many eat less. The problem, therefore, is not eating too much. Rather it is eating too much for the energy expended. The generally low level of physical activity that appears to be characteristic of American youth and the consequent low caloric need make increased activity an essential part of the regimens for obesity prevention and control. At these low levels of energy expenditure, basal or metabolic requirements become a large proportion of the total energy need. Over time, even the customary ± 20 percent considered as a "normal" basal metabolic rate could make a significant difference in the energy balance.

As long ago as 1932, Wait and Roberts[13]

in a careful study of the total energy needs of girls 10 to 16 years of age found that energy requirements peaked just before puberty and then dropped rapidly because of the basal metabolic component. More recently Heald et al.[14] confirmed this observation.

The shortcomings inherent in studies of noninstitutionalized individuals must be noted. In the studies cited, methods of assessing overt activity were of necessity crude, periods of observation were understandably short, and behavior may have been influenced by the fact that it was observed. Errors doubtless occurred in some of the estimates.

Nutrient Intake

In our study the intakes of protein, calcium, iron, thiamine and riboflavin tended to parallel caloric intake (table 2). As is usual in dietary studies, intakes of vitamins A and C tended to be more independent of caloric intake. Mean intakes of most nutrients studied approximated the levels recommended at that time,[15] exceptions being calcium, iron and thiamine intakes by girls. Judging from the detailed dietary records, however, some individual subjects tended to have consistently low intakes. Roughly half of the girls ate less than two-thirds of the recom-

Table 3. Average Daily Caloric Intakes of Lean, Average and Obese Girls of Same Age and Matched for Height and Lean Body Weight

Subject	Weight (kilograms)		Height (decimeters)		Lean Body Weight (kilograms)		Four Seven-Day Periods (calories per day)			
	Grade 9	Grade 12	Grade 9	Grade 12	Grade 9	Grade 12	1	2	3	4
A.F. (lean)	51.40	52.10	16.20	16.42	47.49	50.06	2,304	2,304	1,570	2,580
B.C. (average)	57.90	56.80	16.20	16.12	48.18	49.01	2,434	2,679	2,841	2,857
D.C. (obese)	67.60	74.80	15.76	15.88	46.48	50.57	724	1,201	1,335	1,332
B.A. (lean)	46.50	45.70	16.66	16.92	46.50	47.97	1,860	1,528	2,003	2,246
C.B. (average)	56.90	58.70	15.94	15.98	47.01	47.00	2,271	1,571	2,135	2,021
E.D. (obese)	63.90	63.40	16.10	16.21	46.62	45.76	1,620	1,854	1,657	1,701
F.K. (lean)	36.90	41.80	15.58	15.90	36.84	42.74	1,607	2,139	1,766	1,744
G.H. (average)	56.80	51.90	15.92	15.98	45.70	43.84	2,094	2,083	1,517	1,758
I.J. (obese)	68.20	65.50	15.82	15.92	47.57	43.42	2,075	1,853	2,408	1,853
K.F. (lean)	48.20	48.10	15.97	16.03	44.00	45.00	2,732	2,248	1,920	2,517
H.G. (average)	58.20	57.00	15.78	16.15	45.12	47.23	2,221	1,581	1,889	1,955
J.I. (obese)	60.80	64.70	15.68	15.97	44.52	46.71	1,450	1,175	1,165	1,993
L.P. (lean)	45.50	50.05	16.07	16.20	44.72	47.71	2,948	2,778	2,900	1,659
M.N. (average)	53.70	54.80	15.54	15.68	44.18	44.27	1,918	1,162	1,055	1,731
O.P. (obese)	56.70	64.10	15.32	15.40	40.82	45.23	1,546	810	811	2,009
P.L. (lean)	60.50	54.70	17.17	17.44	56.37	58.02	1,900	2,356	2,196	1,917
O.N. (average)	63.10	65.30	17.30	17.43	53.03	55.72	2,079	2,123	2,476	1,750
P.R. (obese)	74.70	81.70	17.16	17.30	54.78	57.78	3,216	2,680	2,498	2,247

mended amounts of calcium and iron, and one-sixth had low intakes of vitamins A and C. Of the boys, roughly one-third reported eating less than two-thirds of the recommended amounts of vitamin C, one-fifth had low calcium intakes, and about one-tenth had low intakes of iron and thiamine. Except for a few whose caloric intake was low, the girls had a protein intake in line with or higher than the recommended level.

Eppright and Roderuck[16] reported lower nutrient intakes, along with lower calorie levels, for overweight girls than for girls of medium build. These observers also found that almost half of the girls had low iron intakes (less than two-thirds of the recommended amounts[17]) and that the intakes of calcium and ascorbic acid by both girls and boys were commonly low. Studies made of adolescents in eight states during the period from 1947 to 1958 and summarized by Morgan[18] showed intakes of the same nutrients to be low. It will be interesting to compare these findings with those of the recently completed National Nutrition Survey.

Thus, it would seem that a sizable proportion of teen-agers need improved diets. Identification of these individuals and of their particular nutrient needs are important health responsibilities. Particular attention must be given to weight-control diets, because low-calorie diets, unless carefully planned, tend to be low in nutrients. Since weight control is likely to be a lifelong problem,[19] adolescent calorie watchers need to learn nutrient and caloric values.

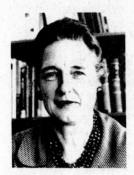

RUTH L. HUENEMANN

Dr. Huenemann is professor
of public health nutrition,
University of California School
of Public Health, Berkeley.

Eating Patterns

It is a common observation that the eating practices of teen-agers are sometimes unusual or even bizarre. A number of studies have tried to determine the extent to which this is true. A common finding already noted[7] is the wide variance of intakes among both the obese and the lean. In our study the lowest individual daily variation noted in the seven-day records was 635 calories and the highest was 4700. For about one-third of the entire group studied, the number of meals and snacks eaten each day and the times when they were eaten varied greatly.[9] Eating frequency averaged four or five times per day. Many irregular eaters did not even mention food in the context of meals. The obese tended to eat less frequently than the subjects in the other groups and omitted breakfast and lunch more often.

Snacking was common to all body-fat classes and ethnic and socioeconomic groups in our study population and generally augmented the protein, mineral and vitamin intake. Hodges and Krehl[12] stated that milk, ice cream, and cheese contributed substantially to the snack items eaten by the subjects in their study. It would seem that snacks are part of our way of life and should be accepted as such, since they can and often do make a significant nutrient contribution.

Hinton and associates[20] made the interesting psychosocial observation that emotional stability, conformity, adjustment to reality, and good family relationships, as determined by the Minnesota Counseling Inventory, appeared to characterize the girls with the better food habits. They found also that the overweight tended to have diets poorer in quality. Knowledge of nutrition was related positively to good food practices.

Vegetarian diets recently have become popular in some parts of the United States. Erhardt[21] has discussed some of these diets and suggested educational approaches suited to this "counterculture." She has found that stressing variety in the diet is one practical way to promote dietary adequacy.

Another interesting development in the area of food practices is the finding of Schachter that obese individuals tend to respond readily to environmental stimuli toward eating while the lean are more likely to obey physiologic urgings to eat.[22]

Adolescents' Views on Food and Body Composition

The popular impression that teen-agers are keenly interested in the size and shape of their developing bodies has been documented by a number of studies.[5, 23, 24] Obesity is commonly a matter of concern. In our study group, for example, the proportion of girls who considered themselves fat increased from 43 percent in the ninth grade to 56 percent in the twelfth grade. Only 22 percent of the boys at all grade levels described themselves as fat. These figures contrast sharply with the 12 percent of boys and 16 percent of girls who were classed as "obese" by more objective measures (grade 11, age about 16½ years). About twice as many boys considered themselves too thin as thought themselves too fat. These findings indicate a need for helping teen-agers to develop a better concept of ideal weight and body composition.

Does their concern motivate teen-agers to action? Dwyer, Feldman and Mayer[24] in a study of 416 twelfth-grade girls found that

60 percent had been on reducing diets at some time and 30 percent were on diets at the time of interview. In our study, about 50 percent of the boys and 65 percent of the girls in the ninth grade were trying either to gain or to lose weight. The results of these efforts were far from satisfactory. For example, we learned from the questionnaires that 69 of 91 girls who dieted to lose weight in the ninth grade were still trying to lose weight in grade 12.

It was also evident from the questionnaires that the social aspects of food (companionship, freedom, environment at mealtime) were quite as important as the food itself to girls of all ages and to both boys and girls in grades 11 and 12. Unfortunately, these aspects are not always given consideration by persons responsible for teen-age diets.

Summary

From the data available, it is evident that adolescent eating practices vary highly among groups and individuals and over time for the same groups and individuals. This appears to be true for the obese and the nonobese. Evidence also indicates that the obese may eat fewer calories than the nonobese and that their nutrient intakes are therefore likely to be lower. Snacking is common and appears to make a worthwhile nutrient contribution. Low physical activity apparently is characteristic of adolescence.

Because teen-agers vary greatly in their eating practices, treatment of every weight-control patient should begin with an assessment of his problem.

REFERENCES

1. Mayer J: Obesity: Etiology and pathogenesis. Postgrad Med 25:623, 1959
2. Johnson ML, Burke BS, Mayer J: Relative importance of inactivity and overeating in energy balance of obese high school girls. Am J Clin Nutr 4:37, 1956
3. Stefanik PA, Heald FP, Mayer J: Caloric intake in relation to energy output of obese and nonobese adolescent boys. Am J Clin Nutr 7:55, 1959
4. Bullen BA, Reed RB, Mayer J: Physical activity of obese and nonobese adolescent girls appraised by motion picture sampling. Am J Clin Nutr 14:211, 1964
5. Huenemann RL, Shapiro LR, Hampton MC, et al: A longitudinal study of gross body composition and body conformation and their association with food and activity in a teen-age population. Views of teen-age subjects on body conformation, food and activity. Am J Clin Nutr 18:325, 1966
6. Hampton MC, Huenemann RL, Shapiro LR, et al: A longitudinal study of gross body composition and body conformation and their association with food and activity in a teen-age population. Anthropometric evaluation of body build. Am J Clin Nutr 19:422, 1966
7. ____: Caloric and nutrient intakes of teen-agers. J Am Diet Assoc 50:385, 1967
8. Huenemann RL, Shapiro LR, Hampton MC, et al: Teen-agers' activities and attitudes toward activity. J Am Diet Assoc 51:433, 1967
9. ____: Food and eating practices of teen-agers. J Am Diet Assoc 53:17, 1968
10. Behnke AR: Quantitative assessment of body build. J Appl Physiol 16:960, 1961
11. Eppright ES, Coons I, Jebe E: Very heavy and obese school children in Iowa. J Home Econ 48:168, 1956
12. Hodges RE, Krehl WA: Nutritional status of teen-agers in Iowa. Am J Clin Nutr 17:200, 1965
13. Wait B, Roberts LJ: Studies in the food requirement of adolescent girls. I. The energy intake of well-nourished girls 10 to 16 years of age. J Am Diet Assoc 8:209, 1932
14. Heald FP, Daugela M, Brunschuyler P: Physiology of adolescence. N Engl J Med 268:192; 243; 299; 361, 1963
15. Food and Nutrition Board, National Academy of Sciences, National Research Council: Recommended Dietary Allowances, 6th Revised Edition. Publication 1146, 1964
16. Eppright ES, Roderuck C: Diet and nutritional status of Iowa school children. Am J Public Health 45:464, 1955
17. Food and Nutrition Board, National Academy of Sciences, National Research Council: Recommended Dietary Allowances, Revised. Publication 302, 1953
18. Morgan AF: Nutritional status U.S.A. Calif Agr Exp Sta Bull, 1959, p 769
19. Abraham S, Collins G, Nordsieck M: Relationship of childhood weight status to morbidity in adults. Public Health Rep 86:273, 1971
20. Hinton MA, Eppright ES, Chadderdon H, et al: Eating behavior and dietary intake of girls 12 to 14 years old. J Am Diet Assoc 43:223, 1963
21. Erhardt D: Nutrition education for the "now" generation. J Nutr Educ 2:135, 1971
22. Nisbett RE: Determinants of food intake in obesity. Science 159:1254, 1968
23. Deisher RW, Mills CA: The adolescent looks at his health and medical care. Am J Public Health 53:1928, 1963
24. Dwyer JT, Feldman JJ, Mayer J: Adolescent dieters: Who are they? Physical characteristics, attitudes and dieting practices of adolescent girls. Am J Clin Nutr 20:1045, 1967

Obesity in Adolescence

Frank Carrera, III, M.D.

■ The demand for psychiatric, diagnostic and therapeutic services for adolescents has increased markedly over the past few years and projective studies indicate that these clinical demands will continue to increase. It becomes imperative, then, as recommended by the APA Committee on Psychiatry of Childhood and Adolescence, for child psychiatrists and general psychiatrists to enhance their effectiveness in dealing with the emotional problems of adolescents. How to best approach the evaluation of that group of adolescents who present with obesity is the purpose of this paper.

Obesity among adolescents seems to be a significant clinical problem. Garell's (1965) survey of 55 hospitals in the United States and Canada revealed that 16 of these hospitals had special adolescent clinics. He reported that the majority of adolescents who were seen in these adolescent specialty clinics were seen because of obesity and that in ten of these clinics obesity was listed as the most frequent diagnosis. That obesity in teenagers often interferes with healthy personality development is agreed upon by anyone who has even had a casual relationship with an obese adolescent. Yet it seems that child psychiatry clinics see relatively few of these patients. If they are referred, they frequently get lost in clinic waiting lists. This is probably due to two main factors: the pressures for child psychiatrists to focus on other more urgent and dramatic psychiatric problems, and general clinical experience that obese adolescents are "poor therapy" candidates.

This lack of exposure to obese adolescents on the part of psychiatrists seems to result

too often in a stilted "classical" view of the problem—namely, that all obese adolescents are "fixated in the oral stage of psychosexual development." It seems relevant, then, in view of the prevalence of the problem, to review the recent literature on obesity which seems pertinent to a more up-to-date understanding of obesity in adolescence, and which seems to define the role of the clinical psychiatrist in his work with obese adolescents.

The old basic physiological mechanism in obesity of a positive energy balance still remains basic today in our physiologic understanding of how obesity begins and how it is maintained, i.e., obesity results when a person takes in more calories than he uses. But Bruch (1958) noted that this basic physiological mechanism is part of the symptomatology and *not* an explanation of the underlying factors.

Over the past 25 years the scientific view of childhood and adolescent obesity has changed from one of "it's all soma" or "it's all psyche" to the more reasonable present view that there are multiple etiological factors and probably a variety of obesities. Factors reported in the literature which influence food intake and energy output include social, economic, somatic, emotional and genetic elements. Relevant to the focus of this paper is that this present view of obesity points to the necessity for the psychiatric clinician to focus on the individuality of each obese adolescent he sees and that any tendency to lump all obese adolescents in one formulation frame would put him at least ten years behind the times.

Although some of the literature on the natural history of obesity in children and adolescents points to this imperative to individualize our diagnostics with obese teenagers, the literature in most other instances still reflects the old view of lumping all obesity together. This fact seems to define for the

---

Dr. Carrera is Assistant Professor of Psychiatry, College of Medicine, University of Florida, Gainesville.

Presented at the Regional Meeting of the Academy of Psychosomatic Medicine, March 17, 1967, Gainesville, Florida.

present the primary role of the clinical psychiatrist with obese adolescents as one of researcher, data-gatherer, or "fact-finder." I would propose, then, the following checklist to be used during the history taking and physical examination of every obese adolescent. The data obtained would serve as either an important bit of information for a differential diagnosis of obesity based on our present knowledge, or would provide more research data to clarify certain issues which are still unresolved.

1. *Birth Weight*. Heald (1966) recently reported conflicting evidences regarding whether obese children or adolescents are obese at birth or tend to have higher birth weights. It is likely that this contradictory evidence reflects the heterogeneity of the obese adolescent population. The importance of obtaining birth weight information on each obese adolescent becomes clearer when we consider the next bit of data on our checklist.

2. *Age of Onset*. The age of onset of the obesity would seem to be a particular valuable factor in differential diagnosis. Unfortunately, very few studies have focused on the age of onset specifically. However, Forbes (1964), studying body compositional changes in adolescents, was able to identify two types of obesity when the lean body mass was determined by the whole body potassium counter. Interestingly, and of great significance, is the fact that each of these two types of obesity had *different* ages of onset. Forbes' work suggested the following *two* types: Type I, characterized by an increase in lean body mass, a tendency to tallness, advanced bone age and a history of overweight since infancy; Type II, showing no increase in lean body mass, normal growth characteristics, with obesity developing during the childhood years. This data suggests that a number of sub-groups exist among obese youngsters and that they are obese for different reasons. In view of this, the necessity for intensive and detailed history taking concerning life events and the general family milieu during the time of age of onset becomes critical. It would help differentiate between a Type I juvenile obesity as Forbes suggests in which psychological factors may play a relatively minor role, and a Type II juvenile obesity whose ages of onset may be largely determined by psychological and social factors.

3. *Rates of Growth and Maturation*. Wolff (1955), in reviewing the literature on the relationship between obesity and height in children, reported that obese children tended to be above average height during childhood but Lloyd, et al. (1961), reported that the ultimate height of these same youngsters after puberty was significantly below the standard height. They then concluded that what appeared to be accelerated growth during childhood seemed to be really accelerated maturation. These cases would seem to correspond to Forbes' Type I of childhood obesity characterized in part by a tendency to tallness and advanced bone age.

It would appear that the heterogeneity of obese children again explains the contradictory reports in the literature concerning the age of menarche in obese girls. This should be part of the checklist in adolescent girls' evaluations in order to provide more data concerning this event's relationship to obesity and particularly to possibly differentiate sub-types of obesity. It would seem reasonable to assume that for this Forbes I type of accelerated maturer, the psychological effects of menarche may play a lesser role in obesity than in Forbes Type II where the psychological factors centering around the menarche may play a more prominent role.

4. *Body Types*. A recent study by Seltzer and Mayer (1964), of the somatotypes and anthropomorphic measurements of obese adolescent girls and non-obese teen-age girls, demonstrated that obesity did not occur in all the varieties of physical types but occurred in greater frequency in some physical types than in others. Their findings suggest that a prime prerequisite for the development of obesity in the group of adolescent girls they studied is a physique with at least a moderate degree of endomorphy under normal conditions, the endomorphy predisposing to the laying on of additional quantities of fat *unless* excessive activity, disease or voluntary weight control supervened (Mayer 1966). The theoretical implication of this last statement which makes detailed history-taking important is that the phenotypic expression of a somatotypic genotype may be altered by environmental factors such as the eating patterns in the family, by psychological factors or even by other constitutional factors such as differences in temperament as Stella Chess proposes, par-

ticularly the individual child's characteristic activity level which she has reported persists from infancy into childhood. This study of the role of somatotype on the subsequent development of obesity in adolescent girls may best be considered as another evidence of the significance of constitutional and genetic factors in the predisposition to obesity.

5. *Family Occurrence.* It has been reported many times that a high incidence of obesity in one or both parents is associated with the development of obesity in the child. Familial occurrence of obesity in some of these studies ranges from 69 per cent to 80 per cent of obese children having had one or both parents obese. In the diagnostic evaluation of obese adolescents it would be important to inquire not only into the incidence of obesity in the family but also to obtain a detailed history of family life in order to better evaluate the relative weight of genetic factors versus other factors such as family eating patterns and family attitudes toward food which are operating, interacting, and possibly modifying the genetic components.

6. *Activity versus Inactivity.* Evaluation of the obese adolescent's usual activity level pattern is of major importance in the differentiation of obesity at the very basic physiological level as regards the concept of positive energy balance. Two broad types of obesity in childhood and adolescence appear in relation to this physiological factor: a) the hyperphagic type of obesity in which the imbalance seems primarily due to excesses at the intake end of this equation, and b) the low activity type in which the imbalance in the equation seems to be on the output side of the equation.

It is difficult to estimate from the literature the relative frequency of the hyperphagic type in childhood and adolescence since these are reported primarily in the form of clinical case studies. A recent survey however, conducted by the Department of Agriculture of adolescents in Iowa (1961), reported that only 4 per cent of the obese teenagers they studied ate excessively. By comparison, the low activity type of obesity in children and adolescents has been reported many times. Bruch (1940) had called attention to the relative inactivity of many obese children back in 1940. More recently Johnson, et al. (1956), compared 28 obese high school girls with 28 aver-age weight controls and reported that the obese girls ate *less* than the controls but that they spent ⅔ less time than the controls in active pursuits. Stefanik, et al. (1959), also called attention to this phenomenon in 14 obese adolescent males as compared to 14 non-obese controls. Bullen (1964), using photographic time-motion studies, also noted that the average obese adolescent girl expends far less energy than the average non-obese adolescent girl during scheduled exercise periods. This inactivity which seems to be most characteristic of obese adolescents may be the result of physiological factors, constitutional factors, or psychological factors. A possible physiological explanation for the inactivity comes from the study of Wenzel, et al. (1962), in which he noted that among an outpatient clinic adolescent population the obese youngsters had a significantly lower serum iron (with normal serum hemoglobin) than did non-anemic, non-obese controls. Whether this lower serum iron represents a physiological basis for the inactivity or whether it is a concomitant effect of the inactivity is yet to be determined.

For another possible interpretation of this relative inactivity we could refer again to Chess' work concerning individual differences in temperament, particularly activity level present at birth and stable through early childhood. Since these subjects in Chess' follow-up study have not yet reached adolescence no definite connection between these two factors can yet be made. The psychodynamic factors in personality formation which may tend to result in a child's "passive" solution to stresses and which may also directly affect activity level is another factor which must be investigated.

It appears important from these studies that urging these obese teenagers to increase their activity level seems imperative in treatment. How to best promote this change from their usual low activity level will depend to a large extent on the specific etiology and/or attached meanings of this behavioral manifestation in the individual, pointing to the need for individualized, focused interviewing.

7. *Hunger and Satiety Sensations.* In evaluating obese teen-age patients, we can no longer fall back comfortably on old and familiar formulations derived from classical

drive theories—formulations which assumed that all obesity was the result of an increased drive to eat and in which the concept of orality was used across the board in understanding obesity and the obese individual.

Research data does not support this exclusive reliance on these classical drive theory assumptions.

Brobeck (1955) demonstrated in his animal studies that there were two anatomically and behaviorally distinct centers in the hypothalamus, the one regulating feeding and the other regulating satiety. Since then it has been repeatedly demonstrated in animals that experimental obesity due to overeating may result from either increased activity of the feeding centers with an apparent increase in the "hunger drive" *or* from decreased activity of the satiety centers with a resultant disorder in satiety mechanisms. The point to be emphasized is that the one behavior, overeating, may result from two quite different mechanisms at hypothalamic cellular level. Stunkard (1958) and others have reported many instances in obese adult humans in which the associated overeating seemed to be due to disturbances in satiety mechanisms. Monello (1965) recently reported that in adolescent obesity, satiety abnormalities also occur and, in fact, suggested that they were more prevalent than differences in hunger among the obese adolescent girls he studied. In comparing hunger and satiety sensation differences between obese teenage girls and non-obese controls, his preliminary findings indicate that at the end of the meal, obese subjects require more conscious will power to stop eating even though they report more frequently than controls that they experience sensations of discomfort at the end of the meal, particularly distention and nausea. Increased hunger and disturbed satiety appear to be two different mechanisms leading to overeating and obesity. As clinicians we should identify the type of overeating in the individual patient.

8. *Psychological Factors.* That we cannot approach an obese adolescent with preconceived fixed psychodynamic notions is reflected in Glucksman's (1966) recent statement that "all we do know is that obese patients do not have a common personality structure and their obesity does not have a common meaning." However, the necessity of a close look at psychological-emotional factors is evident from common clinical knowledge that among obese adolescents there seems to be a clear connection between heightened emotional tension, eating behavior and weight gain.

Bullen, et al. (1963), reported that in the 115 obese adolescent girls he studied, the majority stated they went on eating sprees when they felt bad, tense, nervous, depressed, bored, worried, etc. However, the underlying mechanisms mediating this relationship of psychic tension to increased eating have not been elucidated although it is likely that learned patterning in reaction to stress plays a part.

Along these lines, Bruch (1961) reformulated her thinking about the etiology of certain cases of obesity in terms of learning theory when she noted that these patients seemed to suffer from an inability to identify their bodily sensations correctly, in particular, hunger and satiation. Her hypothesis is that the deficit occurred as the result of disturbed early mother-child interactions in which the mother would repeatedly feed the child inappropriately when he was *not* hungry—so that the child never learned the significance of the stimuli arising from his own stomach.

Bruch describes other psychological characteristics of this type of "I can't feel when I'm hungry" obese adolescent which indicate a more general lack of a sense of basic trust in their own feelings and in their ability to identify their own feelings. Her patients in this group frequently made statements like "Mother always knew how I felt when I myself did not know it." She concluded that a prerequisite for psychotherapy with any lasting success with obese adolescents of this type must focus on this conceptual disturbance—the therapy directed to helping the patient express how he feels right now rather than an approach that suggests in any way how he *should* feel.

It would seem then, that on the basis of our present information, among certain obese adolescents psychological factors leading to overeating may form distinct sub-groups which are themselves distinct from those where psychological factors lead to inactivity, and distinct from those where psychological factors lead to disturbances in satiety mechanisms.

A quantity of research showing the interplay between emotions and obesity has been done. When we look to the literature for the prevalance of significant emotional illness occurring in obese adolescents we find a broad range reported. Tolstrup (1953) reported evidence of significant psychological disturbances in 45 per cent of 40 obese children and adolescents studied. Bruch (1955) reported that 40 per cent of her obese child patients who were seen in 20 year follow-up remained obese *and* significantly emotionally maladjusted. Ostergaard (1954) reports an even higher prevalence of 81 per cent emotional disorders among 58 obese children. These studies underscore the danger of underestimating the significant psychological disorders associated with obesity in children and adolescents. A recent study by Monello and Mayer (1963) of 100 adolescent obese girls compared to 65 non-obese controls focuses our attention on how serious the psychological maladjustments tend to be in the adolescent obese female group specifically. The results of 3 projective tests administered to these girls revealed that the obese teenage girls showed personality characteristics strikingly similar to the traits of ethnic and racial minorities: a) "obsessive concern" with heightened sensitivity and preoccupation with status, b) "passivity," withdrawal, sense of isolation and feeling of rejection by their peers; c) "acceptance of dominant values" and considered obesity—and therefore their own bodies—as undesirable and somewhat harmful.

Stunkard and Mendelson (1961) had reported similar minority group personality characteristics in a small percentage of obese adult female subjects who also demonstrated distorted body images.

The three prerequisites for the development of a distorted body image in his study were: the person developed obesity in childhood or adolescence; the person suffers from an emotional disturbance; the obesity was the focus of derogatory parental concern.

Since these serious psychological problems all carried into adulthood, it appears that prolonged intensive psychotherapy is indicated for those obese adolescents who demonstrate these particular characteristics.

Bruch (1958) reported on her more than twenty-year study on obese children whose onset occurred before puberty. She found a high correlation between a congenial family environment and a favorable outcome, i.e., with normal weight (15%) or a stable condition of overweight (20%) and good social adjustment in adulthood. These were the families in which there was little anxious or punitive overconcern with the child's obesity.

In contrast, the follow-up on children whose families showed unrelenting preoccupation with the excess weight and were resistant to reassurance revealed an unfavorable outcome in adulthood, with progressive obesity (40%) or artificially maintained thinness (25%) and poor total adjustment including psychotic reactions in those cases where the psychopathological relationships with the parents had been intense.

Bruch (1958) concluded that of practical importance for making fairly accurate predictions concerning the outcome of childhood obesity and for purposes of determining when intensive psychiatric intervention is definitely indicated, that the diagnostic evaluation should include the following data: a) an evaluation of the emotional status of the child, b) the child's interraction with the family and in particular the parental attitudes toward the child's obesity, c) an evaluation of the weight curve including its stability or fluctuations.

The need to study the family in depth is also reflected in the results of the following study. Disturbances in family relationships were the rule in those obese adolescent girls in Bullen's, et al. (1963) study who were having rather total adjustment difficulties of adolescence. The family relationship disturbances were characterized by a low degree of sociability among family members and by much fighting between siblings. The poorly adjusted obese adolescent girl was more dependent on the family, had conflict over separating from the mother, had a great concern with sex on the fantasy level with a concomitant lack of heterosexual interests at the reality level. They typically used passive responses like avoidance or denial, seemingly clinging to the status quo, and gave evidence of disturbances in body image. It would seem imperative then that these psychological symptoms be part of our checklist, since their presence indicates the need for psychotherapeutic intervention which must involve the parents whenever unhealthy emotional parental attitudes concerning the child's obesity are present.

We will proceed now to some other factors for our checklist which specifically have to do with treatment of the obese adolescent. It is clear from the literature that the best treatment for obesity and the accompanying emotional disturbance in 65 per cent of the cases is preventive work done early. Mullins (1958) reported that one third of the adult patients in his survey had a history of juvenile obesity. He also reported that juvenile obesity persisting into adult life tended to be more severe and more difficult to treat than adult onset obesity (Heald, 1966). It is obvious that the "he'll grow out of his fatness" attitude is false and that much of our previous treatment for the obesities of childhood and adolescence has been less than adequate.

Stunkard and Mendelson (1961) attempt to explain why treatment has been inadequate when neurosis and obesity become intertwined. They propose that obesity is the only condition which involves at the same time a disturbance in body image and a disturbance in impulse control. The simultaneous occurrence of both these problems makes each more malignant. In view of this, if we consider the naturally occurring body image changes and impulse control disturbance of the average adolescent state, it is no wonder that the treatment of obesity in adolescents is difficult and that preventive intervention is imperative.

The presence of deviant eating patterns seem to affect prognosis and treatment methods. Stunkard reports that binge eaters are usually able to carry out a weight reduction program successfully. However, obese patients with the night eating syndrome (morning anorexia, evening hyperphagia and insomnia) are poor therapeutic candidates and frequently become highly emotionally disturbed when they try to diet. Although the obese person with the night-eating syndrome seems fairly resistive to psychotherapy, recent evidence shows that they do respond to anti-depressants. Further experimental studies of the "night-eater" may eventually elucidate

more clearly the relationship and mechanisms between depression and eating behavior. This night-eating syndrome has not been reported in adolescents, but since its presence has prognostic significance, it should be included in the checklist.

In summary, it seems evident that the use of this proposed checklist with obese adolescents would provide the kinds of data essential for the clinical child psychiatrist's important role as researcher-fact finder in his attempt to differentially diagnose the obesities in adolescence. In addition, such a checklist does appear to provide the clinician also with information useful in determining the indications for psychotherapy.

For the child psychiatrist evaluating obese teenagers the presence of the following factors obtained from the patient interview and from history-taking would seem, from the literature review, to constitute indications for psychotherapy: evidence of a pathological child-parent relationship; hypercritical family attitudes regarding the patient's obesity; seemingly "compulsive" eating in response to a variety of moods and affects; eating seems to be the only comfort in an otherwise sterile existence; the withdrawal—"hate my body"—increased sensitivity triad is present and seems to represent a way of life; eating patterns include the night-eating syndrome at which time psychotherapy plus anti-depressant drug therapy would be indicated; evidence that the teenager is not attuned to his own feelings including his own bodily sensations of hunger and satiety; a lack of closeness among family members with coexistent difficulties for the obese teenager in separating from the family; an attitude of preference for the status quo reflected in delayed involvement with the tasks of adolescence: developing a sense of individual identity, a growing independence and self reliance, involvement in heterosexual orientation, and participation and involvement in the peer culture.

In conclusion, the data reviewed would tend to suggest that there are multiple etiological factors involved in adolescent obesity and that they may be different for obese persons with early age of onset than for those with late onset. In other words, obesity is a symptom which is the end-product of many syndromes:

1. The environment plays a permissive role in that food has to be available in sufficient quantity for a constitutional predisposition to manifest itself.

2. Inactivity seems to be an important factor in the development and maintenance of adolescent obesity.

3. Overeating may be a primary mechanism and may be due to psychological or physiological factors.

4. Inactivity may be the primary mechanism involved and it, too, may be due primarily to physiological and/or psychological factors.

5. It would appear that abnormalities in satiety might be more prevalent in adolescent obesity than difference in hunger.

6. It appears dangerous to underestimate the psychological effects of the pressures of society on the obese child and on the obese female adolescent in particular.

7. It would appear that a psychotherapeutic orientation aimed at proving the psychogenicity of obesity in a teenager is contraindicated, ineffective and out-dated.

It is obvious that in order to understand obesity in adolescence and to understand the obese teenager himself the child psychiatrist must approach him in the highly individualized fashion that has traditionally characterized the child psychiatrist's view of the child and his family. But in addition to this helping approach, it is obvious because of the confusion and lack of information in the literature that one of the primary roles of the clinical child psychiatrist with the obese teenager is that of fact finder and researcher.

BIBLIOGRAPHY

Bruch, H. and Touraine, G.: Obesity in Childhood: V. The Family Frame of Obese Children. *Psychom. Med.*, II, No. 2:141, Apr. 1940.

Juel-Nielson, N.: On Psychogenic Obesity in Children. II. *Acta Paediat.*, 42:133, Mar. 1953.

Quaade, F.: On Psychogenic Obesity in Children. III. *Acta Paediat.*, 42:191, May 1953.

Tolstrup, K.: On Psychogenic Obesity in Children. IV. *Acta Paediat.*, 42:289, July 1953.

Ostergaard, L.: On Psychogenic Obesity in Childhood. V. *Acta Paediat.*, 43:507, Nov. 1954.

Bruch, H.: Obesity. *Ped. Clin. N. Amer.*, 613, Aug. 1958.

Apley, J. and MacKeith, R.: *The Child and His Symptoms: A Psychomatic Approach.* Blackwell, Oxford 1961.

Stunkard, A.: *Research on a Disease: Strategies in the Study of Obesity.* Roseler R. and Greenfield, N. S., Ed., Physiological Correlates of Psychological Disorder, Chap. 11, Univ. of Wis. Press, 1961.

Stunkard, A. and Mendelson, M.: Body Image of Obese Persons. *J. Amer. Dietet. Ass.*, 38:328, 1961.

Bullen, B. A., Monello, L. F., Cohen, H. and Mayer, J.: Attitudes Towards Physical Activity, Food and Family in Obese and Non-Obese Adolescent Girls. *Amer. J. Clin. Nutr.*, 12, No. 1:1, Jan. 1963.

Masterson, J. F., Jr., Tucker, K. and Berk, G.: Psychopathology of Adolescence IV: Clinical and Dynamic Characteristics. *Amer. J. Psychiat.*, 120, No. 4:357, Oct. 1963.

Shirley, Hale F.: *Pediatric Psychiatry.* Harvard Univ. Press, 1963.

Coddington, R. D., Sours, J. A. and Bruck, H.: Electrogastrographic Findings Associated with Affective Changes. *Amer. J. Psychiat.*, 121, No. 1:41, July 1964.

Offer, D., Sabshin, M. and Marcus, D.: Clinical Evaluation of Normal Adolescents. *Amer. J. Psychiat.*, 121, No. 9:864, Mar. 1965.

Garell, D. C.: Adolescent Medicine. *Amer. J. Dis. Child*, 109:314, April 1965.

Silverstone, J. T. and Solomon, T.: Psychiatric and Somatic Factors in the Treatment of Obesity. *J. Psychosomatic Res.*, 9:249, 1965.

Mayer, J.: Inactivity as a Major Factor in Adolescent Obesity. *Ann N. Y. Acad Sci.*, 131, Art. 1:502, Oct. 1965.

Monello, L. F., Seltzer, C. C. and Mayer, J.: Hunger and Satiety Sensations in Men, Women, Boys and Girls: A Preliminary Report. *Ann. N. Y. Acad. Sci.*, 131, Art. 1:593, Oct. 1965.

Christakis, G., Sajecki, S., Hillman, R. W., Miller, E., Blumenthal, S. and Archer, M.: Effect of a Combined Nutrition Education and Physical Fitness Program on the Weight Status of Obese High School Boys. *Fed. Proc.*, 25, No. 1:15, Jan.-Feb. 1966.

Heald, F. P.: Natural History and Physiological Basis of Adolescent Obesity. *Fed. Proc.*, 25, No. 1:1, Jan.-Feb. 1966.

Huenemann, R. L., Hampton, M. C., Shapiro, L. R. and Behnke, A. R.: Adolescent Food Practices Associated with Obesity. *Fed. Proc.*, 25, No. 1:4, Jan.-Feb. 1966.

Mayer, J.: Physical Activity and Anthropometric Measurements of Obese Adolescents. *Fed. Proc.*, 25, No. 1:11, Jan.-Feb. 1966.

Seltzer, C. C. and Mayer, J.: A Review of Genetic and Constitutional Factors in Human Obesity. *Ann. N. Y. Acad. Sci.*, 131, Art. 2:688, Feb. 1966.

Masterson, J. F., Jr. and Washburne, A.: The Symptomatic Adolescent: Psychiatric Illness or Adolescent Turmoil? *Amer. J. Psychiat.*, 122, No. 11:1240, May 1966.

Lorber, J.: Obesity in Childhood: A Controlled Trial of Anorectic Drugs. *Arch. Dis. Child.*, 41, No. 217:309, Jun, 1966.

London, A. M. and Schreiber, E. D.: A Controlled Study of the Effect of Group Discussions and an Anorexiant in Outpatient Treatment of Obesity. *Ann. Int. Med.*, 65:81, July 1966.

Kessler, J.: *Psychopathology of Childhood.* Prentice-Hall, 1966.

A. P. A. Committee on Psychiatry of Childhood and Adolescence: Position Statement on Psychiatry of Adolescence. *Amer. J. Psychiat.*, 123, No. 8:1031, Feb. 1967.

College of Medicine
University of Florida
Gainesville, Florida

Health is proudly related to one's way of thinking, to one's sense of values, and physical well being. . . . The chemistry of the body is not independent of the condition of the inner man. . . .

Diet, physical exercise, are (both) important, but so are the capacity to praise, the power to revere, self-discipline and the taste of transcendence, qualities of being human.

Sickness, while primarily a problem of pathology, is a crisis of the total person. . . . At a moment when one's very living is called into question, the secretions of character, commitments of the heart, the modes of answering the ultimate question of what it means to be alive are of supreme importance. . . .

Sickness ought to make us humble. In a world where recklessness and presumption are the style of living, and callousness dominates relationships . . . sickness is a reminder of our own neediness . . . an opportunity for the cynic to come upon the greatness of compassion.

—RABBI A. J. HESCHEL, "The Patient as a Person." Read before the 113th Annual Convention of The A.M.A., San Francisco, June 21, 1964.

Obesity in childhood is relatively common and usually is not a cause of major concern to either the child or his parents. Obesity in the teens is equally if not more common and frequently gives rise to intense concern on the part of the teen-ager and the parents, particularly when the teen-ager is a girl. Because this common abnormality of body composition occurs during a period of rapid biologic and psychologic changes, the impact of adolescence on the therapeutic approach to human obesity merits considerable thought and discussion. In order to understand better the rationale for treating obesity in adolescence, it is well to keep in mind characteristics of normal growth and development during this period.

In biologic terms the teen-age growth period is characterized by rapid linear growth, almost a doubling of body weight in boys, and a lesser weight gain in girls. During the peak year of growth, the weight gains vary from 5 to 10 kg. Therefore, one of the characteristics of adolescence is rapid weight gain. This fact becomes important in attempting to differentiate normal weight gain and excessive gain in adipose tissue in an obese adolescent.

The increments in body composition are generalized in that all organs and compartments of the body participate in the growth spurt, with two exceptions. Lymphoid tissue decreases in absolute amounts in both boys and girls, and body fat decreases in amount in boys. Specifically, growth of adipose tissue organ obviously begins in utero and continues during infancy and child-

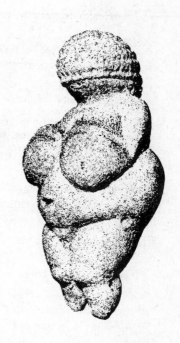

Treatment of Obesity in Adolescence

Rapid weight gain is normal in adolescence. In an obese teen-ager, triceps skinfold measurements help in determining how much of this weight is excess fat. Conventional weight-control methods are notable for their lack of success in this age group. Severe caloric restriction, besides being inherently risky from a metabolic standpoint and inadvisable for psychologic reasons, is a wholly unworkable approach. Cutting food portions to prevent further fat gain is realistic.

FELIX P. HEALD, M.D.
University of Maryland School of Medicine
Baltimore

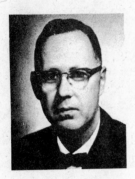

FELIX P. HEALD

Dr. Heald is professor of
pediatrics and head, division
of adolescent medicine,
University of Maryland School
of Medicine, Baltimore.

hood. In infancy girls have somewhat more fat than boys; this difference persists throughout growth. During late childhood and early adolescence, the amount of body fat increases at a similar rate in boys and in girls. In early adolescence, however, deposition of fat in girls accelerates, whereas during mid-adolescence boys actually become leaner and have less body fat. These changes in body fat appear to be physiologic and under hormonal rather than environmental control. Therefore, one could predict that a girl who is obese during childhood or as she enters adolescence will become fatter during adolescence. Over the years I have consistently observed this prediction to be valid, although supporting data are not available.

Accompanying these dramatic biologic changes are profound increases in caloric and protein requirements. It has been clearly shown that the increase in body mass brings an almost parallel increase in caloric requirements for both boys and girls. A large sex difference in requirements of calories and nutrients, related probably to size and possibly to activity, becomes apparent in mid-adolescence, boys requiring about 1000 more calories per day.

Among the complex psychologic aspects of adolescence, one of particular importance in a discussion of obesity in teen-agers is their intense concern about their bodies. Their body image appears to solidify during adolescence. Any distortions of body image de-

veloped in adolescence will persist into adult life and may create difficult and disturbing psychologic functioning. In treating obese teen-agers, it is well to keep in mind the possibility of distorted body image.

Some items of the clinical history deserve emphasis. One should be careful to note whether or not there is a strong family history of obesity. A greater likelihood of obesity in children of obese than of nonobese parents appears to be borne out clinically. The time of onset of the obesity is another important item. In my experience, obesity developing very early in life is likely to persist into adolescence and be more severe and resistant to treatment than obesity developing later.

Any psychologic factors associated with early-onset obesity are less obvious and may be secondary rather than primary. On the other hand, a youngster whose parents and siblings are thin and who becomes obese during childhood is more likely to have a clear-cut psychologically determined hyperphagia underlying his obesity than is a youngster who has a strong family history of obesity and becomes obese earlier in life. The obese youngster in a thin family often will have disturbances in other aspects of his life.

It is useful to inquire into the dietary habits of the obese teen-ager and the family. Although the physician can do this on a screening basis to elicit evidence of abnormal and bizarre eating habits, often a nutritional survey is best done by an experienced nutritionist. If there is true hyperphagia, causes such as neurotic, familial or ethnic food patterns should be explored.

Eating patterns should be organized so that these young people have enough to eat on a regular basis. Sufficient protein during rapid growth is particularly important. Excesses of carbohydrates should be avoided.

Two points concerning the physical examination should be stressed. (1) Whenever possible, particularly in mild to moderate obesity, triceps skinfold should be measured for diagnostic and follow-up purposes. The standards published by Mayer will suffice as guides. Frequent use of the skinfold calipers will be helpful later in determining whether weight loss is fat or other body components. (2) Because of the amount of adipose tissue in the arm, blood pressure elevation may be recorded and a diagnosis of hypertension entertained. It has been clearly shown that these are falsely high readings; direct arterial measures of blood pressure in such individuals are normal.

In the differential diagnosis, a normal rate of growth rules out endocrine deficiency. Hormonal deficiency states such as hypothyroidism in children or adolescents are always associated with slow or absent growth. Occasionally, Cushing's disease is a factor in the differential diagnosis, but again cessation of growth is characteristic in this disease, along with other phenomena such as virilization, hypertension, and glucose intolerance. In my experience, endocrine disturbances rarely become a cause for concern in obese adolescents.

Before considering the subject of caloric restriction in growing teen-agers, it would be well to review some features of their energy metabolism. A pound (454 gm) of adipose tissue is about 87 percent fat and would yield 395 gm of fat with a caloric value (9.5 calories per gram) of approximately 3,770 calories. It has been shown that carbohydrates and proteins retain three or more parts of water when stored in the body, whereas anhydrous fat is stored almost water-free. A gram of storage fat has a caloric value of about 9, while a gram of glycogen or protein in storage provides about 1 calorie due to obligatory dilution with water. For every pound of fat catabolized, a pound of weight will be lost. For every pound of protein or of carbohydrate catabolized (caloric value 1,850), there will be a weight loss of 4 lb due to the concurrent water loss.

It is clear that weight loss will be more rapid with a lesser caloric deficit if only protein and carbohydrate are preferentially metabolized. It is equally clear that this is undesirable, particularly during a period of growth; the aim is to reduce the amount of body fat, not lean body mass. Ideally, if protein and carbohydrate equilibrium were attained, all catabolic energy would be derived from fat stores. Unfortunately, there is little evidence to suggest that this goal is fully attainable even in adults.

In view of the unusual intensity of anabolism during adolescence, unusual sensitivity to caloric restriction is predictable. One study showed that even a moderate caloric restriction could not keep obese adolescents in positive nitrogen balance. Negative nitrogen balance of any appreciable duration can and does limit growth. Achieving the ideal of reduction of body fat without loss of lean body mass may be difficult or impossible during growth, particularly during pubescence.

In early to middle adolescence, when growth is still intense, sharp restriction of calories may result in relatively large losses of lean body mass. For this reason and because of the metabolic complications inherent in nutrient restriction and the psychologic stress generated by food withdrawal, severe caloric restriction for long periods is not recommended for children or adolescents. Only a restriction of clear excesses through portion control is advisable.

The child or adolescent being treated for obesity needs reinforcement from the family in fostering a positive attitude toward food restriction. These youngsters can eat what the rest of the family eats, but less of it. Deprivation of foods especially enjoyed by these young people, such as pie and pizza, should be avoided. These foods can be allowed, *in small portions*.

An additional factor in weight control is physical activity. While some investigators feel that this is a key variable in the production of excessive adipose tissue, to date no one has presented convincing evidence that at the practical level of patient care an increase in exercise alone will adequately control weight. Although exercise should be encouraged, obvious success in weight control can come only through long-term moderate reduction of caloric intake.

A rigid approach to weight control based on parental enforcement of diet and exercise must be studiously avoided. Particularly in early adolescence, parental coercion may so intensify the normally strained parent-teen-ager relationship that the product of a well-intentioned therapeutic endeavor is a sullen, angry, rebellious youngster who is gaining rather than losing weight. No matter how hard they try, adults cannot control teen-agers' food intake; food is easily obtainable outside the home.

A thorough explanation of the complexities of weight control in early and middle adolescence is frequently helpful. The teen-ager and the parents must understand that all adolescents gain weight while growing. Increased adipose tissue is the problem and must be separated from normal weight gain. As I mentioned earlier, gains or losses in adipose tissue can be monitored by measuring the triceps skinfold.

Neither the literature nor my experience gives any evidence to suggest that conventional methods for weight control are successful in teen-agers. It is therefore counterproductive to raise the parents' expectations and expose the teen-ager to the risk of failure by expecting large amounts of fat to be lost. This just does not happen. A more realistic goal in early to middle adolescence is the prevention of further gains in body fat. This can be done by moderation in eating habits. In late adolescence, particularly in girls who are well motivated, weight loss will occur and usually without supervision.

It is quite clear that when teen-agers are well motivated, they are able to withstand the biologic and psychologic stresses of food deprivation for the long periods required for weight loss. These factors should be emphasized to the parents so that they may understand the complexities of weight reduction in early to middle adolescence and will not be too demanding. Some parents, when made aware of the complexities of the problem, express relief that it is "really not our fault."

Psychotherapy is never indicated for simple obesity. There must be other indications of disturbance such as poor schoolwork or disordered peer, sibling or parent relationships to justify this form of treatment. An evaluation directed toward eliciting such disturbance should give particular attention to the teen-ager's self-concept. One might ask the following questions: What do you see when you look in the mirror? How do you think you look to other people? What do you think of your body? If a teen-ager views his or her body in a consistently disparaging way, one must explore further to determine the depth of the psychologic difficulties. A physician experienced in the care of adolescents can do this easily, or specific psychologic evaluation can be requested. Psychotherapy may be indicated but not because of obesity.

The treatment of obesity is less than satisfying to a physician who expects loss of large amounts of weight as the primary goal. If the goal is more realistic, such as preventing further increments of fat and being supportive in a situation difficult for both teen-ager and parents, then much can be achieved with these unhappy youngsters. Only with a better understanding of the pathogenesis of obesity can a more rational and successful approach be devised for treating the obese teen-ager.

REFERENCES

1. Heald F: Obesity in children and adolescents. In Gardner LI (Editor): Endocrine and Genetic Diseases of Childhood. Philadelphia, WB Saunders Company, 1969, pp 979-990
2. Mendelson M: Psychological aspects of obesity. Med Clin North Am 48:1373, 1964
3. Stunkard AJ: Eating patterns and obesity. Psychiatr Q 33:284, 1959
4. Wishnofsky M: Caloric equivalents of gained or lost weight. Am J Clin Nutr 6:542, 1958

WEIGHT CONTROL IN A COLLEGE SITUATION

As a group, college students display intelligence, candor, and a keen awareness of the importance of weight control. These and other attributes favor success in treatment of obesity, but special pressures and circumstances of college life tend to offset them. Even though success as measured in the usual terms is not outstanding, early failure often turns into success when situations change and students are able to put to good use what they learned through nutritional counseling.

POSTGRADUATE MEDICINE

CHARLOTTE M. YOUNG, Ph.D.
Cornell University
Graduate School of Nutrition
Ithaca, New York

At Cornell University the medical nutritionist is an integral part of the staff of the student health service and clinic. Some of my experience in that capacity, now spanning 30 years, has been described in previous publications.[1-3] The nutritionist keeps regular hours at the clinic and sees students by appointment. Some of the students seek this help voluntarily, while others are referred by clinic physicians, other members of the university community, or family physicians.

By access to the medical record of each patient, the nutritionist is informed of pertinent items in the medical history. A careful dietary history is taken, and advice is given on the basis of the referring physician's recommendations, the nutritionist's insights gained from the interview, and the student's eating habits. Individual plans suitable to the immediate situation are drawn up during the conference, and if needed, appointments for subsequent visits are scheduled. The nutritionist's comments are incorporated in the student's medical record; in addition a more detailed card file is kept by the nutritionist. In a 12 year period the nutritionist saw nearly 1400 students for a total of more than 5600 visits.[3] All types of nutritional problems may be referred, but the majority are related to weight control, with a ratio of overweight to underweight of three to one.

The university's medical clinic is the logical place for nutrition counseling, a service which is part of total health care. Physicians who are interested in both mental and physical health are available for mutual interchange. The nutritionist has expertise to offer and can give the physician more time to devote to other purposes.

To work successfully with the weight problems of students, the nutritionist must be armed not only with knowledge of nutritive and caloric values of food and of energy needs and expenditures of individuals under various circumstances but also with a thorough orientation to the many nonmetabolic, nonnutritional uses of food. In addition to obtaining a good diet history, she focuses much of her attention on finding out what food means to the individual being treated and why he tends to eat too much or too little. She tries to help the overweight patient to gain insight as to why he eats excessively and to find better means of satisfying his needs.

Weight problems I have observed tend to fall into three broad groups. For some students the difficulty is just poor eating habits readily correctable by a little discreet counseling, but a fair proportion of weight problems have some emotional basis. The nutritionist can help many of these students develop insight, can give them emotional

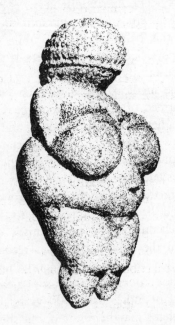

support, and can help them cope with the actual hunger phase. The third group is made up of problems so deep-seated that without competent psychiatric help the nutritionist can be of little service.

The nutritionist also is responsible for other phases of the nutrition program for students. Dietary studies[4,5] have been carried out to build a representative picture of the actual eating habits on campus and relative adequacy of nutrient intake. These have aided persons concerned with health counseling as well as those responsible for student feeding. Currently, because of the rapidly changing student culture, there is need for new studies of eating. In the past a "special diet table" was operated as a service to students with difficult dietary problems and as an educational tool in helping students to adjust to new diets. Now the same facilities are used as an ambulatory metabolic unit for nutritional research.[6,7] With increasing student interest in nutrition, a course in general nutrition without prerequisites is being given.

Particular Characteristics of College Students

College students are curious mixtures of adolescent and adult. At one moment the student wants to be grown up and independent and to make his own decisions. In the next, he wants someone to be very supportive and to let him be dependent without calling attention to his dependence. The person counseling him needs to be flexible and able to meet the student where he is at the moment. The student wants acceptance, honest and straightforward answers to questions, and freedom to accept or reject advice.

There are particular joys in working with college students. They are intelligent, intellectually honest, and quite frank to admit what they have done, and they engage in less fantasy than do adolescents or older persons seen in similar clinical situations.[8] They have the intelligence and often the means to achieve the desired goals if they can be motivated to make the effort, and they are at a stage of life when correction of a weight problem can be extremely important, and they realize this. Often they feel strongly the cultural condemnation of obesity, yet threats of the future penalties of obesity mean little. They are likely to seek help with marginal weight problems and thus are easier to help. With a nutritionist available, the student may have help if he wishes; frequent follow-up observation is possible if desired.

Problems of Weight Control Peculiar to College

College life requires many adjustments. While some of these favor weight control, others are unfavorable in this respect. Emotional pressures are involved in the maturing process, in seeking acceptance by peers, and in the need to achieve in a highly competitive setting. Social patterns involve eating, drinking, and many irregularities. For many students, physical activity decreases. Long hours of night study are punctuated by snacking as

---

To be realistic, the student must come to regard weight control as a lifetime proposition.

---

a means of diversion; students are likely to skip breakfast and instead eat high-calorie snacks between classes.

In the past, when campus housing arrangements included compulsory meal contracts, obese students found it difficult to select a low-calorie diet and were tempted to eat what had been paid for, with frequent weight gain. Now this temptation may be gone, but other problems have taken its place. There appears to be much more eating of high-calorie snack items by students in their rooms and less eating of meat, fruit and vegetables. With no scheduled lunch hour, there is a tendency for classes to continue through

lunchtime; consequently, students tend to consume most food in a few evening hours.

Many graduate students suddenly find their weight increasing as their physical activity is limited by hours of study. Students from other countries present a special problem stemming from the easy availability of food and the development of fondness for new high-calorie sweets, along with other problems of adjustment. Still another special problem is unusual fat distribution in non-obese students. Therapeutic efforts in the latter cases should concentrate on bringing understanding to the patient, guarding against vain attempts to get rid of the offending fat deposits by excessive dieting, and helping him to learn to live with the situation.

Some Points in Treatment

An attitude of acceptance of and interest in the obese student as he is, without criticism or judgment, is very important. Initially, emphasis is on establishing rapport and listening without censure. Once the student is comfortable with the nutritionist, the interview can proceed quite rapidly. One looks not at weight alone but at relative fatness, and there is a chance to give an understanding of body composition, body build, and differences between overfatness and overweight.

One tries to determine the underlying cause of the obesity. Often in a directed conversation the student will be able to identify and verbalize the root of his problem toward which treatment should be directed. The nutritionist should make it quite clear that the problem is the patient's to solve and that the therapist will do all that she can to help by sharing information, by helping him with adjustments, and by support. He should not be misled to believe that the task will be easy. The only person who believes that weight reduction is easy is one who has never had to reduce. The satisfactions from weight loss must be greater than the momentary satisfactions from eating or from inactivity and withdrawal. To be realistic, the student must come to view weight control as a lifetime proposition; the sooner he is able to start, the better.

Role of Nutritionist

The nutritionist serves several roles in her contacts with the patient. After assessing his situation, she gives much of her initial effort toward helping him to find a motivation meaningful to him for undertaking weight reduction, for this is a prime factor in success. Among motivations of particular value are personal attractiveness and the weight requirement of a job. The motivation must be the student's. The nutritionist helps him to examine his problem and to see where the best adjustments can be made. Each person is an individual; there can be no stereotype handling. It is best to be nonthreatening, because threats mean little and may increase anxiety, thereby causing the student to remove himself from the anxiety-producing situation and hence therapy.

The nutritionist adjusts dietary suggestions to meet the patient's current patterns insofar as is consistent with therapeutic purpose. The tendency is to stress the choice of a nutritionally adequate diet, with limitation of foods highest in calories. The emphasis is on moderation, not abstinence, how to accommodate a reduction regimen to the stresses of college life, and the place of treats on special occasions. The high-protein, moderate-fat, somewhat low-carbohydrate type of diet often lends itself well to these purposes because it is high in satiety value, can easily be adequate in all nutrients, is easy to obtain almost anywhere, and fits the way of eating preferred by many persons.

The nutritionist gives the student someone to answer to until he makes adjustments and can see self-motivating results. Amount of weight loss is less important than continuous progress in the right direction. In

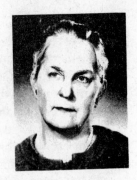

CHARLOTTE M. YOUNG

Dr. Young is professor of medical nutrition, Cornell University Graduate School of Nutrition, Ithaca, New York.

many cases weekly visits initially are helpful. The nutritionist also can prepare the student for the reactions of family and friends and can encourage him to have clothes adjusted as weight is lost in order to avoid the traps of excessive self-satisfaction and of self-pity.

Probability of Success

In my experience, success in weight-reduction programs for college students is not much greater than the success achieved with other groups in spite of the more favorable aspects of treatment in the college setting. This means that we are still a long way from solving the problems of the obesities and have not yet been able to tackle effectively the roots of the problems. A prime factor in success would appear to be personal motivation for weight loss. Emotional stability would appear to be the second most important factor. The immediate life circumstances are important, for times of stress are not times to undertake the added discipline of weight reduction. Age of onset of obesity is a factor, for obesity originating in childhood is particularly refractory to treatment. All these factors relate to an individual's ability to exert the will power to control such fundamental human behavior as eating, drinking and activity patterns.

The counseling of obese college students usually does accomplish an educational job in that the student gains insight into his problem, whether or not he can do anything about it. Perhaps at the time meaningful motivation cannot be aroused or circumstances are too unsettled for him to make progress. But many times one sees the ultimate results in the same student. Suddenly the right motivating force is exerted or changes take place in the student's life, and he is able to exert more self-control and discipline. He is intelligent, and he remembers what to do, does it, and is very pleased with himself. Thus, nutrition counseling in the student clinic is more effective than statistics derived from initial contacts might indicate.

Impressions of Current Trends

Certain impressions neither confirmed nor refuted by reliable statistics have come out of my experience in counseling college students. It would appear that gross obesity among college students is decreasing. There appears to be more involvement in food faddism and fad diets. There seems to be more concern with adequacy of diet for most efficient operation, perhaps a reflection of faddism. The cultural condemnation of obesity is being felt more than it was in the past. More students come to the nutrition counselor on their own initiative for information. There seems to be more interest in prevention. Relatively speaking, more men than women seem to be seeking advice.

The services of the medical nutritionist in the Gannett Medical Clinic and Sage Infirmary at Cornell University are made possible through continuing support of the Frank E. Gannett Newspaper Foundation, Inc., Rochester, New York.

REFERENCES

1. Young CM: The role of the dietitian in a college nutrition program. J Am Diet Assoc 20:590, Oct 1944
2. ____: The nutritionist in the student medical clinic. Student Med 1:25, Apr 1953
3. Waldner B, Pilcher HL, Young CM: Twelve years of nutrition counseling in a student medical clinic. Student Med 4:20, Oct 1955
4. Young CM: Dietary study of Cornell University women. J Am Diet Assoc 22:25, Jan 1946
5. Young CM, Einset BM, Empey EL, et al: Nutrient intake of college men. J Am Diet Assoc 33:374, Apr 1957
6. Young CM: Weight reduction using a moderate-fat diet. J Am Diet Assoc 28:529, 1952
7. Young CM, Scanlan SS, Im HS, et al: Effect on body composition and other parameters in obese young men of carbohydrate level of reduction diet. Am J Clin Nutr 24:290, Mar 1971
8. Young CM, Moore NS, Berresford BK, et al: What can be done for the obese patient? Am Pract Dig Treat 6:685, May 1955

Obesity surgery aids four adolescents

Fat melts away after jejunoileal bypass, and youngsters have no complications

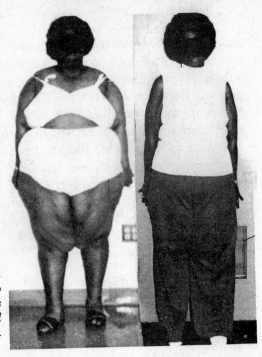

After her intestinal bypass operation, this 16-year-old lost 234 lb in 18 months, dropping from 437 lb to 203 lb. She and three other youngsters in the study are back in school now, unrestricted in activity and diet.

Four massively obese adolescents have lost some of their bulk and gained some personality improvements since last year, when they became the first nonadults to undergo jejunoileal bypass for weight reduction. One boy even grew four inches taller, say physicians at the National Medical Center in Washington, D.C.

Furthermore, Drs. Judson G. Randolph, William H. Weintraub, and Andrew Rigg told the American Academy of Pediatrics meeting in Chicago, the carefully selected adolescents have not suffered—so far—the infections, severe biochemical derangements, urinary tract oxalate stones, and liver problems that have plagued adults undergoing this operation (MWN, Sept. 7, p. 34).

The children were three girls aged 15, 15, and 16 who weighed respectively, 318, 404, and 437 lb, and an 11-year-old boy with Prader-Willi syndrome, who weighed 195 lb at a height of 4 ft, 4 in.

The six criteria the group used to select the patients for the operation included extreme obesity (more than twice the ideal weight for at least two years); failure of at least a year's trial of dietary treatment; absence of any contributory disease, especially hypothyroidism or Cushing's disease; absence of any unrelated disease that might increase risk of operation; assurance by parents that they would cooperate in management of their child's condition before and after the operation; and evidence of psychological stability as determined by an attending psychiatrist.

In each case, Dr. Randolph says, the attending surgeon resected a segment of the patient's jejunum, then restored intestinal continuity by uniting the now-shortened jejunum to the terminal ileum. The removed segment of the jejunum, however, was left in the patient's body to make possible the re-establishment of normal bowel function and anatomy, should the need arise. One end of this removed section of jejunum was closed and anchored to the patient's mesocolon, to prevent intussusception, and the other was united with, and allowed to drain into, the transverse colon in two patients, the sigmoid flexure of the colon in another, and the cecum in the fourth.

After operation the four patients had diarrhea for one to three months, but all now pass two to six formed or semiformed stools a day without antidiarrheal medication. All of them are taking a multivitamin preparation.

A year after operation the three girls had lost 90 lb (28% of preoperative weight), 134 lb (33%), and 179 lb (40%), and the little boy 57 lb (30%). Six months later the heaviest girl had lost another 55 lb, for a total weight loss of 234 lb. The patients' weight loss is now leveling off.

Postoperative metabolic studies yield normal findings except for the obvious effects of altered absorption.

Thus, the physicians point out, decreased absorption is reflected in a flattening of the results of glucose and xylose tolerance tests, marked increase in fecal losses of fat and nitrogen, and in lower serum levels of triglycerides and cholesterol. Vitamin A serum levels are lower "as might be expected with depressed fat absorption," they note.

Analyses of serum samples yield normal results, however, for electrolytes, calcium, magnesium, blood urea nitrogen, creatinine, total protein, and albumin. And the patients, all of whom had fatty infiltration of the liver at operation, have not had any hepatomegaly since, the physicians note.

Postoperative x-ray studies of each patient show that the anatomy of each remained as created by surgery, without significant lengthening or change in bowel caliber. Transit time from stomach to colon is 15 minutes or less in each patient. However, the girl whose bypassed segment drains into her cecum has some reflux into the bypassed loop, and her weight loss has been "less impressive" than the others'. But Dr. Randolph and his colleagues see no apparent interference with skeletal growth, and they point to "an improvement in personality concomitant with gradual weight loss" in each patient. All four patients' appetites have gradually decreased, and all are back in school, unrestricted in activity and diet. ∎

Part V: Dynamics of Weight Control *

The treatment of obesity is one of the most exasperating experiences in clinical and preventive health.

Expressed in its simplest terms, treatment of human obesity of whatever type involves greater energy expenditure than energy intake.

Good clinical judgment is needed to determine the desirable weight for an individual. This should be based on 1) actual weight, 2) physical appearance and 3) subcutaneous fat disposition.

Because the treatment of obesity is often a frustrating task, it is not surprising to see the plethora of "treatments" that are published each year by physicians and laymen. Unfortunately, most of these regimens are directed toward accelerating weight loss which is not necessarily the same as accelerating fat loss. Recognition of this discrepancy, coupled with the realization that the problems of the obese are not restricted to the area of caloric intake, begins to establish a foundation upon which to approach this disorder.

There are strong physiological arguments in favor of preventing obesity rather than correcting it after it occurs.

Recent work on experimental animals suggests that once an animal subject has become obese, it becomes obese more easily and more rapidly a second time, even when food intake is the same as in the previous period of weight gain. This increased deficiency in food utilization may be partly responsible for the lack of "staying quality" noted in many weight reduction results.

The frequent weight gains and losses indulged in by the many obese patients who practice what one writer calls the "rhythm method of girth control" may be actually more harmful than maintenance of a steady weight at a high level. For example, it has been shown that serum cholesterol levels are elevated during periods of weight gain, thus increasing the risk of deposition. We have no evidence to show that once cholesterol is deposited it can be removed by weight reduction. It is possible that a patient whose weight has fluctuated up and down a number of times has been subjected to more stress than a patient with stable though excessive weight. Animal experiments have shown that animals of normal weight have a longer life expectancy than obese animals. If an animal has once been obese and then has been repeatedly reduced, it will have a shorter life expectancy than the obese animal which has never been reduced—adding further question to the advisability of weight reduction that cannot be sustained.

Inactivity is a major factor in the etiology of many—perhaps most—obese patients. The lack of ease and the discomfort which accompanies the moving of a body mass when it is too large, and the resulting fatigue, particularly in individuals not highly motivated to exercise in the first place, are likely to further decrease voluntary motion.

The decrease in energy expenditure tends not only to trip the caloric balance toward the positive side, it may do so to such an extent that the food intake which would keep the subject in balance is too small to satisfy a minimum appetite.

It is well to remember the remarks of Plato who said in effect that the human animal consists of a body and a soul and when one doesn't function well neither does the other.

As Hutton suggests: no two of us are alike in our fingerprints. Obesity is more complex than fingerprints; consequently, no one method of treating obesity is likely to be suitable for every fat person.

This section is a review of weight control methods and programs as presented by some of the foremost authorities in the field. They range from discussion of weight control through diet and exercise to behavior modification and jejuno-ileal surgery.

*Excerpts from: *Obesity and Health*, U.S. Public Health Service Publication No. 1485.

The Myth of Diet in the Management of Obesity[1,2,3]

George A. Bray

OBESITY IS A WIDESPREAD MALADY in our society, yet its underlying cause still eludes medical science and its therapy is, therefore, empirical. Many therapeutic approaches have been tried including diets of all kinds, total and intermittent starvation, health spas, exercise machines, and medication of various types. Recent information provides some insight into the generally disappointing results that have been obtained using a dietary approach.

Obesity exists when fat makes up a greater than normal fraction of total body weight. Overweight, on the other hand, is defined in relation to tables of ideal weight that have usually been prepared by life insurance companies. It is fair to say that obese people are usually overweight, but that not all overweight people are obese. Since it is easy to measure weight, but more difficult to quantitate fatness, most of the epidemiological data implying that obesity is a hazard to health are in fact derived from studies of "overweight." When the abnormality in weight exceeds the ideal for height and age by more than 30% in the

nonathletic individual, overweight is almost assuredly due to excess fat. The prevalence and significance of obesity can best be conveyed from the following statistics. The United States Public Health Service indicates that 25–45% of the adult American population over 30 years of age is more than 20% overweight (1). In childhood, obesity, defined as 40% or more above the median weight for height, occurred with an incidence of 2–15% (1). This burden is not borne equally among all segments of society. A study in Manhattan has shown that obesity is 7 times more common in the lowest socioeconomic group as compared with the highest group (2). The medical importance of corpulence is clear from the increased mortality and morbidity associated with overweight. In the Framingham Study of factors related to heart disease, obese subjects were more prone to angina pectoris and to sudden death than were people of normal weight (3). In addition, diabetes mellitus, gall bladder disease, and respiratory disease are all more common in the overweight patient.

RATIONALE FOR DIETARY MANAGEMENT OF OBESITY

In the simplest terms, obesity occurs because the caloric value of ingested food is greater than the daily requirements. Excess

[1] From the New England Medical Center Hospitals and Department of Medicine, Tufts University School of Medicine, Boston, Massachusetts.

[2] Supported by National Institutes of Health Grants AM 09897 and FR-52.

[3] Based on a lecture given to the New England Dairy Council, April 1, 1970.

calories not used each day are converted to fatty acids and are stored in adipose tissue cells because this site can be expanded almost without limit. Excess fat can accumulate in persons continuing normal food intake if energy expenditure is reduced. Evidence for this mechanism in obese teenage girls has been presented by Bullen and colleagues (4), who utilized motion pictures to document that obese girls were measurably less active than their thin contemporaries. Chirico and Stunkard (5), using pairs of obese and lean subjects of the same sex and occupation, showed that activity was less in the obese member of most pairs. The most striking example of obesity due to reduced energy output, however, was the report by Wilkins and his co-workers from the Johns Hopkins Hospital (6). They reported a 6-year-old child who became almost completely paralyzed and gained weight whenever daily intake exceeded 500 kcal.

A second way in which an imbalance between calorie intake and expenditure can occur is by increasing food consumption while maintaining normal activity. To learn whether calorie intake was excessive or energy expenditure diminished, we quantitated the energy expenditure of a group of grossly obese adult patients (7). Measurements of oxygen consumption were made and used to calculate energy needs. Samples of expired air were collected on each patient several times a day for a period of 6–12 days and analyzed for their content of oxygen and carbon dioxide. Energy expenditure has been measured by this technique in more than 30 obese patients. In general, heavier patients have greater requirements for oxygen. Total oxygen consumption (energy expenditure) among patients had a high correlation with total body fat, surface area, and body weight but a much less significant correlation with measures of lean body mass, such as total body water, exchangeable potassium, and creatinine excretion. The data relating oxygen consumption with surface area in 18 of our obese patients had the slope of 1,100 kcal/m^2 (7). This means that for each additional square meter of surface area an extra 1,100 kcal, on the average, is required just to maintain body weight. This relationship between oxygen consumption and surface area in obese patients is essentially the same as the one for lean individuals, indicating that obese and lean people have the same calorie requirement per unit surface area. From this information we can calculate that, to gain weight, an individual with a surface area of 2 m^2 would require in excess of 2,200 kcal daily. As most of our obese patients were between 2 and 3 m^2 (corresponding to 250–450 lb.), a diet containing 3,500 kcal should produce only a slight weight gain in individuals in this group. When we placed six obese patients on a diet of 3,500 kcal for 1 week, there was no significant increase in weight, thus supporting our conclusion that obese patients require a large number of calories to maintain weight and even more to gain weight. Conversely, we would expect that if restriction of calorie intake were adequate, weight loss would ensue. This fact has been demonstrated many times (8).

RESULTS OF CALORIE RESTRICTION IN THE MANAGEMENT OF OBESITY

Clinics employing dietary management in the treatment of obesity have generally achieved poor results. Stunkard and McLaren-Hume (10) reviewed the experience of a number of nutrition clinics that have treated obesity, and some of these data have been summarized in Fig. 1. The number of patients in each study is shown at the bottom of the figure and the percentage of patients achieving a weight loss of 20 or 40 lb. is shown by the height of the bars. There was some variability from one study to another, but in general the percentage losing 20 lb. or more was less than 30% (mean = 24%). When one looks at the percentage achieving a 40-lb. weight loss the outlook is considerably less satisfactory. Here the aver-

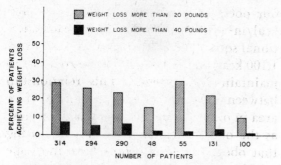

FIG. 1. Weight loss in patients treated with diet. Number of patients in each study is listed below each pair of bars and the percentage losing 20 or 40 lb. is indicated by the height of the bars. The references for columns 1–7, reading from left to right are 11, 12, 13, 14, 15, 16, 10.

age was only 9%. Such a method of presenting data on weight loss has its limitations. There are always patients for whom a weight loss of 20 or 40 lb. would bring them very close to their desired weight and other patients for whom such weight losses would be trivial. To make some correction for these factors, Young et al. (16) evaluated weight loss in relation to the amount of excess weight. Thus, patients were divided into six groups and the successes evaluated in relation to the weight to be lost. With increasing initial weight, the success rate fell, yet it is the heavier patient for whom weight loss is more important (Table I).

These observations indicate that dietary treatment of obesity is more likely to succeed in patients who are only modestly overweight. For these patients the companionship of similarly afflicted individuals may provide an additional incentive to lose weight. It is this technique that such groups as the TOPS (Take Off Pounds Sensibly) Clubs have used with reported success. Several other groups, including Diet Kitchen, Diet Workshop, and Weight Watchers, have added an additional monetary incentive to weight reduction by dietary means. In patients with marked obesity, however, the outlook would appear bleak for any of these methods. In a follow-up study of 199 patients who were 50% or more overweight, Glennon (17) found that only one individual approached normal weight, another 12% were able to achieve a weight loss of more than 20 lb. but only 6% lost more than 40 lb.

Unfortunately, for the obese patient each new diet produces its temporary weight loss, but this is usually followed by a relapse, with weight returning to the same or higher levels. Mayer (9) has aptly described this as "the rhythm method of girth control." If there was an effective diet, there would be no need for the continuous introduction of new diets: the "Grapefruit diet," the "Drinking Man's diet," "the "Air Force diet," the "Mayo diet," the "Quick Weight Loss diet," and so on. It seems obvious from the number of diets that have been made available and are continuing to appear, none of them provides the answer to obesity.

ADIPOSE CELLS IN OBESITY

Two areas of investigation have provided a partial explanation for the failures of calorie restriction in the treatment of obesity. Accretion of fat can occur by either enlarging the existing fat cells to accommodate the extra fat, increasing the total number of fat cells, or by a combination of both (18). We have measured the size of subcutaneous fat cells under a microscope after dispersing the cells by incubating them in collagenase (19). The size of subcutaneous fat cells in a

TABLE I

Weight reduction in relation to initial weight[a]

Initial weight range, lb.	Criteria of success (pounds to be lost)	Number of successes	
		Total number	%
Under 150	10	11/25	44
151–175	15	11/36	31
176–200	20	13/47	28
201–225	25	3/22	14
226–250	30	1/15	7
Over 250	35	2/11	18
Total		41/156	26

[a] Modified from the data of Young et al. (16).

group of obese and control patients is shown in Fig. 2. Subcutaneous fat cells from the control subjects (patients undergoing laparotomy) were about one-third the size of the fat cells from the obese subjects. Indeed, the one fat patient with the smallest cells had lost 120 lb. prior to his biopsy. From this comparison we would conclude that obese patients have considerably larger subcutaneous fat cells than control subjects. In the control group there was a positive correlation ($P < 0.05$) between the volume of fat cells and body weight. Thus, we would conclude that heavier patients had larger fat cells and that the accumulation of fat is accompanied in part by enlargement of subcutaneous fat cells.

We have estimated the total number of fat cells by two methods. In the obese patients we measured the total body water from the distribution of tritiated water and used these data to calculate the total amount of fat (7). In the control patients it was not possible to measure their total body water by isotopic methods and, therefore, we calculated body fat from height and weight. In the obese subjects the two estimates of body fat had a correlation coeffi-

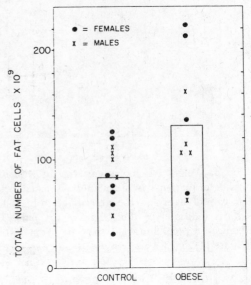

FIG. 3. Number of fat cells in control and obese patients.

cient of greater than $+0.90$ ($P < 0.01$). We have assumed that subcutaneous fat cells are representative of all fat cells.[4] It would appear that many grossly obese individuals have an increased number of fat cells as well as enlarged fat cells (Fig. 3). The increased number of fat cells limits the effectiveness of dietary therapy in the treatment of obesity. This is so because fat cells, once formed, are apparently removed very slowly. Indeed the fat person with an increased number of fat cells has no way of destroying these cells by any currently available medical technique. During weight loss, the size of individual fat cells shrinks, but the total number appears to remain constant. Thus, even when the size of individual fat cells returns to normal, the patient is still overweight from the extra cell mass. The one obese patient whose fat cells were at the upper limits of normal (Fig. 2) still weighed 270 lb. The control patients with cells of this size were only 220 and 225 lb.

EFFICIENCY AND CALORIC EXPENDITURE

A second reason why the use of dietary therapy as the sole treatment of obesity is

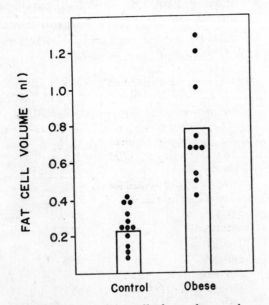

FIG. 2. Volume of fat cells from obese and control patients. Reproduced by permission of the Annals of Internal Medicine.

[4] Total number of fat cells $= \dfrac{\text{body fat} \times 10^9}{0.92 \text{ fat cell volume}}$.

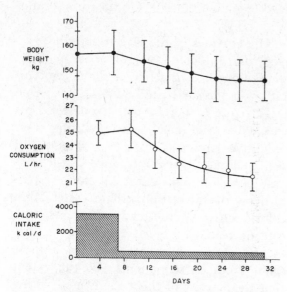

FIG. 4. Oxygen consumption of six obese patients during calorie restriction. From *Lancet* by permission of the publisher.

often unsuccessful is related to the adaptive changes in energy expenditure that occur with calorie restriction (20, 21). We noted earlier that obese patients require in excess of 1,100 kcal/m² to maintain their weight. During calorie restriction this figure drops so that obese patients on a weight-reducing regimen may require less than 900 kcal/m² to maintain weight.

After calorie intake was abruptly lowered there was a gradual reduction in calorie expenditure that amounted to more than 15% during the 2 weeks of observation (Fig. 4). This might result simply from the decreased food intake in that digestion and absorption of food increases energy requirement, the so-called specific dynamic action of foods. The time course of the adaptation is against this interpretation, however. For the first 2 days after food intake was reduced the oxygen consumption showed little change. The decline came over the subsequent days of the experiment. The importance of this observation to the "dieter" is clear. It simply means that the usual basis for estimating the quantity of calories that need to be restricted to produce a given loss is underestimated. This is illustrated in

Table II. Thus, a patient requiring 2,500 kcal for maintenance would be expected to lose 2 lb. weekly on a 1,500-kcal reduction diet. However, considering the reduced calorie requirement, a weight loss of less than 1 lb./week would ensue. If the diet were reduced to 1,000 kcal/day, the rate of weight loss would increase to 900 kcal daily, still less than 2 lb. a week. Thus, it requires considerably greater calorie restriction to produce a meaningful weight loss than most currently published data would lead us to think.

It is apparent from what has been described that any technique for increasing energy expenditure would accelerate weight loss. Regular exercise provides one such avenue to increasing the caloric deficit. Exercise would also appear to reduce food intake. This finding was clearly shown in studies by Mayer and his colleagues (22, 23).

TABLE II

Calculation of expected weight loss

Classic method (1 lb. = 3,500 kcal)	
Total kilocalories needed for weight maintenance	
Basal	1,700
Activity	800
Total	2,500
Kilocalories in prescribed diet	1,500
Daily deficit	1,000 kcal/day
Weekly deficit	7,000 kcal = 2 lb.
Considering reduced requirements (1 lb. = 3,500 kcal)	
Total kilocalories needed for weight maintenance	
Basal	1,400
Activity	500
Total	1,900
Kilocalories in prescribed diet	1,500
Daily deficit	400
Weekly deficit	2,800 = 0.80 lb.

In animals and in human beings very low levels of activity actually increased food intake, whereas modest degrees of activity seemed to reduce food intake. Thus, increasing activity in obese patients in spite of the difficulties has a place in helping to control food intake and accelerate weight loss.

Obesity occurs because the number of calories ingested is greater than the number required. These calories measure the total amount of heat produced during the oxidation of foodstuffs. The same number of calories are produced whether the foodstuffs are oxidized in the body or outside the body, provided that a correction is made for the fact that nitrogen-containing foods are incompletely oxidized in the body. From the physiological point of view, however, it is not the total number of calories that is important, but the fraction of these calories that can be used for metabolic needs. As is well known, part of the calories produced during metabolism are retained temporarily in high energy intermediates such as ATP. When glucose is metabolized, for example, a maximum of 45% of the total calories in this molecule can be converted to ATP. The efficiency of metabolic processes in the body may be reduced below this level by several mechanisms, one of which is the glycerophosphate cycle. When the activity of these enzymes is increased, the efficiency of biological oxidations would be reduced, and conversely, low activity of this cycle would lead to greater efficiency in the formation of ATP (26).

The enzymes in the glycerophosphate cycle from adipose tissue of obese patients were about half as active as the enzymes in fat from normal individuals (24). One might expect, therefore, that obese people would be more efficient in coupling their oxidative processes to the formation of ATP. Of particular importance for the present discussion is the effect of calorie restriction on the glycerophosphate cycle. With calorie restriction there was a further significant decrease in the activity of the enzymes in the glycerophosphate cycle in adipose tissue from obese patients. To the extent that the activity of this cycle is modulating the efficiency of food utilization, these obese patients would produce relatively more ATP when eating less. Indeed, it is possible that the decline in total energy expenditure observed with calorie restriction may reflect the increased efficiency that could result from decreased activity of this cycle. Since the activity of the glycerophosphate cycle is lower in obese patients and declines further with calorie restriction, there may, therefore, be some truth in the oft-repeated statement of fat patients that "Doctor, everything I eat turns to fat."

ALTERNATIVE APPROACHES

Since dieting is a safe but often ineffective treatment for obesity, what alternative avenues of therapy are open? One approach was suggested by the finding that the glycerophosphate cycle was underactive in adipose tissue from obese patients. In experimental animals, the activity of these enzymes are controlled in part by the level of thyroid hormones (25). This observation has led us to reevaluate the effects of thyroid hormones in obese subjects (26). Eight obese patients were fed a high calorie diet followed by calorie restriction (Fig. 5). During the period of restricted intake these subjects were treated with triiodothyronine. With the reduction in calorie intake, the activity

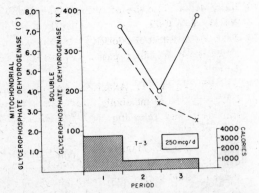

FIG. 5. Effect of calorie restriction and triiodothyronine on the activity of the enzymes in the glycerophosphate cycle in eight obese patients.

of the enzymes in the glycerophosphate cycle declined. When triiodothyronine was added the activity of the mitochondrial enzyme increased to the level at which it had been before the low calorie intake was started. As this enzyme is the rate-limiting one in the glycerophosphate cycle, the activity of the entire cycle would appear to be increased by thyroid hormones. This increase was accompanied by a corresponding rise in total oxygen consumption. From our previous discussion it would appear that the level of activity of the glycerophosphate cycle may be inversely related to the efficiency with which foodstuffs are oxidized. When the activity of the cycle is increased, as it was during the administration of triiodothyronine, efficiency is reduced and more substrate required to produce the same quantity of ATP.

It must be emphasized that these last two studies with thyroid hormone have been conducted under the carefully controlled conditions of a metabolic ward. Moreover, the doses used would be considered large by the usual criteria of what is required for treatment of hypothyroidism. However, they do suggest that some therapeutic modalities that have come under recent criticism may need reevaluation as potential agents in our search for more effective ways of dealing with obesity.

REFERENCES

1. U. S. Public Health Service. Obesity and Health, p. 19 and 20.
2. Moore, M. E., A. Stunkard and L. Srole. Obesity, social class and mental illness. *J. Am. Med. Assoc.* 81: 962, 1962.
3. Kannel, W. B., J. E. LeBauer, T. R. Dawbert and P. M. McNamara. Relation of body weight to development of coronary heart disease. The Framingham Study. *Circulation* 35: 734, 1967.
4. Bullen, B. A., R. B. Reed and J. Mayer. Physical activity of obese and nonobese adolescent girls appraised by motion picture sampling. *Am. J. Clin. Nutr.* 14: 211, 1964.
5. Chirico, A-M., and A. J. Stunkard. Physical activity and human obesity. *New Engl. J. Med.* 263: 935, 1960.
6. Wilkins, L., R. M. Blizzard and C. J. Migeon. *The Diagnosis and Treatment of Endocrine Disorders in Childhood and Adolescence* (3rd ed.). Springfield, Ill.: Thomas, 1965, p. 565.
7. Bray, G. A., M. Schwartz, R. R. Rozin and J. Lister. Some relationships between oxygen consumption and body composition in obese patients. In press.
8. Kinsell, L. W., B. Gunning, G. P. Michaels, J. Richardson, S. E. Cox and C. Lennon. Calories do count. *Metab. Clin. Exptl.* 13: 195, 1964.
9. Mayer, J. *Overweight: Causes, Cost and Control.* Englewood Cliffs, N. J.: Prentice-Hall, 1968, p. 2.
10. Stunkard, A., and M. McLaren-Hume. The results of treatment for obesity. *Arch. Internal Med.* 103: 79, 1959.
11. Gray, H., and D. C. Kallenbach. Obesity treatment: results on 212 outpatients. *J. Am. Dietet. Assoc.* 15: 239, 1939.
12. Fellows, H. H. Studies of relatively normal obese individuals during and after dietary restrictions. *Am. J. Med. Sci.* 181: 301, 1931.
13. Harvey, H. I., and W. D. Simmons. Weight reduction: a study of the group method. Report of progress. *Am. J. Med. Sci.* 227: 521, 1954.
14. Munves, E. D. Dietetic interview or group discussion—decision in reducing. *J. Am. Dietet. Assoc.* 29: 1197, 1953.
15. Osserman, K. E., and H. O. Dolger. Obesity in diabetes: a study of therapy with anorexigenic drugs. *Ann. Internal Med.* 34: 72, 1951.
16. Young, C. M., N. S. Moore, K. Berresford, B. M. Einset and B. G. Waldner. The problems of the obese patient. *J. Am. Dietet. Assoc.* 31: 1111, 1955.
17. Glennon, J. A. Weight reduction—an enigma. *Arch. Internal Med.* 118: 1, 1966.
18. Hirsch, J., J. L. Knittle and L. B. Salans. Cell lipid content and cell number in obese and nonobese human adipose tissue. *J. Clin. Invest.* 45: 1023, 1966.
19. Bray, G. A. The size of human fat cells. *Clin. Res.* 17: 608, 1969.
20. Bray, G. A. Effect of caloric restriction on energy expenditure in obese patients. *Lancet* 2: 397, 1968.
21. Grande, F., J. T. Anderson and A. Keys. Changes of basal metabolic rate in man in semi-starvation and refeeding. *J. Appl. Physiol.* 12: 230, 1958.
22. Mayer, J., N. B. Marshall, J. J. Vitale, J. H. Christensen, J. H. Mashayahi and F. J. Stare. Exercise, food intake and body weight in normal rats and genetically obese adult mice. *Am. J. Physiol.* 177: 544, 1954.
23. Mayer, J., P. Roy and K. P. Mitra. Relation

between caloric intake, body weight, and physical work in an industrial male population in West Bengal. *Am. J. Clin. Nutr.* 4: 169, 1956.

24. GALTON, D. J., AND G. A. BRAY. Metabolism of α-glycerol phosphate in human adipose tissue in obesity. *J. Clin. Endocrinol. Metab.* 27: 1573, 1967.

25. LEE, Y-P., AND H. A. LARDY. Influence of thyroid hormones on L-α-glycerophosphate dehydrogenases and other dehydrogenases in various organs of the rat. *J. Biol. Chem.* 240: 1427, 1965.

26. BRAY, G. A. Effect of diet and triiodothyronine on the activity of sn-glycerol-3-phosphate dehydrogenase and on the metabolism of glucose and pyruvate by adipose tissue of obese patients. *J. Clin. Invest.* 48: 1413, 1969.

Management of the Obese Patient

Jonathan J. Braunstein, M.D.[*]

Obesity is the most common nutritional disorder confronting the physician in this country today. It has been estimated that approximately 30 per cent of our adult population is more than 20 per cent overweight. There is evidence that the obesity is associated with an increase in morbidity and mortality which can be lessened by weight reduction.[13] It is because of the prevalence and health risks associated with obesity that the management of the obese patient should be of interest to all physicians.

Unfortunately, the results of the treatment of the obese patient are often discouraging; not only does the obese patient often fail to lose weight but when therapy is initially successful the patient frequently relapses to his former state within a short time. Perhaps because of these poor results, physicians have become discouraged with the management of the obese patient and, occasionally, in the place of rational medical therapy, less reputable forms of therapy have sprung up.

This paper will review some general concepts with regard to the management of the obese patient, including: diagnosis, underlying causes, complications, and therapeutic programs for weight reduction. It is only by such a systematic approach to the management of each obese patient that a better understanding of this complex condition and better therapy will result.

DIAGNOSIS OF OBESITY

The diagnosis of obesity is generally made on simple inspection of the patient. There are instances clinically and for research purposes when a more exact qualitative and quantitative definition of the obese state is necessary. It is important to keep in mind that body weight is contributed to by all of the body tissues (water, muscle, other fat-free protoplasm, skeleton, and adipose tissue) and that an alteration of any of these can influence the total body weight.

Obesity is the excessive accumulation of body fat or adipose tissue which is usually associated, but not synonymous, with the overweight

[*]Assistant Professor of Medicine, University of Miami School of Medicine

state. For example, there are the well known situations in which the excessive accumulation of fluid (as in the edematous states) or muscle tissue (as in the muscular athlete) result in an abnormal increase in weight without excess adipose tissue or obesity being present. For usual purposes, however, excess weight in the adult is a reflection of the deposition of excess adipose tissue.

The diagnosis of obesity is, therefore, made by weighing the patient and comparing the actual weight to an ideal or desirable weight as determined from weight tables in which body proportions, height, and sex are taken into consideration. A body weight greater than 20 per cent of the ideal or desirable weight is felt to represent a significant degree of obesity. More exact measurement of the degree of obesity can be made by determining the skin-fold thickness in certain body areas using a specially designed caliper. This method is based on the fact that the subcutaneous fat deposits reflect the overall body content of adipose tissue.[9]

The greater the degree of obesity, the more serious the condition, both in terms of associated morbidity and mortality, and in terms of difficulty in treatment. The prognosis for the very overweight patient is much poorer than for the mildly obese individual.

THE UNDERLYING CAUSES OF OBESITY

Obesity is a very complex disorder in which multiple causative factors are potentially operative in any given patient (Fig. 1). It is only by a careful and comprehensive evaluation of the individual patient that the particular causes present in a given situation can be determined.

The fundamental metabolic disturbance in the obese patient is a

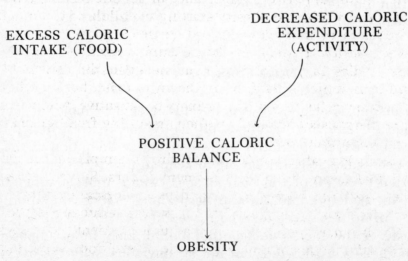

UNDERLYING FACTORS:

Genetic, metabolic, psychological, social, environmental, underlying disease

EXCESS CALORIC INTAKE (FOOD)

DECREASED CALORIC EXPENDITURE (ACTIVITY)

POSITIVE CALORIC BALANCE

OBESITY

Figure 1. Cause(s) of obesity.

positive caloric or energy balance in which the calories ingested exceed those expended by the patient at some time during his life. This is generally the result of both excessive caloric intake in the diet and decreased caloric expenditure in the form of physical activity in the usual obese patient. The excessive caloric intake of obese patients has been greatly emphasized and rightly so, but it has become increasingly evident that reduction in physical activity also plays a significant role in the positive caloric balance.[5]

The underlying factors responsible for this positive caloric or energy balance are multiple and differ from patient to patient. These should be sought for and determined in each case, if possible, for the correction of these underlying pathogenetic factors would form the most rational approach to the correction of the caloric imbalance. These underlying factors include genetic, metabolic, psychological, social, and environmental factors.

Obesity is properly thought of not as a disease but as a symptom or sign of positive caloric balance; as such, it requires that a careful search be made for the underlying causative factors (genetic, metabolic, psychological, social, and environmental) which can lead to a positive caloric balance.

The vast majority of obese patients do not have an underlying disease to account for their overweight state. Conditions such as hypothyroidism, hyperadrenalcorticism, hypogonadism, insulinoma, and hypothalamic disease may be associated with obesity, but these are unusual and account for less than 1 per cent of all obese patients. Nevertheless, a consideration of these secondary causes of obesity should be given, if only because therapy in these instances would be, of course, directed toward the underlying disease.

As noted, most patients with obesity have idiopathic or primary obesity, in that no underlying disease can be demonstrated to be present. However, a good deal of evidence has been accumulated to support the role of genetic, metabolic, psychological, social, and environmental factors in the pathogenesis of the condition. For example, Mayer has presented data to support the importance of genetic factors in obesity,[14] and it is generally felt that obesity starting in childhood is a much more difficult problem in management and carries a poorer prognosis than adult-onset obesity. Recent literature summarized by Bortz[7] shows numerous studies in which significant metabolic differences between obese and lean subjects have been shown to exist, but whether these differences are a reflection of the primary or causative factors in obesity or they are merely secondary phenomena resulting from the obese state has yet to be determined.

The psychological factors in obesity are as complex as the condition itself and have been the subject of many papers. Suffice it to say that some obese patients have deep seated psychological dysfunction and, in these individuals, the prognosis for weight reduction is poor, compared with the more psychologically adjusted patients. The social and environmental factors influencing caloric intake and caloric output in our modern affluent society are so obvious that they hardly need mentioning. The social emphasis in recent years of the cosmetic attractiveness of leanness in this country has tended to offset these otherwise strong socioeconomic factors leading to obesity.

COMPLICATIONS OF OBESITY

Obesity is associated with certain medical complications which form the basis of the increased morbidity and mortality attributed to the overweight state. The more severe the obesity, the more prominent are these complications. First, as mentioned above, there are numerous metabolic abnormalities which characterize the obese patient when compared with the lean individual (Table 1). It is probable that many of these are the result of the obesity, as they may remit with weight reduction and correction of the obese state.[3]

There are a number of diseases which are clinically associated with obesity: diabetes mellitus, atherosclerosis, cholelithiasis, and hypertensive cardiovascular disease. In addition, there is the cardiopulmonary syndrome associated with extreme degree of obesity, the Pickwickian syndrome.

Obese patients are said to be more accident prone and have a higher rate of complications following surgical procedures than lean patients. There are a number of medical conditions in which the obese state plays an aggravating role and in which weight reduction is a major therapeutic goal: spine and hip joint disease, congestive heart failure, etc.

The psychologic and social effects of the overweight state may also be considered important complications of obesity in that they may interfere with the overall adaptation of the individual. In summary, it would be fair to state that a significant degree of obesity carries with it a risk to health, certainly enough to warrant an attempt at prevention and therapy.

THERAPEUTIC APPROACH

As may be inferred from the preceding discussion, the management of the obese patient begins with a thorough general medical evaluation, one in which the underlying causative factors and complications of obesity are carefully considered. A critical part of this evaluation is a

Table 1. *Metabolic Abnormalities in Obesity*

Increased fat utilization
Decreased glucose utilization
Increased blood levels of glucose, amino acids, triglycerides, and cholesterol
Increased plasma free fatty acid level and turnover rate (fed state)
Increased insulin secretion and plasma level
Insulin resistance
Increased cortisol secretion and turnover rate
Decreased growth hormone secretory responsiveness

detailed dietary history and assessment of the physical activity pattern of the patient, present and past. Other historical information includes the age of onset of the obesity (childhood or adult) and the psychologic makeup of the individual, as these aspects form important therapeutic and prognostic guides. The degree of motivation of the patient to reduce weight is a key factor to assess, as this will ultimately form the basis of the success or failure of any therapeutic plan. As in most chronic ills, an important part of any therapeutic program is patient education with regard to certain of the basic concepts of the illness. The patient's understanding is necessary for good motivation and cooperation. This education is a continuing process and built on at subsequent visits.

Finally, the physician must be fully aware that the management of the obese patient will require prolonged therapy with close and frequent follow-up visits, and that relapses may occur as in any chronic illness. He must realize that his understanding and guidance are strong factors in the success of any program. Assistance for the physician may come from the dietician and, when indicated, from the psychiatrist or psychologist.

The basic concept underlying all therapy for obesity is the production of a negative caloric or energy balance, so that the patient is forced to burn his excess body fat as a source of energy (Fig. 2). This can be accomplished by a reduction of caloric intake in the diet or an increase in caloric expenditure in the form of physical activity. In most instances, a combination of these is most effective. The production of a negative caloric balance by these means will result in a loss of adipose tissue in the obese patient which will be reflected by a loss of weight.

It is important to emphasize once again that total body weight is contributed to by all the body tissues and that body water content is particularly prone to fluctuations quite apart, at times, from calorie balance. These day to day fluctuations in body water may initially mask a reduction in adipose tissue weight resulting from a negative caloric balance, but over a longer period of observation, an overall weight loss will occur in response to a negative caloric balance. The physician and his patient must thoroughly understand these basic concepts to avoid the discouragement that sometimes occurs with a patient who faithfully follows a therapeutic program which produces a negative caloric balance, but despite this fails to lose weight, or even gains weight owing to fluid retention. To emphasize again, this is usually a transient phenomenon which will correct itself over a period of time.

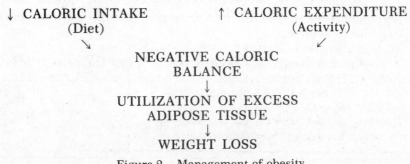

↓ CALORIC INTAKE   ↑ CALORIC EXPENDITURE
(Diet)   (Activity)

NEGATIVE CALORIC
BALANCE
↓
UTILIZATION OF EXCESS
ADIPOSE TISSUE
↓
WEIGHT LOSS

Figure 2. Management of obesity.

Dietary Management

The basic concept of the dietary management of obesity is the production of a negative caloric balance by providing in the diet fewer calories than are utilized by the patient. In addition to the quantitative caloric aspects, the qualitative aspects of the diet are also important: protein, carbohydrate, fat, salt, and vitamin content.

In general, there are several degrees of calorie restriction that may be used in dietary therapy (Table 2).

1. "Common sense" reduction in calories. Here, no specific count of calories is made, but the patient merely eliminates or reduces from his usual diet, on a "common sense" basis, obviously high caloric foods, particularly those high in carbohydrate and fat content. While not a quantitatively exact diet, this is a rational approach to therapy in which the patient learns to eat fewer calories in a diet which is familiar and usual for him. This may be effective in weight reduction for the mildly overweight person whose obesity began in middle or late life.

2. 1000 calorie deficit. In this diet the number of calories required by the patient for daily living (basal caloric requirement plus the calories necessary for daily activity) is determined, and 1000 calories subtracted from this figure. For an active young man this may represent a reducing diet of 1500 to 2000 total calories a day or more, and for a woman, from 1200 to 1500 total calories. In this diet, there is a deficit of 1000 calories a day or 7000 calories per week, resulting in a theoretical weight loss of about 2 pounds during this time provided that the activity pattern is unchanged. A weight loss of 1 to 2 pounds a week is an ideal rate of reduction, and avoids the weakness that sometimes occurs with more rapid loss of weight.

3. 1000 to 1200 calorie diet. This is just a stricter reduction in calories than in (2), and while it is quite satisfactory and effective for the middle-aged or elderly patient who is relatively inactive, it may not be as acceptable to the active young working patient, because the weakness which sometimes occurs with this diet may prevent necessary daily activities from being carried out.

4. Intermittent fasting. In this form of therapy of total caloric restriction popularized by Duncan,[10] the patient is fasted for 1 to 2 days a week, or for a 7 to 14 day period while in a hospital under the supervision of a physician experienced in this therapy. A period longer than 7 to 14 days should not be used, and even this period of fasting should be reserved for the severely and intractably obese patient for whom the other more conservative programs have not been successful. It should be noted, however, that the fast is well tolerated and accepted by the patient, who

Table 2. *Dietary Therapy. Control of Calorie Intake*

1. "Common sense" reduction
2. 1000 calorie deficit
3. 1000 to 1200 calorie total
4. Fasting

is actually anorexic and euphoric during the absolute fast and does have the great psychological advantage of the rapid induction of weight loss.

The fact that most of this weight loss is, in fact, water and lean body tissue rather than adipose tissue, as several studies have indicated,[1,2,6] is important to recognize, and certainly detracts from the physiologic effectiveness of the diet. Also, side-effects do occur, some serious, and there are definite contraindications to the use of this therapy (pregnancy, labile diabetes, liver disease, etc.).

As regards the qualitative aspects of the diet, the following are important points for the physician to keep in mind.

The composition of the diet should be planned to allow sufficient protein content (at least 1 gm. per kg. of body weight in the adult), and adequate carbohydrate content; finally, the amount of fat is added to make up the desired final caloric content. The different foods (i.e., protein, carbohydrate, and fat) are completely interchangeable on the basis of 4 calories per gram of protein and carbohydrate and 9 calories per gram of fat, and with the exception of the points listed below there is no advantage in terms of weight reduction in altering the usual distribution of calories in the diet.

It has been observed that carbohydrate ingestion is associated with the retention of salt and water to a greater degree than with protein or fat, and that a sodium diuresis may occur with carbohydrate restriction.[4] Also, protein is said to have a "high satiety value" and does have a higher specific dynamic action than the other foods. From these points, it might be argued that a diet somewhat higher in protein and lower in carbohydrate would be more effective in inducing weight loss. In the practical planning of meals, the diabetic exchange lists may be of great help to the physician and patient in the conversion of calories to actual food equivalents in the diet.

The spacing of meals has been shown to affect the metabolic influence of the diet on body composition in animal experiments.[8] If animals that usually feed by continuous nibbling during the day are forced to ingest the same number of calories in one or two large meals they will become obese, despite the fact that the number of calories ingested is the same in both instances. This has not been demonstrated to occur in patients, and the rate of weight loss is the same whether the reducing diet is consumed in three meals a day or six small frequent feedings, provided that the total number of calories is the same.

Activity

Activity is a very important part of any therapeutic program for the obese patient. As previously noted, studies have shown that obese children and adults are less active than their lean counterparts and that this inactivity does play a significant role in their positive caloric or energy balance. Further, because a good deal of energy is expended in moving the heavier obese body, a significant loss of energy can be induced by encouraging increased physical activity in the obese patient. This increase in activity can be in the form of brisk walking or engaging in sports such as swimming, golf, or tennis, but it should be emphasized that any program of activity should begin with a small increase over the usual activity pattern and a gradual progressive increase to the desired amount. The activity should be a regular, habitual event, occurring daily at the same time.

Salt and Water Metabolism

It is well known that obese patients following a reducing diet will gain and lose weight on an irregular basis, at times having no apparent relation to caloric balance. This forms the basis of the frequent complaint of the patient who faithfully follows the reducing diet but despite this either fails to lose or actually gains weight. These discrepancies are due to gains or losses of salt and water and are related to the metabolism of sodium in the obese patient.

The tendency to sodium retention in the obese patient can be dealt with by the physician in several ways. First, the restriction of sodium in the diet and reduction in carbohydrate intake may result in sodium and water diuresis and weight loss. Secondly, if necessary, a diuretic agent may be used to promote this diuresis and weight loss. The influence of sodium and water metabolism on the response to dietary therapy in the obese individual is emphasized again, principally because of the psychological effect on the patient. In terms of the goal of therapy, the loss of excess adipose tissue, these fluctuations in weight due to fluid gains and losses have no real importance. What is important in the therapy of obesity is the reduction of excess adipose tissue and weight loss due to this.

Miscellaneous Therapy

Little will be said here about the role of drugs in the therapy of obesity, because they certainly play a secondary role in management. The anorexigenic agents (derivatives of amphetamine) do have a temporary appetite-suppressing effect, but this effect abates over several weeks as tolerance to the drugs develops. While they can be helpful in some patients in curbing the appetite, they are not usually major determinants in the success or failure of any program. Also, they have side-effects which may be quite significant, particularly in the obese patient.

Diuretic agents have been alluded to previously and may be of psychological value in promoting a salt and water diuresis with resulting weight loss in a patient who has failed to lose weight while following the calorically restricted diet. It would be much better, however, first to attempt dietary sodium restriction for this effect before prescribing a drug. Tranquilizing agents have been used to aid an emotional patient in coping with anxiety that may promote excessive eating or anxiety associated with dietary restriction, but frequent visits to a supportive and understanding physician may be more effective than a drug in these instances. Needless to say, the thyroid analogues have no role in the therapy of obesity unless, of course, the patient is hypothyroid.

Surgery for obesity, in the form of intestinal shunt operations, has been performed with a resulting loss of weight. This is obviously a drastic form of therapy with significant morbidity and possible mortality, and one yet to be evaluated adequately. It should be limited to those medical centers in which there is experience and in which studies are being undertaken to evaluate its effectiveness, and to those patients with extreme degrees of obesity, intractable to medical therapy, in whom obesity is a serious hazard to health.

EFFECT OF MANAGEMENT AND ROLE OF THE PHYSICIAN

The goal in the management of the obese patient is the loss of excess adipose tissue and the return of body weight to the level desirable for that patient. The real effectiveness of any therapeutic program for obesity, however, should be measured with regard to the long-term maintenance of any weight reduction and not the achievement of a temporary loss of weight, followed, all too often, by a relapse in a short time to the former state of obesity.

Regardless of the form of therapy used in obesity, the results of treatment have been relatively poor, particularly as regards the long-term maintenance of weight reduction. The effectiveness of self-help groups (TOPS, Weight Watchers) appears to be as good as the record of many physicians in dealing with this problem.

Although the overall prognosis for successful management is not good, certain general guidelines can be used to predict the response of the individual patient (Table 3). Those patients whose obesity had its onset in childhood, those with extreme degrees of obesity, those with serious psychological problems, and those who are poorly motivated in terms of following a therapeutic program will generally not respond well to therapy; those with the onset of obesity of middle and late life, those with mild degrees of obesity, those in whom no significant emotional problems exist, and those who have good motivation are more likely to lose weight and maintain the reduced weight as a result of management.

In any case, the role of the physician should be that of helping the patient to achieve weight reduction with a therapeutic program in keeping with the magnitude of the medical problem. Although the effects of obesity have been emphasized, there are those physicians who are not so convinced of the ill effects of mild to moderate degrees of obesity.[12]

In the vast majority of instances, this means that simple and conservative management, consisting of mild to moderate caloric restriction coupled with increased physical activity, will suffice; extreme forms of therapy such as extended periods of fasting and surgery have no place in the management of the usual mildly to moderately obese patient.

Table 3.   *Management of Obesity. Prognostic Factors*

Age of onset
Emotional state of patient
Degree and duration of obesity
Motivation of patient
Past history of response to therapy

As emphasized by a recent editorial,[11] the physician must always keep a clear perspective in the management of the obese patient. We would like to correct a potentially harmful condition but certainly not by accepting a risk of injury to the patient out of proportion to the original medical problem.

SUMMARY

The management of the obese patient is the commonest and one of the most difficult nutritional problems confronting the physician in clinical practice. Obesity is associated with an increased risk of morbidity and mortality which warrants therapeutic attempts at weight reduction.

The fundamental cause of obesity is a positive caloric or energy balance occurring at some time in the patient's life, with the resultant deposition of excess adipose tissue; but the underlying factors leading to this imbalance are complex and differ from patient to patient. The starting point in the management of the obese patient is a thorough medical evaluation, in which an attempt is made to define these underlying causes and, if possible, to correct them.

Management of the overweight patient consists of dietary restriction of calories and a program of increased physical activity in an effort to induce a negative caloric balance with resultant weight loss. Proper attention should be given to fluctuations in salt and water metabolism, which are often the cause of weight changes apparently unexplained by caloric balance. Above all, the physician must exercise discretion in the treatment of the obese patient, avoiding drastic therapeutic programs in the management of the usual mild to moderately overweight patient.

As in many chronic illnesses, the results of the treatment of obesity are often discouraging with frequent relapses even if initial weight reduction is successful. The physician must be prepared for long-term treatment with frequent follow-up visits, in which his role as a supportive and understanding figure will be a major factor in the success of any program.

REFERENCES

1. Ball, M. F., Canary, J. J., and Kyle, L. H.: Comparative effects of caloric restriction and total starvation on body composition in obesity. Ann. Intern. Med., 67:60, 1967.
2. Benoit, F. L., Martin, R. L., and Watten, R. H.: Changes in body composition during weight reduction in obesity. Balance studies comparing effects of fasting and a ketogenic diet. Ann. Intern. Med., 63:604, 1965.
3. Berkowitz, D.: Metabolic changes associated with obesity before and after weight reduction. J.A.M.A., 187:103, 1964.
4. Bloom, N. L., and Azar, G. J.: Similarities of carbohydrate deficiency and fasting. I. Weight loss, electrolyte excretion and fatigue. Arch. Intern. Med., 112:333, 1963.
5. Bloom, W. L., and Eidex, M. F.: Inactivity as a major factor in adult obesity. Metabolism, 16:679, 1967.
6. Bolinger, R. E., Lukert, B. P., Brown, R. W., Gurvara, L., and Steinberg, R.: Metabolic balance of obese subjects during fasting. Arch. Intern. Med., 118:3, 1966.
7. Bortz, W. M.: Metabolic consequences of obesity. Ann. Intern. Med., 71:833, 1969.

8. Cohn, C. J., and Joseph, D.: Role of rate of ingestion of diet on regulation of intermediary metabolism (meal eating vs. nibbling). Metabolism, *9*:492, 1960.
9. Cook, G. H., Bennett, C. A., Norwood, W. D., and Mahaffey, J. A.: Evaluation of skin-fold measurements and weight chart to measure body fat. J.A.M.A., *198*:157, 1966.
10. Duncan, G. G., Jenson, W. K., Fraser, R. I., and Cristofori, F. C.: Correction and control of intractable obesity. Practical application of intermittent periods of total fasting. J.A.M.A., *181*:99, 1962.
11. Editorial: Drastic cures for obesity. Lancet, *1*:1094, 1970.
12. Hollifield, G., and Parson, W.: Corpulence, calories and confusion. *In* Ingelfinger, F. J., Relman, A. S., and Finland, M., eds.: Controversy in Internal Medicine. Philadelphia, W. B. Saunders, 1966, p. 443.
13. Marks, H. H.: Influence of obesity on morbidity and mortality. Bull. New York Acad. Med., *36*:296, 1960.
14. Mayer, J.: Genetic factors in human obesity: Ann. N.Y. Acad. Sci., *131*:412, 1965.

Department of Medicine
University of Miami School of Medicine
P. O. Box 875, Biscayne Annex
Miami, Florida 33152

A Three-Dimensional Program
for the Treatment
of Obesity

Richard B. Stuart†

The University of Michigan, Ann Arbor, Michigan, U.S.A.

Summary—Obesity is seen as a consequence of a positive balance of energy consumed over energy expended. The reduction of obesity is accordingly sought through the reduction in the amount of food eaten coupled with an increase in the rate at which energy is expended. Both the reduction in the rate of eating and the increase in the rate of exercise are sought through management of critical aspects of the environment. Specific recommendations are made for the behavioral treatment of obesity, with the success of the treatment seeming to depend upon the effectiveness with which environmental stimuli are brought under control rather than depending upon motivational or other personal characteristics of the overeater. Pre-test data generated by the use of this procedure, coupled with the results of several recent studies appear to indicate uniquely positive results for the behavioral control of overeating.

WHETHER overweight is determined by gross body weight (Metropolitan Life Insurance Company, 1969) or skin-fold measurement (Seltzer and Mayer, 1965) even when differences in fat as a proportion of body weight are controlled (Durnin and Passmore, undated, p. 137), at least one in five Americans is found to be overweight (United States Public Health Service, undated). The social and economic costs of being overwieght are staggering and are complicated by greatly increased vulnerability to a broad range of physical diseases, including cardiovascular and renal diseases, maturity-onset diabetes, cirrhosis of the liver, and gall bladder diseases, among many others (Mayer, 1968).‡ Despite the history of concern with obesity and the magnitude of the problem, little uncontested knowledge has been accumulated with respect to its etiology and treatment. Mayer (1968) has suggested that genetic factors may contribute to the onset of a small number of cases, while an additional small number of cases can be explained on the basis of injury to the hypothalamus, hormonal imbalance and other threats to normal metabolism. The exact role of genetic and physiological factors has, however, remained a mystery, and there has been little evidence to countermand an early observation by Newburgh and Johnston (1930) that most cases of obesity are:

Portions of this paper were presented at the annual meeting of the American Bariatrics Society, Washington, D.C., November 1969, and at the Fourth Annual Meeting of the Association for the Advancement of Behavior Therapy, Miami, Florida, 6 September, 1970. The author wishes to express his gratitude to Barbara Davis, Judith Braver and Merrilee Oakes who contributed significantly to the development and testing of the approach which is described, and to Lynn Nilles for editorial assistance in the preparation of this manuscript. A more detailed description of the procedures may be found elsewhere (Stuart and Davis, in press).

† Requests for reprints should be sent to Richard B. Stuart, School of Social Work, University of Michigan, 1065 Frieze Building, Ann Arbor, Michigan 48104.

‡ It has been argued that the relationship between obesity and such illnesses as cardiovascular diseases depends in part on the way in which fat is accumulated. For example, "People who become fat on a high carbohydrate, low fat diet are much less prone to develop atherosclerotic and thrombotic complications than those on a high fat diet (Cornell Conferences on Therapy, 1958, p. 87)."

. . . never directly caused by abnormal metabolism but (are) always due to food habits not adjusted to the metabolic requirement—either the ingestion of more food than is normally needed or the failure to reduce the intake in response to a lowered requirement (p. 212).

Therefore most obesities can be attributed to an excess of food intake beyond the demands of energy expenditure, and a major objective in treating obesity is a reduction in the amount of excess food consumed.

Just as there is uncertainty concerning the etiology of obesity, there is great confusion over the role of psychological factors in overeating and its management. Some authors have contributed various useful typologies; for example, Stunkard (1959a) classified eating patterns as night eating, binge eating and eating without satiation, while Hamburger (1951) classified the triggers of excessive eating as either external or intrapsychic. Despite Suczek's (1957) observation that "single psychologic factors may not relate to either degree of obesity or ability to lose weight (p. 201)," other authors have sought to identify specific psychological mechanisms associated with obesity. For example, Conrad (1954) postulates that specific intrapsychic factors, such as efforts to prevent loss of love and to express hostility or efforts to symbolically undergo pregnancy and to ward off sexual temptations, underlie obesity. In a similar vein, while eating has been seen as a means of warding off anxiety (Kaplan and Kaplan, 1957), it has also been seen as a depressive equivalent (Simon, 1963). Furthermore, while writers have suggested that "depression, psychosis . . . suicide (Cappon, 1958, p. 573)" and other stress reactions have accompanied weight loss (Cornell Conferences on Therapy, 1958; Glucksman et al., 1968), other studies have shown that: (a) the so-called "depression" associated with weight loss by some people is actually just a function of lowered energy due to reduced food consumption (Bray, 1969); (b) negative psychological reactions are frequently not found (Cauffman and Pauley, 1961; Mees and Keutzer, 1967); and (c) a reduction in anxiety and depression may actually accompany weight loss (Shipman and Plesset, 1963). Despite this evidence, Bruch's (1954) admonition that treatment of overeating which does not give "psychologic factors . . . due consideration (can lead) at best to a temporary weight reduction (while being) considered dangerous from the point of view of mental health (p. 49)" is still influential in dissuading experimenters and therapists from undertaking parsimonious treatment of overeating.

While the research pertaining to physiological and psychological concomitants of obesity has led to some paradoxical conclusions, Stunkard's (1968) review of environmental factors related to obesity has demonstrated a clear-cut connection between obesity and socioeconomic status, social mobility and ethnic variables. It is interesting to note, however, that where comparative data are available, the differences ascribed to each of these factors are stronger for women than men. One explanation of this sex difference may be that the physical expenditure of energy in work may reduce the tendency toward adiposity of lower class, socially nonmobile men while the women, faced with relative inactivity, may show a more direct effect of high carbohydrate, low protein diets common at lower socioeconomic strata (Select Committee on Nutrition and Human Needs, 1970).

The literature describing the treatment of obesity is dismal and confusing. One authoritative group noted:

. . . most obese patients will not remain in treatment. Of those who do remain in treatment, most will not lose significant poundage, and of those who do lose weight, most will regain it promptly. In a careful follow-up study only 8 per cent of obese patients seen in a nutrition clinic actually maintained a satisfactory weight loss (Cornell Conferences on Therapy, 1958, p. 87).

Failure has been reported following some of the most ambitious and sophisticated treatments (e.g. Mayer, 1968, pp. 1–2; Stunkard and McLaren-Hume, 1959), while success has been claimed for some of the more superficial "diet-clinic"-type approaches (e.g. Franklin and Rynearson, 1960). The role of drugs has been extolled by many writers, while others have cautioned that their side effects strongly contraindicate their use (American Academy of Pediatrics, 1967; Gordon, 1969; Modell, 1960). Fasting has been shown to have a profound effect upon weight loss (e.g. Bortz, 1969; Stokes, 1969), but the results have been shown to be short-lived as the patient is likely to quickly regain lost weight when he leaves the hospital setting (MacCuish et al., 1968). Claims of success have also been advanced for individual and group psychotherapy (e.g. Kornhaber, 1968; Mees and Keutzer, 1967; Stanley et al., 1970; Stunkard et al., 1970; Wagonfield and Wolowitz, 1968) and hypnosis (Hanley, 1967; Kroger, 1970), although these reports are typically not supported by controlled investigation. Finally, positive outcomes have been reported for behavior therapy techniques ranging from token reinforcement (Bernard, 1968), aversion therapy (Mayer and Crisp, 1964) and covert sensitization (Cautela, 1967) through complex contingency management procedures. Illustrative of the latter approaches are the work of Stuart (1967), which has been replicated in controlled studies by Ramsay (1968) and Penick and his associates (Penick et al., 1970), and the work of Harris (1969), which included control-group comparisons in the original research.

It is probably true that behavior therapy has offered greater promise of positive results than any other type of treatment. This paper will present a rationale of and description for the treatment of overeating based upon behavioral principles.

RATIONALE

The treatment of obesity has typically attempted to stress the development of "self-control" by the overeater whose self-control deficit is often regarded as a personal fault. Conceding that behavior modifiers recognize first that self-control is merely the emission of one set of responses designed to alter the probability of occurrence of another set of responses (Bijou and Baer, 1961, p. 81; Ferster, 1965, p. 21; Holland and Skinner, 1961, Chapter 47; Homme, 1965, p. 504), and second, that self-controlling responses are acquired through social learning (e.g. Bandura and Kupers, 1964; Kanfer and Marston, 1963), most behaviorists still appear to regard self-control as a personal virtue and its absence a personal deficit (Stuart, 1971). For example, Cautela (1969, p. 324) is concerned with the individual's ability to manipulate the contingencies of his own behavior while Kanfer (1971) offers among other explanations for the breakdown of self-control "the patient's commitment to change," a presumed index of the patient's degree of motivation, or "the patient's prior skill in use of self-reward or self-punishment responses for changing behavior," a presumed index of the patient's capacity to utilize treatment.

In any event, the relevance of the concept of self-control to the management of overeating may be questioned in the light of many recent studies. The most basic of these is the work of Stunkard (1959b) who demonstrated that in comparison with nonobese subjects, obese subjects are far less likely to report hunger in association with "gastric motility." Thus the cues for hunger experiences of the obese may be tied to external events. Several ingenious studies have contributed to this possibility. First, Schacter and his associates demonstrated that obese subjects are less influenced than nonobese subjects by manipulated fear and deprivation of food (Schacter *et al.*, 1968), while they are more influenced by the time they think it is than by the actual time (Schacter and Gross, 1968). In addition it was shown that when the cues of eating are absent, as on religious fast days, obese subjects are more likely to observe dietary restrictions than nonobese subjects (Schacter, 1968). In a similar vein, Nisbett (1968) and Hashim and Van Itallie (1965) showed that obese subjects are more influenced by the taste of food than are nonobese subjects when the duration of food deprivation is controlled. These varied studies and others suggested that the first of two requirements for the treatment of overeating must stress environmental management rather than self-control because the cues of overeating are environmental rather than intrapersonal.

The second requirement for the management of obesity must be a manipulation of the energy balance—the balance between the consumption of energy as food and the expenditure of energy through exercise. If all of the energy which is derived from the consumed food is expended in exercise, then gross body weight will remain constant. Any excess of food energy consumption over energy expenditure, however, is stored as adiposity at the rate of approximately one pound of body fat for each excessive 3500 kcal (Gordon, 1969, p. 148; Mayer, 1968, p. 158). Weight can therefore be lost through: (1) an increase in the amount of exercise, holding food intake constant; (2) a decrease in the amount of food intake, holding exercise constant; or (3) both an increase in exercise and a decrease in food intake.

It has been well-demonstrated that the rising problem of obesity is associated with decreasing demands for exercise. Mayer (1968) suggested that "inactivity is the most important factor explaining the frequency of 'creeping' overweight in modern societies (p. 821)," while Durnin and Passmore (undated, p. 143) revealed that food intake is typically not adjusted to reduced exercise. Recent evidence adduced by the Agricultural Research Service (1969, pp. 22–24) demonstrated that the diets of young men in higher-income brackets include 20 per cent more kcal than the diets of those with smaller incomes and presumably more physically taxing occupations, and this is most likely to result in some measure of obesity among middle-class males. Increase in the rate of exercise can, however, have a profound effect upon body weight although the amount of exercise necessary is greater than generally expected.* Furthermore, given the fact that an obese person actually expends *less* energy than a nonobese person doing the same amount of work (e.g. a 250-pound man walking 1.5 mph expends 5.34 kcal per min, while a 150-pound man walking at the same rate and carrying a 100-pound load expends 5.75 kcal per min [Bloom and Eidex, 1967, p. 687]), planned programs for exercise are particularly important. In addition to aiding in the management of gross body weight, exercise programs for the thin as well as the obese seem definitely to reduce the risk of certain cardiovascular diseases (Mayer, 1967).

Just as it is important systematically to increase the amount of exercise, so too is it important to reduce the amount of food or change the nature of foods eaten. Mayer (1968) recommends:

* Stuart (unpublished data) asked a group of obese women to estimate the amount of exercise required to work off the weight gain attributable to such common foods as donuts, ice cream sodas and potato chips. Comparing their answers with the estimates based upon Konishi's (1965) figures for a 150-pound man walking at the rate of 3.5 miles per hr (29, 49 and 21 min respectively), they were found to underestimate the true work required by from 200 to 300 per cent.

A balanced diet, containing no less than 14 per cent of protein, no more than 30 per cent of fat (with saturated fats cut down), and the rest carbohydrates (with sucrose—ordinary sugar—cut down to a low level) ... (p. 160).

Apart from its nutritional advantages, it is important to include a substantial amount of protein in the diet because smaller amounts of protein as opposed to carbohydrates produce satiety and because a portion of the caloric content of protein is used in its own metabolism (Gordon, 1969, p. 149), leaving a smaller proportion as a possible contributor to adiposity. Conversely, it is important to reduce the amount of carbohydrates consumed because a higher proportion of its caloric content is available for adiposity, because at least certain carbohydrates—e.g. sucrose (Yudkin, 1969)—are associated with increased incidence of certain cardiovascular diseases to which obese persons are vulnerable, and because "carbohydrate food causes the storage of unusually large amounts of water (Gordon, 1969, p. 148)"—typically a special problem faced by obese individuals.

The foregoing observations lead to several basic considerations for weight reduction programs. First, it is essential to design an environment in which food-relevant cues are conducive to the maximal practice of prudent eating habits. This is required by the fact that overeating among obese persons appears to be under environmental control. Also, training the patient in the techniques of environmental control will probably reduce the gradual loss of therapeutic effect found in certain (e.g. Silverstone and Solomon, 1965) but not all (Penick et al., 1970) other programs. Second, it is essential to plan toward a negative energy balance. In doing this, however, it is essential to avoid exercise or dietary excesses. They are unlikely to be followed, and if they are followed each may result in iatrogenic complications. Excessive exercise might lead to overexertion or serious cardiovascular illness. Unbalanced diets might lead to physiological disease, while insufficient diets might lead to enervation and physiologically produced depression. It is therefore essential to plan gradual weight-loss programs associated with progressive changes in the energy balance, as these are both safer and more likely to meet with success (Wang and Sandoval, 1969, p. 220). The exact determination of these levels must be empirically determined for each patient, beginning with tables of recommended dietary allowance (e.g. Mayer, 1968, pp. 168–169), adjusting these for the amount of exercise, carefully monitoring weight and mood changes as time on the program progresses, and being careful to make certain that the degree of weight loss provides sufficient motivation for the patient to continue using the program.

TREATMENT

Translation of the above rationale into a set of specific treatment procedures sometimes requires an arbitrary selection of intervention alternatives derived from contrary or contradictory conclusions in the basic research literature. For example, while Gordon, (1969) repudiated his earlier contention that a patient's eating several smaller meals each day would necessarily result in greater weight loss than his eating only the three traditional meals, others (e.g. Debry et al., 1968) have shown that with caloric intake held constant patients who eat three meals daily may not only maintain their weight but may actually gain weight, while the same patients dividing their caloric allowance into seven meals lose weight precipitously. As another example, Nisbett and Kanouse (1969) demonstrated that obese food shoppers actually buy less the more deprived of food they are while nonobese shoppers increase their food buying as a function of the extent of food deprivation. In contrast, Stuart (unpublished data) demonstrated that when a group of obese women confined their food shopping to the hours of 3:30–5:00 p.m., they purchased 20 per cent more food than when they postponed their food shopping until 6:30–8:00 p.m. Thus the therapist reading the Gordon and Nisbett studies would have his patients eat three meals and delay their food shopping until they were at least moderately deprived of food, while the therapist familiar with the work of Debry *et al.* and Stuart would do just the reverse. The therapist familiar with both must decide which recommendations to follow, framing his decision as a reversible hypothesis which can be invalidated in response to patient-produced data.

The treatment procedures which have been used in this investigation fall into three broad categories. First, an effort is made to establish firm control over the eating environment. This requires: (a) the elimination or suppression of cues associated with problematic eating while strengthening the cues associated with desirable eating patterns; (b) planned manipulation of the actual response of eating to accelerate desirable elements of the response while decelerating undesirable aspects; and (c) the manipulation of the contingencies associated with problematic and desirable eating patterns. A sample of the procedures used in the service of each of these objectives is presented in Table 1.

TABLE 1. SAMPLE PROCEDURES USED TO STRENGHTHEN APPROPRIATE EATING
AND TO WEAKEN INAPPROPRIATE EATING

Cue elimination	Cue suppression	Cue strengthening
1. Eat in one room only 2. Do nothing while eating 3. Make available proper foods only: (a) shop from a list; (b) shop only after full meal 4. Clear dishes directly into garbage 5. Allow children to take own sweets	1. Have company while eating 2. Prepare and serve small quantities only 3. Eat slowly 4. Save one item from meal to eat later 5. If high-calorie foods are eaten, they must require preparation	1. Keep food, weight chart 2. Use food exchange diet 3. Allow extra money for proper foods 4. Experiment with attractive preparation of diet foods 5. Keep available pictures of desired clothes, list of desirable activities

↓	↓
Reduced strength of undesirable responses	Increase strength of desirable responses
1. Swallow food already in mouth before adding more 2. Eat with utensils 3. Drink as little as possible during meals	1. Introduce planned delays during meal 2. Chew food slowly, thoroughly 3. Concentrate on what is being eaten

↓	↓
Provide decelerating consequences	Provide accelerating consequences
1. Develop means for display of caloric value of food eaten daily, weight changes 2. Arrange to have deviations from program ignored by others except for professionals 3. Arrange to have overeater re-read program when items have not been followed and to write techniques which might have succeeded	1. Develop means for display of caloric value of food eaten daily, weight changes 2. Develop means of providing social feedback for all success by: (a) family; (b) friends; (c) co-workers; (d) other weight losers; and/or (e) professionals 3. Program material and/or social consequences to follow: (a) the attainment of weight loss subgoals; (b) completion of specific daily behavioral control objectives

Second, an effort is made to establish a dietary program for each patient on an individual basis. The first step in the development of a diet is completion by the patient of a self-monitoring food intake form. Because patients frequently claim to exist on unbelievably small quantities of food, only to lose weight rapidly when their diet is regulated at amounts two or three times greater than originally claimed, it is helpful to provide some social monitoring of the use of the monitoring sheets to ensure accuracy. Procedures such as those employed by Powell and Azrin (1968) have proven helpful. When validated eating records have been obtained for a 14-day period, adjustments in food intake can be planned based upon recommended caloric levels, balanced diet planning and adjustments for the level of food intake in light of the patient's exercise. In dietary planning, "food exchange" recommendations are made (Stuart and Davis, 1971) rather than recommendations for specific food choices. In food exchange dieting, foods in each of six food categories (e.g. milk, fruit, meat, etc.) are grouped according to similar caloric levels (e.g. one egg has approximately the same caloric value as one slice of bread). Selections are made according to food exchanges and this greatly increases the ease and precision of meal planning. Furthermore, when this is done as a means of increasing the probability that the diet will be followed, the unavailability of specific foods frequently leads to a termination of the entire dietary program.

Third, an effort is made to develop an individualized aerobics exercise program based upon walking in most cases (Cooper, 1968). In introducing the need for exercise, the patient is offered a choice between adherence to a punishing diet which may lead to chronic discomfort throughout the day and a more permissive diet coupled with exercise which may lead to discomfort for an hour or less per day. When an exercise program is developed, an effort is made to weave the exercise activity into the normal fabric of the patient's day to increase the likelihood that it will be followed. For example, a patient might be asked to park his car 10 blocks from the home of friends he is about to visit, to avoid elevators and walk up to his destinations, and to carry each item upstairs as needed—rather than allowing several items to accumulate—as a means of increasing the number of steps necessary.

RESULTS

The pilot investigation reported here reflects the treatment of six overweight, married, middle-class women (171–212 pounds) between the ages of 27 and 41. Each woman requested treatment on a self-referred basis. Treatment was offered on an individual basis, but women were randomly assigned to one of two cohorts. Both groups of three patients were asked to complete the Sixteen Personality Factor Questionnaire (Cattell and Eber, 1967) and to keep a 5-week baseline of their weight and food intake. The first group was then offered treatment twice weekly (average 40 min per session) for a 15-week period, while the second group was asked to practice "self-control" of eating behavior. The self-control subjects were given the same diet planning materials and exercise program that the treatment group was offered. They were not, however, given instruction for the management of food in the environment. At the conclusion of the 15-week period, the treated group was asked to continue the treatment program and the second group was offered 15 weeks of the same treatment. Approximately 6 months following the termination of treatment of Group 1 and 3 months following the termination of treatment of Group 2, follow-up data were collected including weight, eating patterns and the readministration of the Cattell 16 P.F. The results including follow-up data are presented in Fig. 1. It will be seen that patients in Group 1 lost an average of 35 pounds while those in Group 2 lost an average of 21 pounds. These results are consistent with the objective set for gradual weight loss approximating one pound per week. It will also be seen that the mere collection of baseline self-monitoring data was associated with mild weight loss in both groups, although these gains were dissipated as time progressed for the second group. Finally, comparison of the pre- and post-test personality test results reveal little change other than small improvement in "ego stability" and tension (Factors C and Q4) of the 16 P.F.

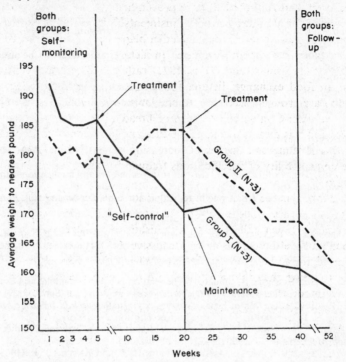

FIG. 1. Weight changes in two groups of women undergoing behavior therapy for overeating.

The results provide suggestive evidence for the usefulness of a threefold treatment of obesity stressing environmental control of overeating, nutritional planning and regulated increase in energy expenditure. The sample size was too small to permit generalization, and the superiority of the initially treated (Group 1) over the initially untreated (Group 2) patients may be due to an inclination among the latter group to be casual about weight reduction. To forestall this possibility, every effort was made to make the treatment appear "official" but no validation of the success of this effort was undertaken. Furthermore, it is perhaps noteworthy that the results were obtained with no evidence of psychological stress in a patient population which was regarded as "well-adjusted" at the start and termination of treatment.

To validate these procedures in any definitive manner, extensive replication is needed using careful experimental control procedures applied to a far more diverse population than was used in this pilot study. Research such as that recently completed by Penick *et al.* (1970) has made important strides in this direction. It is only through such experimentation that the vast amount of "faddism and quackery (Gordon ,1969, p. 148)" which characterizes the broad field of obesity control can be replaced by a scientifically validated set of procedures.

REFERENCES

AGRICULTURAL RESEARCH SERVICE, U.S. DEPARTMENT OF AGRICULTURE (1969) *Food Intake and Nutritive Value of Diets of Men, Women and Children in the United States, Spring* 1965: *A Preliminary Report.* (ARS 62-18), Washington, D.C.: United States Government Printing Office.

AMERICAN ACADEMY OF PEDIATRICS, COMMITTEE ON NUTRITION (1967) Obesity in childhood. *Pediatrics* **40**, 455–465.

BANDURA A. and KUPERS C. J. (1964) Transmission of patterns of self-reinforcement through modeling. *J. abnorm. soc. Psychol.* **69**, 1–9.

BERNARD J. L. (1968) Rapid treatment of gross obesity by operant techniques. *Psychol. Rep.* **23**, 663–666.

BIJOU S. W. and BAER D. M. (1961) *Child Development I: A Systematic and Empirical Theory.* Appleton-Century-Crofts, New York.

BLOOM W. L. and EIDEX M. F. (1967) The comparison of energy expenditure in the obese and lean. *Metabolism* **16**, 685–692.

BORTZ W. (1969) A 500 pound weight loss. *Am. J. Med.* **47**, 325–331.

BRAY G. A. (1969) Effect of caloric restriction on energy expenditure in obese patients. *Lancet* **2**, 397–398.

BRUCH H. (1954) The psychosomatic aspects of obesity. *Am. Practnr Dig. Treat.* **5**, 48–49.

CAPPON D. (1958) Obesity. *Can. Med. Assoc. Jl* **79**, 568–573.

CATTELL R. B. and EBER H. W. (1957) *Handbook for the Sixteen Personality Factor Questionnaire.* The Institute for Personality and Ability Testing, Champaign, Ill.

CAUFFMAN W. J. and PAULEY W. G. (1961) Obesity and emotional status. *Penn. Med. Jl* **64**, 505–507.

CAUTELA J. R. (1967) Covert sensitization. *Psychol. Rep.* **20**, 459–468.

CAUTELA J. R. (1969) Behavior therapy and self-control: Techniques and implications. In *Behavior Therapy: Appraisal and Status* (Ed. C. M. FRANKS). McGraw-Hill, New York.

CONRAD S. W. (1954) The problem of weight reduction in the obese woman. *Am. Practnr. Dig. Treat.* **5**, 38–47.

COOPER K. H. (1968) *Aerobics.* Bantam Books, New York.

CORNELL CONFERENCES ON THERAPY (1958) The management of obesity. *N. Y. S. J. Med.* **58**, 79–87.

DEBRY G., ROHR R., AZOUAOU G., VASSILITCH I. and MOTTAZ G. (1968) Study of the effect of dividing the daily caloric intake into seven meals on weight loss in obese subjects. *Nutritio Dieta* **10**, 288–296.

DURNIN J. V. G. A. and PASSMORE R. (undated) The relation between the intake and expenditure of energy and body weight. *Problemes Actuels D'Endocrinologie et de Nutrition* (Serie No. 9), 136–149.

FERSTER C. B. (1965) Classification of behavior pathology. In *Research in Behavior Modification* (Eds. L KRASNER and L. P. ULLMANN). Holt, Rinehart & Winston, New York.

FRANKLIN R. E. and RYNEARSON E. H. (1960) An evaluation of the effectiveness of diet instruction for the obese. *Staff Meet. Mayo Clin.* **35**, 123–124.

GLUCKSMAN M. L., HIRSCH J., McCULLY R. S., BARRON B. A. and KNITTLE J. L. (1968) The response of obese patients to weight reduction: A quantitative evaluation of behavior. *Psychosom. Med.* **30**, 359–373.

GORDON E. S. (1969) The present concept of obesity: Etiological factors and treatment. *Med. Times* **97**, 142–155.

HAMBURGER W. W. (1951) Emotional aspects of obesity. *Med. Clin. N. Am.* **35**, 483–499.

HANLEY F. W. (1967) The treatment of obesity by individual and group hypnosis. *Can. Psychiat. Ass. J.* **12**, 549–551.

HARRIS M. B. (1969) Self-directed program for weight control—A pilot study, *J. abnorm. Psychol.* **74**, 263–270.

HASHIM S. A. and VAN ITALLIE T. B. (1965) Studies in normal and obese subjects with a monitored food dispensary device. *Ann. N. Y. Acad. Sci.* **131**, 654–661.

HOLLAND J. G. and SKINNER B. F. (1961) *The Analysis of Behavior.* McGraw-Hill, New York.

HOMME L. E. (1965) Perspectives in psychology: XXIV. Control of coverants, the operants of the mind. *Psychol. Rec.* **15**, 501–511.

KANFER F. H. (1971) Self-monitoring: Methodological limitations and clinical applications. *J. consult. clin. Psychol.* in press.

KANFER F. H. and MARSTON A. R. (1963) Conditioning of self-reinforcement responses: An analogue to self-confidence training. *Psychol. Rep.* **13**, 63–70.

KAPLAN H. I. and KAPLAN H. S. (1957) The psychosomatic concept of obesity. *J. nerv. ment. Dis.* **125**, 181–201.

KONISHI F. (1965) Food energy equivalents of various activities. *J. Am. Diet. Ass.* **46**, 186–188.

KORNHABER A. (1968) Group treatment of obesity. *G.P.* **5**, 116–120.

KROGER W. S. (1970) Comprehensive management of obesity. *Am. J. clin. Hypnosis* **12**, 165–176.

MACCUISH A. C., MUNRO J. F. and DUNCAN L. J. P. (1968) Follow-up study of refractory obesity treated by fasting. *Br. Med. J.* **1**, 91–92.

MAYER J. (1967) Inactivity, an etiological factor in obesity and heart disease. In *Symposia of the Swedish Nutrition Foundation, V: Symposium on Nutrition and Physical Activity* (Ed. G. BLIX). Almqvist & Wiksells, Uppsala, Sweden.

MAYER J. (1968) *Overweight: Causes, Cost and Control*. Prentice-Hall, Englewood Cliffs, N.J.

MEES H. L. and KEUTZER C. S. (1967) Short term group psychotherapy with obese women. *NW Med.* **66**, 548–550.

METROPOLITAN INSURANCE COMPANY (1969) New weight standards for men and women. *Statistical Bulletin* **40**, 1–8.

MEYER V. and CRISP A. H. (1964) Aversion therapy in two cases of obesity. *Behav. Res. & Therapy* **2**, 143–147.

MODELL W. (1960) Status and prospect of drugs for overeating. *J. Am. Med. Ass.* **173**, 1131–1136.

NEWBURGH L. H. and JOHNSTON M. W. (1930) The nature of obesity. *J. clin. Invest.* **8**, 197–213.

NISBETT R. E. (1968) Taste, deprivation, and weight determinants of eating behavior. *J. person. soc. Psychol.* **10**, 107–116.

NISBETT R. E. and KANOUSE D. E. (1969) Obesity, food deprivation, and supermarket shopping behavior. *J. person. soc. Psychol.* **12**, 289–294.

PENICK S. B., FILION R., FOX S. and STUNKARD A. (1970) Behavior modification in the treatment of obesity. Paper presented at the annual meeting of the Psychosomatic Society, Washington, D.C.

POWELL J. and AZRIN N. (1968) The effects of shock as a punisher for cigarette smoking. *J. appl. Behav. Anal.* **1**, 63–71.

RAMSAY R. W. (1968) Vermageringsexperiment, Psychologisch Labratorium van de Universiteit van Amsterdam, *Researchpracticum* **101**, voorjaar 1968.

SCHACHTER S. (1968) Obesity and eating. *Science* **161**, 751–756.

SCHACHTER S., GOLDMAN R. and GORDON A. (1968) Effects of fear, food deprivation, and obesity on eating. *J. person. soc. Psychol.* **10**, 91–97.

SCHACHTER S. and GROSS L. P. (1968) Manipulated time and eating behavior. *J. person. soc. Psychol.* **10**, 98–106.

SELTZER C. C. and MAYER J. (1965) A simple criterion of obesity. *Postgrad. Med.* **38**, A101–A106.

SHIPMAN W. G. and PLESSET M. R. (1963) Anxiety and depression in obese dieters. *Archs gen. Psychiat.* **8**, 26–31.

SILVERSTONE J. T. and SOLOMON T. (1965) The long-term management of obesity in general practice. *Br. J. clin. Pract.* **19**, 395–398.

SIMON R. I. (1963) Obesity as a depressive equivalent. *J. Am. Med. Ass.* **183**, 208–210.

STANLEY E. J., GLASER H. H., LEVIN D. G., ADAMS P. A. and COOLEY I. C. (1970) Overcoming obesity in adolescents: A description of a promising endeavour to improve management. *Clin. Pediat.* **9**, 29–36.

STOKES S. A. (1969) Fasting for obesity. *Am. J. Nurs.* **69**, 796–799.

STUART R. B. (1967) Behavioral control of overeating. *Behav. Res. & Therapy* **5**, 357–365.

STUART R. B. (1971) Situational versus self control. In *Advances in Behavior Therapy* (Ed. R. D. RUBIN). Academic Press, New York, in press.

STUART R. B. and DAVIS B. (1971) *Behavioral Techniques for the Management of Obesity*. Research Press, Champaign, Ill., in press.

STUNKARD A. (1959a) Eating patterns and obesity. *Psychiat. Q.* **33**, 284–295.

STUNKARD A. (1959b) Obesity and the denial of hunger. *Psychosom. Med.* **21**, 281–289.

STUNKARD A. (1968) Environment and obesity: Recent advances in our understanding of regulation of food intake in man. *Fed. Proc.* **6**, 1367–1373.

STUNKARD A., LEVINE H. and FOX S. (1970) The management of obesity. *Archs intern. Med.* **125**, 1067–1072.

STUNKARD A. and MCLAREN-HUME M. (1959) The results of treatment for obesity. *Archs intern. Med.* **103**, 79–85.

SUCZEK R. F. (1957) The personality of obese women. *Am. J. Clin. Nutr.* **5**, 197–202.

UNITED STATES PUBLIC HEALTH SERVICE (undated) *Obesity and Health*. (Publication No. 1495), United States Department of Health, Education and Welfare, Washington, D.C.

UNITED STATES SENATE, SELECT COMMITTEE ON NUTRITION AND HUMAN NEEDS (1970) *Nutrition and Human Needs*—1970. Parts I, II & III. U.S. Government Printing Office, Washington, D.C.

WAGONFIELD S. and WOLOWITZ H. M. (1968) Obesity and self-help group: A look at TOPS. *Am. J. Psychiat.* **125**, 253–255.

WANG R. I. H. and SANDOVAL R. (1969) Current status of drug therapy in management of obesity. *Wis. Med. J.* **68**, 219–220.

YUDKIN J. (Spring, 1969) Sucrose and heart disease. *Nutrition Today* **4**, 16–20.

Treating obesity: three approache

Conflicting views on the management of obesity abound, even among physicians who treat it. Most agree that the problem is a complex one and that low-calorie diets alone do not provide a long-range solution. For this In Consultation article, MWN has recruited three experts with divergent opinions. If they share a common theme, it is simply this: To lose weight and not regain it, the obese patient has to change some of his basic living habits.

Dr. James B. Sidbury is professor of pediatrics and director of the clinical research unit at Duke University in Durham, N. C. Dr. Robert J. Westlake is assistant professor of clinical psychiatry at the University of Pennsylvania and director of the psychiatric inpatient service at the Hospital of the University of Pennsylvania in Philadelphia. Dr. George V. Mann is associate professor of biochemistry and medicine at Vanderbilt University in Nashville, Tenn., and a Career Investigator for the National Heart and Lung Institute.

As a pediatrician, Dr. Sidbury gets first crack at treating obesity. His program is based on a low-calorie diet, but it also relies heavily on family cooperation and re-education:

Q. How do you involve the family in your program?

Dr. Sidbury: Initially, we bring the child into the hospital for four days. On the first we do a glucose tolerance test and other chemistries. Then the child fasts until the urine begins to show ketones. At this point we put him on a high-protein diet of about 300 calories and send him to physiotherapy for vigorous exercise, which speeds the development of ketosis.

The effect is to depress the child's appetite, and the parents are astonished when they see a child who has been stuffing at home actually turn away food in the hospital. The hospital period also allows time for the dietician to indoctrinate the mother about the diet and food equivalents. We explain, too, the importance of maintaining ketosis after the child goes home, and instruct the mother to do a daily dipstick test for ketones in the urine.

When the other members of the family are fat, as is often the case, we convince them that it would be much easier for the patient if everyone would diet with him. Then we can set up a family program and the mother can prepare one meal for the group with the amounts adjusted for age and activity level. The initial cost of the family program is more than compensated for by the savings in food that result, which is a big factor in

these days of high medical costs.

Q. How long do you maintain the child on the high-protein diet?

Dr. Sidbury: For the first three or four months. We want to reduce carbohydrates because obese individuals tend to release excessive amounts of insulin in the presence of carbohydrates. These high blood levels of insulin drive the carbohydrates into the adipose tissue, and also inhibit the release of fat from adipose cells. Maintaining some degree of ketonemia seems to decrease the efficiency of in-

sulin and allow for mobilization of fat from adipose deposits.

Q. Do you have problems with maintaining ketonemia once the child goes home?

Dr. Sidbury: Both the child and the mother understand that if the ketones disappear from the urine the child has to fast until they return. We don't call this punishment, but the child soon learns that fasting is the direct consequence of cheating on his diet.

Q. Do you require children to exercise after they leave the hospital?

Dr. Sidbury: Yes. We urge them to walk or bicycle. We have the mothers make weighted belts—five pounds of sand in four pockets—and ask the child to wear these while climbing up and down stairs for 15 or 20 minutes a day. A child can do this on a rainy or snowy day.

Q. Can the child resume a normal diet after four months?

Dr. Sidbury: As his weight approaches normal, we do liberalize the diet more and more. The deprivation diet may be needed for as long as six

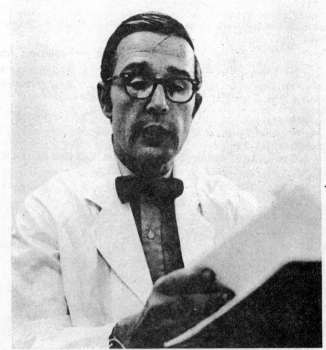

Dr. Sidbury involves family in measuring ketones as child is maintained on low-calorie diet for four months or so, and then in monitoring intake afterward.

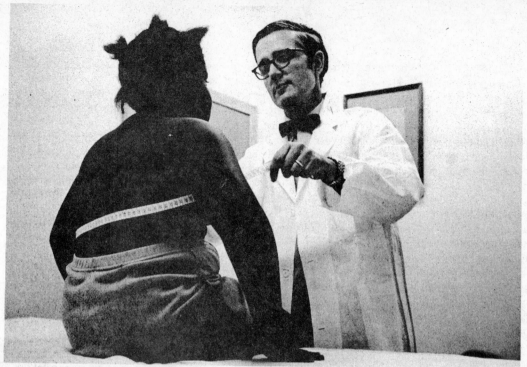

Children in the program often lose chest and abdominal girth before losing pounds, and the Duke pediatrician explains to them that muscle mass is replacing fat as they exercise.

months, though. Then the things we stress most for the long term are a reduction in carbohydrate intake and control of total calories.

Q. Do you impose any other dietary restrictions?
Dr. Sidbury: We avoid table salt. The body retains water in retaining salt, and the child gets discouraged because he thinks he's not losing weight.

Q. How do you measure weight loss in children?
Dr. Sidbury: In addition to the loss in pounds, we measure the loss in chest and abdominal circumference. Frequently, children lose in these two measurements before they've actually lost much weight; so this is one way we can give them encouragement. And we explain to them that when they begin to exercise they build up muscle mass at the expense of fat tissue and that this is not necessarily reflected in an immediate loss of weight.

Q. What about eating between meals?
Dr. Sidbury: *Verboten.* Everybody in the family has to give up snacks. No cookies, no soft drinks. We do allow room for some exchanges so that the child doesn't feel left out of things his friends are doing. For instance, if the rest of the kids are having ice cream, the dieter can have some sherbet—remembering that the sherbet counts as

a part of the day's total food.

Q. Do you think TV advertising of snacks, etc., affects obese children?
Dr. Sidbury: Yes. I didn't realize this, not being food-oriented. With me it goes in one ear and out the other. But for children on diets, it's pure agony, and particularly for adolescents. They say they have to stop looking at TV until they get into equilibrium.

Q. What about holiday eating?
Dr. Sidbury: If the family has bought our method they'll feel guilty about overeating. But we don't want to take away all their pleasures. So, if they break out at Thanksgiving, we tell them to fast afterward and catch up.

Q. How long have you followed up patients who have lost weight on this regimen and what has your success rate been?
Dr. Sidbury: Follow-up has been about 18 months to two years and our success rate has been about the same as you get with any other formal treatment. But failures have been due to poor compliance at home. In the six-to-eight-year-old group—children with whom we had uniform failure before—we now get successes in the neighborhood of 80%. And I think the rate will go up as more family members are involved.

In children with incipient Pickwickian syndrome, alertness increases and attention span improves. One boy's IQ went from 110 to 121

during the year and he got an award for making the greatest improvement in school. His personality is completely changed; he's on the move all the time, where before he literally had to sit because he couldn't move. His whole attitude toward life has changed, and that's very gratifying.

Q. Do you ever prescribe amphetamines?
Dr. Sidbury: No. The long-range results are poor and some experimental evidence is developing to suggest that the ill effects are far-reaching. If parents ask for amphetamines, we explain that we don't want to encourage the child to join the drug culture—and that usually settles the question.

Q. Is your regimen adaptable for use by the family physician?
Dr. Sidbury: Absolutely. It's the simplest regimen you could use, the problems are minimal, and very little physician time is required. A nurse could see these people on a weekly basis to take blood pressure, make measurements, check on diets, and answer dietary questions. All that's needed is a trained supervisor who cares.

Q. Do you think obesity in children could be prevented?
Dr. Sidbury: Yes, in large part. But it means re-educating parents through the family physician, the pediatrician, and the public health nurse. We have to get away from the idea that the chubby baby is the healthy baby;

it's the well-proportioned baby we should aim for. Instead of allowing a baby to develop "baby fat" it would be much wiser to reduce the fat intake and switch them early from animal fats to unsaturated fats. You can do this very easily by changing over from cow's milk to skimmed milk or a commercial formula.

At the University of Pennsylvania Hospital, Dr. Westlake sees obesity that has become well entrenched. "Our people have been to many doctors, followed many diets, and lost and gained thousands of pounds collectively," he says. Working with Dr. Leonard S. Levitz, an instructor in psychiatry and co-director of the hospital's day treatment center, Dr. Westlake is applying an approach based on behavioral psychology:

Q. What is behavioral therapy and how do you use it in the treatment of obesity?
Dr. Westlake: It's a new branch of psychiatric treatment based on learning psychology evolved from the work of Pavlov, Skinner, and other theorists. It applies rewards for proper behavior and, in some instances, punishments to extinguish undesirable behavior. One of its principles is that any behavior you regularly repeat is probably rewarding to you. The application to eating is very important because eating behavior is learned, and maladaptive aspects of eating behavior can therefore be unlearned.

Basically, the eating problem is one of too much input and too little expenditure. But in terms of behavior, the varieties and forms of excessive input are endless. Eating too fast is one of these maladaptive patterns. When you eat, a certain amount of time must elapse before the feeling of satiety sets in. If you eat too rapidly, you're liable to take in too many calories before your satiety mechanism has time to tell you, "Hey, that's enough!" That many meals take no more than five or ten minutes may not matter to the normal-weight person, but for the obese person it means trouble.

Q. What type of patient benefits from behavioral therapy?

Dr. Westlake: Behavior modification in obesity can be used with almost any patient because its principles are simple and basic. However, patients who are intrigued by the idea of a learning approach usually do best in our program. Some obese people have a psychological set in their lives that says, "I want something suddenly and I want it done *for* me." These patients often do less well. But even this attitude can shift during the program, as a patient experiences success and becomes self-motivated.

Q. How is this therapy conducted?
Dr. Westlake: Patients meet in groups of about ten once a week for ten weeks. We take both men and women and include all ages from late adolescence up through the fifties. We have scheduled two programs: One runs for a full six hours and includes a lunch prepared by the patients; the second, designed primarily to meet the needs of students and businessmen, takes only one afternoon a week.

Q. What happens during the sessions?
Dr. Westlake: First, each patient is weighed privately. There's no public embarrassment, no public discussion of their weight. Then a nurse and a mental health worker or a nutritionist meet with the group and discuss various issues—nutrition, caloric content of foods, spacing of meals, etc. During that time, I and my associate, Dr. Levitz, go over the daily food intake records compiled by each patient during the week. Next, we have a formal session on behavior modification; in each session we introduce two or three new behavioral techniques. During the afternoon the patients exchange their food records for review and comment. At the end, each patient gets his record back, along with a written comment from me and from one group member.

Q. What behavioral techniques are discussed?
Dr. Westlake: One is cue elimination. For the obese, many things have become cues to start eating. For example, a lot of people eat while they're watching television. If you

pair eating with TV long enough, when you sit down to watch you're going to feel like eating. But that's an inappropriate cue; it's got nothing to do with hunger or the state of your nutrition. We try to reduce the number of cues by suggesting that the patient eat in only one place. We ask them to pick a place at home that's comfortable—their kitchen or dining room—and stick to that.

In our full-day sessions that include lunch we practice many of the things

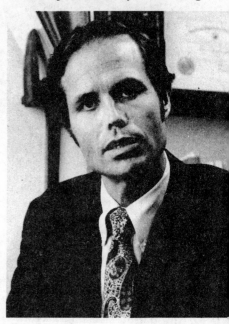

Fast eaters take in extra calories before satiety catches up
—Dr. Westlake

we teach: slowing the pace of eating; planning a pause during the meal; never preparing the next bite while you're eating the last; never having anything in your mouth while you have something on your fork; putting the fork down between bites. Everybody has been taught by his parents to clean his plate because of all the people starving in the world; we've learned that so thoroughly that a clean plate has become the cue for the end of a meal. We try to introduce the opposite notion—that the end of a meal is signaled by some food left on the plate. We ask people to select a small portion of something they like, set it aside at the beginning of the meal, and leave it there. That's hard to do, and even staff members take forever to learn it, but eventually it becomes a habit.

We limit our lunches to 300 calories and try to show that eating only that much can be an interesting experience. We've compiled a booklet of "gourmet" recipes used by patients in preparing these lunches.

Q. Are all the behavioral techniques related to eating habits?
Dr. Westlake: Most of them are, but we also stress habits related to activity. We try to help the patient re-program his usual activities so that he uses more energy in what he does. For example, instead of looking for the parking space nearest to where he's going, we try to get him to park farther away and do some walking.

Q. Do you use group pressure to shame or punish transgressors?
Dr. Westlake: We've discussed that with our patients, and our conclusion has been that if embarrassment, punishment, or adversive stimuli—such as warnings about the medical consequences of obesity—could help them, they would have been helped before they came to us. These people have had so much criticism and pressure put on them because of their weight problems that it's more profitable, we think, to use only a positive reward system in our program.

Q. What are these rewards?
Dr. Westlake: There's losing weight, of course, and gaining control over behavior. Also, our people contract with themselves to practice the techniques we have discussed. If they complete one of these successfully, they reward themselves by doing something they enjoy—something unrelated to eating. It may be playing a musical instrument, doing needlepoint, gardening, or any other activity they like but have had to put off for lack of time.

Q. How do the families of patients react to the new regimen?
Dr. Westlake: We've recently introduced a family night—a two-hour session every other week—to which group members are encouraged to bring at least one relative or friend, hopefully someone they eat with. We get great turnouts. The families learn that the problem is behavioral and may involve them all. They become very positive about the program and sometimes these guest observers are even moved to try out some of the techniques themselves.

Q. Has the program been operating long enough for a report on results?
Dr. Westlake: The first University of Pennsylvania program was an experimental one under the direction of Dr. Sydnor Penick. His patients averaged a 20-pound weight loss in ten weeks and almost all those who lost weight maintained the loss. When we started the program on a regular clinical basis, the weight loss also averaged about 20 pounds in ten weeks.

That's not sensational, but we weren't looking for sensational results. We're more concerned about what happens at the end of the program. If behavior has really been modified, the loss should be sustained. Of the patients who completed the program six months ago, almost all have sustained the weight loss and about half have continued to lose.

Compared with other weight-loss programs, that's a very good result.

Q. What method of follow-up do you use?
Dr. Westlake: We hold group sessions of an hour and a half, first at two-week intervals and then at one-month intervals for a year. At these, we review the techniques and look for trouble spots.

Q. What are some of the common trouble spots?
Dr. Westlake: Holidays and social gatherings. We emphasize that there are other things besides eating that families can do together on holidays. Also, we try to get them to preplan what they will eat at social gatherings and restaurants.

Unlike Drs. Sidbury and Westlake, whose programs are designed specifically for the obese, Dr. Mann works with patients who are likely candidates for heart attacks. His approach to prevention is a program for attaining physical fitness through systematic exercise, and he advocates a similar regimen for combating obesity.

Q. Are you suggesting that exercise alone can conquer obesity?
continued

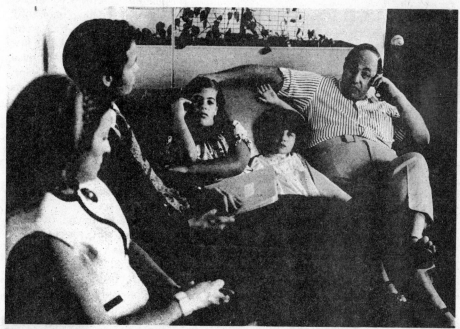

Dr. Westlake (dark suit) employs group sessions in which patients can unlearn 'maladaptive' eating habits and learn new behavior techniques.

Dr. Mann: Many fat people say plaintively to the doctor, "I don't eat as much as my husband and he only weighs 129 pounds." And everybody nods and says to himself, "You're lying in your teeth. It can't be." But it *can* be and probably often is. The difference between lean and fat children is that the lean ones are playing ball, climbing, running, jumping, and the fat ones are sitting under a tree reading a book. It's the difference in expenditure that makes the difference in weight. I think this is the most underrated aspect of obesity.

Q. What is your program for physical conditioning?

Dr. Mann: It includes a series of calisthenics, running, and jogging. The calisthenics are designed for limbering and to strengthen the shoulder-girdle muscles. After a warm-up with calisthenics, our people go out and sprint—up to their predetermined physical limit—and then slow to a walk, and repeat the process. This kind of spurting effort maximizes the effect of training and cuts down the time required for conditioning. The process may take six to ten weeks, at three sessions a week. But once fitness is attained, one can maintain it with as little as two 30-minute sessions a week.

Q. Do you have a method for measuring fitness?

Dr. Mann: For this purpose we use a step-test performed at a constant speed, stepping up to successively higher levels, and continuing until the pulse rate reaches 85% of its predicted maximum, as determined by age-scaled tables. The step-height reached before the pulse rate accelerates to that point is an accurate measure of fitness.

Q. Is this test for use in the physician's office?

Dr. Mann: A patient can do it at home if he knows how to count his pulse, a simple matter to learn. The step apparatus is a handsome-looking piece of furniture that could stand in the living room. If it's raining you could use it as a workout device—in lieu of running in place or doing calisthenics. But the important point here is that

people need to be taught how to quantitate the effects of their exercise, because this is very reinforcive.

Q. Is this type of training suitable for women?

Dr. Mann: Yes. Housewives have been able to follow the same routines as men and make the same rates of progress. Husbands and wives should usually exercise separately, however, to avoid an aggravating competition. Fitness should be thought of as a very personal accomplishment.

Q. Can other types of exercise be substituted for those you outline?

Dr. Mann: Oh, sure. There are almost innumerable possibilities. But we do find that as you become fit you've got to depend more and more on your big running muscles. Three quarters of your muscles are in your calves, thighs, and lower back. So, to get a workout as you become fitter, you've got to bring your major muscles into play. That's what's wrong with most of the health studio programs, with all their emphasis on massaging and vibrating.

Q. Don't obese people have problems with increased appetite as they exercise?

Dr. Mann: Not always, particularly if they're genuinely interested in attaining some goal like improving their appearance. And after all, we're not asking them to diet. We're just asking them to keep as close as possible to what they're eating now. With these daily exercise regimens they expend an additional 500 kcal to 900 kcal a day. If they do that five days a week and don't increase their intake, they'll lose weight.

Q. Do you recommend that an exercise program be supervised by the family physician?

Dr. Mann: He's too busy. In some cases, he's fed up with the fat problem, or he makes a moral judgment on it and in effect throws the patient out at the start. Besides, doctors and nurses don't know about fitness themselves; they need to be taught.

Q. Where is this fitness concept being taught?

Dr. Mann: It isn't. The schools are the ideal place for it, but the teachers' colleges are turning out people indoctrinated with health notions left over from 1910. You know—sleep with your windows open and drink six glasses of water a day. And yet explaining to children the ABCs of calorie balance and how to keep fit is really quite simple. Children—particularly between the ages of ten and 16—are of-

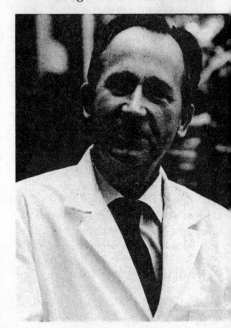

Fat elimination via vibration or massage is an absurd notion
—Dr. Mann

ten preoccupied with health, are often *more* apprehensive about poor health than their parents.

Q. Has the President's Commission on Physical Fitness been useful?

Dr. Mann: It's simply a flop. Commissioners seem to have been appointed on the basis of their public image, not because of any special ability to teach fitness or to communicate health science.

Q. Do you think doctors—and patients—need nutrition training?

Dr. Mann: Yes, but there aren't many good courses or textbooks on the subject. As a result people, even intelligent, educated people, fall into the hands of quacks and food faddists.

Q. What do you think of the various group therapies?
Dr. Mann: They have a place. Groups like Weight Watchers and TOPS are doing a good job. They provide the kind of support people need—a group that *cares* whether you are doing well, or whether you slipped a little this week.

Q. Do you think amphetamines are indicated in treating obesity?
Dr. Mann: Doctors use amphetamines as an escape mechanism to get obese patients off their backs. And they don't work. But it's much easier and much more profitable to give somebody a pill than it is to sit down and spend some time discussing alternative solutions.

Q. What do you think of the use of human chorionic gonadotropin injections in treating obesity?
Dr. Mann: There isn't any valid scientific evidence that that scheme works. Nor do we know anything about the action of the hormone that would lead us to expect it to work.

Q. Is there any valid method of reducing that redistributes body fat?
Dr. Mann: Fat distribution is conditioned by genetics and sex. The notion the health studios perpetuate— that you can eliminate fat by vibration or massage—is absurd. But now that women are throwing away their bras and girdles, they seem to be beginning to accept the idea that bodies come in a variety of shapes. The youngsters, at least, are feeling less hung up about the fact that they don't look like those android females fashion designers seem to like.

Q. Is there ever a problem with nutritional deficiencies resulting from stringent dieting?
Dr. Mann: There is an iron-deficiency problem in women during the reproductive years. These women need 18 mg of iron a day, and to get this amount from the diet one would have to eat 2,500 calories. So, when they cut down to 1,500 calories in a struggle to look like Twiggy, the result is a cohort of starved, iron-deficient women.

Q. Is obesity a factor in causing heart attacks?

Dr. Mann: It becomes a factor, I would say, when a person is 25% or more overweight.

Q. Are there some patients who should not undertake the conditioning program you describe?
Dr. Mann: We turn them down if they have high blood pressure. When they get their blood pressure under control with the standard medications they can start training.

Q. Do you think the current emphasis on unsaturated fats in weight-loss diets will help cut down heart attacks?
Dr. Mann: Despite the American Heart Association's official stand that coronary heart disease is caused by an excess of saturated animal fats, there is no sound basis for this position. The Masai tribesmen of East Africa eat more milk and meat than we do and they have cholesterol levels around 120. They don't get heart attacks, and we think the main reason is that they keep fit. The vegetable oil industry, with some help from science adventurists, has taken the citizenry down the garden path on this unsaturated fat issue. ■

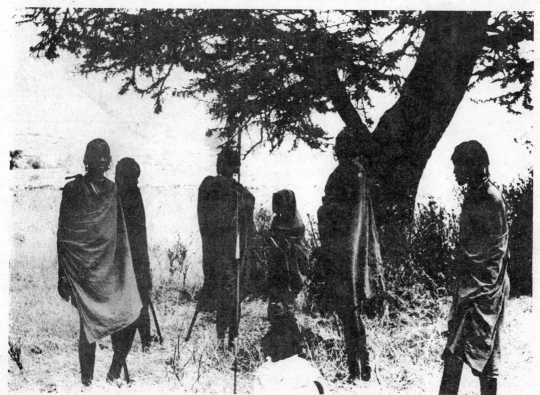

If saturated fats are a threat to figure and heart, how come these Masai herdsmen of East Africa, who subsist on meat, blood, and milk, remain lean and stouthearted? Dr. Mann answers his own question: 'They keep fit.'

59 ways to help patients lose weight

Prepared in consultation with:

W. L. Asher, M.D.
Englewood, Colo.

Mason R. Baker, M.D.
Evansville, Ind.

P. C. Black, M.D.
Oakland

Francisco M. Canseco, M.D.
Laredo, Texas

Philip J. Cecala, M.D.
Houston

William P. Corr, Jr., M.D.
Riverside, Calif.

William H. Fee, M.D.
Alameda, Calif.

Bernard P. Harpole, M.D.
Portland, Ore.

T. Reginald Harris, M.D.
Shelby, N.C.

William J. Hossley, M.D.
Deming, N.M.

Norman W. Jankowski, D.O.
Northfield, Ohio

Harold B. Kaiser, M.D.
Minneapolis

Jesse P. Kuperman, M.D.
Dayton

David P. Lauler, M.D.
Boston

Warren T. Longmire, M.D.
Hitchcock, Texas

James W. Manier, M.D.
Minneapolis

Michael J. Moore, M.D.
Roanoke, Va.

Theodore R. Reiff, M.D.
Baltimore

Ronald R. Roth, M.D.
Waterloo, Iowa

Roy J. Thurn, M.D.
Duluth, Minn.

Tennyson Williams, M.D.
Delaware, Ohio

George T. Wolff, M.D.
Greensboro, N.C.

Charlotte M. Young, Ph.D.
Ithaca, N.Y.

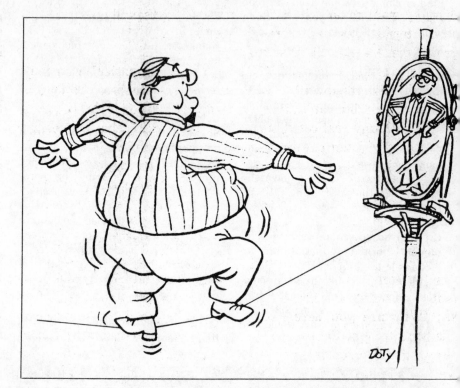

The most recent significant milestone in treatment of obesity probably was the discovery that patients must eat less to lose weight. The next real breakthrough appears to be a long way off.

However, obesity continues to be a major medical problem and a challenge in every family practice. To help you meet the challenge, Patient Care asked a number of your colleagues—listed above—to explain what works for *them* in helping their patients reduce.

The best way to handle the overweight person, of course, is to deal with the problem *before* it gets out of hand. Once obesity is a fact,

nearly all physicians agree that unless a patient wants to lose weight, he won't. A few believe *they* can motivate a patient to make the initial commitment, but most won't attempt to treat the obese patient unless he is already committed, or nearly so.

You'll find tips (sometimes contradictory) on diet, weighing and scheduling, encouraging the patient, and, most important, motivating him. Here is what the respondents to our survey say works for them:

The will to lose

"People who are really motivated to lose weight can tell yo

why they want to do it in rather specific terms—they are short of breath, don't feel well, tire too easily, etc. Often a patient who isn't really motivated will *tell* you he wants to lose, but can't give his reasons with any real conviction. You've got to listen carefully if you want to avoid the futile task of working with a patient who isn't really committed to losing weight."

"When an overweight patient says 'Doctor, I'm too heavy, I want to do something about it,' I ask: 'Why are you here *now*?' This helps me put the patient on the spot and determine if the motivation is really there."

"Much of the initial time I spend with an obese patient is devoted to finding a reason for losing weight which is meaningful to the patient. It may be something as insignificant as being in a wedding the next month. Until you find some such specific motivation, you're not going to make much progress."

"You can usually convince people who need to lose weight for reasons of health to eat less, even if they hadn't foreseen this necessity when they came in. Self-motivation builds when they begin to realize that being over-

weight is personally dangerous to them."

"The obese patient who must lose weight because of a specific medical condition is rarely a problem. All that is usually necessary with these people is an easy low-calorie diet, an anorexiant before meals, regular checkups and encouragement."

"Ask the overweight man who is in good health now but could have trouble later to hop 25 times on each foot. Frequently, he'll be short of breath, his pulse and blood pressure will go up, and he'll spontaneously ask 'I'm not in very good shape, am I?' Your reply should be: 'No, you're not. Are you interested in doing something about it?' "

" 'What do you want out of life, and how are you getting it?' These are the questions an obese patient must answer if he hopes to lose weight. Overeating invariably occurs because the patient lacks something essential in his life, or is responding in an unhealthy way to an emotional or environmental pressure. The physician has to help the patient explore his situation and accept its realities."

"The physician has to help the patient find acceptable gratifica-

tion substitutes for eating. Sometimes this can be done by working out solutions to the problems that are driving the patient to eat. For example, a woman who has an unsatisfactory sex life may start overeating. What she needs is a substitute for food in the form of better sex. A businessman may develop an expense-account waistline because he's worried about his job performance. What he needs is to substitute self-confidence for food."

"Emphasis must be put on long-term weight loss. A program that lasts for only a month or two invariably fails, even though the patient loses weight while the program is going on."

"In some cases, it may be necessary to find some external activity that gives the patient as much pleasure as eating which will substitute for it. While a change in diet is important, a change in life style may be critical."

Candidates for success and failure

"I've found that a goal-oriented person has the best chance of succeeding in a weight reduction program and I try to appeal to this quality."

"In assessing whether I can help an obese patient, I watch him

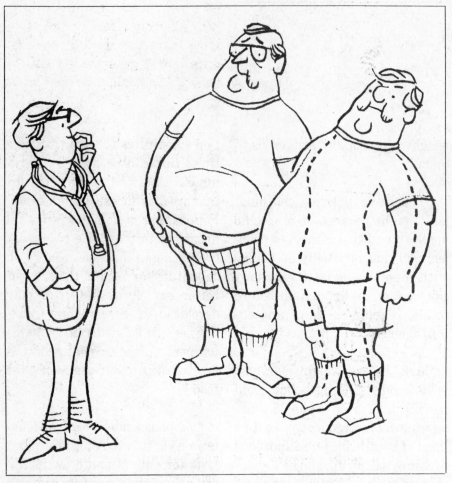

carefully while I'm taking the initial food history. I watch his hands and his facial expressions to see if he is becoming defensive or belligerent. If he squirms, chain smokes or crosses his arms and withdraws from the situation, I'm probably not going to be able to help him much."

"Prime candidates for motivation and treatment are those for whom it is almost too late. A man who has had a heart attack is really motivated and will succeed in getting the pounds off; six months prior to the attack he wouldn't have tried."

"You can hope to succeed with the man in good health who wants to forestall future trouble, providing he understands that it will be hard work which demands determination and perseverance. Be sure to bolster his resolve with a discussion of why his decision is medically wise."

"Usually, it doesn't pay to try to force someone to lose weight against his will. Such patients flout their inability to lose, as if they want to punish me."

"To be successful, the obese patient has to personally request the physician's help. If the weight loss isn't his idea, success is unlikely."

"Usually, I don't press the point with overweight ladies unless they've decided they want to lose weight on their own. In theory, while overweight people ought to get the pounds off, there are many unhappy patients who have failed on diet after diet, and I often counsel them to learn to live with their obesity."

"For many patients, obesity is a crutch which, if suddenly knocked out from under them, can trigger a psychic reaction that is much more serious than being overweight. This is frequently the case with women who complain for reasons of vanity. She is, in effect, daring the doctor to make her lose weight. In these situations, I first determine that the obesity doesn't constitute an imminent danger to the patient's health, and that it isn't caused by glandular imbalance. Then I put the decision on her shoulders. She can lose weight *if* she's willing to go hungry, and diet."

Helping the patient through the ordeal

"Warn your patient not to tell anyone he's on a weight-reducing diet. There's something about human nature that makes others take this as a challenge to tempt the overweight individual to 'fall off the wagon.' Consequently, it's wise to advise the patient to tell

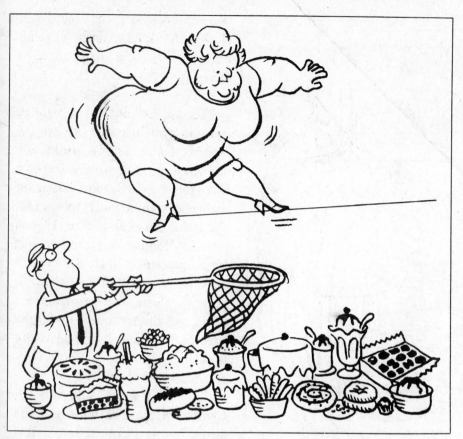

—I show great interest in the 'why' of his progress, or lack of it. If he is convinced about my concern, it will generate his self-interest. Above all, I never berate him."

"The patient losing weight will be helped if he *feels* well. Exercise can help physical fitness and in mild simple form will also help relieve some of the tensions previously relieved by food."

"Telling a patient to say to himself 'I'm going to eat it, but not right now' is bad advice, I think, since it keeps what may be an irresistable temptation constantly before the patient. It's just like telling an alcoholic to keep a drink in front of him."

people that his doctor has ordered him to lose weight because of high blood pressure, a heart condition, colitis, or some other disorder. Once the diet has succeeded, the patient can reveal the truth about himself."

"I'm often asked: 'How do I resist the temptation to eat something I shouldn't?' Rather than to tell himself he won't eat it, I advise the patient to say to himself 'I'm going to eat it, but not right now.' If he keeps putting it off long enough, he'll forget about it."

"Set goals that are reasonable —1-1½ pounds per week—and then insist that the patient meet them."

"The patient has to realize that weight loss seldom occurs in a straight line since fluid retention often masks fat loss. I tell my patients that if they're following an eating plan faithfully and their clothing is becoming looser, the scale will soon show that they really are losing weight."

"I praise my patients as often and as enthusiastically as I can, even if they have only lost a little or have remained stable. Rarely do I scold, unless a patient is using an anorexiant and gains weight anyway. Then I re-investigate his motivation."

"No matter how little weight the patient loses—even if it is none

"There are patients who want and perhaps need a supportive policeman-father image to monitor their program. With them the cajoling or quarreling approach may be successful."

"If the patient slips, I tell him to forget his failure and start again, pointing out that very few things in life are the products of instant success. I never scold patients if they are not losing weight. If you must resort to negative reinforcement in order to motivate the patient, the chance of long-term success is poor."

"Like the alcoholic the obese patient needs support, not punishment or judgment."

▶

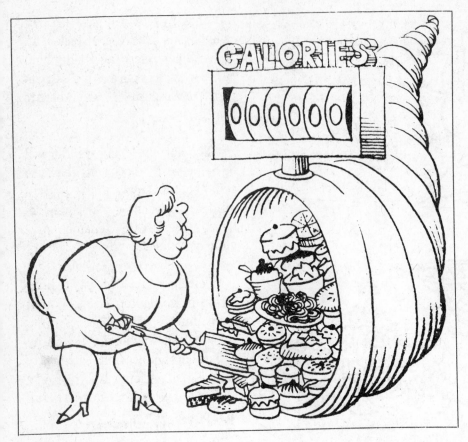

"Get away from the concept that obesity is a moral issue and that we must sit in judgment of overweight patients. There's no one more upset than the patient himself when he hasn't followed orders. He needs support, not chastisement."

"One of the great crimes in handling patients is to lump them into a group and treat them alike. Every overweight patient is an individual and should be treated as such."

Diet and dieting
"When I set a diet, I usually tell the patient to stick to it five days out of seven and to take the weekends off and eat what he wants as long as he doesn't exceed the stipulated maximum weekly calorie count. For example, if a patient is restricted to 7000 calories a week, suggest that he keep his intake below 800 calories a day during the week, then splurge with 1500 calories a day on the weekend."

"Ask the patient to keep a record of everything he eats, including foods he shouldn't, and to bring it to you. Often people don't realize how often and how much they eat, and the record helps them and you control their eating habits. They are often amazingly ignorant about which foods are fattening. For example, a patient may say that he hasn't been eat-

ing any bread, yet the record will show that he's been eating crackers twice a day or corn flakes for breakfast."

"I give the patient a calorie counter and ask him to keep a record of his calorie intake for one week on a day-to-day basis. I then recommend a diet based on this report. Invariably, this is just about the same as a diet I'd prescribe without the gimmick, but for some reason patients seem to have more faith in it. Counting normal calorie intake for a week also gives the patient a vivid picture of just how much he really *is* eating."

"The diet must suit the patient's taste, pocketbook and life situation. It is absurd to tell a construction worker to eat cottage cheese for lunch."

"Whatever diet is selected should be adapted as closely as possible to the patient's usual habits yet gradually retrain him. It should allow him to eat without feeling set apart from other people either at home or away and keep him reasonably hungerfree and with a feeling of well-being. Also, the diet should help maintain the reduced weight."

"The standard, balanced, nutritional diet is precisely what so many patients have tried and repeatedly failed. For the short run, I will accept *any* kind of diet as long as caloric intake is restricted

—even if it comes out of a martini pitcher."

"There is a group of patients who think about food all day. The liquid formula diets can make life easier for these people by eliminating decisions about what foods they can or cannot eat."

"Explain that high carbohydrate diets actually prompt overeating by producing marked changes in blood sugar. Each time the level falls, appetite increases. In contrast, a high protein diet keeps blood sugar at a more constant level and thus helps to control appetite."

"I have rarely known a patient who was physically hungry if a fair proportion of his calories came from protein. Something in the relationship of fat and protein seems to keep a person from feeling hunger."

"Warn patients about eating too fast. Most fat people are fantastically fast eaters, and are apt to clean their plates before anyone else at the table, thus setting themselves up for seconds."

"Also warn against the tendency to be 'human disposals.' They've got to fight against the habit—taught to them as children —of 'cleaning the plate.' "

"Tell patients how to recognize fatty foods by putting a little of the food on a piece of paper. If the paper becomes translucent, the food is fatty."

"Each meal should be prepared, served and eaten at one time. The food should be assembled all at once, and that's all the patient should eat."

"I point out that one pound equals 4,000 calories, and that the patient will lose one pound when his caloric intake is 4,000 less than what he uses."

"Once the patient has decided to restrict his diet, he should be helped by keeping the pantry locked or empty and by buying no more than is needed each day. Between-meal snacks simply shouldn't be in the house."

"Starchy vegetables can be identified by the 'pinch test.' If the vegetable is pinched and the pulp is left, it is starchy (potatoes, corn). If water and fiber are left, it's not (celery, beets)."

"The patient's physical activity is critical in planning a diet. A maximum of 1,200 calories a day is appropriate for the sedentary; the limit for those who do heavy work may reach 1,800 or more calories a day."

"I often put my obese patients on one or two 'fast' days a week and limit their intake to water, black coffee, tea, diet soda, diet gelatin, lettuce and diet dressing."

Drug therapy

"You must watch for the obese patient who seeks an anorexiant for the wrong reason. Often, these people are really after the stimulation which the drug gives them without even realizing it. Frequently such a patient may tell you she feels much better now that she's lost some weight when really the drug is responsible."

"When I prescribe an anorexiant, I tell the patient that it's only a crutch and that he'll only lose weight by reducing his calories, not because of any pill!"

"I don't think anorexiants should ever be prescribed for obese patients since they are potentially habit forming, and have a dangerous effect on the cardiovascular system."

Weighing and scheduling

"Patients should not weigh themselves between office visits. One or two pounds a week registers as a few ounces a day and can be very discouraging. Also, they should avoid counting calories. Doing so just doesn't seem to work, and there are many who wonder why they fail to lose weight on 1,000 calories a day. The content of the diet is the essential."

"I expect a patient to lose an average of two pounds a week. I like to have him record his weight every morning upon arising and to bring or mail the records to me every two weeks. This educates the patient in showing him that weight loss is never a straight-line decline and also dramatizes the effects of cheating."

"After the initial visit, I see the patient again in two weeks. If he's losing at a rate of one pound or more a week, I then see him once a month. If the loss drops below a pound a week, I see him every two weeks. If this doesn't work, between visits to me he comes in to be weighed by my nurse."

"During the initial visit, we find out what deviation exists between our scale and that of the patient, if any. We ask him to go home, weigh himself, record the results, and return to the office within the hour to be weighed on our scale."

Keeping it off

"I use an 'alarm weight' which is 4-5 pounds above normal. If the patient hits that weight, I want him to see me and resume dieting."

"Educate the patient to come back to you if he slips. Explain that maintaining weight can be difficult, and not to feel guilty if he starts to regain a few pounds.

If so, he's apt to stay away from you until the problem is out of control."

"From the very beginning, I stress that obesity is a chronic disease like diabetes, which can never be cured but only controlled by a lifetime change in eating habits. I tell my obese patient that when his weight is down he's not a thin person, but an obese person in a thin body. As such, he'll never be able to eat the way he once did if he expects to stay thin."

Vanity is probably the most common reason why patients seek medical help to lose weight. In our society, excess weight is socially undesirable, particularly in women. Medical complications are a second reason and are particularly relevant for a middle-aged man who is overweight at the time of his first heart attack and is advised to reduce his weight. Weight reduction is also indicated in diabetes mellitus, osteoarthritis, and problems with vascular insufficiency. Whatever the reason, a high degree of motivation to achieve and maintain weight loss is essential for success with any form of therapy. One of the primary responsibilities of a physician who undertakes to treat obesity is to motivate the patient and to provide continuing sympathetic understanding for accompanying emotional and medical ills.

Factors in Development of Obesity

Management of obese individuals must be based on an understanding of the factors that lead to the development of obesity. Studies of experimental animals have provided a classification of etiologic factors in some forms of obesity which serves as a useful framework for consideration of human obesity (table 1).

Obesity associated with hypothalamic injury[1] is relatively rare in man but has been an extremely useful experimental tool. A more common form of obesity in man is that induced by endocrine imbalance. Endogenous production of excess cortisol (Cushing's disease) or its exoge-

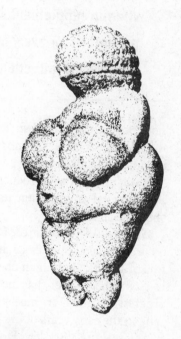

Clinical Management of the Obese Adult

In most instances, obesity in adults represents increased food intake and decreased energy expenditure. In the management of these patients, increased physical activity is just as important as dietary restriction. The preferred diet is one that produces a deficit of 500 to 1000 cal per day and contains 30 to 50 gm of carbohydrate. There is good evidence that eating five or six small meals a day is a better schedule than one or two larger meals.

GEORGE A. BRAY, M.D.
University of California School of Medicine
Los Angeles

nous administration produces a plethoric face and typical truncal obesity. Treatment consists of removing the excess cortisol, if this is possible.

Hyperinsulinemia can also induce obesity. The frequent association of obesity with a nonketotic type of diabetes in adults suggests that insulin may play a significant role in development of some forms of obesity in man as it does in the experimental animal.

Because caloric restriction can lead to vitamin deficiencies, a vitamin supplement should be prescribed for every patient on a weight-reduction diet.

This possibility is further supported by the absence of obesity in most patients with juvenile-onset diabetes.

A high-fat diet will produce obesity in some experimental animals, but its role in human obesity is not clear.

Genetically transmitted forms of obesity occur in several species of animals,[2] but the role of genetics in human obesity is less clearly established. I feel that many patients with progressive gross or morbid obesity beginning in the early years of life have a genetically transmitted disorder. However, the biochemical basis for this corpulence is not clear.

Most forms of human obesity probably represent the interaction of several factors including both genetic and environmental components. Important environmental components include the ready availability of tempting foods and the steady decrease of physical activity resulting from increasing use of the automobile. From a practical point of view, the approach to obesity requires investigation to rule out treatable causes. The group in whom treatable causes cannot be identified (making up more than 95 percent of the total) present a continuum extending from only modest obesity through gross obesity (more than 100 percent of ideal weight).

The obese state in its simplest form represents an imbalance between caloric intake and caloric expenditure. When intake increases relative to expenditure, excess fat is stored. The available evidence suggests that obesity in most instances represents a combination of increased food intake and decreased energy expenditure. In general, the efficiency with which calories are stored is increased in obesity. This is demonstrated most clearly in experimental animals[2] by a relatively greater weight gain per unit of food consumed. However, the available data on human obesity lead to a similar conclusion. For example, Mayer[3] showed that although obese adolescent girls consumed only a little more food than did their lean contemporaries, energy expenditure in the former was significantly lower, leading to greater conservation of food.

Reduction in Caloric Intake

These observations in man and in animals suggest that the approach to weight control must involve a reduction in caloric intake and, equally important, an increase in caloric expenditure. The National Academy of Sciences in 1968 estimated the caloric requirements of a "reference man" and a "reference woman" 22 years of age weighing 70 kg and 58 kg to be 2800 and 2000 cal, respectively.[4] These estimates are lower than corresponding figures published five years earlier and are probably still somewhat high for most Americans.

Intakes of less than 2000 cal would meet the needs of most normal women, and just over 2000 cal would suffice for many men. Adjustments must be made for body size, since larger individuals need more calories.

Table 1. A Classification of Obesity

1. Hypothalamic injury
2. Endocrine imbalance
   a. Cushing's syndrome
   b. Hyperinsulinemia
3. High-fat diet
4. Genetic transmission
5. Unknown etiology

Table 2. One Dietary Approach to Obesity

1. 1000 cal diet

   Carbohydrate, 40 gm or less
   Fat, 60 gm
   Protein, 75 gm

2. All foods weighed (postage scale) or measured

3. Several small meals

   Breakfast, 200 cal
   Lunch, 200 cal
   Snack, midafternoon, 100 cal
   Dinner, 400 cal
   Snack, evening, 100 cal

4. Regular exercise

5. Vitamin supplement if needed

Table 3. Equivalent Units of Exercise*

Walking 3 mi
Bicycling 6 mi
Running 1½ mi
Swimming 800 yd
Playing 36 holes of golf

*From Cooper.[10] The point value for each of these exercise units is 6. A desirable level of physical fitness is achieved by a cumulative score of 30 points weekly.

The requirements must also be adjusted for climate, activity and age. A warmer climate and sedentary living lower the caloric requirements, and greater physical activity raises them. There is convincing evidence that caloric requirements decline progressively with age. Thus, an older person in a sedentary occupation and a warm climate may need substantially less than 2000 cal per day to maintain weight.

In the treatment of obesity, restriction of caloric intake should be sufficient to produce a negative caloric balance of 500 to 1000 cal per day. Loss of a pound of adipose tissue requires a loss of 3500 cal from the body. Since the usual intake is 2000 to 2800 cal per day, total starvation would produce a weight loss of less than a pound per day. However, starvation is an impractical and probably a hazardous means of weight loss for all but the grossly obese patient, and requires hospitalization. With a diet of 1000 cal, the net caloric deficit is 1000 to 1800 cal per day. This level of caloric intake will provide a slow, but steady, weight loss (table 2).

What kinds of food should be included in the 1000 cal diet? Careful studies reported from two laboratories indicated that variations in the distribution of calories among carbohydrate, protein and fat did not alter the rate of weight loss when total caloric intake remained the same.[5,6] However, carbohydrate intake was not severely restricted in these studies, and a recent study suggests that severe carbohydrate restriction is important.[7] A 1200 cal diet containing 30 gm of carbohydrate was compared with a similar caloric intake containing either 60 or 104 gm of carbohydrate. Weight loss, as fat, was greatest with the lowest carbohydrate intake.[7] It is my current feeling, therefore, that a 1000 cal diet with restriction of carbohydrate to 30 to 50 gm is preferred. Protein intake should be moderate, 70 to 100 gm per day.

Increasing evidence suggests that the size and number of meals eaten can influence lipid metabolism and body weight.[8] Small meals eaten at frequent intervals are associated with a significant reduction in cholesterol and a greater tendency to weight loss in obese subjects. Conversely, one or two larger meals consisting of the same total amount of food are accompanied by elevation of cholesterol, impairment of glucose tolerance, a tendency toward obesity, and augmented lipogenesis in adipose tissue.[8] It would appear prudent to divide the caloric intake of any diet into a minimum of three meals or, preferably, into five or six small meals each day (table 2). This division tends to distribute both the caloric intake and the satiety value throughout the entire day.

The social milieu is another factor in the therapy of obesity. Some individuals have

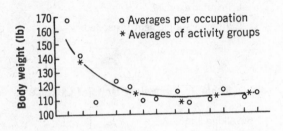

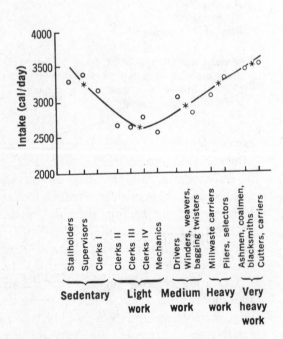

Figure 1. Body weight and caloric intake in relation to activity. Adult males were grouped according to their work. Of note is the rise in body weight and caloric intake of men with sedentary occupations.

Reproduced with permission from Mayer J, Roy P, Mitra KP: Am J Clin Nutr 4:169, 1956.

sufficient motivation to lose weight successfully on their own initiative. For many others, the initial joy of weight reduction is not sustained, rigorous adherence to caloric restriction fades, and weight is regained. There is convincing evidence that weight loss is more effectively achieved in a group of similarly affected persons than alone.[9] This is why some of the self-help groups have succeeded.

Increase in Caloric Expenditure

Complementary to the reduction of caloric intake is an increase in caloric expenditure. Experimental and clinical studies show that food intake increases with physical activity over a wide range (figure 1). Of more importance to the obese patient is the fact that food intake also increases as energy expenditure falls to very low levels. These observations not only suggest that a certain minimum amount of daily exercise can actually reduce the desire to ingest food, but also underline the importance of exercise in any approach to obesity. Indeed, in my clinical experience the most striking examples of prolonged weight loss have been seen in grossly obese patients who voluntarily undertook regular and vigorous exercise.

One of the most convenient ways of achieving an optimum of exercise is set forth in the book "Aerobics."[10] This approach was developed by determining the amounts of various kinds of exercise which produced comparable degrees of physical fitness in air force personnel (table 3). Running 1½ mi in 15 minutes, for example, is equivalent to walking 3 mi in 35 to 40 minutes, riding a bicycle 6 mi, or swimming 800 yd. A point value is assigned to each of these units of exercise. A satisfactory level of physical fitness is achieved by gradually increasing exercise to a goal of 30 points each week. Since running 1½ mi in 15 minutes equals 6 points, this exercise performed on five days of a week is enough to achieve the goal of 30 points. This system has the obvious advantage of providing a quantitative comparison of various forms of physical activity and a way of achieving optimal levels of exercise within the limitations of modern life and individual preferences.

Pharmacologic Therapy

In addition to dietary restriction and increased exercise, several groups of pharmacologic agents may have roles as adjuncts in treatment of obesity. Among them are vitamin supplements, anorectic drugs, and thyroid hormone. In view of convincing evidence that caloric restriction can lead to vitamin deficiencies, it would seem prudent to give a vitamin supplement such as a decavitamin preparation to every patient on a weight-reduction diet.

The use of anorectic drugs is controversial. Their use has recently been criticized because of their potential for drug abuse. They have been shown to be effective in increasing the rate of weight loss during the early period of treatment for obesity, and their usefulness lies in this initial phase of therapy. For most patients the transition from their usual eating habits to a 1000 cal diet is difficult. Use of an anorectic for two to six weeks will often facilitate adaptation to the new eating pattern and strengthen the relationship between doctor and patient.

Use of thyroid hormone is also controversial. In low dosages this calorigenic hormone replaces endogenous thyroid hormone. At higher dosages it initiates its own sequence of pharmacologic actions, including increased oxygen utilization, increased lipolysis with elevation in plasma free fatty acids, and increased breakdown of protein. The catabolism of protein can represent one-third or more of the extra caloric expenditure during treatment with thyroid hormone[11] and indeed may partially explain the effectiveness of thyroid hormone in the induction of weight loss.

The caloric content of fat (including both triglyceride and water-containing portions) is 7 to 7½ cal per gram, whereas the caloric density of protein is only 1½ cal per gram of net weight. This means that 1 gm of fat but nearly 5 gm of protein is lost for every 7 cal expended. Thus, catabolism of small amounts of protein will appear as a much greater weight loss than catabolism of a calorically equivalent quantity of fat. The duration of the negative caloric-nitrogen balance associated with a reduced caloric intake sup-

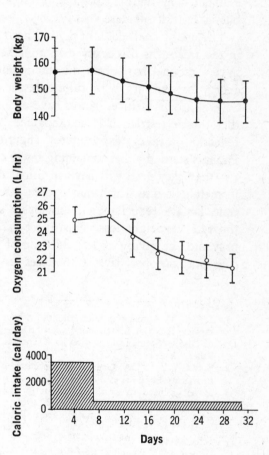

Figure 2. Effect of caloric restriction on energy expenditure and body weight. Beginning two to three days after the lowering of the caloric intake, there was a gradual and significant decline in oxygen utilization which approximated 15 percent.

Reproduced with permission from *The Lancet*.[12]

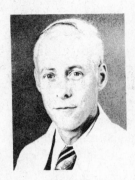

GEORGE A. BRAY

Dr. Bray is associate professor of medicine, University of California School of Medicine, Los Angeles (Harbor General Hospital Campus, Torrance), and director of the Clinical Research Center, Harbor General Hospital.

plemented by thyroid hormone is unknown but is at least 30 days.[11]

The use of small doses of thyroid hormone in the treatment of obesity may nonetheless have a rational basis from the standpoint of energy expenditure with caloric restriction. Several groups of investigators have observed that caloric restriction is accompanied by a reduction in energy expenditure[12] (figure 2). Patients starting a diet containing fewer calories than they need will have an initial drop in metabolic rate which may exceed 20 percent. Such a reduction will obviously slow the rate of weight loss. This effect can be prevented by giving 180 to 240 mg of thyroid hormone per day. With doses in this range, there is little likelihood of untoward effects from thyroid hormone.

Combined Therapy

Regimens of dietary restriction and nutritional reeducation, combined with increased exercise and the use of pharmacologic adjuncts, may be helpful for patients with moderate degrees of obesity but have generally been ineffective for those who are grossly overweight. The available data indicate that the success of any weight-reducing program declines as the degree of overweight increases.[13] Thus, the usual methods of treatment are unlikely to succeed in grossly obese patients.

Jejunoileal Shunting

In a number of clinics, jejunoileal shunting is being tried as a method of reducing the absorption of food from the gastrointestinal tract. A review of reports on this mode of therapy suggests a cautious optimism about its possible use for that group of patients who are grossly obese and for whom more conventional treatment has been unsuccessful.[14]

Dr. Bray's address is Harbor General Hospital Campus, 1000 West Carson Street, Torrance, California 90509.

REFERENCES

1. Frölich A: A case of pituitary tumor without acromegaly. In Major RH (Editor): Classic Descriptions of Disease. Springfield, Ill, Charles C Thomas, Publisher, 1932
2. Bray GA, York DA: Genetically transmitted obesity in rodents. Physiol Rev 51:598, 1971
3. Mayer J: Inactivity as a major factor in adolescent obesity. Ann NY Acad Sci 131:502, 1965
4. Recommended Dietary Allowances. Publication 1694. Washington, DC, National Academy of Sciences, 1968
5. Kinsell LW, Gunning B, Michaels GD, et al: Calories do count. Metabolism 13:195, 1964
6. Pilkington TR, Rosenoer VM, Gainsborough H, et al: Diet and weight-reduction in the obese. Lancet 1:856, 1960
7. Young CM, Scanlan SS, Im HS, et al: Effect on body composition and other parameters in obese young men of carbohydrate level of reduction diet. Am J Clin Nutr 24:290, 1971
8. Fabry P, Tepperman J: Meal frequency—a possible factor in human pathology. Am J Clin Nutr 23:1059, 1970
9. Howard AN: Dietary treatment of obesity. In Baird IM, Howard AN (Editors): Obesity: Medical and Scientific Aspects. Edinburgh, E & S Livingstone Ltd, 1969
10. Cooper KH: Aerobics. New York, M Evans & Company Inc, 1968
11. Bray GA, Raben MS, Londono J, et al: Effects of triiodothyronine, growth hormone and anabolic steroids on nitrogen excretion and oxygen consumption of obese patients. J Clin Endocrinol Metab 33:293-300, 1971
12. Bray GA: Effect of caloric restriction on energy expenditure in obese patients. Lancet 2:397, 1969
13. Young CM, Moore NS, Berresford K, et al: Problems of obese patient. J Am Diet Assoc 31:1111, 1955
14. Salmon PA: The results of small intestine bypass operations for the treatment of obesity. Surg Gynecol Obstet 132:965, 1971

Etiology of Obesity — The QQF Theory*

GEORGE EDWARD SCHAUF, MD**

Riverbank, California

ABSTRACT: The QQF theory for the etiology of obesity is contrasted with the traditional caloric theory. QQF represents (Q) the quality of food as well as (Q) the quantity of food, and (F) the frequency of ingestion. The QQF approach to the treatment of obesity (over 900 cases) is based on the differential between lipogenesis and triglyceride storage on the one hand, and lipolysis and fatty-acid oxidation on the other.

Obesity has presented a continual challenge to the medical profession throughout its long history. Traditionally the approach to the basic cause of obesity has focused upon a consideration of energy input versus energy output.

According to the first law of thermodynamics, heat energy and work energy are interchangeable in a constant ratio; therefore the calorie, a unit of heat, was chosen as the common denominator for expressing energy gained or expended by the body. The principle of conservation of energy states that energy is neither created nor destroyed. Hence the *Caloric Theory* — if caloric input exceeds caloric output, body weight is gained; if caloric input is less than caloric output, body weight is lost — was taken as a basic postulate upon which the etiology of obesity was based.

It is the purpose of this paper to present data which form the basis for the *QQF Theory* that obesity is related to the quality (Q) as well as the quantity (Q) of food and the frequency (F) with which it is ingested.

In recent years new research findings along with the elucidation of fat and carbohydrate metabolic pathways have provided a more specific basis for the etiology of obesity.

With the development of new analytic techniques, it has become possible to determine accurately the percentage changes in body components during variations of dietary intake. In short-term starvation, the lean tissues contribute a greater percentage of the weight loss than does fat. In recent experiments involving use of volumetric analysis and the whole-body radioactive spectrometer, it was demonstrated that in periods of total abstinence from food ranging from ten to seventeen days, the lean tissues contributed 59-66 per cent of the weight loss (1-3). Since lean tissues oxidize free fatty acid as a primary energy, dietary regimens which cause loss of lean tissue will proportionately decrease the body's capacity to oxidize and lose fat.

The traditional treatment of obesity based upon the caloric concept, has placed major emphasis upon creating a caloric deficit in the diet. Bray (4) and others have noted that unqualified caloric restriction will cause a decline in energy expenditure. Of necessity, if more fat is to be lost as energy, the energy expenditure must be increased. Therefore it would appear that the method of unqualified caloric restriction may have been working contrary to the goal in the treatment of obesity, i.e., losing more fat.

The terms obesity and overweight should not be used synonymously since obesity pertains specifically to the excess accumulation of body fat whereas the term overweight includes the total weight of the three general body compartments, lean tissue, fat, and water. Moreover, there seem to be two basic classifications of obese people: 1) the overnourished obese, with excess adipose tissue and a full lean-mass complement, and 2) the undernourished obese, with excess adipose tissue but with concurrent

* Presented at the 47th Anniversary Congress of the Pan American Medical Association, Family and General Practice Section, Miami Beach, Florida, November 20, 1972.
** Diplomate of the American Board of Family Practice.
Address: George Edward Schauf, M.D., 3443 Atchison Street, Riverbank, California 95367.

depletion of the lean-mass tissue and resultant anemia, fatty infiltration of the liver, thin flabby musculature, and poor resistance to infection.

QUANTITY OF FOOD AND TIMING

The Caloric Theory has in effect equated all foods by translating them into a common denominator, the calorie. It does not specify whether the energy consumed will become cellular structure, hormones, enzymes or blood cells; or will be stored as triglyceride or glycogen; or oxidized as free fatty acid, glucose, or ketone bodies; or lost in the process of thermogenesis; or excreted as waste materials. It appears that the quality of the diet — proportion of protein, fat, and carbohydrate — is a crucial determinant of the destiny of ingested food, the particular interest being whether it will be stored as fat or synthesized into essential lean tissues.

The quantity, the number of calories in the diet, is important if the specific kind or kinds of calories promote increased fatty-acid synthesis and triglyceride storage.

Animal studies by Tepperman and Tepperman (5) and Friend (6) have indicated that when daily rations are forced upon rats within a short period, the animals sacrifice lean tissue to lipogenesis and triglyceride storage. When experimental rats are forced to consume the entire daily caloric intake in one meal, after several months they become obese, with a marked increase in adipose tissue but a simultaneous serious depletion of the lean mass. My analysis of this finding is as follows: When the daily caloric ration is consumed by the animal within a short time (e.g., one hour), the ceiling capacity of the liver to store glycogen is exceeded; this produces hyperglycemia, insulin response, and an increased production of lipogenic enzymes with resultant adaptive hyperlipogenesis. Hollifield and Parson (7) have demonstrated an increase of C^{14}-labeled acetate in the body fat of rats fed one large meal a day. This increase was twenty-five times the amount found in the carcass fat of rats allowed free access to their food.

Within a few hours after one large meal, the glycogen stores in the liver (rarely exceeding 300-400 calories in the human) become depleted. During the several subsequent fasting hours before the next large meal, homeostatic serum glucose levels are maintained chiefly by the conversion of protein to glucose (there being little net conversion of fat to glucose in mammalian species) through the process of gluconeogenesis in the liver. Therefore, each day in the foregoing experiments the rats gained in increments of fat while losing in increments of lean tissue. From these animal experiments, it would appear that the frequency of meals is an important factor in the etiology of obesity.

LIPOGENESIS AND TRIGLYCERIDE STORAGE VERSUS LIPOLYSIS AND FATTY-ACID OXIDATION

Obesity is always caused by a sustained differential favoring lipogenesis (the formation of fatty acid) and triglyceride storage over lipolysis (the mobilization of fatty acids from the fat cell) and oxidation of free fatty acids.

Lipogenesis occurs in the liver and at the membrane of every fat cell. Previously the fat cell was considered to be an inert storage depot but now is known to be a most dynamic unit where, at the cell membrane, a whole array of metabolic processes take place, the major ones promoting the synthesis of fatty acid from glucose. Insulin is necessary to facilitate lipogenesis from glucose.

Glucose supplies acetyl coenzyme A (from the decarboxylation of pyruvate), a 2-carbon atom fragment built into 12-, 14-, 16- and 18-carbon fatty-acid chains, and donates the hydrogen ions in reduced triphosphopyridine nucleotide (NADPH) necessary for the reduction steps in fatty-acid synthesis. The acetyl coenzyme A derived from the degradation of fat cannot be resynthesized to fat without the energy from NADPH, which comes from the oxidation of glucose.

Glucose is also the major substrate of alpha-glycerophosphate, which is mandatory for the esterification of endogenous and exogenous fatty acids prior to storage as triglyceride in the fat cell.

Glucose appears to play a pivot role in both lipogenesis and triglyceride storage. Ingested fat cannot be stored as fat unless the critical glucose metabolite, alpha-glycerophosphate, is available. In contrast, ingested carbohydrates can be readily converted to fat and stored as triglyceride in the fat cell. Protein from the diet is utilized mainly for lean cell, hormone, and enzyme synthesis but in excess it can be converted to glucose in the gluconeogenic process and in turn be synthesized and stored as fat.

Lipolysis is governed largely by neural and hormonal controls. During circumstances associated with sympatho-adrenomedullary discharge, i.e., stress, fear or rage, norepinephrine secreted from the excitation of sympathetic nerve endings and epinephrine released from the adrenal medulla promote increased lipolysis. Other hormones which promote increased lipolysis are ACTH, growth hormone, thyroid-stimulating hormone, thyroxine, triiodothyronine, cortisol, glucagon, vasopressin and the newly isolated anterior pituitary hormone, lipotropin. These lipolytic hormones activate adenyl cyclase, a fat-cell enzyme, causing the synthesis of cyclic adenosine monophosphate, which has direct lipolytic action.

Physical exercise will promote increased lipolysis and increased oxidation of fatty acid. The major action of thyroid hormone is to promote the oxidation of fatty acid. Insulin is the major antagonist to lipolytic agents.

In the genesis of obesity, new fat cells are synthesized from primitive lipocytes. This formation of new fat cells take place in infancy and hence the seeds of the predisposition toward obesity are planted very early in life. Hirsch et al. (8) found that obese adults have larger fat cells and nearly three times as many fat cells as do their slender counterparts. Therefore the obese apparently have an increased capacity to synthesize and store fat; each fat cell is a miniature "fat factory."

The energy system of the human body is dichotomous. The brain, nervous system, adrenal medulla, germinal layers of the gonads, and erythrocytes during glycolysis only, are obligatory users of glucose, whereas the main lean-mass tissues (muscle, kidney, heart, and liver) use free fatty acid as a primary energy. Secondary energy sources are stored glycogen in the muscles, used mainly in states of oxygen debt, and ketone bodies formed in the liver during glycogen depletion states from the partial oxidation of fatty acids. Ketones are oxidized by the lean tissues and apparently to some extent by the brain during prolonged starvation.

The traditional approach to the cause and treatment of obesity (energy input versus output) should be replaced with a more specific approach oriented toward the differential between lipogenesis and triglyceride storage on the one hand and lipolysis and fatty-acid oxidation on the other. Reducing it to the most fundamental concept — when fat is being stored in the fat cell, obesity is promoted whereas when fatty acids are leaving the fat cell and being oxidized by the muscles and other lean tissues, obesity is diminished.

QUALITY OF FOOD

The total number and individual size of the lean-mass cells and their metabolic rates, are the prime determinants of how much fat is oxidized as expended energy. Therefore, protein and certain fats become essential in the diet for the resynthesis and maintenance of the lean tissues in order to secure the maximal capacity of the lean-mass cells to oxidize fat. Since alpha-glycerophosphate, a glucose metabolite, is essential for the storage of triglyceride in the fat cell, the amount of carbohydrate, particularly sucrose, appears to be a critical determinant regulating the degree of obesity. Marshall et al. (9) demonstrated that sucrose-fed rats gain more fat than do cornstarch-fed rats, and Young et al. (10) showed in college students that weight loss, fat loss, and percentage loss as fat are inversely proportionate to the amount of carbohydrate in isocaloric isoprotein diets. If ingested fatty acids are not esterified by alpha-glycerophosphate and stored as triglyceride they may be bound to albumin and carried to the muscles to be used as energy. This results in an increase in the general metabolic rate, which will promote further oxidation and loss of stored body fat. Gordon et al. (11) demonstrated that the supplementation with polyunsaturated vegetable oil (corn oil) of a low-carbohydrate, moderate-protein diet, would increase the oxidation of stored palmitate by 20-25 per cent.

QQF THEORY

The quality (Q) of food (proportion of protein, carbohydrate and fat at each meal), the quantity (Q) of food (the number of calories in each constituent), and the frequency (F) of ingestion (number of meals per day) are important factors in the etiology of obesity (12).

It follows that the goal in the treatment of obesity should be more specific than loss of weight, and should include: 1) resynthesis and maintenance of the lean-mass tissues, 2) diminished lipogenesis and triglyceride storage, and 3) increased lipolysis and increased oxidation of fatty acids.

RECOMMENDED REGIMEN

The author has treated more than 900 obese patients by means of a diet designed to achieve the foregoing goals. The instructions to patients are:

1. Eat at least three meals per day.
2. Eat animal protein (eggs, meat, fish, fowl or cheese) at each meal (3-4 ounces per serving of meat or fish).
3. Limit carbohydrates to between 15 and 25 grams per meal.
4. Restrict sugar-containing and caffeine-containing[1] foods to breakfast.
5. Do not eat carbohydrates between meals.
6. Ensure an adequate water intake.
7. Use polyunsaturated oils (e.g., corn, safflower, soybean, peanut, and olive oils) as supplements with the noon and evening meals (2-3 ounces per day).
8. Finish each meal feeling nourished and alert, but never "full."

---

[1] Caffeine is restricted in order to decrease the insulin secretion necessary to facilitate lipogenesis.

REFERENCES

1. Benoit FL, Martin RL and Watten RH: Changes in body composition during weight reduction in obesity, Ann Int Med 63: 604, 1965.
2. Ball MF, Canary JJ and Kyle LH: Tissue changes during intermittent starvation and caloric restriction as a treatment for severe obesity, Arch Int Med 125: 62, 1968.
3. Wauters JP, Busset R, Dayer A et al: Effects of various slimming regimens on body composition in simple obesity, Schweiz Med Wchnschr 100: 1272, 1970.
4. Bray GA: The myth of diet in the management of obesity, Am J Clin Nutr 23: 1143, 1971.
5. Tepperman HM and Tepperman J: Adaptive hyperlipogenesis, Fed Proc 23: 73, 1964.
6. Friend DW: Weight gains, nitrogen metabolism and body composition of rats fed one or five meals daily, Canad J Physiol 45: 367, 1967.
7. Hollifield G and Parson W: Metabolic adaptations to "stuff and starve" feeding program. I. Studies of adipose tissue and liver glycogen in rats limited to a short daily feeding period, J Clin Invest 41: 245, 1962.
8. Hirsch J, Knittle JL and Salans LB: Cell lipid content and cell number in obese and non-obese human adipose tissue, J Clin Invest 45: 1023, 1966.
9. Marshall MW, Womack M, Hilderbrand HE et al: Effects of carbohydrates and proteins on carcass composition of adult rats, Proc Soc Exper Biol & Med 132: 227, 1969.
10. Young CM, Scanlan SS, Im HS et al: Effect on body composition and other parameters in obese young men of carbohydrate level of reduction diet, Am J Clin Nutr 24: 290, 1971.
11. Gordon ES, Goldberg M and Chosy GJ: A new concept in the treatment of obesity, JAMA 186: 156, 1965.
12. Schauf GE: The Etiology of Obesity: A More Specific Theory. Scientific Exhibit, 121st Annual Convention of the American Medical Association, San Francisco, Calif., June, 1972.

Nutritional Anarchy:
A Perspective on the
"Atkins Diet Revolution"

S. K. Fineberg, M.D.

"Weight loss is achieved on this diet through the inadvertent reduction of calorie-intake by the dieter. This is due in part to the anorexia produced by the ketosis induced by the malnutrition of carbohydrate deficiency. Weight loss is also caused by the inability of most individuals to adapt to an utterly unbalanced diet consisting of practically all fat and protein. A common reaction, after a short period, is distaste or repugnance."

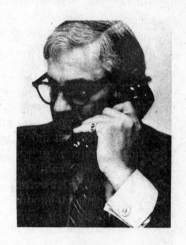

The slight twist of specifically changing the "fat" in the recurring no (or low) carbohydrate, high-protein, high-fat, calories-don't-count, eat-all-you-want, time-worn diets, to "saturated fat" adds just enough of a slow-fuse bomb-threat to qualify this one as *anarchy*. This additional fillip to other unsound, unwise, and nutritionally unbalanced diets is not the least, nor even the most objectionable, feature of the advice found in the book, "Dr. Atkins' Diet Revolution" subtitled "The High Calorie Way to Stay Thin Forever."

Millions of people have already read this book, millions more will read it, and untold numbers will seriously attempt to follow the dietary treatment of obesity which it advocates and which is broadly outlined above. The more successful the attempt or the closer the adherence to the diet, the greater is the possibility of harm to the dieter. This risk or potential for harm to an individual cannot be specifically calculated because it is dependent upon multiple, often invisible, factors, in addition to degrees of adherence. Among these factors are the basic health of the individual, the time span of the diet, and the inborn or genetic capacity of the individual to withstand such metabolic stresses as hyperuricemia and a highly increased intake of cholesterol. The clinical evidence of harm varies from mild, well-tolerated symptoms which are felt by the great majority of those actually on the diet, to the occasional occurrence of a major illness, perhaps even death. Although such extreme reactions may result only rarely, a dietary regimen with this potential can never be accepted or recommended as sound medical advice, especially since it seeks to re-

Dr. Fineberg is a Professor of Medicine at the New York Medical College; Chief, Diabetes and Obesity Clinics, Metropolitan Hospital, New York City; and Director of Medicine and Cardiologist, Prospect Hospital, Bronx, New York.

place a diet which is without similar risks. The primary rule of therapeutics is *Primum Non Nocere.*

The Dangers of Ketosis

Probably the most objectionable characteristic of the Atkins diet is that it is strongly ketogenic, i.e., if its instructions are followed closely, the dieter will quickly develop the abnormal metabolic state of ketosis.[1,2] As the author indicates in his book, he read about the anorexia produced by the ketogenic diet during his attempts to cope with his own obesity. To determine if the dieter is defecting from the diet by the intake of carbohydrates, he is instructed to constantly test his urine for the presence of ketone bodies, acetoacetic acid, and beta-hydroxybutyric acid. If a Ketostix dip test turns deep purple, it indicates ketonuria or the presence of ketone bodies. This serves as laboratory confirmation that the dieter has successfully unbalanced his diet. He has developed "Ketosis," a sign of an illness which in this case is correctly diagnosed as "Malnutrition Secondary to Carbohydrate Deficiency." Other common causes of this type of malnutrition are starvation and very poorly controlled diabetes.[1,2] In starvation, little or no carbohydrate is ingested because of the lack of intake of any nourishment. In uncontrolled diabetes, the metabolic derangement prevents the utilization of sufficient carbohydrates. Should the Atkins dieter find only little or no amounts or ketones in his urine, he is directed to follow the diet more carefully.

The pathological state of ketosis produced by a severe deficiency of carbohydrates can produce many symptoms. The most frequent of these are anorexia, then fatigue, euphoria, dizziness, palpitations of the heart, tachycardia, cardiac arrhythmias, a craving for sweets, nausea, vomiting, postural hypotension, and syncope.[2,3,4] Practically all individuals who develop such malnutrition will have these symptoms; the degree depends upon the severity of the deficiency and individual tolerance. If basic health is good, the symptoms will be mild and possibly annoying, but relatively easily tolerated. The actual threat to a healthy person is really quite minimal, even after a prolonged period of time, *providing his state of health does not decline in the interim.* But who is really healthy?

First, obese people are not in a "state of good health." Besides the many stresses of their obesity, they often have underlying conditions of which they are unaware. Such conditions are frequently outside the capacity of available medical diagnostic skills and facilities to detect. For example, an obese, middle-aged individual may have a considerable degree of atherosclerotic narrowing of one or more coronary arteries without ever having experienced one symptom of heart disease. He may even have registered a perfectly normal electrocardiogram five minutes before having a catastrophic heart attack! Coronary arteriography would have revealed the condition of his coronary arteries only if the disease was in an advanced state. But this invasive technique, while properly indicated in selected patients, is never part of a "thorough physical examination." In an *apparently* healthy person, the relatively mild cardiac and circulatory effects of tachycardia, premature contractions, hypotension, and syncope which occur in ketotic states could very easily precipitate a myocardial infarction. This disastrous sequence has probably occurred thusly an unknown number of times.

In similar, but less dramatic fashion, individuals with underlying, undetected, well-compensated, and therefore symptom-free disease of the heart, kidneys, liver, lungs, or brain, could quite conceivably lose the functional capacity to compensate for impairment and begin to fail. This is precisely the manner in which a *mild* illness such as Carbohydrate Deficiency can plunge the individual into a clinically overt, serious illness, i.e., heart failure, renal failure, coronary insufficiency, or cerebral insufficiency. This can and does occur in apparently healthy obese patients who, in most instances, would easily pass a precautionary preliminary physical examination. Even the mature-onset, obese diabetic classified as "ketosis-resistant," or more properly "ketoacidosis resistant," because the ketosis of *his* carbohydrate deficiency does not usually lead to the acidosis of diabetic coma, is a poor candidate for a ketogenic diet despite the weight loss it may induce. Unfortunately, the diabetic frequently has accelerated vascular disease of the heart, kidney, brain, retina, and peripheral arteries.

Finally, most nutritionists and practicing clinicians firmly believe that a state of "good nutrition" is important, if not essential, for rallying the defense mechanisms of the body. A healthy person who first develops ketosis of carbohydrate deficiency, and then develops an infection with some particularly virulent viruses or bacteria, or is subjected to unexpected surgery or trauma, is believed to be in special jeopardy. The immunologic and hemeostatic defense mechanisms of his body may be impaired by the pre-existence of a severe degree of nutritional imbalance. The evidence for this lowering of resistance is based on experimentation with malnourished animals and many years of clinical observation and experience. Still, it demands serious consideration as a persuasive reason for not gambling with the elective induction of ketosis.

High Saturated Fat and Coronary Heart Disease

Another of the major features of the Atkins diet which is scientifically unacceptable is its specific dictum to freely consume a large quantity ("all you want") of foods containing large amounts of saturated fat, particularly cholesterol. In the face of evidence suggesting a direct association between a high intake of these substances and a distinctly increased risk of coronary heart disease and generalized atherosclerosis, this nutritional directive is foolhardy.[5,6,7]

Preliminary evidence indicates that the faithful and continued consumption of a low-cholesterol diet over a period of years can reduce the coronary attack rate in middle-aged men. Logically, the earlier the diet is instituted, the more effective its protective effect. Many medical scholars and internists not only recommend such a diet prophylactically and therapeutically, but even follow their own advice. This has already resulted in changes in the eating habits of the American public.

Conversely, the author of the "Diet Revolution" seems convinced that a high cholesterol, high saturated fat, severely carbohydrate-deficient diet will actually have a cholesterol- and triglyceride-*lowering* effect on the vast majority of individuals. His conviction, he says, is based on 'data'

collected at various intervals during the eight year course of this diet treatment of 10,000 obese patients, during which time he did not sustain a single failure!

Although the presentation of scientific medical data to the medical profession is usually considered to be the ethical and moral duty of a physician, the reluctance to do so in this instance is understandable. Even Dr. Atkins has, following the publication of his book, publicly expressed regrets that his 'data' was not collected in a 'clean' manner, that is, following a prescribed protocol and in a carefully controlled manner in a properly supervised metabolic research ward. *Uncontrolled observations,* even of such objective findings as determinations of chemical blood levels, especially those made during the course of the very confidential, private practice of medicine, have long since lost their capacity to inspire confidence. Many excellent practicing physicians are untrained and unfamiliar with the necessarily rigid control criteria which governs the modern science of clinical investigation. Even more does the general public find it difficult to understand what is valid scientific evidence. The layman is usually quite impressed by anecdotal, personal observations and mere testimonial evidence. This accounts for much of the confusion and misunderstanding of the public and even such erudite bodies as congressional committees. Most pertinent to the observations of Dr. Atkins is the likelihood that neither he nor his patients ever have more than the roughest approximation of the actual composition of their diets.

It must be concluded from the available evidence that strict adherence to the Atkins' diet will put unknown but probably large

numbers of individuals whose innate susceptibility has been genetically predetermined at high risk of Coronary Heart Disease and accelerated Atherosclerosis.

The Diet's Hoax

The subtitle of the book, "The High Calorie Way to Stay Thin Forever," is deceiving in that calories, of course, do count. This is acknowledged even by the author, who says most people on his diet eat less since they find they *can't* eat as much as before. *Let it be stated clearly and emphatically that many do lose weight rapidly on this diet (but at what risk?) and for exactly the reasons given. No one who loses weight by following the Atkins' diet does so by increasing or even maintaining his previous caloric intake.* No one, including Dr. Atkins, has yet succeeded in repealing the first law of thermodynamics which states that "The energy of an isolated system is constant and any exchange of energy between a system and its surroundings must occur without the creation or destruction of energy."[8]

Weight loss is achieved on this diet through the inadvertent reduction of calorie-intake by the dieter. This is due in part to the anorexia produced by the ketosis induced by the malnutrition of carbohydrate deficiency. Weight loss is also caused by the inability of most individuals to adapt to an utterly unbalanced diet consisting of practically all fat and protein. A common reaction, after a short period, is distaste or repugnance. Most people can only tolerate a reduced amount of calories coming only from these sources. This fact has often been demonstrated under carefully controlled conditions with diets whose actual caloric content was precisely measured. Subjects who were told that they could eat unlimited amounts of meat, fish, eggs, cheese, butter, margarine, and cream, but only these foods, were found to have reduced their calorie intake by 13 to 55%.[9,10]

Conversely, an unknown, but probably considerable, number of seriously obese individuals unfortunately *can* adapt readily to, or are unaffected by, the surfeiting effect of such diets. These individuals *can* probably increase their caloric intake because, as has been demonstrated recently, the "satiety center" in the hypothalamus is less sensitive to the visceral, humoral, neural and psychological stimuli which should signal that a person is full. A relatively inactive or sluggish satiety center, one which does not properly inhibit the appetite center, can result in weight gain and increased obesity. Many obese patients following the Atkins' diet have noted an immediate increase in weight. However, this probably occurs with less frequency than weight loss, particularly when carbohydrate intake is severely restricted and ketosis is present.

The Illusion of Water Loss

The reason for the more rapid weight loss and greater *apparent* success of diets which contain little or no carbohydrates is that they do not promote water retention and, at first, induce diuresis. *The initially greater weight loss resulting from a low-carbohydrate diet of the same number of calories as a balanced, mixed-nutrient diet is due to an additional loss of body water, not of fat.*[12,13,14] Furthermore, a diet that contains carbohydrates, but is still well below the individual's caloric requirement, will often produce a reduc-

tion in scale weight for only a few weeks, especially in women. Then, although body fat continues to decrease, the body retains water, which in turn masks or counterbalances the fat loss. Since the scale measures total weight only and cannot distinguish fat loss from water loss, the patient's weight may register little or no change. This metabolic abnormality of water balance, the cause of which remains unknown, has been demonstrated to be due to the carbohydrate portion of the diet. In such cases, it is not uncommon to see patients on a balanced diet containing only a moderately decreased proportion of carbohydrates, begin to gain weight while sharply decreasing caloric intake. The disturbing and obstructive phenomenon does not occur with diets containing little or no carbohydrates; hence the apparently greater effectiveness of these diets. *It is of extreme practical importance to recognize that uncorrected salt and water retention is often responsible for the failure of obese patients faithfully adhering to a balanced, low-caloric diet to lose weight.*[12] Ignorance of this one fact has probably led to more confusion in dietary treatment of obesity than any other single factor. Unless the individual permanently remains in a severely unbalanced nutritional state, the additional weight loss from the dehydrating effect of carbohydrate deficiency will be regained once carbohydrate intake is increased. Weight losers on the Atkins' diet have become well aware of this fact as they have found the state of carbohydrate deficiency less and less tolerable. Only true fat loss from caloric reduction signifies real progress in the struggle against obesity.

The Trap of Weight-Losing "Crash" Diets

The successful treatment of obesity should be solely concerned with the *permanent* reduction of body fat stores. The proper diet for the treatment of obesity should be calorically restricted and nutritionally balanced. To be balanced, it must contain two or more servings per day from the four basic food groups: the milk, meat, vegetable-fruit, and bread-cereal groups, plus a small amount of unsaturated fat. This is the only basic weight-reducing diet suitable for lifetime control, because *all that is necessary to make it a proper diet for weight maintenance, as opposed to weight reduction, is an increase in the size of portions.* It thus teaches the patient good eating habits which may be used to control his obesity for life. The inability to provide a permanent solution for a lifetime problem is a less obvious, but very serious, deficiency of the Atkins' diet. More obvious is the absurd deception (eat 5,000 calories a day!) that an increased or excessive intake of a strange combination of calories will lead to weight loss, either temporary or permanent.[17]

Long-term experience has indicated that even more important than taking off weight is learning how to keep it off. This is the insidious trap of all "crash diets." A crash diet is one which is severely unbalanced nutritionally and usually severely restricted in calories. Such diets entice the obese public by initially producing a gratifying and rapid weight loss. Aside from the risks involved, frustration is inevitable when the dieter must eventually abandon the diet and return to his former habits. He usually finds himself in worse condition after the diet, for he has the added psychological trauma of regaining all his former weight, plus a little more. Although the Atkins' diet, with its emphasis on "The High Calorie Way," etc., is less obviously a crash diet than most, it does lower calories to induce weight loss, and even its weight-maintaining phase is severely unbalanced. It teaches nothing about caloric content or dietetics, and because of generally poor acceptance in its true form, only the rare individual can comply with its stipulations for an extended period of time.

Probable Reasons for Atkins' Diet Enthusiasm

Beside the involuntary lowering of calories and the lessened tendency to retain water, there is one good reason why many intelligent individuals who are supposedly on the Atkins' diet lose weight with no symptoms other than some hunger. This I refer to as the "John Doe Modification of the Atkins' Diet." Discussions with enthusiasts and perusal of letters from loyal fans of Dr. Atkins has indicated to me that although they may originally closely follow instructions, his followers are no different from others who are improperly motivated. They cheat. They cheat with a 'little' carbohydrate. For this reason, they do not develop the symptoms of carbohydrate deficiency. A 'little carbohydrate' can quickly add 75 to 80 Gms, which will completely prevent ketosis. Also, because they have good sense and want to lose weight, they do not gorge on bacon, butter, bologna, etc., but concentrate on the 'steak and salad' dinner. Even so, they may glory in the illusion that they are "eating all they want" and believe that they are closely adhering to The Diet. Actually, their modifi-

cation of The Diet may roughly approximate a calorically restricted, balanced diet in which the total amount of carbohydrate is reduced, protein is relatively high, though not actually increased, and fat is much decreased.

These are the patients whose cholesterol and triglycerides levels may decrease, as Dr. Atkins claims. It would be difficult, if not impossible, to dispute this explanation retrospectively because of the lack of controls. Unfortunately, although these people lose weight, there is no understanding or knowledge of what they are doing or how they are doing it. Neither does their instructor have sufficient information regarding the diet composition and total food intake. In this situation, the prognosis for the permanent control of obesity, which is the only acceptable goal of diet treatment, is very poor. It is very difficult to convince someone who is losing weight with a minimum of self-discipline and a maximum of ease that his diet should be aimed at discipline—food-intake discipline and educational discipline.

The "Attack" of "Organized Medicine"

The adverse criticism of Dr. Atkins' diet by "organized medicine" has been viewed with suspicion by some laymen and a few members of the press as a personal attack motivated by self-interest. This cynical view is completely unjustified. It was not the politicians, lobbyists, elected delegates, or socio-economic experts of the American Medical Association or its State and County Societies who roused themselves to publicly refute this harmful medical advice. Because the Atkins' diet reached so many people that it warranted consideration as a threat to public

health, statements were made by professors of medicine, consultants, medical scientists, and authorities in nutrition. Such groups compose the scientific committees and councils of the AMA and the scientific organizations which make up the "Medical Establishment." Moreover, no hierarchy dictated or directed this action. This was the *scientific medical world* fulfilling a duty and responsibility to which it was and is clearly obligated. Had it not spoken out, medical science would have, with great justification, become the target of equal, if not as newsworthy, criticism.

The extensive notice given to the refutations or "attacks" in the public media was directly proportionate to, and was caused by, the popularity of the Atkins' diet and book. The denial of merit or validity was not the result of a devious or insidious motivation of scientists who form a distinguished, though little-known, section of "organized medicine" and the "medical establishment." In past years, similar reviews and evaluations of the nutritional nonsense extolled in such books as "Calories Don't Count" by Herman Taller and "The Doctor's Quick Weight Loss Diet" by Stillman, were given little space in the public press and were mostly buried in professional journals. This explanation is in answer to the question, "Why attack Dr. Atkins and not the many who preceded him?" Although these were classical examples of popular fad diets, they certainly never exploded in sales, were aided by massive advertising campaigns, or set publishing history as has the book in question.

To be specific, contrary to the general impression, Dr. Atkins has *not* been singled out for an "attack." It is his undeserved fame which has singled him out. Any authoritative denial of the value of his diet is news because *it* is news. Further, the necessity for medicine to refute poor nutritional advice has become a matter of urgency because of the unceasing series of fad diets and bad books. Another factor is today's tremendous public interest in nutrition and obesity control. The frustration and disappointment caused by the failures of the many previous "miracle" diets may have produced in many an even greater need and desperation to lose weight.

What the American public has never seemed to grasp is that the publication of any book is never a confirmation of its veracity but merely a re-affirmation of the principle of freedom of speech and of the press. We have an unwarranted respect for the printed word. It is quite likely that in some technologically advanced totalitarian state, this book would not have been released from the publisher. I do not condone such an intolerable state of affairs. Obviously, the advantage to be gained by protecting public health by censorship is far outweighed by the disadvantages of the loss of liberty. Still, an appeal to authors and publishers to assume the responsibility of assuring their information and advice be based on scientific facts established by responsible research is so weak that it is no solution at all. It merely constitutes an exercise in futility.

Since none of the existing groups in the field of nutrition have gained the confidence of the American public, a proposed solution is to form a new organization whose membership, chosen from the scientific publishing and other worlds, would be so far above suspicion that its judgement would be accepted by the great majority of the public. The worth of such a body would have to be widely and constantly publicized in order to create an unassailable image of reliability and credibility. A possible first step in this direction would be the formation of a committee designated as "The Committee to Advise and Protect Against Unwise Nutritional practices and Diets."

It is conceivable that one of the first actions of such a committee would be to advise that all copies of the book "Dr. Atkins' Diet Revolution: The High Calorie Way to Stay Thin Forever" be stamped with the legend, "The information and advice in this book may be hazardous to your health." □

References

1. Wohl M. G., et al: *Modern Nutrition in Health and Disease.* Philadelphia, Lea and Febiger, 1964, p 246–247, 806.
2. Kleiner I. S. and Orter J. M.: *Biochemistry.* St. Louis, The C. U. Mosby Co, 1966, p 609–612.
3. Oliver M. F., Korien R. E., Greenwood T. W.: "Relation between serum-free fatty acids and arrhythmias and death after acute myocardial infarction." *Lancet 1*: 710–714, 1968.
4. Kark R. M., Johnson R. E., Lewis J. S.: "Defects of pemmican as an emergency ration for infantry troops." *War Medicine 7*: 345–352, 1945.
5. Joint policy statement of the AMA Council on Foods and Nutrition and the Food and Nutrition Board of the National Academy of Sciences-National Research Council: Diet and coronary heart disease. *JAMA 222*: 1647 (Dec 25), 1972.
6. Report of the Inter-Society Commission for Heart Disease Resources: Primary prevention of the atherosclerotic diseases. *Circulation 42*: A55–A95, 1970.
7. American Health Foundation: Position statement on diet and coronary heart disease. *Preventive Med 1*: 255 286, 1972.
8. White A., et al: *Principles of Biochemistry.* New York, McGraw-Hill Book Co. Inc, 1954, p 9.
9. Yudkin J., Carey M.: The treatment of obesity by the "high-fat" diet. The inevitability of calories. *Lancet 2*: 939–941, 1960.
10. Yudkin J.: "The low carbohydrate diet in the treatment of obesity." *Postgrad Med 51(5)*: 151, 1972.
11. Mayer J. and Thomas W.: "Regulation of food intake and obesity." D. *Science 156/3773*: 328–337, 1967.
12. Elsbach P. and Scwartz I. L.: "Salt and water matabolism during weight reduction." *Metabolism 10*: 595–609 (Aug) 1961.
13. Bloom W. L.: "Inhibition of excretion by carbohydrate." *Arch Int Med 109*: 26–32 (Jan) 1962.
14. Editorial: Inhibition of salt excretion by carbohydrate. *JAMA 179*: 802 (Mar 10) 1962.
15. Fineberg S. K.: "The obesity-diabetes clinic." *JAMA 181*: 862–865 (Sept 8) 1962.
16. Fineberg S. K.: "Massive obesity and water retention." *GP 26*: 104–109 (Apr) 1964.
17. Kinsell L. W., et al: "Calories do count." *Metabolism 13*: 195–204 (Mar) 1964.

Clinical Comment

Ascorbic Acid Deficiency in Drug Addicts

Those who handle drug addicts are often struck by their evident malnutrition. Most of the abused drugs cause anorexia and this, plus various social factors, may produce nutritional deficiency. A recent study evaluated the incidence of ascorbic acid deficiency in seemingly healthy addicts. (See Croft, L. K. American Journal of Clinical Nutrition 26: 1042, 1973.)

Measurements were made of the ascorbic acid levels in the plasma, the buffy coat, and the tongue tissue. It was found that fifty-eight percent of the seemingly healthy addicts had vitamin C deficiency. Since this deficiency may impair intellectual performance and produce depression, its possible role in the maintenance of drug abuse should be studied.

M.D.A.

Are We Not Now Ready for a Diet Revolution?

Counterpoint!

Robert C. Atkins, M.D.

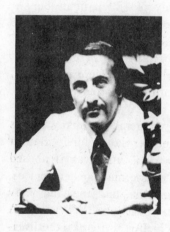

"Perhaps the greatest contribution that an eat-until-you-are-not-hungry diet makes toward the practice of good medicine is that it renders completely unnecessary the use of appetite suppressants, with their potential for harm, diabetogenicity, rebound after-effects, and uniformly poor long-term results. Why consider suppressing the appetite pharmacologically, when it can be done physiologically by removing the insulin-provoking stimuli from the diet?"

I am grateful to Dr. Sidney Fineberg for making such an excellent presentation of the viewpoint of the many "authorities" who have publicly criticized the regimen of carbohydrate-restriction in the management of obesity, and in so doing, exposed the scientific inadequacies of that position. These critics seem to have an unusual concept of the metabolic consequences of a low-carbohydrate diet which is not substantiated by medical literature.

Dr. Atkins is a practicing New York internist whose best selling book, *Dr. Atkins' Diet Revolution*, has been a focal point for controversy on the subject of low carbohydrate dieting for the obese.

The unassailable truth is that the drastic lowering of carbohydrate intake provides an extremely safe and universally effective dietary regimen for the treatment of obesity. This conclusion is based on a) careful clinical observation of more than ten thousand patients; b) communication with other medical centers where similar diets are being studied; and c) a critical view of the medical literature pertaining to low-carbohydrate dieting. Dr. Fineberg's opinion is, of necessity, limited by absence of factual data, inasmuch as a) he has had no first-hand experience with this modality; b) there exists nowhere in the literature he cites any data adverse to

the regimen under question; and c) his own selection of references contains, if anything, only other opinions unsubstantiated by valid first-hand studies.

Are Carbohydrates Essential Nutrients?

In 1972, Dr. Fineberg proclaimed that ketosis "is an abnormal and undesirable metabolic state," [1] and despite dozens of recent studies on this subject, he continues to assert that ketosis represents "Malnutrition Secondary to Carbohydrate Deficiency," indicating that no amount of scientific data can dislodge him from his uniquely-held viewpoint that "carbohydrate is an essential nutrient."[1]

The textbook summary of dietary carbohydrate, in Bondy's words, states: All the necessary sugar units can be manufactured in the body from precursors derived from the amino acids and the glycerol of various fats. As a result, no carbohydrate is required in the diet.[3]

Can a Normal Metabolic Fuel Be Dangerous?

I am further astonished to learn of any "authority" in metabolism, who, writing in 1974, considers the presence of ketone bodies to represent an "illness." Not even Dr. Fineberg's two twenty-year-old textbook references lend support to his thesis that ketosis itself is undesirable or dangerous; they merely point out that ketosis does occur in diabetes and starvation.

One could go back to 1941 and reread the discussion by Wick and Drury:

Our attitude towards the significance of the ketone bodies in metabolism has undergone considerable change in recent years. At one time, the presence of any appreciable amount of these substances in the blood stream would have been regarded as an indication of impaired metabolism. Today we look on such an occurrence as perfectly natural and resulting from a normal mechanism for utilizing fatty acids which consists of a partial oxidation of these substances to form ketone bodies by the liver and distribution of these ketone bodies to the tissues by the blood for complete combustion.[4]

Commenting on this, Dr. Oliver Owen, whose classic studies have done much to elucidate ketone body metabolism, has stated: "It is interesting how the recognition and subsequent confusion pertaining to ketone-body metabolism have occurred, specifically as a consequence of ketotic diets for weight-reduction."[5]

Ketone bodies have been shown to be normal constituents of blood and urine in the fed as well as the fasted state.[2,6,7,8] They not only are used as an effective fuel for metabolic energy needs, but have been shown to be a "preferred fuel" used in preference to glucose in tissues such as the myocardium[9] and skeletal muscle.[10] In a series of studies so significant that they were acclaimed by Van Itallie as causing a "revolution in our thinking,"[11] Owen, Cahill, and associates have shown that *ketone bodies provide the major source of fuel for brain metabolism* in a man subjected to prolonged caloric deprivation.[12]

Moreover, contrary to the accusation, as a major metabolic fuel, ketone bodies do not build up or accumulate, but achieve a steady state on a given diet, being derived from free fatty acids only as the metabolic requirements of the body demand.[13] They were recently shown not to be neurotoxic even in the concentrations found in diabetic coma[14] or in starvation,[15] and they have been administered by intravenous infusion in man with no adverse effects.[5] In short, ketone bodies are the principal metabolic fuel involved in providing the energy derived from stored fat to tissues such as the brain, thus sparing protein gluconeogensis.[16]

Has Anyone Ever Seen These Symptoms?

The acceptance of the hypothesis that the normal metabolic state of ketosis is pathological might be condoned, but Dr. Fineberg's statement that "practically all individuals" in ketosis will develop a long list of symptoms is simply not valid. There is a large body of medical evidence to show that these symptoms never occur. The two notable exceptions are an-

orexia and euphoria, which, you will note, are synonymous with the freedom from hunger and feeling of physical and mental well-being that the overwhelming majority of low-carbohydrate dieters consistently report.

The accusation that ketogenic regimens are associated with tachycardia, premature contractions, hypotension, and syncope appears to be fashioned out of the whole cloth. In my own clinical experience, I have observed, if anything, a decreased incidence of these complications. And Blackburn, in a carefully monitored recent study of 129 patients on an even more austere carbohydrate-free regimen, has reported the total absence of these developments.[17,18] Nor were any such complications reported in the vast clinical experience of the 1920's, when a ketogenic regimen was the treatment of choice for pediatric epilepsy,[19,20] and was used favorably in the management of pediatric asthma, migrane, and genitourinary infections.[20,21]

Dr. Fineberg's use of the Oliver reference is puzzling in this context, since this attempts to indict free fatty acids rather than ketone bodies. But even if free fatty acids were considered to be a risk factor for arrhythmias, Oliver has conceded subsequently that the presence of excessive catecholamines may be the necessary factor for arrhythmia production,[22] and Opie has presented a review which tends to refute this entire concept.[23]

Certainly, the Kark study of the inadequacy of pemmican rations provided to non-obese soldiers on strenuous bivouac in subarctic climates with a caloric deficit of 3,000 per day is not exactly an unerring description of the Diet Revolution program. That both Dr. Fineberg and the AMA Council on Food and Nutrition[24] had to refer to such a study to prove their point against ketosis is an indication of the paucity of medical literature bearing on this point.

Aren't These the Symptoms of Caloric Restriction?

Among the "many symptoms" that Dr. Fineberg asserts "practically all" low-carbohydrate dieters will have are fatigue, dizziness, nausea, vomiting, and a craving for sweets. In each case, these common complaints are seen with far greater frequency on a "balanced" low-calorie diet.[25,26]

An especially noteworthy aspect of the ketogenic diet is the absence of a craving for sweets, which can impede, in afflicted individuals, all dietary progress. This affords perhaps the greatest benefit of all in the day-to-day management of this very distressing type of obese patient. Certainly the statement: "This is the first diet on which I no longer have the craving for sweets" is made by the majority of patients.

I find it incredible that anyone can refer to this eminently safe dietary regimen as "hazardous." Millions of people have been following the diet without any incidence of untoward reactions, despite the AMA's plea to all its members to report on any such case.[24]

Do You Really Expect A Heart Attack?

Nonetheless, Dr. Fineberg has "concluded from the available evidence" that adherence to the diet will put "probably large numbers . . . at high risk of coronary heart disease." But the references he cites are nothing more than a series of position statements of organizations in the business of fundraising. When one analyzes the

fiscal interests of these organizations, as annotated by Pinckney in his excellent book,[27] it is no wonder that they take a position unsupported by scientific evidence.

There has never been a study showing that intake of dietary fats in humans is associated with an increased incidence of coronary heart disease. The Framingham study was unable to make such a correlation.[28] Bruhn and Wolf, in a recent review of 98 studies, concluded that there was no consistent relationship between diet and heart disease.[29]

On the other hand, numerous studies, such as those of the Masai,[30,31] Samburus,[32] Eskimos,[33] etc., have shown cultures in which the intake of saturated fats was high while the incidence of coronary heart disease was low or nil. Cohen, in his classic studies of Yemenite Jews, has presented evidence that the incidence of coronary heart disease more closely parallels the intake of sugar than that of fats.[34] And Altschule has concluded that if there is a dietary cause of atherosclerosis, "it is not dietary fat."[35]

Who Says This is A High Fat Diet?

Perhaps the next point makes the foregoing discussion academic. Dr. Fineberg refers to the Diet Revolution regimen as a high-fat diet, and, at the same time, cites Yudkin's studies showing that dieters on a non-ketogenic low-carbohydrate regimen eat far fewer calories than when following their usual diet. These same studies showed that the dieters reduced their intake of fat by some 20%;[36] and the ketogenic dieter, with his greater anorexia, has an even further reduction of fat intake.

Whether the improvement is a result of the reduction of fats, or calories, or sugar, the fact remains

that a sizable body of data has been gathered from my patient population with regard to serial changes in serum lipid patterns on the ketogenic weight loss regimen. Dr. Fineberg dismisses these data as "uncontrolled observations." But even as a retrospective study, the data are valuable, because there *are* controls, the controls being the baseline studies gathered while the patients were following their usual pre-diet regimen. These data show not only the well-known lowering of the serum triglyceride level, which in many studies has been shown to correlate strikingly well with the restriction of carbohydrate,[37] but a lowering of the statistical mean cholesterol level as well.

When cultures with a high dietary fat intake have been found to have a low cholesterol level, the incidence of heart disease has been very low,[30-34] and no data to the contrary have been offered. Thus, in lowering the levels of cholesterol and triglyceride, we have every right to presume we are lessening, rather than increasing, the incidence of coronary heart disease.

Further, there are recent studies showing that hyperinsulinism may be causally implicated in the etiology of coronary heart disease.[37,38] The restriction of carbohydrates has been reported to reverse the hyperinsulinism of obese patients.[39]

One of the most dramatic types of observation to bear upon this point is the significant decrease in precordial pain and nitroglycerine usage reported by a large majority of exertional angina sufferers who have been followed on this diet.

Can You Ignore Triglycerides?

Whereas the effect of dietary carbohydrates upon the cholesterol level is predictable, their effect upon triglyceride levels is, quite predictably, to elevate them.[40,41,42] Recent studies of hyperlipidemia have emphasized the variations in individual response.[43] In the obese population, particularly, the incidence of type 4 disturbances (triglyceride-formers) is greater than type 2 (cholesterol-formers). Since type 4 patients show a significantly greater improvement in their lipid patterns when subjected to carbohydrate restriction than type 2 patients do on fat restriction, an explanation of the improved serum lipid patterns begins to emerge.

Inasmuch as several studies have shown a tendency toward a reciprocal relationship between serum cholesterol and triglyceride levels, particularly when dietary fats are interchanged for carbohydrates,[44] one must guard against dispensing nutritional advice which will serve to raise triglyceride levels. Albrink has offered considerable evidence to show that triglycerides may have an even greater correlation with coronary heart disease than does cholesterol.[37]

Is It a Hoax to Control Overeating?

I do not understand how the great clinical advantage which a ketogenic diet affords the struggling dieter can be labelled as a "Hoax." The regulating effect upon the abnormal appetite mechanism is so common among obese individuals that it enables them to achieve satiety on a significantly reduced intake of food. Any one can prove this to his own satisfaction by prescribing this diet to a patient with the well-known clinical entity, the "Night-Eating-Syndrome." Within a week, he will report to you a dramatic reduction or cessation of his night-eating or awakening. Try it, too, on a patient with so-called "sugar addiction" and you will see the

emergence of an individual who has achieved control over his eating pattern.

This mastery over the appetite is not achieved through "distaste or repugnance." A meal consisting of shrimp scampi, steak bearnaise, sauted mushrooms, and a tossed green salad with creamy garlic dressing is no more repugnant to the obese dieter who has suffered through a lifetime of cottage cheese, melta toast and carrot strips than it seems to be to you who read about it. Certainly, the popularity of the book was not due to the repugnance of the diet it offers.

Could People Gain on It?

Dr. Fineberg states that "many obese patients following the Atkins diet have noted an immediate increase in weight." Except in the period immediately following a very austere semi-starvation diet, this simply does not occur. I am not stating that a weight gain *could* not occur in a small minority of individuals deliberately stuffing themselves in an effort to disprove the precepts of the diet, but rather that it *does* not occur, partly because the dieter is a motivated individual desirous of losing weight and partly because the very rules of the diet clearly state: "Eat as much of the allowed foods as you need to avoid hunger; don't eat when you're not hungry."[45] Thus, the idea that the book tells the dieter to "eat-all-you-want" is Dr. Fineberg's; it is neither mine, nor is it the words of my book, nor is it the concept gleaned by its readers.

Is the Weight Loss Merely Water?

Dr. Fineberg calls attention to another major clinical advantage in any low-carbohydrate diet—its di-

uretic effect. This fact makes it exceedingly useful in managing patients with obesity complicated by congestive heart failure[46] (for whom I strongly feel that it represents the diet of choice), idiopathic edema of women,[47] or hypertension.[48]

But do not be misled by his innuendo that the weight loss is due to "an additional loss of body water, not of fat." When a subject who is fifty pounds overweight steadfastly follows this diet, he will eventually achieve his normal weight and body configuration.

This loss is virtually all body fat—it does not represent merely dehydration. That the weight lost on the ketogenic diet is virtually all stored triglyceride has been amply demonstrated by Young *et al.*, who were able to show that only 5% of the weight lost on a 30 gram diet was non-adipose tissue, whereas a 104 gram diet produced non-adipose loss nearly five times that amount.[49]

Is There a "Metabolic Advantage?"

In alluding to the third major way in which the diet works, Dr. Fineberg feels that it is an "absurd deception" that the diet also provides a metabolic advantage, which would better explain the phenomenon I have observed many times; that some patients can eat 3,000 to 5,000 calories of non-carbohydrate food daily and show a sustained long term adipose tissue loss. Until energy balance studies can be performed on this sizable group of patients, this remains a true medical controversy, *not* an "absurd deception." Gordon's penetrating essay provides considerable insight as to how differing pathways of metabolic utilization of fuel, particularly that originating as stored triglyceride, *might* provide significant variations in utilization of calories; the caloric balance presumably achieved via increased thermogenesis.[47] Kekwick and Pawan, using carbon excretion data, demonstrated that the metabolic advantage might be achieved, in part, through the excretion of energy-containing substrates.[50] Sims, in his overfeeding experiments,[51] and Kasper, *et al,* in their fat-feeding experiments,[52] provide definite evidence of "Luxus consumption," all tending to refute the theory that a calorie is a calorie is a calorie. The number of potential subjects who would slim down on a high-calorie, all-meat diet is so vast, however, that every practicing physician could demonstrate this to his own satisfaction merely by inviting a small group of obese males with large appetites to follow such a regimen for a few months.

The calorie theory has obstructed the thinking of researchers in the field, even to the point where erroneous conclusions have been reached in otherwise valid studies. An example is the study by Young, *et al,* in which the data clearly show the superior adipose tissue loss of a 30 gram diet compound to a 60 or 104 gram diet, but the conclusion is that the 104 gram diet is to be preferred.[49] And the work of Krehl, *et al,* who were able to demonstrate a 32 pound mean weight loss in 7 obese females in just 10 weeks using a 1200 calories ketogenic low-carbohydrate diet, dismissed this impressive accomplishment with the conclusion that it was "communsurate with caloric restriction."[53] But most studies are similar to those of Kinsell, who concluded that there is no metabolic advantage of a low-carbohydrate diet, despite the fact that only one patient was studied at a level of less than 42 grams.[54] I refer the reader to these studies in

detail so that he may form his own conclusion as to whether this type of study represents merely poor scientific judgment or a deliberate attempt to discredit the diet which poses such an economic threat to the powerful food industry.

Which Interests Did I Offend?

The foregoing may provide some insight into why I feel that Dr. Fineberg is incorrect when he proclaims that the unprecedented public attack upon me, and upon my integrity, was *not* a personal one based on the self-interest of the medical bureaucracy, but rather one which originated from the scientific medical world. I have spent a year seeking the answer to the question of why such a malicious attack, much like the one you see in the accompanying article, has been directed against my clinical results and scientific judgment. I still do not know whose interests I have apparently offended, but I have learned that it is not those of the community of scientists sharing the same fields of interest that I do. For in my discussions with academicians interested in ketone body metabolism or in addressing medical meetings of groups dealing clinically with obesity or carbohydrate metabolism, my dietary recommendations were received enthusiastically.

The purpose of this presentation is to allow the thoughtful reader to question just how "scientific" are the concepts which my critics have enunciated.

What Are My Patients Eating?

I am personally affronted by Dr. Fineberg's twice-repeated statement that I do not have much more than the roughest approximation of the composition of my

patients' diets. I have studied written records of every food and beverage item consumed by thousands of my patients, inasmuch as such record-keeping is a frequent part of the protocol of patient management. It would be difficult for these records to be more than minimally inaccurate, as my staff routinely checks for the presence of the ketonuria and the weight loss proceeds according to the anticipated schedule. The majority of the patients studied have demonstrated ketonuria and certainly an absence of the horrendous side effects to which Dr. Fineberg refers. Thus, his suggestion that my patients who do well are cheating on a 75 gram diet is patently ridiculous since ketopositivity rarely takes place in diets over 60 grams of carbohydrate.

The possibility that my patients are actually following the diet more stringently than their written records reveal is highly improbable. Virtually all inaccuracies of patient reporting have been shown to be in the direction of "non-reporting" of dietary excesses. What patient would state, "I had a helping of mashed potatoes" when, in fact, he did not?

How Safe is the Low-Calorie Diet?

Dr. Fineberg has described the "balanced" low-calorie diet as one "without similar risks." Anyone working with low-calorie dieters knows that they are anything but free of distressing, if not intolerable, side effects, the most prominent of which is hunger in all its biochemical, physical, and psychological manifestations. Serious medical problems, particularly untoward emotional reactions, as well as weakness, nervousness, irritability, and fatigue, have been reported by Stunkard with an all-too-frequent incidence as a consequence of low-calorie dieting.[25] Further, Dr. Fineberg must be aware of these difficulties, for he has himself stated: "The purpose of giving appetite suppressants is to eliminate or reduce the discomfort *which is produced in everyone* by a sharp reduction in calorie intake."[55]

Perhaps the greatest contribution that an eat-until-you-are-not-hungry diet makes toward the practice of good medicine is that it renders completely unnecessary the use of appetite suppressants, with their potential for harm, diabetogenicity, rebound after-effects, and uniformly poor long-term results. Why consider suppressing the appetite pharmacologically, when it can be done physiologically by removing the insulin-provoking stimuli from the diet? *"Primum Non Nocere,"* says Dr. Fineberg. First, do no harm. Is it harmless to provide comfort to the practitioner who prescribes diet pills and the patient who demands them by offering a rationale for their use? And what of the harm, emotional and psychological, that befalls the victim of "severe obesity" when he is prescribed a diet which, in Dr. Fineberg's words, "fails in almost all patients who suffer from massive genetic or metabolic obesity" because "they never really adjust to the extremely low-calorie intake necessary to control the disease."[7] Does not the harm come when "authorities in nutrition" devote full-scale efforts to dissuading these unfortunate victims from solving their obesity problems by following a diet that enables them to achieve their goals with "a minimum of self-discipline and a maximum of ease?" Suppose, for example, a patient comfortably maintaining his weight loss by restriction of carbohydrates comes under the influence of Dr. Fineberg's "teachings" and is convinced that he

must switch to a low-calorie balanced diet. If he happens to have underlying, undiagnosed, but well-compensated congestive failure, his fluid retention might be increased, and this might conceivably precipitate acute pulmonary edema or even death. Far-fetched? Certainly, just as far-fetched as Dr. Fineberg's suggestions. Except that Elsbach and Schwartz, to whom he refers, demonstrated that the tendency of obese subjects to retain water is increased by calorie restriction.[56]

Which Diet Is Easiest to Live On?

On one point Dr. Fineberg and I agree; taking off weight is less important in the long run than learning how to keep it off. I have stated that a low-carbohydrate diet is preferable to a low-calorie diet, both as a technique for losing and a technique for maintaining lost weight. Dr. Fineberg feels this is not so. However, this is in large part a matter of preference but, of necessity, more the patient's preference than the doctor's. I always offer my patients a choice (unless there are medical contraindications) between low-carbohydrate and low-calorie maintenance programs; the overwhelming majority choose a carbohydrate restriction, because it is far more livable and provides a greater sense of physical well-being.

Aren't We Ready for a "Diet Revolution?"

I believe that the arguments against the ketogenic weight-losing regimen have included failure to demonstrate cause-and-effect, specious reasoning, inconsistencies of fact, overlooking of recent medical research, refusal to concede the invalidity of previous utterances, and appeal to statements by au-

thorities, rather than original scientific data.

Keeping this in mind, I hope you will reread the foregoing discussion, refer to the references cited, and reflect on their significance. I hope you will try the program on your more difficult patients. Then, I believe, you will see the Diet Revolution in its true perspective.

References

1. Fineberg, SK: The Realities of Obesity and Fad Diets, Nutrition Today. 7(4):23, 1972
2. Williamson, DH and Hems, R: Metabolism and Function of Ketone Bodies, in Essays in Cell Metabolism. Wiley-Interscience, 1970
3. Bondy, PK: Duncan's Diseases of Metabolism. Phila., Saunders 1969 p. 201
4. Wick, AN and Drury, DR: The Effect of Concentration on the Rate of Utilization of Beta-hydroxy Butyric Acid in the Rabbit. Journal of Biological Chemistry 138:129, 1941
5. Owen, OE: Personal Communication
6. McKay, EM: The Significance of Ketosis, Journal Clinical Endoc. 3:101, 1943
7. Wieland, O: Ketogenesis and its Regulation. Advances in Metabolic Disorders, 3:1, 1968
8. Cahill, GF, Jr., et al: Hormone-full Interrelationships during Fasting. Journal Clinical Invest. 45:1751, 1966
9. Williamson, JR and Krebs, HA: Acetoacetate as a Fuel of Respiration in the Perfused Rat Heart. Biochem. Journal 80:540, 1961
10. Owen, OE and Reichard, GA, Jr.: Substrate Extraction and/or Production by Forearm during Progressive Starvation. Clin. Res. 18:2, 1970
11. Van Itallie, TV: Remarks. Symposium on Childhood Obesity. Institute of Human Nutrition, New York, Nov. 16, 1973
12. Owen, OE, et al: Brain MetabolismClinical Invest. 45:1751, 1966
9. Williamson, JR and Krebs, HA: Acetoacetate as a Fuel of Respiration in the Perfused Rat Heart. Biochem. Journal 80:540, 1961
10. Owen, OE and Reichard, GA, Jr.: Substrate Extraction and/or Production by Forearm during Progressive Starvation. Clin. Res. 18:2, 1970
11. Van Itallie, TV: Remarks. Symposium on Childhood Obesity. Institute of Human Nutrition, New York, Nov. 16, 1973
12. Owen, OE, et al: Brain Metabolism during Fasting. Journal Clin. Invest. 46:1589, 1967
13. Cahill, GF, Jr. and Aoki, TT: How Metabolism Effects Clinical Problems. Medical Time 98(10) 106, 1970
14. Ohman, JL, et al: The Cerebrospinal Fluid in Diabetic Ketoacidosis N.E.J.M. 284:283, 1971
15. Owen, OE: CSF Ketone-body Concentra-

tion during Starvation Metabolism (in press) January, 1974

16. Cahill, GF, Jr., Marliss, EB and Aoki, TT: Fat and Nitrogen Metabolism in Fasting Man. Hormone and Metabolic Res. Suppl. 1,181, 1970

17. Blackburn, GL: Preservation of the Physiological Responses in a Protein Sparing Modified Fast. Clin. Res. (in press) 1974

18. Blackburn, GL: Personal Communication

19. Ellis, RWB: Some effects of Ketogenic Diet. Arch. Dis Child 6:285, 1931

20. Barborka, CJ: The Ketogenic Diet and Its Use. Journal Amer. Dietetic Assoc. 8:471, 1933

21. Helmholz, HF: Therapeutic Results with the Ketogenic Diet in Urinary Infections. JAMA 105:778, 1935

22. Oliver, MF: Metabolic Response during Impending Myocardial Infarction. Circulation 45:483, 1972

23. Opie, GH: Metabolic Response during Impending Myocardial Infarction. Circulation 45:491, 1972

24. American Medical Association Council on Foods and Nutrition: A critique of low carbohydrate reducing regimens, review of "Dr. Atkins' Diet Revolution" JAMA 224:1415, 1973

25. Stunkard, AJ: Dieting Depression. AJM 22:77, 1957

26. Cederquist, DC, et al: Weight Reduction on Low-Fat and Low-Carbohydrate Diets. J. Amer. Dietetic Assoc. 28:113, 1952

27. Pinckney, ER and Pinckney, C: The Cholesterol Controversy Shaerbourne Press. Los Angeles, 1973

28. Kannel, WB: The Framingham Diet Study; Diet and the Regulation of Serum Cholesterol. Pub. Health Service Monograph No. 24 U. S. Gov't. Printing Office, 1970

29. Bruhn, JG and Wolf, S: Studies reporting "Low Rates" of Ischemic Heart Disease; a Critical Review. Amer. J. Public Health 60: 1477, 1970

30. Mann, GV et al: Cardiovascular disease in the Masai. J. Athero. Res. 4:298, 1964

31. Taylor, CB and Ho, KJ: Studies on the Masai. Amer. J. Clin. Nut. 24, 1291, 1971

32. Shaper, AG et al: Cardiovascular Studies in the Samburu Tribe of Northern Kenya. Am. Heart Journal 63:437, 1962

33. Ho, JK et al: Alaskan Arctic Eskimo, Responses to a Customary High Fat Diet. Am. J. Clin. Nut. 25:737, 1972

34. Cohen, AM: Fats and Carbohydrates in Atherosclerosis and Diabetes in Yemenite Jews. Am. Heart Journal 65:291, 1963

35. Altshule, M: The Uselessness of Diet in the Treatment of Atherosclerosis, (in) Controversies in Internal Medicine, Saunders, Phila, 1966

36. Yudkin, J: The Low Carbohydrate Diet in the Treatment of Obesity. Post Graduate Medicine 51:151, 1972

37. Albrink, MJ: The Dietary Prophylaxis of Atherosclerosis Requires the Control of Triglycerides, not of Cholesterol in the Plasma. (In) Controversies in Internal Medicine, Saunders, Phila., 1966

38. Grey, N and Kipness, DM: Effect of Diet Composition on the Hypersinulinism of Obesity. New Eng. Journal of Medicine 285:827, 1971

39. Jensen, SE et al: The Effect of Carbohydrate Restriction on Glucose Tolerance, Serum Insulin-like Activity and Growth Hormone Dependent Sulphation Factor in the Serum of Diabetics Acta Med. Scand. 174:769, 1963

40. Kuo, PT and Bassett, DR: Dietary Sugar in the Production of Hyperglyceridemia. Ann. Internal Medicine 62:1199, 1965

41. Kaufman, NA and Kapitulnik, J: The Significance of Sucrose in Production of Hypertriglyceredemia. Acta Med. Scand, Suppl 542:229, 1972

42. Macdonald, I: Effect on Serum Lipids of Dietary Sucrose and Fructose. Acta Med. Scand, Suppl 542:215, 1972

43. Frederickson, DS, Levy, RI, and Lees, RS: Fat Transport in Lipoproteins. An Integrated Approach to Mechanisms and Disorders. NEJM 276:34, 94, 148, 215, 273, 1967

44. Albrink, MJ: Triglycerides, Lipoproteins, and Coronary Artery Disease. Arch. Int. Med. 109:345, 1962

45. Atkins, RC: Dr. Atkins Diet Revolution, New York McKay, 1972

46. Simonyi, J, et al: The Diuresis Potentiating Effect of a Carbohydrate-Poor Diet in Obese Individuals and in Non-Obese Patients with Chronic Congestive Heart Failure. Cor Vasa 11:251, 1969

47. Gordon, ES: Metabolic Aspects of Obesity. Adv. in Metabolic Disorders 4:229, 1970

48. Adlersberg, D and Porges, O: Dehydration Action of Low Carbohydrate Diet and its Therapeutic Use. Klin. Wochenschr. 12:1446, 1933

49. Young, DM, et al: Effect on Body Composition and other Parameters in Obese Young Men of Carbohydrate Level of Reduction Diet. Am. J. Clin. Nut. 24:290, 1971

50. Kekwick, A and Pawan, GLS: The Effect of High Fat and High Carbohydrate Diets on Rates of Weight Loss in Mice. Metabolism 13:87, 1964

51. Sims, EA et al: Experimental Obesity in Man. Trans. Assoc. American Physicians. 81:153, 1968

52. Kasper, H., Thiel, H and Ehl, M: Response of Body Weight to a Low Carbohydrate, High Fat Diet in Normal and Obese Subjects. American J. Clin. Nut. 26:197, 1973

53. Krehl, WA, et al: Some Metabolic Changes Induced by Low-Carbohydrate Diets. Amer. J. Clin. Nut. 20:139, 1967

54. Kinsell, LW, et al: Calories Do Count. Metabolism 13, 195, 1964

55. Fineberg, SK: Anorexiant Drugs... "Boon or Bust" Nutrition Today (Dec) 67:14

56. Elsbach, L and Schwartz, IL: Metabolic Clin. Exptl. 10:595, 1961

A Critique of Low-Carbohydrate Ketogenic Weight Reduction Regimens

A Review of Dr. Atkins' Diet Revolution

There has been a rekindling of public interest in the low-carbohydrate ketogenic diet touted as a "miraculous" and "revolutionary" approach to weight reduction. A recent example is the publication and extensive promotion of a book, *Dr. Atkins' Diet Revolution*.[1] The Council on Foods and Nutrition of the American Medical Association evaluated the claims made by Dr. Atkins and considered certain general questions concerning the "low-carbohydrate diet."

History of Low-Carbohydrate Diets

The low-carbohydrate diet approach to weight reduction is neither new nor innovative. About a century ago, an English surgeon, William Harvey[2] devised a diet for obesity that specifically interdicted sweet and starchy foods, while permitting meat ad libitum. One of his portly patients, William Banting[3] attested to the efficacy of Harvey's diet in *A Letter on Corpulence, Addressed to the Public*. During the last 20 years, there has been a cyclical recrudescence of similar diets having in common the following major features: (*a*) a low to very low carbohydrate content, (*b*) no restriction of protein and fat, and (*c*) "unrestricted calories." Variants of the diet have been described in 1953 by Pennington[4,5] ("Treatment of Obesity with Calorically Unrestricted Diets"), in 1960 as the Air Force diet,[6]

This statement has been accepted for publication by the Council—Philip L. White, ScD, *Secretary*.

Reprint requests to AMA Council on Foods and Nutrition, 535 N Dearborn St, Chicago 60610 (Dr. White).

in 1961 by Taller[7] (*Calories Don't Count*), in 1964 as *The Drinking Man's Diet*,[8] in 1967 by Stillman,[9] and, most recently, by Atkins[1] (*Dr. Atkins' Diet Revolution*).

Over the years, starting with the "Banting Diet," such regimens have been awarded a succession of eponyms and, from the very beginning, have been proclaimed to the public in glowing terms. If such diets are truly successful, why then, do they fade into obscurity within a relatively short period only to be resurrected some years later in slightly different guise and under new sponsorship. Moreover, despite the claims of universal and painless success for such diets, no nationwide decrease in obesity has been reported.

Physiological Effects

An examination of the claims associated with advocacy of low-carbohydrate diets suggests that, in some instances, the authors found a way of circumventing the first law of thermodynamics, namely: "The energy of an isolated system is constant and any exchange of energy between a system and its surroundings must occur without the creation or destruction of energy."[10] For example, claims have been made that an unlimited calorie intake (excluding carbohydrate) is associated with a consistent and physiologically advantageous loss of weight (which presumably continues as long as the diet is maintained).

Most of the diets focus on diet composition, placing special emphasis on carbohydrate restriction while ignoring the calorie content of the diet.

Some of the authors appear to believe that low-carbohydrate diets generate sufficient ketone bodies (eg, "incompletely burned" fat) to cause urinary losses of ketones in amounts sufficient to account for remarkable rates of weight loss in the face of high caloric intake. Dietary carbohydrate, particularly sugar, is considered by some advocates to be a nutritional "poison" that promotes "hypoglycemia," diabetes, atherosclerosis, and, of course, obesity.

To understand how diets induce changes in body weight, it is necessary to consider their effect on body composition—notably, fat, lean tissue, and water. Obesity is defined as an accumulation of fat in undesirable excess. Such fat can be lost only when calorie expenditure exceeds calorie intake. When water is retained in the body, weight may remain stable or increase even though fat is being lost. When lean tissue is broken down, weight loss may be rapid; however, this kind of weight loss is generally thought to be undesirable. Thus, short-term changes in weight on any diet have little meaning unless the composition of the weight loss is known.

While it is widely understood that calories are obtained from food, it is not as well comprehended that calories (energy) are lost from the body as heat, as excreta and detritus (urine, stools, sweat, etc), in the breath, and as metabolic and mechanical work (the body's metabolic processes and physical activity). There are no other significant pathways of energy loss and no weight reducing regimen can operate without utilizing these channels. No weight reducing diet, including the low-carbohydrate ketogenic diet, can be effective unless it provides for a decrease in energy intake or somehow increases energy losses.

Some observers have suggested that the excretion of large quantities of ketones in the urine might account for the extra weight loss alleged to occur in association with low-carbohydrate ketogenic diets. However, when ketone excretion incident to such diets actually has been measured, it has been found to range between 0.5 and 10 gm/24 hr.[11,12] Studies carried out on starving nondiabetic persons indicate that at most about 20 gm of ketones per day may be excreted in the urine.[13,14] And, as Folin and Denis[15] have shown, the total acetone excretion with the breath is quantitatively insignificant; at most, 1 gm/day. Since the caloric value of ketones is about 4.5 kcal/gm, it is clear that, in subjects on ketogenic diets, ketone losses in the urine rarely, if ever, exceed 100 kcal/day, a quantity that could not possibly account for the dramatic results claimed for such diets.

Another claim made by proponents of the low-carbohydrate high-fat diet has been based on observations by Kekwick and Pawan[16] in 1956 that obese patients on extremely high-fat diets of 1,000 kcal (90% of calories from fat) lost weight more rapidly over an eight- to ten-day period than when they were on an isocaloric diet containing a similar proportion of carbohydrate. To explain their findings, these authors suggested that "obese patients must alter their metabolism in response to the contents of the diet." However, when Pilkington and associates[17] studied the effect of similar diets for periods of 18 to 24 days, rate of weight loss was the same for both diets.

During the first few days of their study, Pilkington et al did observe differences in rate of weight loss similar to those reported by Kekwick and Pawan; however, they concluded that these temporary differences were due chiefly to changes in water balance. Olesen and Quaade,[18] conducting similar studies, reported observations and conclusions similar to those of Pilkington et al. Finally, it should be

mentioned that some years earlier, Werner[19] studied subjects on the Pennington version of the low-carbohydrate diet and found that, apart from transient changes in water balance, the rate of weight loss in obese subjects on the low-carbohydrate diet that restricted calories was similar to that of a "balanced" diet of equal caloric value.

The excretion of sodium and water from the body can be inhibited by dietary carbohydrate.[20,21] Bloom[22] has shown that the weight loss of fasting can be decreased or abolished by the sodium and water retention that occur after ingestion of 600 kcal of carbohydrate. This effect on weight occurs even while the subject remains in negative caloric balance. It should also be pointed out that diets devoid of or very low in carbohydrate tend to promote a temporary sodium loss from the body. In addition, a diet very high in protein content places an extra solute load on the kidneys necessitating an increase in excretion of urinary water; thus a low-carbohydrate diet, by several mechanisms, may cause dehydration, if suitable precautions are not taken. Patients whose renal function is already compromised may have difficulty in handling the extra burden placed on their kidneys by such a diet.

Basis for Weight Loss

No scientific evidence exists to suggest that the low-carbohydrate ketogenic diet has a metabolic advantage over more conventional diets for weight reduction. The fact remains, however, that some patients have lost weight on the low-carbohydrate diet "unrestricted in calories." Why is this so? Yudkin and Carey[23] have reported experiments that provide an adequate explanation of the long-term weight loss that can occur when a "ketogenic" diet is consumed. These workers studied six obese adults who were carefully instructed in the weighing and recording of their complete diets. They were told to eat their usual food for two weeks. At the end of this time, they were asked to reduce the carbohydrate in their diets to about 50 gm/day for an additional two weeks and to eat as much protein and fat as they liked. Specifically, the subjects were told that they could eat unlimited amounts of such foods as

meat, fish, eggs, cheese, butter, margarine, and cream. The intake of calories, protein, fat, and carbohydrate from the daily dietary records was then calculated.

In all subjects, there was a reduction in calories ranging from 13% to 55% during the time they were consuming the low-carbohydrate diet. Interestingly, none of the six subjects ate more fat, and three of them showed a significant reduction of fat intake, ranging from 22 to 35 gm/day. It was concluded that weight lost on such diets was principally due to the consumption of fewer calories.

When obese patients reduce their carbohydrate intake drastically, they are apparently unable to make up the ensuing deficit by means of an appreciable increase in protein and fat. This is especially noteworthy when one considers the fact that carbohydrates comprise 45% or more of the average American's diet.[24] It is difficult to unbalance a diet to this extent and continue to consume the same calories as before. However, for persons who are adapted to a diet virtually devoid of carbohydrate it is not hard to maintain body weight. Tolstoi[25] and McClellan and DuBois[26] studied two normal men who maintained their usual weight for one year on a diet that consisted exclusively of lean and fat meat. The two men consumed about 120 to 130 gm of protein and enough fat to provide a total intake of 2,000 to 3,000 kcal/day. Thus, the weight reduction that occurs in obese subjects who are shifted to a low-carbohydrate diet seems to reflect their inability to adapt rapidly to the marked change in dietary composition. There appears to be no inherent reason why body weight cannot be maintained on a diet devoid of carbohydrate if the other essential nutrients are provided.

At the other extreme, a majority of human beings, particularly those in Asia and Africa, remain lean on diets extremely high in carbohydrate (by American standards) and correspondingly low in fat.[27,28] Thus, there is equally no inherent reason to associate a diet rich in carbohydrate with obesity.

Potential Hazards

What are the potential hazards of a

diet very low in carbohydrate and rich in fat? Perhaps the greatest danger is related to hyperlipidemia, which may be induced by such a regimen. Hypercholesterolemia and hypertriglyceridemia are associated with an increased risk of developing coronary heart disease.[29,30] A diet rich in cholesterol and saturated fat could be responsible for accelerating artherosclerosis, particularly in susceptible persons. The two subjects reported on by Tolstoi[25] developed a visible lipemia on their all-meat (low-carbohydrate) diets, and their plasma cholesterol rose to high levels (in one subject up to 800 mg/100 ml).

Ketogenic diets also may cause a significant increase in the blood uric acid concentration. It appears that, by competing with uric acid for renal tubular excretion, elevated blood ketones can promote hyperuricemia. In patients with a gouty diathesis, the increment in hyperuricemia induced by such a regimen could exacerbate the underlying disease.

Bloom and Azar[31] have reported that all of the subjects whom they studied on "carbohydrate-free diets" complained of fatigue after two days on the diet. "This complaint was characterized by a feeling of physical lack of energy [and] was brought on by physical activity. The subjects all felt that they did not have sufficient energy to continue normal activity after the third day. This fatigue promptly disappeared after the addition of carbohydrate to the diet."

Another observation made by Bloom and Azar was that the subjects on the low-carbohydrate diets developed postural hypotension. The average systolic pressure fell 30 mm Hg and the diastolic 15 mm Hg when the subjects assumed an upright position after being supine.

Evaluation of Dr. Atkins' Diet Revolution

In light of these facts, some of the claims in *Dr. Atkins' Diet Revolution* can be examined. It is alleged that ". . . carbohydrates—not fat—are the principal elements in food that fatten fat people. They do this by preventing you from burning up your own fat and by stimulating your body to make more fat. . . . Protein and fat combinations alone do not do this."[1(p7)]

How does this thermodynamic miracle take place? It is stated that the diet promotes the production of "fat mobilizing hormone" (FMH) ". . . and the production of FMH is the whole purpose of this diet—and the reason it works when all other diets fail."[1(p16)] But, according to Dr. Atkins, "FMH releases energy into your bloodstream by causing the stored fat to convert to carbohydrate. Thus, the fatigue clears without having to call upon the defective insulin mechanism."[1(p73)] Accordingly, ". . . this is the diet revolution; the new chemical situation in which ketones are being thrown off—and so are those unwanted pounds, all without hunger."[1(p13)]

As for a "fat mobilizing hormone" (FMH), no such hormone has been unequivocally identified in man. Fat is mobilized when insulin secretion diminishes.[32] Also, it is recognized that growth hormone and catecholamines stimulate fatty acid mobilization from the fat depots; however, neither of these substances is known to physicians and scientists as "FMH." Thus, the existence and physiological role of a putative FMH in man remain to be established.

The assertion that carbohydrates are the principal elements in food that fatten is, at best, a half-truth. In point of fact, human subjects can gain weight by increasing their intake of fat, the most concentrated source of calories available. This was the rationale for the successful use of oral fat emulsions in the treatment of underweight persons.[33] Also, obesity is prevalent in North America, where the proportion of fat in the diet is higher than that in most other countries,[34] whereas obesity is relatively rare in large areas of the world where the "hidden sugar" of rice starch comprises a very high proportion of the total daily food intake.[35]

Body fat is burned in increasing quantity when total calorie intake is inadequate—regardless of the quantity of carbohydrate in the inadequate diet. Body fat is made from dietary fat as well as from dietary carbohydrate. This fact is obvious when one considers that the linoleic acid in the body's fat depots (usually 10% to 12%) cannot be made in the body but is derived entirely from the diet. Indeed, the fatty acid pattern of

fat in the body's adipose stores tends to reflect the pattern of fatty acids in the diet.[36]

The notion that sedentary persons, without malabsorption or hyperthyroidism, can lose weight on a diet containing 5,000 kcal/day is incredible. No reliable nutritional studies have been reported to support such a claim. Nor is it possible to explain the alleged weight loss in the presence of a high calorie intake on the basis of ketonuria.[11-15]

With respect to ketosis, it is of particular interest to consider the experience of the Canadian Army during World War II with pemmican (dehydrated prime beef with added suet) as an emergency ration for infantry troops. In the Canadian study,[37] the pemmican derived 70% of its calories from fat and 30% from muscle. Thus, the ration was essentially free of carbohydrate.

The performance of the troops using pemmican and tea as the sole components of their ration deteriorated so rapidly as to incapacitate them in three days. When carbohydrate was added to the ration the men recuperated to a reasonably high level of performance.

While on the carbohydrate-free diet, the men complained of nausea and several of them vomited. Pathologic fatigue was evident. On the morning of the fourth day of the diet, physical examination disclosed a group of listless, dehydrated men with drawn faces and sunken eyes, whose breath smelled strongly of acetone. Because of anorexia and water loss the men had lost weight rapidly.

Throughout Dr. Atkins' book, the statement is made that fat is readily converted to carbohydrate; this is biochemically incorrect. Available biochemical evidence indicates that the even-numbered carbon chain fatty acids stored in adipose tissue triglycerides cannot be used for appreciable net synthesis of carbohydrate.[38] Essentially all stored fat is composed of even-numbered carbon acids. The glycerol released during hydrolysis of triglyceride is potentially available for carbohydrate synthesis; however, glycerol is not a fat. In addition, glycerol in adipose tissue is derived entirely from circulating glucose. It comprises about 10% of the calories available when triglycerides are broken down and their components oxidized. There is no evidence that the fatty acid released from stored triglyceride ". . . stabilizes the gyrations in your blood sugar level."[1(p73)]

The book vigorously condemns carbohydrates as being nutritionally pernicious. Dr. Atkins states that "It is important, then, to understand that sugar has antinutrient properties. . . . Starch is the major source of hidden sugar."[1(p57)] To describe starch as the major source of hidden sugar is naive. All carbohydrates in the diet must be converted to "sugar" by the digestive processes prior to their absorption by the intestine. To refer to sugar as having "antinutrient properties" is inaccurate. Although the thiamin (vitamin B₁) requirement increases somewhat when dietary carbohydrate increases, this does not mean that sugar is an "antinutrient" any more than is linoleic acid, a dietary constituent that may increase the body's requirement for vitamin E.

The book also puts great stress on "hypoglycemia" and its alleged relationship to obesity: "Hypoglycemia is undersuspected and underdiagnosed to an extent without parallel in medicine."[1(p71)] Dr. Atkins' position on hypoglycemia should be considered in the light of the following statement[39] recently published Feb 5 (223:682, 1973) in THE JOURNAL.

Recent publicity in the popular press has led the public to believe that the occurrence of hypoglycemia is widespread in this country and that many of the symptoms that affect the American population are not recognized as being caused by this condition. These claims are not supported by medical evidence. Because of the possible misunderstanding about the matter, three organizations of physicians and scientists (the American Diabetes Association, the Endocrine Society, and the American Medical Association) have issued the following statement for the public concerning the diagnosis and treatment of hypoglycemia:

"Hypoglycemia means a low level of blood sugar. When it occurs, it is often attended by symptoms of sweating, shakiness, trembling, anxiety, fast heart action, headache, hunger sensations, brief feelings of weakness, and, occasionally, seizures and coma. However, the majority of people with these kinds of symptoms do not have hypoglycemia; a great many patients with anxiety reactions present with similar symptoms. Furthermore, there is no good evidence that hypoglycemia causes

depression, chronic fatigue, allergies, nervous breakdowns, alcoholism, juvenile delinquency, childhood behavior problems, drug addiction or inadequate sexual performance. . . ."

It is curious that hypoglycemia does not appear to be a problem in parts of the world where carbohydrate provides up to 80% of dietary calories. Indeed, it is of interest that in those same high-carbohydrate areas diabetes mellitus is less common than in the United States.[27] Also, it has been shown[40] that diabetic patients consuming a diet low in cholesterol (100 mg/24 hr), high in carbohydrate (64% of total calories), and low in fat (20% of total calories) maintained good to excellent regulation without an increase in insulin requirements and with a decrease in plasma cholesterol levels. Plasma triglycerides did not increase.

According to Dr. Atkins, most overweight people are hypoglycemic. A majority of physicians probably would not agree with this statement since it is well known that obese patients tend to be resistant to their own insulin. Moreover, there is no sound evidence to suggest that Dr. Atkins' recommendations of ". . . megadoses of B-complex, C, and especially E vitamins"[1(p153)] will help keep blood sugar at an even level. The blood sugar remains remarkably stable without the help of unphysiologic doses of vitamins.

The diet encourages a high intake of saturated fats and cholesterol. The possible hazards of this practice are shrugged off with statements such as: "Studies have shown that you cannot absorb more cholesterol than is in two eggs each day."[1(p282)] This is not entirely correct. It is not impossible to increase the plasma cholesterol level somewhat further by increasing the intake of egg cholesterol beyond this quantity.[41-44] More to the point, when they are added to a low cholesterol diet, two egg yolks per day can cause an undesirable increase in the plasma cholesterol concentration. Moreover, a rise in plasma cholesterol is not necessarily "compensated for" by a concurrent decrease in triglycerides. Indeed the most ominous type of hyperlipidemia, from the standpoint of coronary heart disease, is the form in which the plasma cholesterol concentration is elevated while the tri-

glyceride level is normal (Type II).[45]

When a person consumes a diet very high in fat, he tends to develop an exaggerated alimentary lipemia.[46,47] Some persons may already suffer from an inability to clear fat properly. There is also preliminary evidence to suggest that elevated levels of free fatty acids (such as would occur in patients consuming a low-carbohydrate ketogenic diet) may promote both vascular thrombosis and cardiac arrhythmias.[48-55]

An elevation of the plasma uric acid level is a frequent, if not invariable, concomitant of the low-carbohydrate ketogenic diet. If it becomes necessary to prescribe a drug like allopurinol to counteract such diet-induced hyperuricemia, then the risk of untoward side effects from the drug[56] is added to the nausea, anorexia, and fatigue that so often occur during adaptation to a diet virtually devoid of carbohydrate.

In summary, the approach to treatment of obesity recommended by Dr. Atkins is to restrict carbohydrate intake to less than 40 gm/day thus inducing a state of ketonuria as measured by means of a dipstick.

Summary of Critique of Dr. Atkins' Diet Revolution

The material cited appears to be more than sufficient to make the following points clear:

1. The "diet revolution" is neither new nor revolutionary. It is a variant of the "familiar" low carbohydrate diet that has been promulgated for many years.

2. The rationale advanced to justify the diet is, for the most part, without scientific merit. Furthermore, no evidence is advanced that controlled studies were ever carried out to validate the observation that weight can be lost by sedentary subjects who consume a carbohydrate-poor diet providing 5,000 kcal/day.

3. The Council is deeply concerned about any diet that advocates an "unlimited" intake of saturated fats and cholesterol-rich foods. In persons who respond to such a diet with an elevation of plasma lipids and an exaggerated alimentary hyperlipemia, the risk of coronary artery disease and other clinical manifestations of atherosclerosis may well be increased—particularly if the diet is maintained

over a prolonged period.

4. Any grossly unbalanced diet, particularly one which interdicts the 45% of calories that is usually consumed as carbohydrates, is likely to induce some anorexia and weight reduction if the subject is willing to persevere in following such a bizarre regimen. However, it is unlikely that such a diet can provide a practicable basis for long-term weight reduction or maintenance, ie, a life-time change in eating and exercise habits.

5. It is unfortunate that no reliable mechanism exists to help the public evaluate and put into proper perspective the great volume of nutritional information and mis-information with which it is constantly being bombarded. The Council believes that, in the absence of such a mechanism, members of the media and publishers as well as authors of books and articles advising the public on diet and nutrition have a unique responsibility to ensure that such information and advice are based on scientific facts established by responsible research. Bizarre concepts of nutrition and dieting should not be promoted to the public as if they were established scientific principles. If appropriate precautions are not taken, information about nutrition and diet that is not only misleading but potentially dangerous to health will continue to be conveyed to the public.

6. Physicians should counsel their patients as to the potentially harmful results that might occur because of adherence to the "ketogenic diet." Observations on patients who suffer adverse effects from this regimen should be reported in the medical literature or elsewhere, just as in the case of an adverse drug reaction.

References

1. Atkins RC: *Dr. Atkins' Diet Revolution: The High Calorie Way to Stay Thin Forever.* New York, David McKay Inc Publishers, 1972.

2. Harvey W: *On Corpulence in Relation to Disease.* London, Henry Renshaw, 1872, pp 109, 122.

3. Banting W: *Letter on Corpulence, Addressed to the Public* (London, 1863) ed 2. London, Harrison, 1863, p 22.

4. Pennington AW: An alternate approach to the problem of obesity. *J Clin Nutr* 1:100-106, 1953.

5. Pennington AW: Treatment of obesity with calorically unrestricted diets. *J Clin Nutr* 1:343-348, 1953.

6. *Air Force Diet.* Toronto, Canada, Air Force Diet Publishers, 1960.

7. Taller H: *Calories Don't Count.* New York, Simon and Schuster Inc Publishers, 1961.

8. Jameson G, Williams E: *The Drinking Man's Diet.* San Francisco, Cameron and Co, 1964.

9. Stillman IM, Baker SS: *The Doctor's Quick Weight Loss Diet.* Englewood Cliffs, NJ, Prentice-Hall Inc, 1967.

10. White A, et al: *Principles of Biochemistry.* New York, McGraw-Hill Book Co Inc, 1954, p 9.

11. Grande F: Energy balance and body composition changes: A critical study of three recent publications. *Ann Intern Med* 68:467-480, 1968.

12. Azar GJ, Bloom WL: Similarities of carbohydrate deficiency and fasting. II. Ketones, nonesterified fatty acids, and nitrogen excretion. *Arch Intern Med* 112:338-343, 1963.

13. Lusk G: *The Elements of the Science of Nutrition.* New York, W. B. Saunders Co, 1906, p 63.

14. Deuel HJ Jr, Gulick M: Studies on ketosis. 1. The sexual variation in starvation ketosis. *J Biol Chem* 96:25-34, 1932.

15. Folin O, Denis W: On starvation and obesity, with special reference to acidosis. *J Biol Chem* 21:183-192, 1915.

16. Kekwick A, Pawan GLS: Calorie intake in relation to body weight changes in the obese. *Lancet* 2:155-161, 1956.

17. Pilkington TRE, et al: Diet and weight reduction in the obese. *Lancet* 1:856-858, 1960.

18. Olesen ES, Quaade F: Fatty foods and obesity. *Lancet* 1:1048-1051, 1960.

19. Werner SC: Comparison between weight reduction on a high-calorie, high-fat diet and on an isocaloric regimen high in carbohydrate. *N Engl J Med* 252:661-665, 1955.

20. Gamble JL, Ross GS, Tisdall FF: The metabolism of fixed base during fasting. *J Biol Chem* 57:633-695, 1923.

21. Hervey GR, McCance RA: The effects of carbohydrate and sea water on the metabolism of men without food or sufficient water. *Proc R Soc (Biol)* 139:527-545, 1952.

22. Bloom WL: Inhibition of salt excretion by carbohydrate. *Arch Intern Med* 109:26-32, 1962.

23. Yudkin J, Carey M: The treatment of obesity by the "high-fat" diet. The inevitability of calories. *Lancet* 2:939-941, 1960.

24. *Recommended Dietary Allowances,* 7th ed, publication 1964. National Academy of Sciences, Washington, DC, 1968, pp 9-10.

25. Tolstoi E: The effect of an exclusive meat diet on the chemical constituents of the blood. *J Biol Chem* 83:753-758, 1929.

26. McClellan WS, DuBois EF: Prolonged meat diets with a study of kidney function and ketosis. *J Biol Chem* 87:651-668, 1930.

27. West KM, Kalblfleisch JM: Glucose tolerance nutrition, and diabetes in Uruguay, Venezuela, Malaya and East Pakistan. *Diabetes* 15:9-18, 1966.

28. McLaren DS, Pellet PL: Nutrition in the Middle East, in Bourne GJ (ed): *World Review of Nutrition and Dietetics,* vol 12. Basel, Switzerland, S. Karger, 1970, pp 43-127.

29. Kannel WB, et al: Serum cholesterol, lipoproteins, and the risk of coronary heart disease: The Framingham Study. *Ann Intern Med* 74:1-12, 1971.

30. Brown DF, Kinch SH, Doyle JT: Serum triglycerides in health and in ischemic heart disease. *N Engl J Med* 273:947-952, 1965.

31. Bloom WL, Azar GJ: Similarities of carbohydrate deficiency and fasting. I. Weight loss, electrolyte excretion, and fatigue. *Arch Intern Med* 112:333-337, 1963.

32. Cahill GF Jr: Physiology of insulin in man. *Diabetes* 20:785, 1971.

33. Shoshkes M, et al: Fat emulsions for oral nutrition; use of orally administered fat emulsions as caloric supplements in man. *J Am Diet Assoc* 27:197-208, 1951.

34. *Obesity and Health. A Source Book of Current Information for Professional Health Personnel,* publication 1485. Washington, DC, US Public Health Service, Division of Chronic Diseases, 1966.

35. Insull W, Oiso T, Tsuchiya K: Diet and nutritional status of Japanese. *Am J Clin Nutr* 21:753-777, 1968.

36. Christakis G, et al: Effect of a cholesterol-lowering diet on fatty acid composition of subcutaneous fat in man. *Circ* 26:648, 1962.

37. Kark RM, Johnson RE, Lewis JS: Defects of pemmican as an emergency ration for infantry troops. *War Medicine* 7:345-352, 1945.

38. West ES, et al: *Textbook of Biochemistry,* ed 4. New York, The Macmillan Co Publishers, 1967, pp 1050-1052.

39. Statement on hypoglycemia, editorial. *JAMA* 223:682, 1973.

40. Stone DB, Conner WE: The prolonged effects of a low cholesterol, high carbohydrate diet upon the serum lipids in diabetic patients. *Diabetes* 12:127-132, 1963.

41. Beveridge JMR, et al: Dietary cholesterol and plasma cholesterol levels in man. *Canad J Biochem Physiol* 37:575, 1959.

42. Bronte-Stewart B: Lipids and atherosclerosis. *Fed Proc* 20 (pt III, suppl 7):127-134, 1961.

43. Connor WE, Hodges RE, Bleiler RE: The serum lipids in men receiving high cholesterol and cholesterol-free diets. *J Clin Invest* 40:894-901, 1961.

44. Inter-Society Commission for Heart Disease Resources, Atherosclerosis and Epidemiology Study Groups. Primary prevention of the atherosclerotic disease. *Circ* 42:A-55-A-95, 1970.

45. Fredrickson DS, Levy RI, Lees RS: Fat transport in lipoproteins—An integrated approach to mechanisms and disorders. *N Engl J Med* 276:34-42, 94-103, 148-156, 215-225, 273-281, 1967.

46. Brunzell JD, Porte D Jr, Bierman EL: Evidence for a common saturable removal system for removal of dietary and endogenous triglyceride in man. *J Clin Invest* 50:15a, abstract #48, 1971.

47. Connor WE: Effect of dietary lipids upon chylomicron composition in man. *Fed Proc* 18:473, abstract #1861, 1959.

48. Greig HBW: Inhibition of fibrinolysis by alimentary lipaemia. *Lancet* 2:16-18, 1956.

49. Merigan TC, et al: Effect of chylomicrons on fibrinolytic activity of normal human plasma in vitro. *Circ Res* 7:205-209, 1959.

50. Philip RB, Wright HP: Effect of adenosine on platelet adhesiveness in fasting and lipaemic bloods. *Lancet* 2:208-209, 1965.

51. Farbiszewski R, Worowski K: Enhancement of platelet aggregation and adhesiveness by beta lipoprotein. *J Atheroscler Res* 8:988-990, 1968.

52. Oliver MT, Yates PA: Induction of ventricular arrhythmias by elevation of arterial free fatty acids in experimental myocardial infarction, in Moret P, Feifar Z, (eds): *Metabolism of the Hypoxic and Ischaemic Heart.* Basel, Switzerland, S. Karger, 1972, p 359.

53. Oliver MF, Kurien VA, Greenwood TW: Relation between serum-free fatty acids and arrhythmias and death after acute myocardial infarction. *Lancet* 1:710-714, 1968.

54. Hoak JC, Warner ED, Connor WE: Effects of acute free fatty acid mobilization on the heart, in Bajusz E, Rona G (eds): *Myocardiology: Recent Advances in Studies of Cardiac Structure and Metabolism.* Baltimore, University Park Press, 1972, vol 1, pp 127-135.

55. Hoak JC, Connor WE, Warner ED: Toxic effects of glucagon-induced acute lipid mobilization in geese. *J Clin Invest* 47:2701-2710, 1968.

56. *AMA Drug Evaluations,* ed 1. Chicago, American Medical Association, 1971, pp 196-197.

We often forget that there are two essential features in the reduction of excessive weight by means of diet: the individual and the diet. The individual must have sufficient incentive to adhere to the diet; the diet must be constructed so that it provides fewer calories but adequate nutrients. These two features are clearly interrelated, for anything that makes the diet difficult to follow tends to counteract incentive. These considerations, I believe, make the low-carbohydrate diet the diet of choice in the treatment of obesity. It reduces excessive caloric intake; it is likely to contain a better supply of nutrients than do other calorie-restricted diets; it is intrinsically palatable; it is socially acceptable; it is not costly; and for all these reasons it can become a permanent eating pattern to maintain weight at a reasonable level.

Caloric Intake

Since calories are produced from protein, fat and carbohydrate, it is obvious that reduction in caloric intake must be achieved by reduction in one or more of these constituents. Reducing protein to half the average consumption of about 100 gm a day would save only about 200 cal; at the same time it would reduce the palatability of the diet, and more importantly, it would introduce the hazard of protein inadequacy. Reducing fat to about half the average intake would save more calories, something like 500 a day. This would certainly not be hazardous, but for most people it would result in an unacceptably un-

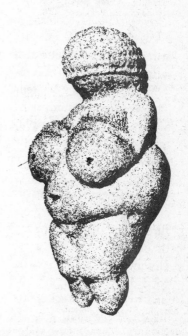

The Low-Carbohydrate Diet in the Treatment of Obesity

Obese patients are not likely to follow a diet that is unpalatable and unsatisfying. With the low-carbohydrate diet, patients limit carbohydrate to about 50 or 60 gm a day and eat as much protein and fat as they want. This plan gives palatability, satisfaction of hunger, good nutrition, and a deficit of 1000 cal a day or more. Moreover, the patient does not need to know caloric values of foods.

JOHN YUDKIN, M.D.
Queen Elizabeth College
University of London

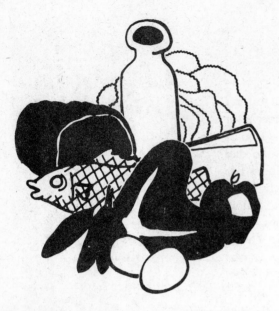

attractive diet and one that would not be as satisfying in terms of hunger.

What then if we reduce carbohydrate? The average consumption is about 350 gm a day; however, many people take much more than this. On the other hand, it is quite possible to construct acceptable diets containing 50 to 60 gm of carbohydrate a day, thus producing a saving of 1000 cal or more.

There is, moreover, one remarkable feature of the diet containing this small amount of carbohydrate. For reasons that I do not clearly understand, restricting carbohydrate to a daily amount of 50 to 60 gm allows one to take as much protein and fat as one likes. As we shall see, this is not the same as saying that one eats an unlimited amount of these dietary constituents, but it certainly simplifies dietary instruction.

As an alternative to the reduction of calories in one of the three major dietary constituents, one can, of course, reduce any two of them or all three. Many physicians, in fact, say to their patients (usually the more sophisticated ones) that they should simply eat less: "Leave the table before you are really satisfied." Certainly some people can do this, but I do not believe that it is at all a popular way of weight reduction or weight control.

Nor do I believe that it is usually the most desirable nutritionally, since it assumes that the excessive intake of calories is matched by an excessive intake of all nutrients.

Nutritional Value

The main carbohydrate-rich foods are sugar, candy, cakes, cookies, soft drinks, ice cream, bread, potatoes and pasta. Since sugar contributes about 450 cal a day to the average American diet, and since it is free from any nutrients whatever, it is clearly the first choice for curtailment or elimination in a diet that is to be rich in nutrients but reduced in calories. It is true that some nutrients accompany sugar in preparations such as ice cream and cakes, but the quantities are small in relation to the number of calories.

So much for theory. What in practice is the nutrient content of a low-carbohydrate diet? As far as I know, the only studies of what people eat on this regimen are the two that Carey, Stock and I[1,2] published in 1960 and 1970. In the first, we were concerned to show that the low-carbohydrate diet is not a high-fat diet, a designation frequently and incorrectly ascribed to it. In our second study we also looked at the nutrient intake, for by then there were claims that the low-carbohydrate diet was accompanied by a hazard of deficiency in calcium, thiamine, riboflavin, folic acid, and ascorbic acid.

We determined the usual dietary intake in our subjects from their diaries of weighed food and drink over a period of 14 days. They were then told that they could eat as much as they wished of foods very low in carbohydrate (meat, fish, cheese, butter, and green leafy vegetables). They were to have between 10 and 20 oz of whole milk a day; otherwise they were free to choose up to 50 gm of carbohydrate-containing foods daily. Details of the diet are given elsewhere.[3] Again, subjects kept a record of the weight or measure of everything they ate or drank for the following two weeks.

The first study showed that the diet decreased average caloric intake by about 35 percent, almost entirely a reduction in carbohydrate. There was no increase in protein intake, and there was a small decrease in fat intake. The second study gave almost precisely the same results: a fall in calories, no change in protein, and a slight decrease in fat (table 1). We decided that the best way of assessing the nutritional value of the diet was to compare the nutrient intake with what would have been achieved if our subjects had reduced all their food and drink by the same amount, about 35 percent.

In this way, we calculated that of a possible 99 items (nine nutrients for each of 11 subjects), the low-carbohydrate diet provided a higher nutrient intake in 87 items and an insignificantly lower intake in most of the 12 other items. However, we have to take into account that some of the other nutrients are more available from the foods eaten on the low-carbohydrate diet than from those eaten on the ordinary diet. Thus, iron and niacin are poorly available in cereal foods, which provided a sizable proportion of these nutrients on the usual diet, whereas they are more available from meat, which provided a higher proportion of the nutrients on the low-carbohydrate diet.

Thus, the low-carbohydrate diet significantly reduces calories while in almost every instance improving intake of nutrients. I cannot think of any other practical regimen for reducing caloric intake that will have a similar beneficial effect on the nutrient intake.

Social Acceptability

Looked at in terms of particular meals, the low-carbohydrate diet follows the normal pattern so closely that it requires little deviation from what is being eaten by the rest of the family or by one's hosts at a party. Think of just one meal, the main meal of the day. You take no bread with your soup; you take one small potato or none with your helping

Table 1. Comparison of Normal and Low-Carbohydrate Diets*			
	Normal	Low-Carbohydrate	Difference
Calories	2,340	1,390	−950
	2,330	1,560	−770
Protein, grams	77	80	+3
	84	83	−1
Fat, grams	122	99	−23
	124	105	−19
Carbohydrate, grams	206	65	−141
	216	67	−149

*The upper figure in each instance is from the study reported in 1960 (six subjects),[1] and the lower figure from the study reported in 1970 (11 subjects).[2]

of meat and vegetables, nor need you trim the fat off the meat or avoid putting butter on the string beans; you have a piece of fruit after the main course and, if you are still hungry, a piece of cheese with perhaps a small cracker. You do not, of course, take sugar in your coffee, and you avoid soft drinks unless they are sugar-free. For most individuals, the party occasion demanding a helping of blueberry pie does not happen often enough to undermine the principles of following the low-carbohydrate diet in everyday life.

The low-carbohydrate diet should be followed permanently, of course, because it is nothing more than a good, sound, nutritious eating pattern. Nor would the diet harm the rest of the family, obese or nonobese, child or adult, for there is nothing wrong in reducing the amount of carbohydrate-rich foods, especially those rich in sucrose. In this connection it is important to impress on the patient that the low-carbohydrate regimen is not a universally weight-reducing regimen; it will only reduce excessive weight. Since it allows people to eat to satiety, it does not need to be modified for "maintenance" as do diets in which calories are counted.

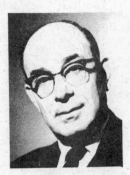

JOHN YUDKIN

Dr. Yudkin is emeritus professor of nutrition, Queen Elizabeth College, University of London.

A major reason for the acceptability of the diet is that it does not require knowledge of the caloric values of food items. Since only carbohydrate is restricted, instruction can begin with the psychologically impressive statement, "You may eat as much as you like of all these foods: meat, fish, eggs, cheese, butter, margarine, oils, cream, leafy vegetables." You then need to point out that it is important to take moderate quantities of milk. After that, simply give a list of foods with their carbohydrate content. It is absurd to do this with any pretense of precision, since people will not wish to weigh every item; for this reason I give a list in terms of "carbohydrate units," each of 5 gm, and tell the patient to take no more than 8 to 10 units a day. Thus, I say that an apple contains 2 units, a thin slice of bread 3 units, and a small bottle of cola drink 3 units. Calculated in this fashion, the total intake of carbohydrate will not be precisely 50 gm a day, but it will approximate that achieved with more meticulous calculation and be sufficiently near for practical purposes.

Expense

I am often told that this diet is a high-protein diet and therefore must be costly. We have seen that it is not a high-protein diet. Nor must it be expensive. First, it is not necessary to think of protein entirely in terms of T-bone steak or lobster; there are other sorts of meat, other sorts of fish. And the cheese need not be imported Brie or Stilton; cheddar is nutritionally just as good. Second, people rarely realize just how much they spend on carbohydrate-rich foods. They think of how little they will save on bread and potatoes but forget how much they will save on soft drinks, ice cream, candy, cakes and cookies. In fact, on comparison, many people find that the low-carbohydrate regimen is less expensive than their usual regimen. One of my patients found that he was saving nearly one-third of the cost of his food after he made the change.

Comment

I should like to make one final point. A few years ago the National Livestock and Meat Board[4] published a critical survey of the low-carbohydrate diet. The report is an example of the danger of drawing conclusions from theoretical considerations rather than from practical experience. It said, for example, "Low carbohydrate diets are unavoidably high in both protein and saturated fats." As we have seen, this is just not true. It also mentioned effects, such as ketosis, which have been shown to occur in persons whose diet is completely free from carbohydrate. But the low-carbohydrate diet is not the same as a highly experimental carbohydrate-free diet, and it certainly does not produce ketosis. I have no doubt that in practice the low-carbohydrate diet will be found to be the most effective and, nutritionally, the most desirable for the management of obese patients.

REFERENCES

1. Yudkin J, Carey M: The treatment of obesity by the "high-fat" diet. The inevitability of calories. Lancet 2:939, 1960
2. Stock AL, Yudkin J: Nutrient intake of subjects on low carbohydrate diet used in treatment of obesity. Am J Clin Nutr 23:948, 1970
3. Yudkin J: This Slimming Business. Ed 3. London, Penguin, 1971
4. National Livestock and Meat Board: Characteristics of Low Carbohydrate Diets. Chicago, Ill, 1966

Rational Diet Construction for Mild and Grand Obesity

I. Frank Tullis, MD, Memphis

Rational diet construction for obesity requires understanding of two facts: (1) energy expenditure must be considered along with diet and (2) psychological incentive must be maintained.

Ironically, time may prove that diet construction in the present day sense will play a minor role in obesity correction. It has become progressively more apparent that psychological and behavioral characteristics of the individual represent the true etiological factors in obesity. Correction of these depends on successful behavior modification of the individual. The best current concept is that diet and exercise are fundamental for obesity control, but also that behavior modification is the underlying essential for long-term regulation.

Physiologically and psychologically, mild and grand obesity are different. In mild obesity the problem is usually one of insidious, often slight shift of caloric balance to one beyond weight maintenance over a prolonged period. Dietary intake and energy expenditure are both usually involved in the change of balance. Psychological factors enter the picture in mild to moderate obesity, most often as behavioral responses to stressful life situations.

In grand obesity the positive caloric balance is the result principally

of prolonged high caloric dietary intake, often in the range of 3,000 to 4,500 calories daily. The larger body mass and surface area increase the basal metabolic expenditure appreciably but not sufficiently to balance the caloric intake. Diminished overall physical activity contributes to the balance picture as the individual progressively retreats from social contact. Psychologically individuals with grand obesity characteristically exhibit striking emotional abnormalities. They may show such deviations as distorted body images, manic-depressive or depressive personality patterns, or pathological dependency. Both "night-eating" and "binge-eating" are more common among those severely obese persons.

Observations by psychologists suggest that obese persons are influenced more by external cues or stimuli in their eating habits rather than by the normal physiological hunger signals. As long as food is before them they tend to keep eating and are more sensitive to the taste of food. Obese persons as a group eat little or no breakfast, usually a light lunch, and then the bulk of their food at dinner, often snacking in the afternoon and in the evening.

Basic Dietary Adequacy

For any diet plan to be rational it must be nutritionally adequate. For purposes of this discussion, only healthy adults are considered who do not have special nutritional requirements. Guidelines for a diet can be

outlined in simple broad terms, as follows:

Nutritionally Adequate Diet
1. Lean meat, fish, or fowl twice daily plus three or four eggs weekly.
2. Cereal or bread three times a day.
3. Green or yellow vegetables twice daily.
4. Fruit or fruit juice twice daily (one citrus).
5. Milk or cheese twice daily.

Rules for the Obese
1. Sufficient calories to permit physical vigor.
2. Minimum of 300 calories at each of three or four meals daily, without snacking.
3. Reasonable size servings without second servings.
4. Increase in daily physical exercise.

The Mild to Moderate.—It is reasonable to hope that the positive caloric balance of some persons can be shifted successfully by a very simple regimen. Such persons likely would be those only 10% to 15% above desirable weight who have unsuspectingly drifted into positive caloric balance. For these persons, a reasonable approach would be a simple caloric control plan as outlined here:

1. Always observe the factors of the essential diet (previous list).
2. Broil, boil, bake, or roast meat, fish, and poultry; remove visible fat from meat and use only natural juice instead of thickened gravy.
3. If low-fat milk is used, a small amount of margarine (preferably corn-oil type) may be used to season vegetables.
4. Cook vegetables without fat and add allowed margarine after cooking; flavor cooking water with herbs or bouillon cube.

From the University of Tennessee College of Medicine, Memphis.
Reprint requests to Sanders Clinic, 20 S Dudley, Memphis 38103.

5. Favor green, yellow, or red vegetables over starch vegetables.
6. Use low-calorie dressings, lemon, or vinegar on salads.
7. Favor plain fruit over pastries for dessert.
8. To avoid "empty calories," sweeten with sugar substitutes and use only sugar-free soft drinks.
9. Eat meals at about the same hour each day to allow a consistent interval between them.
10. Take little or no alcoholic beverages.

Depending on the level of previous caloric excess, this regimen would usually provide negative caloric balance sufficient to produce fat loss at the rate of half kilogram every two to three weeks. This rate is slow, but even so it is frequently faster than the rate of previous fat gain, and obviously it will be effective if followed long enough.

If all mildly and moderately obese persons should decide to follow the above plan, it is certain a great many would fail to continue the regimen the full period necessary to reduce body fat to ideal level. For such persons a more rigid program is mandatory, either to provide negative caloric balance of greater degree or to enhance psychological incentive sufficiently to make the program effective. The crucial ingredients at this level are personalization and substantial support of psychological incentive. These are best provided by a diet prescription, a physical activity prescription, and participation in a group effort as a means for generating incentive and modifying behavior.

The ideal diet is one constructed by a professional dietitian having several key features in mind. There should be at least 300 calories at each meal. Emphasis should be placed on a daily caloric intake that will permit a vigorous physical activity program. Generally this will be at least 1,200 calories. The dietitian also should evaluate and capitalize on personal characteristics of the individual. In the design of such variations, the positive value of encouraging the individual to continue the program is more important than achieving greater caloric restriction. The ideal physical activity prescription is the one the patient will follow regularly. Determining that regimen necessitates discussion and deliberation with the patient and can be done by the physician, the dietitian, or a group leader. The third essential ingredient is a plan to keep up enthusiasm and psychological drive. All recent indications are that this can be supplied best by some type of group effort.

An even more effective approach that deserves much more trial than is presently available is organized group therapy with active behavior modification programs under professional control and guidance. In medical centers of reasonable size, an ideal plan would be the organization of groups of 20 to 35 persons with a trained group leader, the general physician, the psychiatrist or clinical psychologist, and the dietitian as consultants and participants.

The Severe.—In many respects there is no rational diet for the severely obese person (two or three times his optimum weight). The very finding of this degree of obesity should serve as immediate warning that the person requires far more important therapeutic measures than a diet plan or exercise prescription. It is equally unlikely that such patients will respond effectively to incentive bolstering and behavior modification via group effort. Instead they need careful psychiatric evaluation and appropriate psychiatric treatment. It is reasonable for the practicing physician to accomplish general medical evaluation, to construct a diet with no fewer than 1,600 calories daily for women and 2,000 calories for men, and to explore means for increasing regular outdoor physical exercise. At some point along the way, however, the opportunity must be seized to insist that such patients have good psychiatric evaluation and treatment.

In selected cases, with joint care by seriously interested internists and psychiatrists, it is possible that initial fasting in the hospital or intestinal bypass surgery such as jejuno-ileostomy, might fill a role of getting the patient started toward body-fat change. In these instances, from the medical point of view, it must be remembered that nearly 50% of weight loss in fasting is water, and most types of jejuno-ileostomy likely provide benefit only up to two to three years.

In summary, rational diet construction for both mild and grand obesity necessitates broad understanding of the disorder, categorizing of patients according to the seriousness of their problems, and applying appropriate treatments.

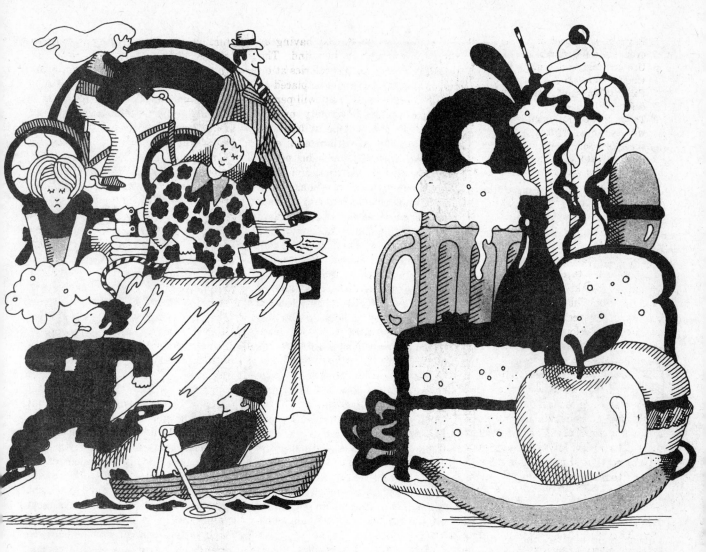

An hour of exercise vs. A pound of flesh

By PROF. JEAN MAYER

Most of us eat much less than our grandfathers did. A respectable dinner on an ordinary Saturday night used to consist of ham and chicken, white potatoes and sweet potatoes, several choices of vegetables, fresh homemade bread and hot rolls with plenty of sweet country butter, and the inevitable pie and cake. Those who wanted ice cream went to the kitchen to fetch it themselves.

Yet our grandparents were not noticeably more obese than we, the hefty generation.

The reason is simple. To get to the neighbor's house for that dinner, Grandpa had to walk for some distance, even in the dead of winter. If there was old-fashioned dancing afterward, it was gen-

erally more strenuous than the modern variety, including rock. If Grandfather farmed, nothing more need be said about how rapidly he worked off the hot rolls. And if he had a factory job, his daily hours and his work week were considerably longer than our 40 hours going on 35.

I am convinced that inactivity is the most important factor behind the creeping overweight that is shadowing most of us. And our sedentary ways are being encouraged by two widely prevalent myths that have persuaded many people to lie down until the urge to exercise goes away.

The first myth is that it takes a Gargantuan effort to work off a tiny bit of weight or to counteract the effect of just a handful of potato chips. The other is

that exercise is self-defeating because it makes you so hungry you go out and ruin it all by stuffing the yawning hollow you've just created.

If the saga of our forebears isn't persuasive enough to dispel these ideas, perhaps a look at the scientific evidence will be convincing.

The simplest fact is in the standard recommended caloric intake charts prepared by such prestigious organizations as the National Research Council. For sedentary men, some 2,300 calories is considered ideal. But very active men can get by with 4,500 calories. The *only* difference is activity or exercise. Surely, any factor that can double a person's daily food allowance is not to be dismissed lightly.

As the nutritionist on the medical advisory board to the U.S. Olympic team, I have seen athletes at the peak of their preparation eating up to 6,000 calories a day. Obviously, a tired businessman or harassed housewife is just not going to be in shape for that kind of activity. But it makes the point: the more you work, the more you can eat.

Let's consider the caloric expenditure of the simplest kind of effort, the sort of thing most people wouldn't think of as really using any energy to speak of. Just dressing and undressing, depending on how many items you take off and put on,

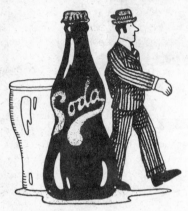

Soda, 106 calories = walking, 20 minutes

or how hard you struggle with zippers, will use up about 40 calories an hour. If you then walk at a moderately fast pace to the office or the train, and it takes you 18–20 minutes, you will have burned up the 96 calories of those two strips of bacon you had for breakfast. Repeat that same walk at night and work off a little lunch. A couple of times up or down a flight of stairs is obviously more trimming than an elevator ride.

It is really that easy, and it has all been accurately charted by having people perform various tasks in a calorimetric chamber. This is a room specially constructed to trap the heat produced by a person's body whenever he does anything, including just lying absolutely still. Because no matter what you do, even breathing, the body uses a certain amount of energy and, as a result, burns up food energy and gives off heat. That's all caloric expenditure means.

It doesn't take so much effort to produce a fair amount of caloric expendi-

ture. Everybody has heard such statements as "It takes thirty-six hours of walking or seven hours of splitting wood just to burn off one pound."

There are several things wrong with such misleading remarks. First, they don't take the person's individual weight into account; it's going to take a thin man longer to use up calories than a fat man doing the same thing. It also assumes that caloric expenditure has to take place all in one continuous period.

Assume that you are an average 150-pound man or 120-pound woman whose caloric intake averages a nice 2,300 or 1,800 a day. If you run for a half hour or wash dishes and sweep and polish the floors for about an hour, you've just used up one-tenth of your day's entire food intake. And you've got 23 hours left over to burn up the rest. Obviously, if you keep to a moderate food intake and just go about your business, you're not likely to put on weight.

But if you loaf through the day, spend a lot of time sitting at a desk, eat large restaurant lunches, then a full dinner, and possibly a bedtime snack, you've got to make some other effort. Playing volley ball all day? This is absurd; it is the kind of suggestion put forth by the enemies of exercise, who persist in maintaining that

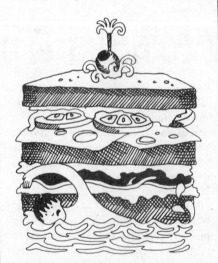

Club Sandwich, 590 calories = swimming, 1 hour

exercise has to be done in one uninterrupted stretch to do any good. The energy expended in physical activity gets spent regardless, whether you do it in

five-minute bursts at a time or three hours at a stretch. Splitting wood for seven hours would be difficult for anyone but Paul Bunyan. Splitting wood for a half hour is not only possible for the

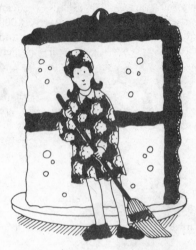

Layer cake, 356 calories = sweeping, 4 hours

average healthy man but surprisingly pleasant if it's a nice fall day. If a man split wood for 30 minutes every day, it would add up to the equivalent of 26 pounds of body fat neatly worked off in the space of a year.

The amount of energy that can be used up in most types of activity, which involve only certain parts of the body, is directly related to how much a person weighs in the first place. A tennis player, for instance, uses up very few calories moving his racket. Most of the calories are burned up moving himself. And since it takes a lot more effort to move a 200-pound object around a tennis court than it does to move a 150-pound one, a heavier man is going to get rid of more calories in an hour than his average-weight opponent. As a result, he would lose more weight—unless, of course, he ate more. So, the heavier the person, the more results he will get from the same activity.

On the average, walking for an hour will use up between 100 and 300 more calories than just sitting still; bicycling, up to 500 calories; swimming and skating, up to 600; skiing, up to 900. If you are a well-trained athlete, rowing can get you up to a caloric expenditure of some 1,300 calories as a clock ticks off an hour.

You do not have to knock yourself out. An expenditure of 500–600 calories in one hour is about the limit that the average out-of-condition adult can handle without discomfort. If you spread this out in half-hour periods, you can manage a good deal more—say, 1,000 calories in one day. And that's over and above the calories you use up just getting from breakfast through the day and back to bed.

It can be put another way, perhaps more meaningfully to those who are food-oriented. Thirty minutes of an activity that uses up calories, such as riding a bike, is the equivalent of a small piece of cherry pie.

This raises the specter of the other long-surviving myth: namely, if you burn up 500 calories in an hour, you will be so famished you'll have to have a snack to tide you over until mealtime—and the whole effort will have been wasted. There is just enough truth in this myth to have helped keep it alive far beyond its useful life expectancy. Most adults remain at about the same weight level because, when they exert themselves more, their

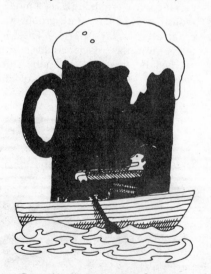

Beer, 114 calories = rowing, 6 minutes

appetite switches on and they eat more to compensate. The two things—effort and eating—remain in balance. But this applies strictly to the average person, whose weight is normal, whose activity and food intake remain *generally* the same over a long period, even though it may fluctuate a good deal in any given

day or week. For a number of rather complicated reasons, it does not apply to people who drastically change their eating habits without changing their activity, or vice versa.

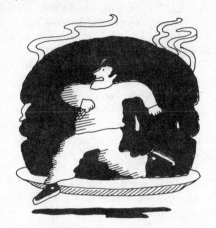

Hamburger, 350 calories = running, 18 minutes

A sedentary life just seems to lead to excessive eating. Studies of people suddenly immobilized by fractures or blindness show that they usually gain weight. And people who work and exercise harder may eat more than they did when they were lazier, but they don't get fatter. Generally, the extra food eaten as a result of exercise is not so great as the amount of calories burned up.

Recent studies involving young people underscore this point nicely. A number of years ago, Dr. Mary Louise Johnson and I did some research on high school girls in a Massachusetts town. When we examined the eating habits of equal groups of overweight and normal-weight girls, the same age and height, we found that the fatter girls divided into two groups. The larger group included girls who actually ate a little less than the normal-weight girls but who exercised much less. They preferred sitting activities to walking or active sports, and they watched TV four times as many hours as the girls in the normal-weight group. There were also a few overweight girls who ate more and exercised as much as the normal group. They were red-cheeked, cheerful, and significantly more muscular than the others. So while they were considered overweight, they were not so overfat as the sitters.

Looking more closely at what these

girls were calling exercise, we unearthed some revealing facts. When the fat girls supposedly exercised, they were in fact spending much less time in motion than the normal-weight girls. Motion pictures of these girls swimming or playing volley ball or tennis showed that the overweight ones moved only a fraction of the time that the normal-weight girls moved. In terms of calories spent, they used up much less energy, despite their energy-consuming burden of extra fat.

Studies of boys at summer camp, furthermore, showed that when overweight youngsters increased their activity, they didn't eat as much as normal-weight boys who were also exercising more. The normal-weight boys tended to gain weight, the fat ones to lose.

The inescapable conclusion, it seems to me, is that our inactive way of life is what's putting on most of the extra weight. Although it is difficult to work exercise into our schedules, it is the only way out of the sit-and-eat cycle.

If there is still any lingering doubt, I can only point to the field of animal husbandry for dramatic proof. Trainers of race horses rely on exercise to keep their winners fleet, trim, and supple. But the farmer keeps his young hogs, geese, and steer cooped up in pens so they won't walk off their valuable poundage. It's well known that the first step toward producing lard or *pâté de foie gras* is to prevent the animals from using up any energy in unhampered wandering. ∎

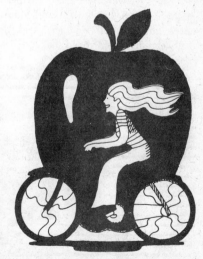

Apple, 101 calories = cycling, 15 minutes

We use the word "exercise" to describe activities that are almost as varied as the foods we eat. But unlike food, which we often describe at rapturous length, we seldom bother with the details of exercise. "I got a lot of exercise last summer," we will say, or, "Now that summer is here, I hope to exercise again."

Descriptive? Not at all. But somehow it seems to suffice. Even the medical profession is careless in its use of the word. "You ought to lose some weight, say ten to fifteen pounds—and try to exercise regularly" is a common piece of medical advice. A very vague reference, I'm sure you'll agree, for a multitude of extraordinarily diverse activities, with very different effects on health.

Let me go through the different types of exercises—and explain the benefits and risks we can expect from each one.

Exercises to Control Your Weight

First, as I have often pointed out, physical activity is an essential element in appetite and weight control. When you are inactive, the appetite, normally a marvelously precise guide of how much you should eat, no longer functions accurately. In other words, you will eat more than you actually expend, with a corresponding increase in weight.

This problem of underexercising is particularly significant for children and adolescents. Our studies of overweight schoolchildren in the Boston area show that excessive weight gains usually begin in the late fall and winter, and almost never during good weather. And the overweight children spend strikingly less time in physical activities than their slimmer counterparts. Likewise, we found that on the average, the overweight youngsters ate less, not more, than the normal-weight children. So the answer to the weight problems of these children was to increase their exercise, rather than decrease their food intake.

The same theory applies to adults. Indications are that our average caloric intake in this country has decreased since 1900, even though our problems of overweight have increased. Of course, since 1900 the automobile has replaced walking, and all sorts of mechanical aids have lightened our toil in the factory, on the farm, and around the home. In the past few years, even such small residual exercise as shifting car gears or pressing the keys of a non-electric typewriter have been eliminated. And that extra telephone extension in the kitchen may save you steps, but it's also worth a few pounds of fat a year.

A pound of fat is the equivalent, on the average, of 3500 calories. Even a surplus of 100 calories a day—an apple or a serving of potato chips—will grow into 10 pounds of fat a year! But those 100 calories could be used up by walking 20 minutes a day. Remember that exercise does consume an appreciable number of calories, and if you're inactive, you will still eat that small but, in the long run, deadly surplus each day. Walking, bicycling, swimming—any exercise done at however moderate a rate—will bring your appetite back under control if you do it long enough. (See the accompanying chart for precise activities to burn off the calories in various foods.)

Exercises That Help Your Heart

But what about the more vigorous exercises—working out at the gym, jogging, or swimming at a moderate pace? Such exercises, if done with sufficient intensity and duration, are of great benefit to your heart. Dr. Ernst Jökl of the University of Kentucky has demonstrated that an hour of vigorous exercise each day can help lower the blood pressure of men suffering from hypertension.

What's more, prolonged vigorous activity—up to several hours a day—seems to lower blood cholesterol levels, even for people on a high-fat diet. Studies on lumberjacks in Finland first suggested this finding. Then a Swiss physician, Dr. Daniella Gsell, and I confirmed it by comparing the cholesterol levels of the extremely hard-working population of an isolated Swiss village and a control group in Basel, a modern industrial Swiss city. Both groups were ethnically similar—German-speaking Swiss. But the village could not be reached by truck or automobile, and everything—lumber, large cans of milk

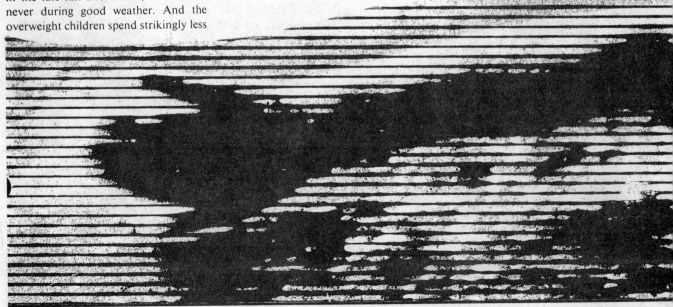

Enough...

You're a weekend golfer, and you've just taken up archery. Is this exercise? Not necessarily, says this noted nutritionist, who explains different kinds of exercises and tells how they keep you fit   BY DR. JEAN MAYER, Professor of Nutrition, Harvard University

for cheese making, millstone-like Gruyere cheeses, bales of hay and bags of potatoes—had to be carried in by mules or by the villagers themselves. People in the village had a high-fat intake, and they consumed 100 calories more each day than the urban dwellers. However, the serum cholesterol levels of the physically active men and women in the village were much lower than those of the Basel residents.

The value of physical activity in warding off heart disease has been demonstrated over and over again in other careful studies. For example, a survey of London bus drivers, who sit all day at their wheel, showed that they had more frequent and more severe coronaries than the bus conductors, who do a great deal of stair climbing each day in the double-decker London buses. Of course, it can be argued—and it was—that the drivers are under greater stress than the conductors. So a second study was conducted, comparing English rural mail postmasters and clerks with rural delivery mailmen. Again, the walking mailmen had fewer coronaries and a much lower mortality rate from coronary disease than did the group who spent their day sitting. In this study, neither group was under any great stress (what is more peaceful than the English countryside?). And if there was any stress, it was among the walking

mailmen who have to cope with hazards such as overzealous watchdogs.

The story is the same on this side of the Atlantic. A study comparing mortality from heart disease among railroad employees again showed the importance of activity. The section hands, who do the heavy labor of repairing the roadbed, had a much better record than switchmen (light activity, walking), who, in turn, did much better than the sitting clerks.

The rate of physical activity of the Swiss villagers or railroad section hands—several hours every day—is obviously more than can be expected of the average professional or business person in this country. An hour a day is much more compatible with the 1973 American way of life. Actually, there is mounting evidence that three or four 15-minute sessions of intense exercise a week (by intense I mean enough to send your pulse racing to 110–120 beats a minute) are enough to keep your heart and its vessels elastic. And if deposits of cholesterol plaque have narrowed the coronary vessel, this vigorous exercise helps open up additional vessels—what

is known technically as "collateral circulation," increasing your chances of survival should you suffer a heart attack.

Of course, these periods of vigorous exercise can take many forms, but if you swim and have access to a pool, this is one of the best all-round exercises. Jogging or running up stairs also are good "intense exercises."

Exercises for Strength and Grace

So far, I have spoken of exercise solely in terms of health. There are, of course, other values to exercise. You may want to develop strength, an important attribute in bygone days and still a useful asset. Lifting weights or climbing ropes will strengthen your arm and back muscles, and help prevent lower-back pain later in life. However, before embarking on such strenuous exercises, make sure you're not afflicted with some structural weakness, such as a tendency to hernia or slipped disks, and be careful not to overdo.

Then there are exercises to "limber up" and to improve coordination. These make you feel better, and improve your looks, grace, and ease of movement. Still other exercise will help you to keep your stomach flat, a *(continued)*

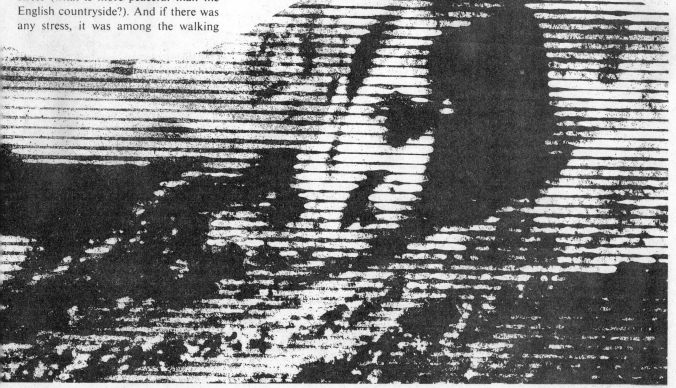

Burning Off Those Extra Calories

The idea that you can't lose weight by exercising is one of those completely false myths that dies very hard. But you can see for yourself that exercise does burn off those extra calories. Just look at the chart below. The number of calories needed for optimum health varies from person to person. For example, an average male executive needs about 2400 a day, while an active farmer requires 3500. Women need 1600 to 2800, depending upon individual routines. If you do "splurge" a bit now and then, you can burn off the extra calories with a few minutes of physical activity. The following chart tells you exactly how much exercise is needed.*

		Minutes of Activity				
Food	Calories	Walking[1]	Riding bicycle[2]	Swimming[3]	Running[4]	Reclining[5]
Apple, large	101	19	12	9	5	78
Bacon, 2 strips	96	18	12	9	5	74
Banana, small	88	17	11	8	4	68
Beer, 1 glass	114	22	14	10	6	88
Bread and butter	78	15	10	7	4	60
Cake, 2-layer, 1/12	356	68	43	32	18	274
Carbonated beverage, 1 glass	106	20	13	9	5	82
Carrot, raw	42	8	5	4	2	32
Cereal, dry, 1/2 c. with milk, sugar	200	38	24	18	10	154
Cheese, Cheddar, 1 oz.	111	21	14	10	6	85
Chicken, fried, 1/2 breast	232	45	28	21	12	178
Cookie, plain	15	3	2	1	1	12
Cookie, chocolate chip	51	10	6	5	3	39
Doughnut	151	29	18	13	8	116
Egg, fried	110	21	13	10	6	85
Halibut steak, 1/4 lb.	205	39	25	18	11	158
Ham, 2 slices	167	32	20	15	9	128
Ice cream, 1/6 qt.	193	37	24	17	10	148
Ice cream soda	255	49	31	23	13	196
Malted milk shake	502	97	61	45	26	386
Milk, 1 glass	166	32	20	15	9	128
Milk, skim, 1 glass	81	16	10	7	4	62
Orange, medium	68	13	8	6	4	52
Orange juice, 1 glass	120	23	15	11	6	92
Pancake with syrup	124	24	15	11	6	95
Peach, medium	46	9	6	4	2	35
Pie, apple, 1/6	377	73	46	34	19	290
Pizza, cheese, 1/8	180	35	22	16	9	138
Pork chop, loin	314	60	38	28	16	242
Potato chips, 1 serving	108	21	13	10	6	83
Club sandwich	590	113	72	53	30	454
Hamburger sandwich	350	67	43	31	18	269
Tuna salad sandwich	278	53	34	25	14	214
Sherbet, 1/6 qt.	177	34	22	16	9	136
Shrimp, French fried	180	35	22	16	9	138
Spaghetti, 1 serving	396	76	48	35	20	305
Steak, T-bone	235	45	29	21	12	181
Strawberry shortcake	400	77	49	36	21	308

[1]Energy cost of walking for 150-lb. individual = 5.2 calories per minute at 3.5 m.p.h. [2]Energy cost of riding bicycle = 8.2 calories per minute. [3]Energy cost of swimming = 11.2 calories per minute. [4]Energy cost of running = 19.4 calories per minute. [5]Energy cost of reclining = 1.3 calories per minute. *From: Konishi, F. "Food energy equivalents of various activities," **J. Amer. Dietetic Assoc.,** 46 (1965), 186. Used by permission.

healthful as well as an aesthetically important feature. These types of conditioning exercises often are taught in special-movement exercise or ballet classes, or may be found in any number of exercise books.

Sports and Games of Skill

Then we have team sports. These have been praised to the sky in this country, both as educational tools and for their value in teaching sportsmanship. Be that as it may. Let me add that some team sports expend a great deal of energy and are, therefore, good body conditioners—for example, soccer, lawn hockey, and basketball. But some sports, while quite entertaining to players and spectators, do not call for a high, constant expenditure of energy. At the risk of being immediately deported, let me say that neither baseball nor football is, by itself, a good body conditioner. And let me add certain games of skill to this list, games that are great entertainment but are no longer physical exercise. For instance, if you play golf out of a golf cart, or shoot at clay pigeons on a rifle range, or take up archery, you are not really exercising; you're just playing.

So where does all this leave us? If those of us who are middle-aged recognize that we can't lower our cholesterol levels by 6–10 hours of hard labor a day, unless we happen to be railroaders or isolated Swiss villagers. But we can walk half an hour to an hour every day to control our weight, and find 15 minutes three times a week for more vigorous exercise. Or we can run up the stairs every opportunity we get, and practice more active sports—hiking in the neighboring hills or tennis or swimming—on weekends and during vacations. (All of this, of course, presupposes that you have had a yearly checkup and have the blessing of your physician.)

For children and adolescents, make sure that they have facilities for exercise and are using them. We should encourage them to walk as often as possible, rather than wait to be chauffeured everywhere. Encourage them to develop skills and play team sports if they want, but also try to foster games and sports that they can enjoy throughout life. Football is all very well when a youngster is in high school or even college, but what will that fullback or tackle do after he graduates? Tennis, squash, swimming, mountain climbing, by contrast, last a lifetime, and prolong it as well. ∎

The Caloric Cost of Running

Its Impact on Weight Reduction

Maj Bruce S. Harger, PhD, USAF; Lt Col James B. Miller, MD, PhD, USAF; Maj James C. Thomas, DPE, USAF

• **The purpose of this article is to present a table of caloric expenditure values for running that can be used to augment diet control plans. These values allow the individual to include both energy input and output in his reduction program, thereby increasing the accuracy of obtaining a negative caloric balance. The values were obtained from a formula based on the linear relationship of running speed and energy cost. The data highlight the relatively small caloric expenditure experienced in short bouts of exercise, but it is important to include this contribution in most weight reduction programs. (*JAMA* 228:482-483, 1974)**

THE NATION is currently experiencing a widespread interest in weight reduction programs. The public has become somewhat educated in the art of counting calories, and the most accepted methods center on this approach. The pathway to weight loss by increasing caloric expenditure in relation to caloric intake has become a well-known phenomenon. However, the scientific control of calories has been restricted to published caloric values for various foodstuffs. The individual is taught how to use those charts to determine precisely caloric intake, and the importance of some exercise is then included as an additional but nebulous factor. It seems logical that careful accounting of calories for both input and output would be the most precise means of prescribing a weight control program.

Purpose

The purpose of this report is to present the caloric values for running 2.4 km (1.5 miles) that can be used in determining the exercise portion of a weight reduction program. The 2.4 km distance was selected as a base since it has become a popular jogging distance in accordance with Dr. Kenneth Cooper's aerobics plan.[1] The caloric table values are presented for weight and running speed in order to be specific for individual cases.

Methods

The data presented in the table were obtained from a formula derived by Costill and Fox.[2] This formula resulted from a regression line computed for the relationship between calories per kilogram of body weight (corrected for clothing) and running speed. Following is the equation that was utilized:

$$C = [(RS \times 0.001) - 0.028] \times BW$$

where C indicates calories, RS, running speed, and BW, body weight. The running speed was converted to meters per minute and the body weight was expressed in kilograms. The nude body weight was corrected to clothed weight by adding a constant 2.7 km (6 lb). The equation was employed in a program on a computer (ALGOL language) that produced caloric values for 11 different weights at 16 different running speeds.

Results

The Table presents the energy cost of completing 2.4 km for men of 11 different weights, running at nine different paces. It can readily be seen that pace has very little effect on the caloric cost of running, and thus, individuals in low fitness categories can expend almost as much energy as a similarly sized, conditioned person for a given distance. However, the difference in energy cost when comparing various weights is much more dramatic. For example, a 54-kg (119 lb) man who runs the distance in ten minutes will use 121 calories, while another man weighing 100 kg (220.5 lb), running at the same pace, will burn 219 calories. Therefore, it seems imperative that a weight reduction program that carefully measures

From the Department of Physical Education, Human Performance Laboratory (Dr. Harger), Research Division (Maj Thomas), and the USAF Academy Hospital (Dr. Miller), USAF Academy, Colorado.

The views expressed herein are those of the authors and do not necessarily reflect the views of the US Air Force or the Department of Defense.

Reprint requests to AHP, USAF Academy, Colorado 80840 (Dr. Harger).

Caloric Values for Running 2.4 km									
Weight* kg	Calories/min								
	8	9	10	11	12	13	14	15	16
54.5	125	124	121	120	119	117	116	114	112
59.0	135	133	132	130	128	126	125	123	121
63.6	145	143	141	139	138	136	134	132	130
68.1	155	153	151	149	147	145	143	141	139
72.6	165	163	161	159	156	154	152	150	148
77.2	175	173	170	168	166	164	161	159	157
81.7	185	182	180	178	175	173	171	168	166
86.3	195	192	190	187	185	182	180	177	175
90.8	205	202	199	197	194	192	189	186	184
95.3	215	212	209	206	204	201	198	195	193
99.9	225	222	219	216	213	210	207	204	202

*The weight divisions represent a 10-lb increase at each increment, ranging from 120 to 220 lb.

work output must be based on individual weight. Very often fitness books give a caloric value for running that is based on a single weight, for a period of one hour. We believe this is doubly erroneous since weight is such a large factor in determining cost, and because comparatively few people run for a full hour.

Comment

Running was selected as an exercise medium since most individuals can readily acquire this skill, thus reducing individual differences. Van der Walt and Wyndham[3] have recently concluded that pace length and leg length are not important factors in prediction of energy cost. Margaria et al[4] add that the mechanical efficiency of trained runners is only 5% to 7% higher than that of untrained men. Although walking has recently been shown to be the nation's most popular form of exercise,[5] its energy cost cannot be predicted from a linear relationship. In 1938, Margaria[4] stated that "while the energy cost of walking increases with the speed, the function being given by a progressively steeper curve, the cost of running is a linear function of the speed. ..." It is important to remember that we have shown that speed has little effect on the caloric cost of running, and thus, light jogging can be used instead of walking for the prediction of energy cost. This may help eliminate the fears of those who believe running must be exhaustive if one is to obtain a sufficient energy output.

The caloric expenditure of between 112 and 225 calories for a 2.4-km run seems small when one remembers that an expenditure of 3,500 calories is necessary to lose 0.5 kg (1 lb) of fat. However, if a caloric expenditure of only 100 calories is maintained daily, there will be approximately a 4.5-kg (10 lb) weight loss in a year's time. Another view would suggest that even if a weight level were only maintained constant, at least this would avoid an extra 5 kg (11 lb) being added. Mayer[6] has warned against being fooled by the low daily contributions of exercise, and he, too, emphasizes the importance of maintaining a cumulative record of caloric expenditure.

Although we have pointed up some limitations of exercise as a means of weight reduction, we certainly do not wish to eliminate its important contributions for both caloric balance and personal fitness. Mayer[6] has shown that despite its seemingly small contribution to weight control, exercise is a necessary part of most programs. He also states that his data suggest exercise may be a suppressant rather than a stimulant to appetite.[6] The minimal difference in caloric expenditure between fast and slow times, which was discussed earlier, should not be used as logic for conditioning at a slow pace. It must be remembered that in cardiorespiratory improvement, the individual must be concerned with intensity to obtain the best results.[7-9] In fact, running can be construed as fulfilling two different aspects of preventive medicine. First, cardiorespiratory fitness and, second, as a means of expending calories. Although this article is mainly concerned with weight reduction, it must be said that the ideal program would seek to achieve both benefits running can offer.

Even though the daily effect of exercise may appear small, the proper calculation of work expenditure can provide an enticing variation of an individual's diet plan. It is a very simple procedure. If a person were maintaining a 2,600-calorie diet, he could increase his activity level by 200 calories thus allowing him the luxury of a small piece of cake (or other food containing 200 calories) without his predetermined level of 2,600 calories being altered. Again, over a year's time, without the added calories, a weight loss of 5 to 10 kg (11 to 22 lb) could be recognized. Therefore, through judicious use of the Table, or by applying the formula presented in the text, a person can maintain a more accurate weight control program, because his procedure now includes known values for both work output and caloric intake.

References

1. Cooper KH: *Aerobics.* New York, M Evans and Company, Inc, 1968, pp 27-36.
2. Costill DL, Fox EL: Energetics of marathon running. *Medicine & Science in Sports* 1:81-86, 1969.
3. Van Der Walt WH, Wyndham CH: An equation for prediction of energy expenditure of walking and running. *J Appl Physiol* 34:559-563, 1973.
4. Margaria R, et al: Energy cost of running. *J Appl Physiol* 18:367-370, 1963.
5. Clarke H (ed): *National Adult Fitness Survey, Newsletter.* President's Council on Physical Fitness and Sports, May 1973, pp 1-27.
6. Mayer J: *Overweight: Causes, Cost, and Control.* Englewood Cliffs, NJ, Prentice Hall, Inc, 1968, pp 69-72.
7. Fox EL, et al: Intensity and distance of interval training programs and changes in aerobic power. *Medicine & Science in Sports* 5:18-22, 1973.
8. Astrand P-O, Rodahl K: Physical Training: *Textbook of Work Physiology.* New York, McGraw-Hill Book Co Inc, 1971, pp 389-393.
9. Karvonen MJ: Effects of Vigorous Exercise on the Heart, in Rosenbaum FF and Belknap EL (eds): *Work and the Heart.* New York, Harper & Row, Publishers, 1959, pp 199-210.

WHO CONTROLS
YOUR EATING HABITS?

By John Kelly

Jim Curtin lost seven pounds on a water diet and gained it all back a week later. So he tried a champagne diet. But that didn't work either—and besides, he kept getting the hiccups. An all-steak diet would be his salvation then, he decided. And, indeed, three weeks later, Jim was 12 pounds slimmer and a suit size smaller. Unfortunately, he was also very sick of steak, so he went on a week-long food bender and wound up with a net weight gain of two pounds for the month.

Jim Curtin's experiences with fad diets are not unusual—millions of other Americans have had them too. But what *is* unusual is the way Jim finally resolved his weight problems. It goes by the name of "behavioral control," and it just may be the sanest thing to happen to the American Way of Reducing since the death of the calories-don't-count myth.

It is not, however, a magic formula, nor does it promise "a newer, slimmer you in only 10 days." Behavioral control, in fact, "deliberately tries to steer people away from this all-or-nothing approach," declares University of Pennsylvania psychologist Dr. Leonard S. Levitz. Thus, instead of emphasizing calories and forbidding foods as many fad diets do, it stresses control of the hows, whys, and whens of eating.

The technique's theoretical underpinnings come from some dramatic new findings on the psychology of eating by Dr. Albert Stunkard, a psychiatrist at the University of Pennsylvania School of Medicine, and psychologists Stanley Schachter of Columbia and Richard B. Stuart of the University of Michigan. Their research indicates that overweight people—and in that category they include everybody from the slightly fat to the grossly obese—are very susceptible to what are called external food cues.

"Put a cue—say, a bowl of potato chips —in front of a normal-weight person who's just eaten, and he will ignore them," says Dr. Schachter. "But put that bowl in front of an obese individual

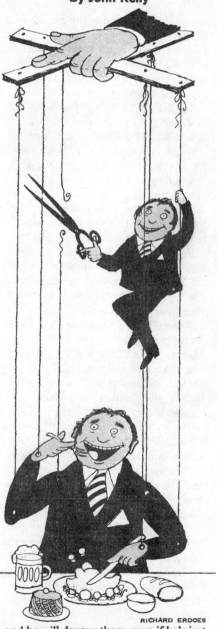

RICHARD ERDOES

and he will devour them, even if he's just gotten up from a large meal." The psychologist doesn't know why the overweight are more receptive to cues, but he believes that a decrease in weight doesn't lead to a decrease in susceptibility. "In all our studies, we observed that former-ly obese people reacted to cues the same

way currently obese individuals did."

Cues can include pizza shops, bakery windows, everybody else's leftovers, that last piece of cheesecake. They are, in short, everywhere. You can even create your own. Watch TV while munching away at a bowl of popcorn and you will soon find that turning on the tube makes you hungry.

Behavioral control will teach you how to spot these cues, eliminate the ones that can be eliminated, and deal with the others in ways that make them less tempting. But it will work only if you stick to it. "It is," says Dr. Richard B. Stuart, "a lifelong program."

Like most of the other psychologists who have begun using the technique, Dr. Stuart works with groups. "This kind of setting provides patients with an extra bit of moral support," he says, "but it isn't essential to the success of the program. The methods can be equally effective on an individual basis, if the person employing them is well motivated and observes the rules closely."

What follows is the core of the behavioral-control program distilled into 10 easy-to-understand steps. Each step is designed to help control your weight problem. But remember, each will only be as effective as you allow it to be.

1. Keep a Food Intake Sheet. You can't correct your bad eating habits unless you know what they are. So begin the program not by dieting, but by keeping a careful record of what you eat for a week or two. Make it as detailed as possible. Write down what you ate, the times you ate, how long it took, where you ate, whom you ate with or if you ate alone, and your mood when you ate.

Dr. Levitz even has his patients record where they sat when they ate "because a person can change his feelings about what he eats by changing the position where he eats."

2. Try to Pinpoint Your Eating Problems. Pay particularly close attention to your eating speed. Dr. Robert Westlake,

Fad diets may help you shed pounds, but they won't help you keep them off. Here's a realistic plan to slim down and stay that way

a colleague of Dr. Levitz' at the University of Pennsylvania, feels this is one of the overeater's most common and harmful problems.

Also check the places where you are doing most of your overeating. Is it in the kitchen, the den, or the bedroom? After analyzing his intake sheet, one of Dr. Westlake's patients, a salesman, was astonished to find that he was doing most of his problem eating in the car between sales calls.

How did you feel when you ate? Were you bored, hungry, depressed? Robert Piasiki, a patient in the Rockefeller University program, managed to shed 150 pounds after he learned how to cope with the depression that triggered his eating. Try also to zero in on the times you ate. Are you, for example, a late-night snacker or an all-day picker?

3. Make Eating a Pure Experience. As we said, people often unconsciously create their own food cues. The reason you've been eating more in the den and bedroom is because you've taught yourself to be hungry in those rooms. The same thing can happen with certain activities. Thus, Dr. Westlake's salesman got hungry on the road because he had begun to pair eating with driving. You snack a lot when you sew because you've conditioned yourself to associate one activity with the other. Sewing, in other words, has become a food cue for you.

When you eat, do nothing but eat. Don't read the newspaper, don't watch TV, don't do anything that will impinge on the pure activity of eating. All this may sound terribly Spartan, but it will train you to become hungry only in certain places and at certain times.

4. Curb Bad Eating Habits. There are a number of ways to slow eating rates. One is to put the fork down after every third bite and leave it down until you've chewed and then swallowed. Another is to pause for five minutes or so in the middle of the meal. Still another is to cut your food into nine or 10 pieces and

thoroughly chew and swallow each piece before going on to the next. If all else fails, try coming to the table five minutes after the rest of the family has begun eating. But promise yourself to stop eating when they stop.

To lick a snacking problem, Dr. Levitz suggests creating an alternate set of activities. If you always sit down with a box of cookies at 4 P.M., begin going for a walk at that time. Or take up a new hobby and devote your midafternoon hours to it. "Just make sure you choose an activity you really like," says the psychologist. "If you force yourself to do it, you are likely to backslide."

You can cure a third common problem—overeating at mealtime—by engaging in a little innocent self-deception. Use a smaller set of plates; it will make your food portions look larger.

5. Reduce Your Temptations. An attractively packaged box of cookies can crumble the sternest dieter's will. But you can avoid this kind of destructive impulse buying: make a shopping list before you market, and take only enough money to buy the items on it.

The list should include lots of moderate-calorie foods, such as fruits, vegetables, lean meats, and snack foods that require preparation. "One is a lot less tempted to eat," says Dr. Stuart, "if he knows he's going to have to spend ten or fifteen minutes preparing the food."

6. Enlist Your Family's Support. By now, it should be clear that the program is going to deeply involve your family. So sit down with them and explain its aims and why you've decided to try it.

Tell them that you'll rely on them for a lot of moral support in the coming months. You may even ask them to make a few sacrifices, such as agreeing to have fewer snack foods in the house.

7. Coping with Emotions. An overweight person almost automatically reaches for food when he's upset. "He uses it as a tranquilizer," says Dr. Joel Grinker, a Rockefeller University psychologist.

Try not to make it yours. Jogging is a healthier way to work off anger. And you're likely to find a phone conversation with a friend a lot more comforting and far less fattening than a piece of pie.

8. Take It Slowly. Don't starve yourself. Aim at a gradual weight loss of one or, at the most, two pounds per week.

Establish how many calories you must restrict yourself to per day to meet that goal, then begin keeping a daily record of your food intake to insure that you are not exceeding the figure. Include items from all the seven major food groups in your daily meal plan, and, of course, go sparingly on high-calorie foods. However, don't feel you have to cut them out completely. "Go on enjoying that doughnut with your morning coffee," says Dr. Levitz, "but from now on just eat half of it."

9. Get More Exercise. If you are athletically inclined, try jogging or calisthenics; if you are not an athlete, try gardening. Whatever your particular choice, the important thing is to stick to it. You are likelier to do that if you have a partner, so try to enlist a friend or relative in your exercise program.

It's a good idea, too, to incorporate more exercise into your daily routine. "I always park my car a quarter of a mile from the office, and walk the rest of the distance," says Dr. Stuart. The psychologist also makes a point of taking the stairs rather than the elevator.

10. Handling Special Situations. The best way to resist the lure of a restaurant menu is not to look at it. Make up your mind what you are going to have before you go out, and order that. Also tell the waiter not to put a bread tray or relish dish on your table.

If you are going to a wedding, party, or church social, eat something substantial before you leave the house, so that you won't arrive at the function hungry. And to avoid temptation while you are there, dance a lot, engage in conversation. In short, keep yourself busy. ∎

Hope for the obese: behavior modification

ALBERT J. STUNKARD, M.D./MICHAEL J. MAHONEY, PhD.

A new treatment for obesity, on the drawing boards for the past several years, is winning the cautious approval of numerous investigators. "Cautious" because the desirability of controlling obesity—coupled with the unrelieved record of failure in its treatment—has rendered both the lay public and the medical profession vulnerable to unwarranted hopes. But now that some carefully controlled studies are in, we can say, unequivocally, that behavior modification represents a significant improvement in the treatment of obesity. We still do not know the potential of this improvement in terms of *initial weight loss* and *weight loss maintained*. But 12 controlled studies carried out within the past five years have all reported results favoring behavior modification over a variety of other treatment methods—an unprecedented example of unanimity among researchers working on this complex and heterogenous disorder.

Behavior modification consists of a variety of techniques with one common denominator – proponents attempt to apply the findings and methods of experimental psychology to disorders of human behavior. The approach postulates that some of the most divergent types of behavior disorder are *learned* responses, and that modern learning theories have much to teach us about the acquisition and extinction of such responses. A complete understanding of behavior modification requires mastery of a large and growing literature. Still, the physician can quickly gain an appreciation for this new therapy and its applications through a description of behavioral control techniques that have proved effective in obesity. We will describe these techniques briefly here; the reader interested in greater detail can find it in a manual, published in 1971, called *Slim Chance in a Fat World: Behavioral Control of Obesity*, by Richard B. Stuart and Barbara Davis (Research Press, Champaign, Ill.).

Interest in behavioral modification in obesity developed as a result of some highly relevant research into environmental influences on the eating and overeating of obese people. Prof. Stanley Schachter and his students at Columbia University found that the obese are far more influenced than are the nonobese by such "external," social/environmental, factors as palatability, time of day, availability of food, and even the ambience of a particular room. On the other hand, they are far less influenced by such "internal," physiologic, factors as hunger, measured both subjectively and by length of time after eating.

That environmental factors largely control the food intake of the obese may help explain both the failure of routine medical management and the relative effectiveness of behavior modification. Because traditional weight-reduction programs fail to teach control of environmental eating cues, they leave the individual unable to cope with his peculiar vulnerability to such cues. By emphasizing specific training in "stimulus control," behavior modification helps him to manage the environmental determinants of his eating.

The first step in most behavior modification programs is to help the patient identify and monitor activities that are contributing to his weight problem: frequent ingestion of sweets, late evening snacking, huge meals, or eating in response to social demands. Once these activities are identified and their significance measured, the patient is given individualized suggestions and homework assignments. Often these involve rearranging eating situations so as to produce more appropriate caloric intake. For example, the housewife who cannot stop nibbling as she prepares the evening meal may be encouraged to prepare as much of this meal as possible right after lunch, when she is satiated. The chronic television snacker is encouraged to separate his snacking from his entertainment; if he wants to drink beer and eat pretzels he can, but only if he leaves the television room. The lonely housewife is encouraged to stop keeping bowls of candy always ready "in case someone drops in," and to replace them with freshly prepared low-calorie snacks such as raw carrots and celery. This kind of change breaks the habitual stimulus-response relationship, which leaves the individual at the mercy of environmental cues, and replaces it with a new one under his direct control.

In addition to stimulus control, the patient is taught to modify the act of eating itself. He is trained to eat more slowly and to put his utensils down periodically during the meal. The patient who feels compelled to finish portions, because they would otherwise go to waste, is taught to leave some food on his plate.

The third target of behavior modification is the patient's motivation to lose weight. A wealth of evidence indicates that a behavior that takes effort is seldom developed or maintained without powerful incentives—rewards or punishments. Rewards generally seem more effective than punishments as motivators of long-term behavior change. Such rewards as improved health, social approval, and physical attractiveness should be enough to maintain the patient's efforts at self-control. However, when weight loss is achieved by altering eating patterns through behavior modification, rather than through the usual drastic dietary changes, weight is lost relatively slowly (approximately one pound per week). Thus the rewards of such gradual loss are often too delayed to effect continued adherence to the program.

To meet this challenge, behavior

INITIAL AND FOLLOW-UP WEIGHT LOSSES

Weight Loss (lb)	Behavior Modification Group (15 subjects)		Control Therapy Group (17 subjects)		Reported Results of Other Methods
	After Treatment	One-Year Follow-Up	After Treatment	One-Year Follow-Up	
40+	13%	33%	0%	12%	5%
30+	33%	40%	0%	29%	—
20+	53%	53%	24%	47%	25%

modifiers have investigated various methods of helping patients to exercise self-control. Group pressure and the therapist's approval seem to be two effective methods. However, as with any antiobesity program, there is always the danger that improvement induced by the influence of the group or the therapist may be reversed when these two sources of motivation are no longer available.

Several researchers have explored the effectiveness of incentives set up by the patients themselves. For example, one of us (Dr. Mahoney) asked patients to award themselves valuable gift certificates for their progress in weight loss. A study compared this *self-reward* strategy with one involving *self-punishment*, in which patients fined themselves an equal amount of money for failing to show improvement. A third group simply recorded their body weight and eating habits. Self-reward was by far the most effective strategy. Its superiority was particularly pronounced in maintaining weight loss after treatment had ended. These findings lead us to believe that self-administered rewards may help patients maintain their modified habits.

Later, Dr. Mahoney demonstrated something that had been generally believed but not previously proved; that self-reward should focus on eating habits, not weight loss. Patients who treated themselves to special privileges or purchases for having attained weekly weight-loss goals were less successful in their long-term weight reduction than patients whose rewards were tied to improvements in their eating habits. Highly significant relationships were found between reported improvements in eating habits and amount of weight lost. Thus the most effective treatment

emphasizes the development of appropriate eating patterns rather than short-term fluctuations in body weight, which can be produced by a variety of transient reducing methods in use today.

In some of the controlled studies previously mentioned, behavior modification not only was more effective than traditional therapies but also, interestingly, produced greater variability in individual weight losses. The greater variability in outcome of treatment carries at least two implications: First, the differences appear to reflect specific treatment effects rather than nonspecific—or placebo—effects of interest and attention. Second, the variability also implies that if we could select which patients are likely to respond to behavior modification, we might further improve our results.

Until recently, treatment of obesity has been so unsuccessful that few attempts at follow-up have been made. With the development of more effective techniques, however, reports of follow-up studies are beginning to appear. A one-year follow-up of patients in the University of Pennsylvania treatment program (table) showed that the excellent results of the behavior modification had per-

sisted. One year later, all eight of the 15 patients who had lost at least 20 pounds through this method had maintained their weight loss, and some had even increased it. These results contrast sharply with the usual experience of successful dieters—prompt regaining of the weight they had lost. To our surprise, our control subjects had also lost further weight after the end of treatment. This is the only study to date in which such continued weight loss was found following traditional therapy.

The difference between behavior modification and more traditional therapies is particularly notable in the demands made on the obese patient in the interval between visits to the doctor. In contrast to the limited demands of traditional therapies, behavior modification requires that the patient invest a great deal of hard work in his treatment. Treatment must help the patient maintain his efforts at self-control, either through group support, physician approval, or training in self-administration of incentives. Some clinically useful suggestions for the latter are presented in *Behavioral Self-Control*, by C. E. Thoresen and M. J. Mahoney (Holt, Rinehart & Winston, in press).

The strong interest researchers are showing in behavior modification for treatment of obesity, and the increasing sophistication with which the research is being carried out, are grounds for hope—that the significant though modest improvement in therapeutic results this method has achieved will not be the end of the story. We feel confident that when results are reviewed next year and the year after, further progress will be evident. 🐾

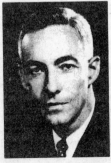

Dr. Stunkard is chairman of the department of psychiatry at the University of Pennsylvania.

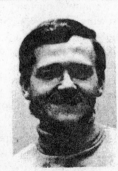

Dr. Mahoney is assistant professor of psychology at Pennsylvania State University.

Behavior therapy in treating obesity[1]

LEONARD S. LEVITZ, PH.D.
Department of Psychiatry,
University of Pennsylvania, and
Philadelphia General Hospital,
Philadelphia

Behavior therapy offers a relatively
new avenue for treatment of obesity. The
author discusses its characteristics and
reports specific techniques for effecting
behavior change which have been
successful in research studies.

Behavior therapy, or behavior modification, has been used successfully in the treatment of a variety of psychologic disorders, notably in the areas of phobic and anxiety states, sexual problems, and mental retardation. In the past five years, attempts to apply behavior modification to the treatment of obesity have resulted in some of the most successful programs reported in the literature (1). The major intent of this paper is to acquaint readers with the distinguishing characteristics of behavior therapy and to describe briefly the type of behavior treatment that has been used in obesity. A second intent is to direct persons interested in the treatment of obesity to source materials providing more detailed descriptions of this approach.

While a number of behavior techniques used in treating obesity may appear simple to describe and apply, it is most important that persons using them understand the rationale for their effectiveness. A primary responsibility of the therapist is to individualize the set of techniques so that they are applicable to a client's particular eating habits; they should form a systematic program and be presented in a logical progression. To fulfill these clinical responsibilities, the therapist should acquire a general background in principles of human learning and behavior theory. Two appropriate sources are Ullmann and Krasner's introduction to *Case Studies in Behavior Modification* (2) and Liberman's *Guide to Behavioral Analysis and Therapy* (3).

It is significant that behavior therapists' interest in obesity was stimulated by the reliable and observable measure of therapeutic success it provided as much as by the medical and social problem it represented. Weight change enabled researchers to compare the effectiveness of various therapeutic techniques (4) and to study general psychotherapy processes (5).

Characteristics of behavior therapy

This original basis of interest in obesity illustrates an important theme that has characterized behavior therapy from its inception, i.e., the focus of attention is on observable behavior and observable behavior change. The therapist is most interested in the dis-

[1] Supported by research grant MH-15383 from the National Institute of Mental Health.

crete behaviors that define the problem and the specific behaviors that should be increased, decreased, eliminated, or instituted to alleviate or solve it. In the area of obesity, the *target behaviors* are the set of habits contributing to excessive caloric intake and decreased energy expenditure. Obesity, or overweight, is seen as the consequence of such habits rather than as a symptom of some underlying psychologic disorder.

A second characteristic of behavior therapy is that efforts are made to measure precisely the target behavior and to assess the degree of change that occurs. In this regard, differences between research and clinical practice become somewhat obscured. Most often, baseline measurements of food intake and habits are taken before behavior techniques are introduced in order to make such an assessment. During therapy, an effort should also be made to determine that weight changes are occurring as a result of some change in eating habits, rather than as a result of simple fasting. The ultimate goal of therapy is to develop a permanent set of appropriate eating habits, the result of which is weight loss and maintenance.

The most distinctive characteristic of behavior therapy is that it attempts to abstract effective clinical techniques from general psychologic principles, primarily from research in human learning and social psychology. For example, independent of the specific technique, a process of *shaping* is implied throughout the therapeutic program. Shaping refers to a process of providing for small, incremental changes in a behavior, with each step more closely approximating the final goal behavior. If eating a particular high-caloric food represents a major habit problem, the final goal —to reach a low level of consumption—would be gradually approached in a series of discrete steps. In working with the overweight person, this principle is also applied to the progression of weight loss. A gradual weight loss of from 1 to 2 lb. a week is generally stated as the criterion for successful progress (6).

In several respects, overeating is one of the most complex behavioral problems that has been approached by behavior therapy. Not only has it proved very resistant to most types of therapeutic intervention, but the physiologic limitations on any intervention are not known. Even barring a physiologic limitation, treatment is complex because it must rely on principles of self-management, which means that the processes of behavior-monitoring and behavior change are under the control of the client. (In many other areas, the same techniques of behavior change have been administered by outside agents—psychotherapists, teachers, psychiatric nurses, or hospital aides.) While there is evidence that self-management can effect behavior changes as profound as those achieved by externally administered treatment (7), there are many questions about self-management that still must be researched (8).

When the success of treatment depends on self-management, the purpose of therapeutic contacts is to provide the client with the techniques for achieving appropriate behavior changes. In the treatment of obesity, an educational approach is taken in which a principal role of the therapist is to teach the client how to analyze his own behavior patterns and how to devise suitable techniques for changing them.

In addition to his function as a teacher, the therapist also serves as a source of social influence to the client, as he does in most systems of therapy. As Krasner pointed out in a recent research review (9), "The technology of behavior therapy becomes effective in modifying behavior only within the context of maximum social influence."

Thus, behavior therapy, as applied to obesity, is characterized by: (a) determination of observable eating and activity habit patterns; (b) measurement of the target behaviors before and during treatment; (c) a series of techniques abstracted from psychologic research in learning; and (d) an educational approach to the development of self-management.

Behavior therapy techniques

The purpose of this section is to provide a basic outline of general techniques which have been used in behavior programs for treating obesity. While reports of research on the use of individual techniques, such as reward contracting (10) and respondent conditioning (11, 12), have been published, most treatment programs have included a variety of techniques. Stuart and Davis have recently published a book (13) which describes a detailed program of behavior techniques for treating obesity. This work extends the behavior analysis of overeating to encompass techniques aimed at promoting change in general nutrition and dietary habits and activity patterns.

INITIAL ASSESSMENT. The first step in a behavior program is a *functional analysis* of the client's eating patterns. The purpose of this analysis is to describe (a) the types of habit patterns and their frequencies or rates of occurrence, (b) the antecedent conditions that appear to signal the occurrence of these habit patterns, and (c) the consequent events that appear to maintain the habits.

A description of maladaptive overeating habits consists of not only the type, quantity, and caloric value of foods a person eats, but also factors such as where and when the person eats, with whom he eats, and social responses to his eating. Other factors that may be important to a functional analysis of eating behavior are the degree of hunger perceived by the person immediately before and after eating; emotional responses, such as anxiety, depression, or boredom which may influence food intake; and self-evaluations of the appropriateness of eating.

The client is generally instructed to keep a careful food record, consisting of his daily food intake and factors such as those listed above. While unreliability in self-reporting is to be expected, it can be reduced to some extent by instructing the client to carry the food record with him at all times so that he can record intake immediately after eating. An initial reduction in food intake as a result of the self-monitoring procedure alone is frequently noted (8).

After a few weeks, the completed food habit records suggest to both the therapist and client some of the major inappropriate eating patterns, the situational and temporal cues which occasion them, and the consequent conditions maintaining the behaviors. Just as important, however, the record also indicates that the client does not overeat all of the time; there is a base rate of appropriate eating behavior. This is useful initially in demonstrating that the therapeutic question is not whether the client is or is not capable of self-control but is discovering what conditions can lead to appropriate eating. Many of the techniques later introduced are aimed at increasing the frequency of existing adaptive habits rather than trying to eliminate maladaptive ones.

Throughout the program, the food habit records are important in determining what habit changes occur. As treatment progresses, they are also used to identify maladaptive sub-habits for which techniques must be devised.

ALTERING EATING BEHAVIOR. After initial assessment, therapy can be devoted to altering specific aspects of eating behavior. One technique of foremost value is the shaping of a more controlled rate of ingestion: the client is instructed to eat more slowly in order to consume less food in a given time. Simply telling a client to "eat more slowly," however, does not provide him with a behavior methodology to accomplish it. Specific new behaviors need to be devised to achieve a slower rate of ingestion.

For example, the client might be instructed to: (a) chew each mouthful thoroughly and slowly; (b) put his eating utensil down after every third bite; (c) swallow food completely before putting more food on the utensil; and (d) plan short delays during the meal. Each behavior change requires practice before a person feels comfortable executing it, but the consequence of eating less food with no accompanying increase in hunger is often a suitable reward and thus increases the probability that the new behavior will continue to be practiced until it becomes fairly habitual.

Another major habit change in behavior therapy programs is alteration of the antecedent stimulus controls of eating. Penick et al. noted (14) that most of their obese patients ate in a wide variety of places in the home and at many different times during the day. Through repeated association with food, such places and times become *discriminative stimuli* for eating; the place or time acts as a signal that a particular behavior (eating) will have rewarding or reinforcing consequences. The result of this process may be habitual eating in the absence of physiologic hunger, and it is important that the client begin to establish different stimulus controls by associating eating only with a particular place in the home at specific times. Penick et al. also encouraged patients to make the dining area as distinctive as possible by using special place settings (14).

The same process also applies to activities that regularly accompany eating, such as reading or watching television; the TV or reading material may become a discriminative stimulus and occasion eating in the absence of physiologic hunger. In this case, the preferred technique is to dissociate the two activities and make eating a "pure experience."

Many other techniques of stimulus control have been described in the literature, particularly by Stuart and Davis (13). Techniques have been designed to alter the stimulus antecedents not only of meals and snacks, but of impulse shopping and food preparation. One technique, using the same principle of discriminative stimulus control, was devised to alter the signal associated with the cessation of eating. Rather than using an empty plate as the cue for the end of the meal, the client is instructed to stop eating when a small amount of food remains on his plate.

PROGRAMMING INCOMPATIBLE BEHAVIORS. In many cases, emotional states, such as boredom, depression, or anxiety, serve as antecedents for maladaptive eating behavior. While it is sometimes necessary clinically to treat the patient's response to the antecedent conditions producing the emotional state, it may be that he has learned to use food as a means of relieving mild anxiety or boredom. In such cases, it is not the *emotional* reaction that differentiates the obese from the normal-weight person, but rather his response to it. This association between an emotional antecedent and eating response can be viewed as a learned maladaptive habit that is susceptible to behavioral change.

During treatment, the concept of programming *incompatible behaviors* is useful in altering this type of habit. Ideally, an incompatible behavior is one which (a) the patient finds engrossing and enjoyable, (b) is readily available, and (c) cannot be engaged in while eating. Patients are instructed to use such an activity, e.g., singing, taking a bath or shower, or art work, as an alternative to eating when they find themselves bored, mildly depressed, or anxious.

The idea of "doing something other than eating" can be extended to include alternate activities that are not necessarily incompatible with eating, giving the patient a wider choice of activities. Errands, hobbies, reading, and work activities can be planned for the times of day when he is most likely to experience boredom. Often a "project list" of short-term household activities provides readily available alternatives to eating in response to a particular feeling.

REINFORCERS. A significant problem encountered in developing self-management of eating behavior is that food is a potent and immediate *positive reinforcer*: this fact tends to increase the probability that the preceding adaptive or maladaptive eating behavior will recur in the future. In weight control, it is important to provide differential consequences for these two classes of eating patterns.

One example of a differential consequence is a written contract that states a contingency between a particular behavior (eating slowly) or behavior result (lowered daily caloric intake or weight loss) and a self-imposed, positively valued consequence. For example, a representative *contingency contract* might involve the self-presentation of a certain amount of money or time in a valued recreational activity, contingent on practicing specific behavior techniques during the day.

For the contract to be used successfully, the positive reinforcement must be meaningful to the person and awarded soon after the appropriate behavior. Because the latter condition is often inconvenient, a token system is frequently employed whereby the client earns a number of points immediately after the performance of an adaptive habit; the points are accumulated and later exchanged for the actual reward. Token systems permit long-term contracts to be established while providing frequent and prompt reinforcements for individual behaviors.

Although most of the emphasis in a behavior therapy program is related to food intake, many of the same principles can be applied to increasing the client's energy expenditure. In the same manner that the patient is not given an inflexible diet, increasing energy expenditure is not accomplished by prescribing a particular set of exercises. Rather, the goal is to alter behavior patterns so that the client must expend more energy in order to engage in his usual activities. One technique suggested by Stuart and Davis (13) is to instruct the client intentionally to park his car farther from his destination; the time spent walking is more productive for the obese client than the time spent looking for the closest parking space. Also, bus-riding behavior can be arranged so that the client gets on or off one or two blocks before his usual stop, and walks the remaining distance. Use of extension telephones, escalators, elevators, and laundry chutes can be programmed gradually so that the patient learns to expend more energy in his everyday activities.

Family member participation

One aspect of the client's environment that is receiving increasing attention is the effect family members can have in a behavior therapy program. At the Day Hospital Obesity Program at the Hospital of the University of Pennsylvania, biweekly family group sessions are scheduled to instruct family members in the behavior approach to overeating, to determine how they can best respond to the client while he is eating appropriately and inappropriately and to enlist their aid in devising and practicing techniques that may be helpful. Often, stimulus control, incompatible behavior procedures, and self-reinforcement contracts necessitate changes in family routines. These techniques are more apt to be successful if other persons affected by the changes understand why they are necessary and in some way can help to achieve them.

There is often a broader reason for including a family member in the therapeutic procedures. Although, on occasion, a family member might deliberately attempt to subvert the patient's weight-loss efforts, more often the problem is that the obesity has become part of the family's stable adjustment pattern. From this viewpoint, behavior change and loss of weight alter the family situation, and the therapist must be prepared to deal with this situation. For example, overweight and overeating may be a strong link between an obese parent and obese child; if the parent begins to lose weight successfully, this link gradually dissolves. In some cases at the Day Hospital, the mother was able to interest the child in applying the techniques she was using to his own eating behavior. The point of common interest was maintained by changing it to one that was more appropriate to both persons.

ADAPTING TECHNIQUES TO THE PATIENT. A behavior program, then, is composed of a wide variety of techniques, each providing a partial solution to the problem habits of obese clients. It must be stressed that the specific techniques introduced to the client must be adapted to his particular habit patterns. While the same underlying principles of learning can be employed, the specific content and order of the program must be defined by the results of the original functional analysis.

In almost all research to date, the clients have been adolescents and adult women. There is little reason to suspect that significantly different principles would be required for adult men, children, or the elderly, or for upper- or lower-class clients. However, the manner in which the program is presented and the formulation of specific techniques would vary for different populations.

Research needs

In the current literature, most research has been conducted by mental health professionals working in individual or small group therapy. An important area of future research is the training of other professionals traditionally involved in weight control in the use of behavior techniques, either in a separate program or one integrated with existing dietary control and general medical programs.

Currently, the applicability of the techniques used in established self-help groups is being investigated. In this issue, Jordan and Levitz report (15) the results of a pilot study in training a self-help group leader in behavior therapy. Stunkard and Levitz are currently engaged in studying the feasibility of training established self-help group leaders in behavioral techniques and assessing their effectiveness relative to professional group leadership.

The question of whether a therapist is necessary has also received some attention. The Stuart and Davis book (13), which includes self-monitoring food intake forms, is arranged for use by a person without the participation of either a self-help group or trained therapist. To date, there has been only one study on the effectiveness of a completely self-managed approach vs. a professional therapy approach (5), but results indicated that with both approaches, college-age women lost significant amounts of weight in comparison with a control group. Furthermore, there was no significant difference between the two treatment modalities.

Behavior therapy represents an approach to the treatment of obesity, which, in the literature to date, has been shown to be effective in promoting gradual weight loss. As the use of behavior therapy is extended by professional and non-professional persons to various client populations, its effectiveness, both during and after treatment, will need to be carefully assessed.

References

(1) STUNKARD, A.J.: New therapies for the eating disorders: Behavior modification of obesity and anorexia nervosa. Arch. Gen. Psychiatry 76: 391, 1972.
(2) ULLMAN, L.P., AND KRASNER, L., EDS.: Case Studies in Behavior Modification. N.Y.: Holt, Rinehart & Winston, 1965.
(3) LIBERMAN, R.: A Guide to Behavioral Analysis and Therapy. N.Y.: Pergamon Press, 1970.
(4) WOLLERSHEIM, J.P.: The effectiveness of group therapy based upon learning principles in the treatment of overweight women. J. Abnorm. Psychol. 76: 462, 1970.
(5) HAGEN, R.L.: Group therapy versus bibliotherapy in weight reduction. Unpublished PH.D. thesis, Univ. of Illinois, 1969.
(6) YOUNG, C.M., MOORE, N.S., BERRESFORD, K., EINSET, B.M., AND WALDNER, B.G.: The problem of the obese patient. J. Am. Dietet. A. 31: 1111, 1955.
(7) KANFER, F.H.: Self-regulation: Research issues and speculations. In Neuringer, C., and Michael, J.L., eds.: Behavior Modification in Clinical Psychology. N.Y.: Appleton-Century-Crofts, 1970.
(8) MAHONEY, M.: Research issues in self-management. Behav. Ther. 3: 45, 1972.
(9) KRASNER, L.: Behavior therapy. Ann. Rev. Psychol. 22: 483, 1971.
(10) MANN, R.A.: The use of contingency contracting to control obesity in adult subjects. Paper delivered at meeting of the Western Psychological Assn., San Francisco, 1971.
(11) STOLLACK, G.E.: Weight loss obtained under different experimental procedures. Psychotherapy: Theory, Research and Practice 4: 61, 1967.
(12) CAUTELA, J.R.: Treatment of compulsive behavior by covert sensitization. Psychol. Record 16: 33, 1966.
(13) STUART, R.B., AND DAVIS, B.: Slim Chance in a Fat World: Behavioral Control of Obesity. Champaign, Ill.: Research Press, 1972.
(14) PENICK, S.B., FILION, R., FOX, S., AND STUNKARD, A.J.: Behavior modification in the treatment of obesity. Psychosom. Med. 23: 49, 1971.
(15) JORDAN, H.A., AND LEVITZ, L.S.: Behavior modification in a self-help group. A pilot study. J. Am. Dietet. A. 62: 27, 1973.

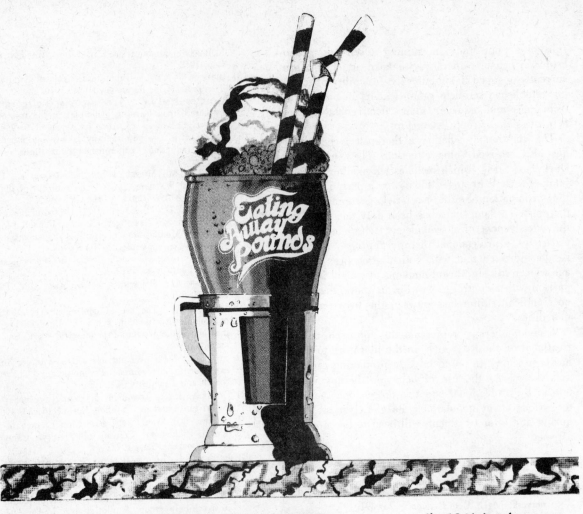

The problem of obesity and its attendant health hazards has been well documented.[1,2] Literally thousands of claims about various treatments have been made in both lay and professional journals. In a thorough review, however, Stunkard and Mc-Laren-Hume[3] found only eight reported studies[4-11] worthy of consideration. These studies document that, in general, medical treatment for obesity has been singularly unsuccessful.

Comparing these studies is not entirely valid but does give some idea of the results of conventional therapies. When pooled, these eight samples provide a population of 1,368. Only 16% lost between 10 and 20

TREATING OBESITY WITH BEHAVIOR MODIFICATION

Behavior modification techniques offer great promise for weight reduction. The system outlined here requires only five 20-minute periods of instruction before the patient applies the principles at home.

DENNIS R. BRIGHTWELL, MD
University of Iowa College of Medicine
Iowa City

lb, 12% lost between 20 and 40 lb, and 5% lost more than 40 lb. These studies were done by investigators, some using highly controlled treatments. The general physician could hardly expect to do even this well in an outpatient setting.

Only some rather heroic measures, such as surgical removal of a portion of the alimentary tract, have generally produced permanent weight loss. Diets and drugs have also been widely used, but on a periodic basis, and weight reduction is temporary. Psychiatrists have used insight psychotherapy aimed at overcoming personality characteristics considered contributory to overeating. When this approach fails, the patient may offer his lack

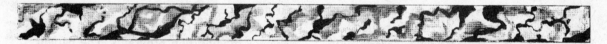

of motivation as his excuse for overeating.

A recently developed approach introduces new methods of changing eating patterns through the principles of behavior therapy. Various systems of behavior modification have been applied to decrease caloric intake and thereby reduce weight.[12-22] However, many of these methods have been too cumbersome and time-consuming to be useful to the general physician.

This article describes a practical method for use of behavior modification in the treatment of obesity. Patients must meet only four criteria: (1) be 10% to 100% over their ideal weight as defined by life insurance statistics,[2] (2) desire to lose weight, (3) be motivated to participate for an extended period, and (4) lack emotional or physical contraindications to weight loss.

Technique

A complete history should be taken and the patient should have a complete physical examination. The actual training for behavior modification occurs in five 20-minute sessions spaced evenly over a two- or three-week period. Subsequently, the patient is seen briefly once a month for follow-up and record checking.

Session 1: The theory—Patients are told both the how-to aspects and the theories that apply to the program. This allows development of the understanding that is necessary if the patient is to cooperate fully in the training, which must be carried out in his own home.

The basic theory of behavior modification can be expressed as $S_d \rightarrow B \rightarrow E$: A discriminatory stimulus (S_d) leads to a behavior (B) that results in an event (E). The stimulus may be any particular sensation that the individual perceives. For example, when a person is hungry, a particular behavior results—eating. This leads to an event—relief of hunger, which positively reinforces this behavior. Therefore, the next time the same stimulus occurs, similar behavior follows more readily.

Most people have more than one discriminatory stimulus for eating. Besides hunger, many emotional states, such as anger, anxiety, depression, boredom, loneliness, and frustration, can be a stimulus to eating. Usually, a patient can offer several examples that apply specifically in his case.

In addition, there are situational stimuli. These arise from the environment in which eating usually takes place. If this is the kitchen, the setting of the kitchen itself can become a stimulus to eating. Although most patients are not aware of all the stimuli that play upon them during the day, nearly all can relate to the theory being discussed.

Before the end of the first session, patients are instructed to begin keeping a thorough record of the time of eating, type and amount of food ingested, and any stimuli bearing on their eating throughout the day, along with a daily note of fasting weight. They must be cautioned not to cut their intake at this time; a base-line record of eating behavior patterns is needed, and any change from their normal pattern will invalidate the results.

Session 2: Failure and success—Many patients have tried several methods to lose weight and are curious about their lack of success. The failure of diet therapy can be easily explained. Most people require a reward for continuing behavior. It is logical to assume that several kinds of rewards may be forthcoming as a result of eating. To want these rewards is normal and healthy, but to obtain them from eating eventually results in unwanted obesity. For example, if a patient is bored and eating occupies his time, boredom is relieved. No one wants to be bored and being occupied is a good thing, although being occupied by eating can have some bad results, eg, obesity.

When a patient becomes too fat, this unwanted state can counterbalance all the positive reinforcements he obtains from eating

and initiate a desire to diet. He begins to lose weight to a point where he does not feel quite as fat, and the objectionable aspects of his obesity are again outweighed by the anticipated rewards resulting from eating. He then stops his diet and his weight creeps back to the point where the fat is again objectionable.

The natural history for most dieters is the roller coaster curve. Their weight goes up and down, sometimes getting lower and sometimes higher, but without permanent reduction. Diet pills are specifically anorectics and their activity is short. In addition, the "buzz" that patients get from these central nervous system stimulants may replace some of the positive reinforcement they formerly got from eating. However, as soon as the pills are withdrawn or tolerance builds up, weight can no longer be lost.

Weight reduction clubs are, in a sense, behavior modification programs. The patient is praised for losing weight and damned for gaining. The berating that is given the patient who gains weight is frequently too much for the obese person to tolerate. He may leave the program for this reason alone, even if he is losing weight most of the time.

Being a dropout from such a club should not prevent a patient from considering the program described here. There is no berating in this program. It is entirely positive, should be as much fun as possible for the patient, and is something in which the patient cannot fail as long as he wants to continue. He may quit, but that is an active decision, not failure of the program. Unlike weight reduction clubs, this program operates in the home, not at a weekly session. The patient should know that this approach has been exceptionally successful with other people and that over the next year he may be able to lose 40 lb if he sticks with it.

The patient's notebook should be reviewed at this and each subsequent session. A commitment should be elicited that the patient will participate in the program for a sufficient period to lose the weight desired at a healthy rate. To expect to lose 30 or 40 lb in less than a year is foolhardy and doomed to failure.

Session 3: The program—The patient's record of eating should first be reviewed for completeness and accuracy. The patient is then instructed to get a different place setting. It does not have to be a new one—an old, odd piece from a discarded set may be used. The purpose of such a setting is to disrupt as completely as possible the situational stimuli and help the patient develop a new way of eating. Preferably, the plate should have an unusual pattern. It should be smaller, if possible, than the one from which he usually eats. Everything the patient eats should come off this plate. He should use a different glass from which all caloric liquids will be drunk, odd silverware that does not match regular utensils, and the gaudiest, most unusual looking place mat he can find.

All eating should take place in the same location, in whatever room is most frequently used at mealtime. Even a candy bar or can of diet pop should be consumed from this place setting.

Practically speaking, there is really nothing that cannot be eaten and there are no specifically forbidden foods. The purpose of this program is not to restrict the patient from anything but to help him learn to take responsibility for what he eats before he consumes it. This can only be done by using a routine such as described. It forces the patient to plan his intake before it enters his mouth. Patients can eventually learn to plan their intake for the whole day.

The special place setting should be used at all meals and all foods should be served before the patient starts to eat. No food should be left on the table during the meal, and all food should be put away completely so that the patient does not have to look at food. For most people, there is no stronger

DENNIS R. BRIGHTWELL

Dr. Brightwell is in the department of psychiatry, University of Iowa College of Medicine, Iowa City.

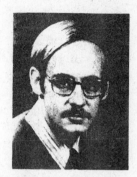

stimulus to eating than a three fourths empty casserole dish. If a second helping is desired, the patient should return to the place where the food is kept, get what he wants, and then put the food away again before starting to eat. No food that can be eaten without preparation should be readily available. Cookies and candy should be put away and not be in a dish in the living room. Many patients are unaware that they almost always have had some food in sight which acts as a stimulus to eating.

For various reasons people may not be able to eat all meals at home. In that event, patients can prepare a meal at home and take it with them. Where this is not feasible, the ingenuity of the patient is the only limiting factor. Some of our patients carry their place mat, silverware, and glass with them. It is indeed amazing what highly motivated patients can do to help themselves. For others, a program can be developed based on limiting what can be spent on the meal and pocketing anything under this as part of the reward system.

Dining out as part of a social gathering presents a more difficult program and is discouraged for at least the first three months of the program. After this time, such eating may take place on a limited basis until it is determined how effectively new eating patterns have been established.

Session 4: The reward system—Since most home scales can detect weight differences of no less than one half pound, the reward system is planned around this measure. This is a practical unit because this amount of weight can be lost usually between one and four times a week. Rewards too distantly spaced seem unreachable and if too frequent, lose their value.

The patient needs to be rewarded as soon as possible after the weight is lost; he should not set his sights on a goal of 10 or 15 lb. This is common in dieting, with weight loss

---

The patient is never, never, never reprimanded for gaining weight. If he gains, the physician should look over the records with the patient and find out why he is failing.

---

itself as the reward, and explains why diets are often a failure. What keeps patients in this program is getting a reward for losing half a pound; they do not have to wait so long before they can feel good about what they are doing.

Rewards might include some household task accomplished for the patient by the spouse. Other patients may wish to put away 25¢ or 50¢ for every half pound lost. The money itself is usually not a sufficient reward, but the patient may agree to spend this money, and only this money, on something he really wants. The symbolic value of the money then increases to the point where it is a suitable reward.

The patient should be encouraged at the end of this session to consider some possible rewards and mention any he has in mind. Finally, another commitment should be solicited from the patient, and he should be encouraged to go ahead with the program.

Session 5: The specifics—During this session, patients should outline a specific reward

they are going to get for losing one half pound. Some patients have trouble getting started. Should they not be a half pound lighter in the morning, it may be suggested that no food be consumed until that weight is lost. This almost always occurs by lunchtime and is usually not too restrictive, although some patients become alarmed at being told not to eat.

Some patients need to set a bigger goal, such as losing 5 lb, before they can be allowed to spend their money. It is conceivable that a patient can lose half a pound one day, gain it the next, and lose it the following, accumulating a large sum of money without getting any lighter. The patient may have a tendency to set this goal too far away: 10 to 15 lb is too distant, and the reward will be meaningless. A goal of 3 to 5 lb is easier to reach and more effective. If the patient loses 2 lb in a week, he may give himself an extra reward; if he loses 7 to 9 lb in a month, he may want something even more special. The reward should not be food. One of the goals of this program is to reduce the value of food as a reward.

A graph is used to chart the patient's weekly average weight or his weight on the day of his follow-up visit. The patient is given a copy, which is updated for him at each session. The physician collects and keeps all pages from the patient's notebook. They should be reviewed in detail with the patient to make sure that all patterns of eating are clear.

By this time most patients are amazed at how much they eat. Just writing down their intake is an eye-opener to them and they are anxious to cut back because they are somewhat ashamed of their involuntary intake. Therefore, they almost always lose weight at the beginning of the program, and this is fine reinforcement for getting them to believe in the program and keeping them committed.

The patient should be seen every two

weeks or once a month. If appointments are spaced farther than a month apart, the patient tends to forget about his record keeping and becomes lax in following his new eating habits.

Subsequent sessions—The eating record should be reviewed and the weight graph updated at each visit. The patient is *never, never, never* reprimanded for gaining weight. If he gains, the physician should look over the records with the patient and find out why he is failing. He should be told that this is to reevaluate the reward system and to discuss in detail what he can do to help turn the program around. Any berating the physician gives the patient who has gained weight is only bound to cause the patient to feel worse than he already does and possibly drop out of the program. He sees no reason to come and get chewed out by the physician for something he already knows is bad.

Many patients have to be reminded frequently that they cannot cheat on this program, that they can eat what they want to eat, as long as it is eaten in the manner specified. If they do not lose weight, it is because the rewards are not sufficient, not because there is anything wrong with the patient. It is frequently helpful to refer back to older records to show the patient how his behavior has changed with time.

Results

In an outpatient clinic at the State Psychopathic Hospital, Iowa City, Iowa, 15 patients under the care of four physicians have begun a program similar to the one described here. One patient came only once; one came four times; two dropped out before completing six months of follow-up. Of the original 15 patients, 8 have completed a one-year program or reached their goal. Three have not completed a six-month program and are still in treatment. Average initial weight at the beginning of treatment was 193 lb with a range of 138 to 250 lb. For those who com-

pleted treatment, the average weight loss was 22.6 lb, with a range of 9 to 46 lb. Three patients had lost more than 20 lb, and one of these more than 40 lb.

Direct comparisons with other studies are difficult. Methods of reporting weight lost are highly variable. What is important is that only 2 of 12 patients voluntarily dropped out. Every patient who remained continued to lose weight at a varying rate. This retention rate alone is atypical, and coupled with the fact that all in the program lost weight (none gained or remained the same for an extended period), the results were truly unusual. We have been able to surpass the best results of conventional treatments lasting up to a year or more. New patients are being added to our program but have not been included long enough for follow-up.

Discussion

Although applying behavior modification to the problem of overeating is a relatively new idea, it would appear that at last a relatively successful method of treating obesity has been developed. Our results at the University of Iowa in a program similar to the one described here are generally in line with those reported by other investigators.[12-22] Such programs help patients learn how to eat properly and take responsibility for their intake. This is something that most obese patients have never done. This program is not a cure-all and it does not work for every patient. Patients must be motivated, but motivation is easier to develop in this program than in most because it is in no way restrictive. There is really nothing patients are not allowed to do, only things they must do in addition to their normal daily behavior. Most people find this easier to tolerate than rules and regulations about what they must avoid. Patients often develop a substantial amount of insight into why they eat and form new patterns of behavior that will serve them well in the future. They begin a new habit of eating which can be with them for the rest of their life. If they find themselves gaining weight after they are through with this program, they can easily reapply its principles.

In this deceptively simple approach, the patient and the physician develop a close relationship. It is an especially trusting one, because the patient knows that the physician believes in him and his desires and abilities. The patient realizes that he will not be criticized or rejected for any failure. This positive outlook and the expectation of success are new ideas to most obese patients and presumably contribute to the good results of such a program.

REFERENCES

1. Mayer J: Overweight: Causes, Cost, and Control. Englewood Cliffs, NJ, Prentice-Hall, Inc, 1968
2. New weight standards for men and women. Stat Bull Metropol Life Ins Co 40:1, Nov-Dec 1959
3. Stunkard A, McLaren-Hume M: The results of treatment for obesity. Arch Intern Med 103:79, 1959
4. Evans FA: Treatment of obesity with low calorie diets. Int Clin 3:19, 1938
5. Feinstein R, Dole V, Schwartz I: The use of a formula diet for weight reduction of obese outpatients. Ann Intern Med 28:330, 1958
6. Fellows HH: Studies of relatively normal obese individuals during and after dietary restriction. Am J Med Sci 181:301, 1931
7. Gray H, Kallenbach DE: Obesity treatment. J Am Diet Assoc 15:239, 1939
8. Harvey HI, Simmons WD: Weight reduction. Am J Med Sci 227:521, 1954
9. McCann M, Trulson MF: Long-term effect of weight-reducing programs. J Am Diet Assoc 31:1108, 1955
10. Murves ED: Dietetic interview or group discussion—decision in reducing? J Am Diet Assoc 29:1192, 1953
11. Osserman E, Dolger H: Obesity in diabetes. Ann Intern Med 34:72, 1951
12. Penick SB, Filion R, Fox S, et al: Behavior modification in the treatment of obesity. Psychosom Med 33:49, 1971
13. Cautela JR: Covert sensitization. Psychol Rep 20:459, 1967
14. Erickson MH: The utilization of patient behavior in the hypnotherapy of obesity. Am J Clin Hypn 3:112, 1960
15. Kennedy WA, Foreyt JP: Control of eating behavior in an obese patient by avoidance conditioning. Psychol Rep 22:571, 1968
16. Harmatz MG, Lapuc P: Behavior modification of overeating in a psychiatric population. J Consult Clin Psychol 32:583, 1968
17. Harris MB: Self-directed program for weight control. J Abnorm Psychol 74:263, 1969
18. Meyer V, Crisp AH: Aversion therapy in two cases of obesity. Behav Res Ther 2:143, 1964
19. Stuart RB: Behavioral control of overeating. Behav Res Ther 5:357, 1967
20. Stuart RB: A three-dimensional program for the treatment of obesity. Behav Res Ther 9:177, 1971
21. Thorpe JG, Schmidt E, Brown PT, et al: Aversion-relief therapy: A new method for general application. Behav Res Ther 2:71, 1964
22. Wollersheim JP: Effectiveness of group therapy based upon learning principles in the treatment of overweight women. J Abnorm Psychol 76:462, 1970

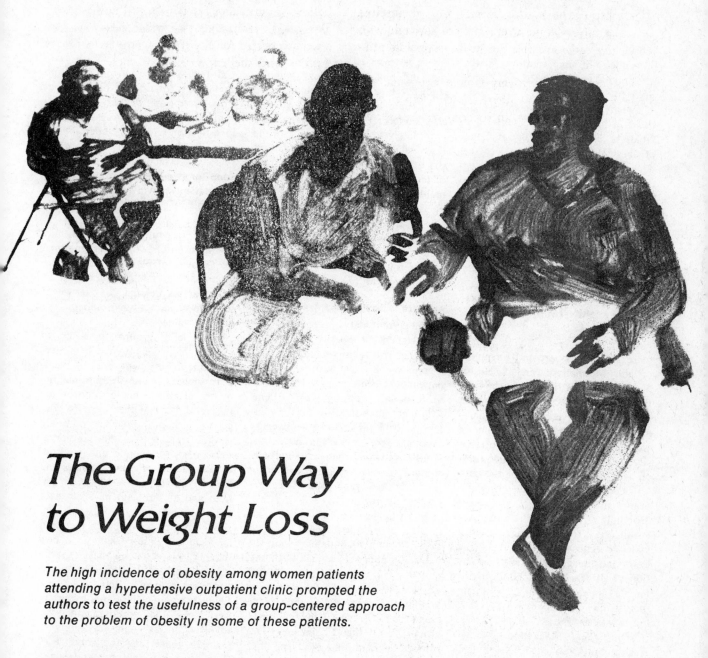

The Group Way to Weight Loss

The high incidence of obesity among women patients attending a hypertensive outpatient clinic prompted the authors to test the usefulness of a group-centered approach to the problem of obesity in some of these patients.

SANDRA SHUMWAY / MARJORIE POWERS

Although the mechanism describing the relationship between obesity and hypertension is not presently known, there are abundant data to illustrate the relationship of obesity to hypertension and coronary artery disease.

In a report of the 1969 White House Conference on Food, Nutrition, and Health, a panel concerned with the problems of hypertension reported that 21 million Americans suffer from hypertension in some de-

gree. Obesity was reported as a major risk factor in hypertension and the prevention and control of overweight was recommended in the management of this disorder. One of the final recommendations of the

Obesity cannot be divorced from the cultural, socioeconomic, and environmental factors which affect eating patterns.

panel was "that the medical profession and the general public be urgently advised that the major approach presently available for the prevention of hypertension is the prevention and control of obesity"(1).

Twenty pounds above the weight listed in height, age, and sex weight tables is usually taken as evidence of obesity. However, because of the wide range of body builds among the general population, it is often difficult to be certain about what is real overweight. Recently, measurement with a skin caliper in standardized regions of the body has been used as a measurement of overweight and it has been suggested that an abdominal skin fold in excess of one inch thickness is a better sign of overweight than measurement on a scale(2).

Obesity also seems to be related to socioeconomic group. The report of the Manhattan Mental Health Survey indicates that, in the population studied, there was an inverse relationship between family incomes and obesity, particularly among women(3,4). The prevalence of obesity in lower economic group women was 30 percent compared with 16 percent in the middle economic group and 5 percent in the upper economic group in this study. According to these findings, obesity was six times as prevalent in the lower income group female population as in the upper income group female population. Findings among men in the population were similar, but to a lesser degree.

While the Manhattan Mental Health Survey indicates a higher prevalence of obesity in lower socioeconomic groups than in middle and upper income groups, Stamler reports that obesity is a common finding in virtually all strata of our society(5,6). His population samples of middle-aged males showed 15

percent or more above desirable weight. He also reports that the grossly obese, those 25 percent or more above desirable weight, constituted between 20 to 50 percent of the different population samples studied. These samples included male and female, black and white. Stamler also found that obese individuals are more likely to be hypertensive, while lean individuals in the populations studied had diastolic blood pressures of less than 80 mm./Hg. The Framingham Heart Study indicates that obesity alone rarely increases the risk of coronary artery disease, but obesity coupled with such other risk factors as hypertension or hypercholesterolemia greatly contribute to coronary disease(7).

Approach to the Problem

The traditional approach to the management of obesity, as well as the other risk factors cited, has been a one-to-one relationship between patient and professional. The health professionals working with patients who were attending the renal hypertension clinic at an urban university hospital were concerned about the large number of these patients who seemed to have a persistent problem with obesity, in spite of the traditional approach.

Chart reviews of all patients attending two clinic sessions revealed that 15 out of 38 patients and 12 out of 64 patients weighed over 180 pounds. Their weights ranged from 180 to 349 pounds in the first analysis and 182½ to 302 pounds in the second chart review. In the latter group, 8 of the 12 patients had gained weight during one year, and only one patient lost more than one pound in that time.

Most of the patients had returned to the clinic on a regular basis every three to four months for a year. They seemed unable to lose weight in spite of regular clinic visits and

in spite of their one-to-one relationships with dietitians, nutritionists, nurses, and physicians. Questions were raised by the professionals as to whether the patients recognized the need to lose weight and about the feasibility of using alternative methods to assist them in losing weight. The professionals suggested using a group approach to resolve the problem.

A review of the current literature on therapy for obesity suggests that most group approaches meet with minimal if any real success(8,9,10). Investigation seldom included follow-up of patients for longer than two years, but even when follow-up was done for two years, it appeared that the patients involved were unable to maintain a weight loss over time (11, 12).

These discouraging findings may be the result of two factors: minimal involvement of patients in group decisions and minimal consideration of such factors related to overweight as socioeconomics, environment, and cultural values.

Only one group approach to overweight, "Weight Watchers," reports the involvement of group members themselves in decision-making or organizational matters concerning the group(13). Other reports concerning group approaches to weight loss do not mention any consideration of socioeconomic and environmental factors or cultural values and tend to isolate treatment of the patient and his problem of overweight from his environment.

We decided to approach the management of obese patients in a new manner. We proposed that a special group approach be included in the treatment plan of selected obese patients attending the renal-hypertension clinic; that group members be involved in as many decisions as possible concerning the conduct of the group; that environmental, socioeconomic, and cultural factors be discussed in group meetings as they related to group members' problems with overweight; and that the approach encourage and use the emotional support that group members could gain from others having to cope with similar problems.

Ten obese hypertensive women from a hypertensive clinic of an urban university hospital were selected for a series of group sessions. Patients were the first 10 referred by physicians or nurses with the exclusion of patients with major psychiatric problems.

Description of the Group

Six of the 10 women selected for the first group attended the first session. Their ages ranged from 30 to 64 years, with an average age of 46 years; five members were under 51 years old and one member was 64. Review of their charts revealed that the average number of visits made to the clinic by group members had been four a year. They had been seen and cared for by a different physician at each visit. To overcome this lack of continuity, arrangements were made with the physician in charge of the hypertension clinic to have patients in the weight group referred to us for primary care. One physician agreed to be available for consultation in reference to medical matters.

Group members had been overweight for various numbers of years; the average was 15.3 years. The distribution of years each had been diagnosed as hypertensive also varied. Chart reviews revealed a range of 1 to 12 years with an average of 4.3 years. With this evidence, it was clear that the prospective group members had longstanding problems and that plans to initiate group therapy should include long-term follow up. The results of only the first 10 group sessions are reported here.

The sessions were conducted over four months. The only structure offered by the co-leaders was a definite starting and concluding time. The co-leaders were joined in the group by a nutrition intern and a nurse's aide. Topics for discussion were chosen by the patients. There was no "lecturing" to patients. Coleaders served primarily to facilitate discussion, to draw attention to commonalities described, and, initially, to open and close the meeting. Reasonably soon, group members handled most of these functions; co-leaders and the nutrition intern were consulted when specific information was needed. The nurse's aide was included in the group meetings primarily because she was black; all of the patients were black and the professional group members, white. We hoped the nurse's aide would help us increase our understanding of black culture.

After each group session, the non-patient group members met to identify problems which had been raised, including those resulting from racial misunderstandings, and to discuss ways in which their recurrence could be prevented. The nurse's aide played a vital role in these post-group sessions by clarifying interpretations. In addition, since she was permanently assigned to the clinic, she also became a vital link in the continuity of care because she was accessible to patients who visited or telephoned the clinic. She relayed many messages to professional group members, thus saving patients much time and frustration.

Initially, the six women were somewhat embarrassed about discussing their specific weight problems. They came to the first group meeting with multiple complaints about physical problems which consisted of bothersome gas pains, feeling bloated, constipation, fatigue, and general sluggishness; most of them used laxatives regularly. One woman had anginal pain associated with periods of stress. All were concerned about their appearances and expressed the desire to be able to wear differently styled clothes. Their appearances suggested that they were trying very hard to be neat; to accomplish this several women declared they had to wear heavy corsets with steel stays in the backs and sides. This presented a problem which the co-leaders had not anticipated: skin breakdown and secondary pressure sores due to tight, rigid girdles. One of the members had reddened areas over the sacrum and redness over an old abdominal scar.

In addition to physical problems, these overweight women had very limited economic resources to use in altering their dietary habits. The values which guided their behavior originated from poverty. Several of the women said their parents had felt a great deal of pride when a child was plump, even though poorly clothed. Being well-fed was a positive symbol for the poor. If we had assumed a traditional nurse-teacher role, we could have corrected this misinformation in a direct manner; however, we felt it would be better for the patients to discover such fallacies for themselves, as indeed they did. Several of the women with growing children expressed the belief that the plump child was not necessarily "good" and that they were not going to force food on their own children. There was lengthy discussion about the difficulty of rejecting their past beliefs.

Changed Behavior

During the first group meeting, a 30-year-old mother of five sons identified one of the problems contributing to her weight as "whenever I am under stress, I eat one cookie after another." Although she recognized this as a problem, she was not able to cope with it. One group member said this was really not such a difficult problem and suggested

MS. SHUMWAY (St. Luke's Hospital School of Nursing; B.S.N., and M.S., Case Western Reserve University, Cleveland, Ohio) is chief of nursing, Hough-Norwood Family Health Care Center in Cleveland and assistant professor of nursing at Case Western Reserve University.

MS. POWERS (St. Peter's Hospital School of Nursing, Albany, N.Y.; B.S.N. and M.S.N., St. Louis University, Mo.) is a full-time graduate student in educational psychology at Case Western Reserve University.

When they did the group work described in the article, both authors were nurse specialists, University Hospitals of Cleveland, and assistant professors in medical-surgical nursing at Case Western Reserve University. The authors acknowledge with grateful appreciation the contributions of Ms. Chiquita English, the nurse's aide (nurse's technical assistant) who participated in the group sessions and Ms. Shelby Smith, coordinator for nursing. Ms. Smith and Ms. English were part of the clinic staff of the University Hospitals of Cleveland. Both are now at the Hough-Norwood Family Health Care Center in Cleveland.

that she put the cookie jar high on a cabinet out of reach, and even suggested that perhaps cookies were not essential to have around the house if the children were taught to eat proper meals on schedule. The woman with the "cookie" problem accepted this advice and started nibbling on carrots instead.

It was difficult and even impossible for some of these women to change their dietary patterns. However, a great deal of positive reinforcement was obtained from the group, and from the disappearance of their physical discomforts. Complete disappearance of the discomforts occurred most dramatically in the oldest member of the group who also lost the greatest amount of weight: 10.75 lbs. She had been accustomed to a large intake of salt in various forms but especially in salted peanuts and in her cooking, which she described as rich. She was accustomed to eating bacon and eggs each morning for breakfast. With great fortitude on her part, this woman simply stopped buying peanuts!

This solved one problem, but eating bacon was more difficult to overcome. When she first came to eliminate bacon from breakfast, she actually had to leave the table and go into another room while her husband ate the rest of his meal. In spite of this difficulty in gaining control of her appetite, this woman continued to eliminate the heavy seasoning and the rich and salty foods in her diet. Although she was able to make significant progress in terms of weight loss, others in the group were unable to progress because of environmental and traditional health problems that had to be solved before they could concentrate on the difficult job of weight loss.

These problems are all too frequently overlooked in a traditional approach to health care delivery, which is often so fragmented that the patients themselves must coordinate their own care. Our approach to the care of these patients included consideration of the whole patient living in a unique environment, and we recognized that major problems other than obesity existed. In many instances, these problems were of such magnitude that they had to be attended to before the patient could concentrate any attention on weight loss. For example, it would have been inappropriate to instruct a 30-year-old woman with severe dental problems about reducing calories, since she probably could not really "hear" the instructions because of severe discomfort. What she needed was immediate information about where to have her teeth cared for. She did not know how to go about this because in the past she had been deterred by misinformation or misdirection.

The patient who lost the least amount of weight also had the least improvement in blood pressure control. She had multiple problems with which to cope since she was the only source of emotional support for all members of her family and had never developed the ability to ventilate her own concerns with any one, even family members. Before she joined the group, her youngest son had been killed in an accident and her husband, who had had a myocardial infarction, was also found to be diabetic. He faced permanent unemployment after having been an active worker and he was depressed by this prospect at an age when most men are settled into a lifetime job. The patient's oldest son was in combat in Vietnam. Although this patient began to seek help from one of us, she was unable to accept the help of other group members.

Our experience has been with only a few women who happen to be obese. Further experience certainly is needed to learn more about identifying and treating concomitant problems if obesity is to be dealt with effectively. It is clear, however, that unless an environment is provided that is conducive to continuity of care, people are not likely to seek services except on an episodic basis.

One of the group members was asked why this group approach seemed so desirable to her. Her reply and the feelings she conveyed were: "You care. . . . Before when I was down and discouraged I would go to see a private doctor. . . . When I needed tests done, even though I did not get the results of the test, I would come here to the clinic because you have all the machines. . . . By having the group, I have come to know the doctors and nurses. I get the answers to my tests and I feel comfortable in coming here."

One result of this project apart from improved care, was a decision to provide graduate students in medical-surgical nursing with an opportunity to participate in group work therapy as one means of providing them with experience in doing primary care; further, it demonstrated to them another method for delivering health care.

References

1. WHITE HOUSE CONFERENCE ON FOOD, NUTRITION AND HEALTH. *Final Report.* Washington, D.C., U.S. Government Printing Office, 1970.
2. REICHLIN, SEYMOUR. The problem obese patient. *J.Med.Sci.* 1:45-53, Oct. 1964.
3. STROLE, LEO, AND OTHERS. *Mental Health in the Metropolis; Midtown Manhattan Study.* New York, McGraw-Hill Book Co., 1962.
4. STAMLER, JEREMIAH. *Lectures of Preventive Cardiology.* New York, Grune and Stratton, 1967.
5. MOORE, M. E., AND OTHERS. Obesity, social class, and mental illness. *JAMA* 181:962-966, Sept. 15, 1962.
6. STAMLER, JEREMIAH, AND OTHERS. Prevalence and incidence of coronary heart disease in strata of the labor force of a Chicago industrial corporation. *J.Chron. Dis.* 11:405-420, 1960.
7. KANNEL, W. B., AND TAVIS, GORDON. *Framingham Study: An Epidemiological Investigation of Cardiovascular Disease.* Washington, D.C., U.S. Government Printing Office. 1968.
8. MUNVES, E. D. Dietetic interview or group discussion—decision in reducing? *J.Am. Diet.Assoc.* 29:1197-1203. Dec. 1953.
9. BOWSER, L. J., AND OTHERS. Methods of reducing—group therapy vs. individual clinic interview. *J.Am.Diet.Assoc.* 29:1193-1196, Dec. 1953.
10. OBESITY and its management. *Dairy Council Dig.* 36:13-16, May-June 1965.
11. BOWSER, L. J., AND OTHERS, *op. cit.*
12. KURLANDER, A. B. Group therapy in reducing. *J.Am.Diet.Assoc.* 29:337-339, Apr. 1953.
13. PASCOE, JEAN. How weight watchers lose weight. *Readers Dig.* 95:143-144ff, July 1969.

An approach to the management of obesity that has received curiously little attention from the medical profession is the self-help group. One such group is TOPS (Take Off Pounds Sensibly), a large and rapidly growing organization with chapters throughout the world. Another organization, Weight Watchers, although commercially sponsored and thus not strictly a self-help group, is also large and thriving. Both are worthy of consideration by physicians who have obese patients.

In order to evaluate the effectiveness of TOPS, my associates and I studied 22 chapters in West Philadelphia and its suburbs. The excellent records kept by these groups greatly facilitated our work. We were able to obtain the age, height, weight on entering TOPS, maximum weight loss, and current weight of more than 95 percent of the 485 members of the sample, an unusually high response rate for this type of study.

From these data a composite picture of the average TOPS member emerged. She is a woman 42 years of age whose ideal weight, calculated from standard tables, is 119 lb. She joins TOPS weighing 188 lb, which is 58 percent more than her ideal weight. She stays in TOPS for 16½ months and loses 15 lb during that time. This picture, although useful as a description of the study group, obscures the wide variability found among members and chapters. This variability is one of the most intriguing aspects of TOPS. Chapter records showed weight losses ranging from mediocre to remarkable.

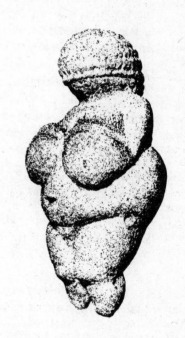

The Success of TOPS, a Self-Help Group

TOPS represents a uniquely successful self-help approach to obesity, with results apparently superior to those of routine medical management. In a study of 22 chapters, the effectiveness of TOPS matched the best reported results of medical treatment. If given the support it deserves from medicine, the organization could be of even greater usefulness in the control of the common problem of overweight.

ALBERT J. STUNKARD, M.D.
University of Pennsylvania
Philadelphia

We compared the chapters with one another and with 14 groups of obese patients treated by medical means.[1,2] The results achieved by the various chapters in our study were strikingly different (figure 1). In the most effective chapter, 62 percent of members lost 20 lb or more, compared with 10 percent in the least effective chapter. When we plotted the 40 lb weight losses, the rank-order of the chapters was similar and again the variation was wide.

For the comparison of TOPS with medical treatment, we divided the 22 chapters into five critical groupings representing the averages of all 22 chapters, the most effective chapter, the least effective chapter, the five most effective chapters, and the five least effective chapters. The last two constitute, in effect, the upper and lower quartiles of the population. These five groupings are depicted in figure 2 as lettered bars. The numbered bars represent the results of medical treatment as given in 14 reports which constitute a large proportion of the total number meeting acceptable standards of reporting.

As is seen in figure 2, the results achieved by the single most effective TOPS chapter (bar A) were better than those of any of the reported medical studies. The five most effective chapters (bar B) ranked with the best in the literature. The average for all 22 TOPS chapters (bar C) was similar to the average achieved by medical treatment. Finally, the five least effective TOPS chapters and the single least effective chapter (bars D and E) ranked with the poorest medical results.

These comparisons offer strong evidence of the effectiveness of TOPS, since the medical results, with one exception, are not those of the average practitioner but were obtained by physicians specializing in the treatment of obesity. The one exception, represented by bar 12, is a study of 100 consecutive obese patients receiving routine treatment in a distinguished teaching hospital. The average of the results achieved in the 22 TOPS chapters is apparently superior to that of routine medical management of obesity. When the criterion used was a 40 lb weight loss, again TOPS was highly successful in comparison with medical regimens.

Our findings were much more favorable than we had anticipated and convinced us that TOPS deserves the active interest of the medical profession.

TOPS was founded in 1948 by Mrs. Esther S. Manz, a Milwaukee housewife with a weight problem. Some 350,000 members are registered in 13,000 chapters in the United States and 24 other countries. Canada has 850 chapters. The organization has grown steadily despite a large but undetermined turnover in membership.

The success of TOPS is especially striking in comparison with other obesity-related groups. A large number of such groups have

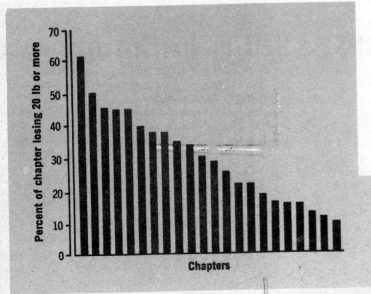

Figure 1. Weight loss in 22 TOPS chapters.

been organized, but most have not lasted long. Membership in one self-help group, for example, dwindled from 162 to six in the nine months of its existence. Some commercial ventures have been transiently successful, but on the whole the durability of these has been as limited as that of the non-profit groups.

Medical auspices often have not improved the outcome of group efforts. One of the few controlled studies of medical therapy of obesity given in groups and individually found that neither method was more effective than no treatment at all. Two of the more ineffective medical studies represented in figure 2 (bars 8 and 11) used group methods. Finally, a psychoanalytically oriented project of group therapy at the University of Pennsylvania enrolled 50 women during its three years of existence, but the highest attendance at any meeting was eight and only five members attended with any regularity.

These studies have made it seem as if obese persons are unable to build the kind of group structure attained in Alcoholics Anonymous. Nevertheless, TOPS, which was modeled in part on AA, proves that obese people can organize to help themselves and can enthusiastically sustain the organization. TOPS' attitude toward the medical profession is a cordial one, yet few physicians seem to know of it, and fewer still, of its therapeutic potential.

TOPS chapters in the United States are distributed according to density of population, with perhaps a slightly higher concentration in suburbs than in urban areas. Outside the United States, members are princi-pally Americans living abroad. Most of the members are female, white, and in the age range from 40 to 60. Male members, comprising about 1 percent, usually join all-male groups such as the successful Sir TOPS chapter in Chicago, which has a membership of 250 business and professional men. Socio-economically, membership appears to be predominantly middle-class, with a small lower-class representation.

The tone and character of TOPS were undoubtedly set by Mrs. Manz, the founder, now in late middle age and still the leader of the organization. A woman of unbounded energy and a lifelong battler with overweight, she identifies easily with the problems of TOPS members and shares her irrepressible optimism with them in the columns of a monthly magazine, *The TOPS News*. She has seen the rise and fall of numerous commercial ventures in the weight-reduction field and is proud that TOPS has withstood the temptation to "go commercial." The steadfast independence of the TOPS leadership, like that of AA, may in part account for the organization's durability.

Growth of the organization has led TOPS to adopt modern business practices such as

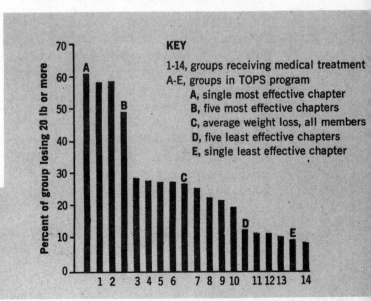

Figure 2. Comparison of effectiveness of TOPS program in 22 chapters with medical treatment of obesity in 14 groups.

KEY

1-14, groups receiving medical treatment

A-E, groups in TOPS program

A, single most effective chapter
B, five most effective chapters
C, average weight loss, all members
D, five least effective chapters
E, single least effective chapter

Percent of group losing 20 lb or more

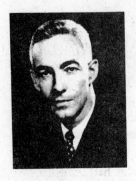

ALBERT J. STUNKARD

Dr. Stunkard was formerly
professor and chairman,
department of psychiatry,
University of Pennsylvania,
Philadelphia. He is now
associated with the Center for
Advanced Study in the
Behavioral Sciences,
Stanford, California.

computer-assisted mailing and automated record keeping. Dues ($6 for the first two years, $4 thereafter) and weight records are dispatched yearly to TOPS International Headquarters in Milwaukee. Members maintain a surprising interest in the activities at "headquarters." They read the organization's magazine regularly and look forward to receiving the bracelet charms that reward successive steps in weight reduction.

While meetings are patterned after those of the first chapter in Milwaukee, TOPS encourages local initiative, and diversity among chapters has naturally developed. We observed certain common features of the meetings of eight chapters in our study. Meetings are held once a week and last for one and a half to two hours. They are conducted by a member elected for a one year term. Two essential activities of each meeting are the weigh-in and the announcement of the weight change of each member. The weigh-in of each member on a professional scale usually takes place before the meeting formally begins. Some members who occasionally cannot stay for a whole meeting will check in just to be weighed. We were told by a number of members that this is the most important factor in their efforts to lose weight.

Each member's weight change is announced as pounds lost or gained during the week, never as total weight. This wise practice seems well designed to prevent discouragement among the heavier members and to focus attention on immediate past performance. The responses to the announcements vary in different chapters, but weight loss is invariably applauded and may be rewarded in other ways, such as with a prize. Announcement of a weight gain may be met with booing or jeering, silence, or expressions of sympathy, but there is always a formal penalty for the member gaining the most weight. It may take the form of payment of a fine or some more personally embarrassing activity.

Emotional control is a central virtue in the TOPS philosophy, which views overeating and overweight as signs of defective control. TOPS members regard each other as intelligent people who have the power to overcome their emotional problems. Along with this emphasis on self-discipline, there was emphasis on competition between individuals in all the groups studied. This competition took the form of contests lasting for a week, a month, or several months. The weekly winners were named "Queen" and often were crowned with a toy crown and given other tokens of recognition of their achievement. All manner of prizes rewarded the winners of longer competitions.

The competition may seem at odds with the cooperation, but both seem to flourish side by side. Members explain that obesity has brought them together and their purpose is to work together for the common good.

Half or more of the meeting may be devoted to discussion, topics including technics of dieting, ideas for self-improvement, and anecdotes about obese people known by members. Some groups, however, spend considerable time discussing other matters, such as appropriation of funds.

On occasion a physician or dietitian may be invited to address the group. The TOPS organization is respectful of medical prerogatives. Individual members' weight goals and the diets to be used are established by their own physicians. A doctor known to have a sympathetic view of the problems of overweight usually is accorded an enthusiastic welcome. On the other hand, members who have experienced both the ineffectuality of medical treatment for obesity and the irritation of their physicians may be expected to be somewhat less than welcoming. In fact, the skits presented at TOPS conventions often portray just this ineffectuality and irritation.

As many as 25 percent of members attend the annual regional meetings. The programs include skits, group singing, and a kind of beauty parade of successful reducers. One by one, these members are presented in the dresses that used to fit them when they entered TOPS. Then they remove the outer dresses to show the new garments they can wear as a result of losing as much as 100 lb.

When members reach their weight goal, they receive diplomas in a graduation ceremony and become members of KOPS (Keep Off Pounds Sensibly). They remain in their original groups, however, and apparently require continued group support in order to maintain their weight loss. They also serve as good examples for the heavier members.

In an effort to learn why this organization is effective and why some chapters are more successful than others, we recently carried out a two year follow-up study of the same chapters. The average weight loss was slightly less than 15 lb, not a statistically significant difference from that found two years before. Thus, this second study supported our initial findings that the average TOPS member loses about 15 lb. However, the chapters that were the most effective in the initial survey did not maintain their high rank. We do not know why they lost effectiveness and are currently searching for an answer. The difference in results could be due to chance; a random distribution of well-motivated members among the chapters probably would lead to results similar to those of our study. In any case, TOPS serves, at the very least, as a way of selecting people who are ready to lose weight. By joining forces to help each other, these people are achieving an enviable record.

Yet doctors, who know well what a frustrating experience the battle against obesity can be, both for their patients and for themselves, have not used the self-help idea to the extent that it deserves. In our study it was the rare TOPS member who had joined at the suggestion of a physician. In another study only 3 percent of members had been referred by doctors.

Comment

As the health care needs in this country expand and tax medical facilities, the traditional systems of delivery of medical care are undergoing great and increasing strain. Paramedical personnel are helping to ease the crisis. However, the possibilities of the self-help approach are still largely unrealized. In the field of obesity, a self-help organization is already functioning effectively and could become more effective with the more active support and guidance of physicians.

If the family physician or internist could confidently turn over to TOPS the jobs of weight monitoring and psychologic support for obese patients, his efforts at controlling obesity could be confined to periodic assessments of their diets and weight goals. We believe that such a plan is feasible and that it would result in larger weight losses for obese patients and in conservation of the physician's time and energy.

Dr. Stunkard's address is Center for Advanced Study in the Behavioral Sciences, 202 Junipero Serra Boulevard, Stanford, California 94305.

REFERENCES

1. Stunkard AJ, Levine H, Fox S: The management of obesity: Patient self-help and medical treatment. Arch Intern Med 125:1067-1072, 1970
2. Stunkard AJ, McLaren-Hume M: The results of treatment for obesity: A review of the literature and report of a series. Arch Intern Med 103:79-85, 1959

A Therapeutic Coalition for Obesity: Behavior Modification and Patient Self-Help

BY LEONARD S. LEVITZ, PH.D., AND ALBERT J. STUNKARD, M.D.

*The effectiveness of a self-help organization for the obese
was significantly increased by behavior modification
techniques. Sixteen chapters of TOPS (Take Off Pounds
Sensibly), with a total of 234 members, received one of
four treatments: behavior modification conducted by a
professional therapist, behavior modification conducted
by the TOPS leader, nutrition education conducted by
the TOPS leader, and continuation of the usual TOPS
program. During the three-month treatment period, behavior modification produced significantly lower attrition
rates and significantly greater weight losses than did the
alternate treatment methods. At nine-month follow-up,
the differences among treatments were even greater.*

SELF-HELP ORGANIZATIONS for weight control are a large
and growing vehicle for the control of obesity. Unfortunately, their effectiveness is limited; most members lose
very little weight (1). Behavior modification seems to be
more effective in treating obesity than any traditional
method, but it has not been widely applied. We designed
this study to see if self-help and behavior modification
could be combined. Behavior modification, we reasoned,
might provide self-help organizations with a more effective treatment. At the same time, the self-help organizations could provide a means for the widespread appli-

A preliminary version of this paper was read at the 126th annual meeting of the American Psychiatric Association, Honolulu, Hawaii, May
7-11, 1973.

Dr. Levitz is Associate in Psychology, Department of Psychiatry, University of Pennsylvania, Philadelphia, Pa. 19174. Dr. Stunkard is Professor and Chairman, Department of Psychiatry, Stanford University
School of Medicine, Stanford, Calif. 94305.

This work was supported in part by Public Health Service grant MH
15383 from the National Institute of Mental Health.

cation of behavior modification.

We asked ourselves four questions:

1. Can behavior modification be used in self-help
groups for the obese?

2. If so, can it produce greater weight loss and/or
lower attrition rates than other treatment approaches?

3. Can self-help group leaders who are given special
training carry out a behavior modification program as
successfully as professional therapists?

4. Are there any predictors of treatment success?

METHOD

TOPS (Take Off Pounds Sensibly) is a 25-year-old
self-help organization for the obese. It has 320,000 members in more than 12,000 chapters nationwide; most are
women. The 16 chapters in our study were selected from
21 chapters in the Philadelphia area whose weight reduction records we had monitored for the previous four
years. Two of the other five chapters had disbanded, two
had fewer than six members, and one chapter declined to
participate.

At the beginning of the study the 16 chapters had 318
members. We deleted from data analysis the records of
20 members who were less than ten percent above their
ideal weight; they had already reached their ideal weight
or had joined TOPS in order to lose only a small amount
of weight. Sixty-four members joined TOPS between the
time the study was announced and its start. Interviews revealed that knowledge of the impending study influenced
at least some of these persons to join TOPS. Accordingly, we analyzed the data from this group separately.
The main sample thus consisted of 234 subjects.

Each of the 16 chapters was assigned to one of four
treatment conditions, with four chapters in each condi-

TABLE 1
Subjects' Characteristics at the Start of Treatment

Condition	Number of Subjects	Current Weight (lb.) Mean ± S.D.	Percent Overweight Mean ± S.D.	Previous Weight Loss (lb.) Mean ±S.D.	Age (Years) Mean ± S.D.	Length of Membership (Months) Mean ± S.D.
Professional behavior modification	73	180.80 ± 15.03	40.4 ± 23.8	10.80 ± 8.76	45.6 ± 10.6	38.2 ± 27.6
Chapter leaders						
Behavior modification	54	181.31 ± 11.27	44.5 ± 19.0	11.00 ± 9.95	48.7 ± 8.7	37.9 ± 20.5
Nutrition education	55	180.40 ± 14.42	42.5 ± 25.1	11.79 ± 11.95	43.3 ± 14.8	35.3 ± 27.4
TOPS control	52	177.50 ± 15.71	42.0 ± 22.1	11.31 ± 9.50	45.1 ± 11.6	33.6 ± 24.9

tion. Active treatment lasted 12 weeks.

Behavior Modification Conducted by a Professional Therapist

Three psychiatric residents and one graduate student in clinical psychology, all men, conducted these groups. At each weekly chapter meeting the therapist introduced two or three behavior modification techniques. Group members were asked to keep detailed records of their food intake. Each time a subject ate, she was asked to record the time, place, and duration of eating; the type, amount, and caloric value of the food consumed; and any associated emotions. At each meeting the therapist taught techniques designed to change any problem habits identified from the food intake records. Among the techniques, which are described more fully elsewhere (2), were: 1) introducing changes in the act of eating, including slowing down the pace and leaving food at the end of a meal; 2) developing control over the stimuli signaling eating, including learning to eat at specific times and in a very limited number of places and removing excess food from the environment; 3) planning food intake well in advance of eating; 4) responding to boredom, fatigue, and emotional states with activities that do not involve eating; and 5) instituting group and individual rewards for behavior change and weight loss. In addition, a special effort was made to help subjects increase physical activity in their daily lives.

Behavior Modification by the TOPS Chapter Leaders

After two preliminary training sessions, each leader and coleader attended 12 weekly training sessions conducted by the investigators. Concurrently, the leaders introduced the previously described behavior modification program to their members at the weekly chapter meetings.

Nutrition Training

TOPS leaders also attended a training program scheduled precisely as above. They were taught general principles of nutrition and in turn taught these principles to their members. The program was designed to control for nonspecific training and therapeutic effects. Attendance and weight records in each of these experimental condi-

tions were given to the investigators each week.

Control Group

In the fourth condition the usual TOPS program was continued. This program, which has been described extensively elsewhere (3), includes a weigh-in, an announcement of weight gains and losses, rewards and sometimes punishments, group singing, and a general discussion of weight-related topics. Each week the chapters' attendance and weight records were mailed to the investigators. Aside from this data collection, the four chapters in this condition had no contact with the investigators and received no information from them.

Following the 12-week active treatment period, the therapist visits and training sessions were discontinued. For the nine-month follow-up period, leaders mailed weekly records of attendance and weights to the investigators.

The homogeneity of TOPS membership made it possible to match the subjects in the different experimental conditions very closely. Table 1 shows the remarkable match in age, current weight, percent overweight, length of membership in TOPS, and previous weight loss in TOPS. The average subject was a 45-year-old woman who had been a member of TOPS for three years and who had lost 5.0 kg. (11 lb.) during her membership. She currently weighed 81.6 kg. (180 lb.), 42 percent above her ideal weight.

RESULTS

Attrition rate

The first major therapeutic problem in obesity is the number of patients who drop out of treatment; attrition rates ranging from 20 percent to as high as 80 percent are reported (4, 5). Figure 1 presents the attrition rates of each experimental condition during the active-treatment and follow-up periods.

During the three months of active treatment fewer TOPS members dropped out of the two behavior modification groups than out of the nutrition education and control groups. At 12 months this difference had become striking. Only 38 and 41 percent had dropped out of the

FIGURE 1
Rates of Attrition in the Four Treatment Groups

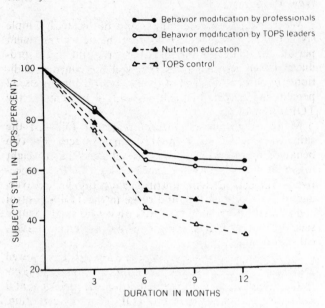

TABLE 2
Mean Weight Change During 12-Week Treatment Period

	Loss or Gain	
Condition	Pounds (Mean ± S.D.)	Kilograms (Mean)
Professional behavior modification	-4.24 ± 2.47	-1.92
Chapter leaders		
Behavior modification	-1.90 ± 1.88	-0.06
Nutrition education	-0.25 ± 1.83	-0.11
TOPS control	+0.71 ± 1.89	+0.32

FIGURE 2
Mean Weight Change During Treatment and Follow-Up

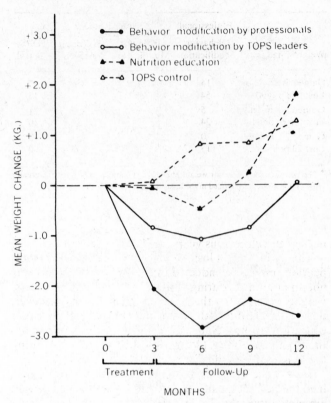

behavior modification groups, compared with 55 and 67 percent for the nutrition education and control groups respectively ($\chi^2 = 12.35$, $p < .01$).

Weight Loss During Treatment

What happened to the subjects who remained in treatment? It must be remembered that their lower dropout rates seriously bias the results against the behavior modification groups. Previous work has shown that poor weight-losers drop out at a more rapid rate than do those who lose greater amounts (1). Decreasing the attrition rates thus means retaining the less successful members.

Despite this bias, groups using behavior modification lost significantly more weight than those in the control conditions (F = 10.7, $p < .001$). The chapters in which behavior modification was introduced by a professional therapist lost a mean of 1.92 kg. (4.2 lb.), significantly more ($p < .001$) than the weight loss in both the nutrition education condition (0.11 kg. or 0.2 lb.) and the

TOPS control condition, in which subjects actually gained 0.32 kg. (0.7 lb.). Chapters in which behavior modification was introduced by professionals lost significantly more weight ($p < .05$) than those taught the same program by the TOPS chapter leaders (0.86 kg. [1.9 lb.]).

Consider now the three conditions in which leadership was provided by the TOPS chapter leaders. The behavior modification program produced significantly greater weight loss ($p < .05$) than did the continuation of the usual TOPS program. The difference between the behavior modification and nutrition education programs was not statistically significant, although the results favored the behavior modification program. The two control conditions did not differ significantly from each other.

Behavior modification thus kept more persons in TOPS during and after treatment. It also produced greater weight losses, despite the bias against weight loss produced by the lower attrition rates.

Weight Loss During Follow-Up

Figure 2 shows the mean weight changes of subjects who stayed in each experimental condition for 12 months. Subjects in the behavior modification groups led by professionals not only maintained their higher weight loss for one year but even increased it slightly. This final mean weight loss of 2.63 kg. (5.8 lb.) was significantly higher ($p < .001$) than that of any of the other conditions. It also represented half the weight lost by these subjects

TABLE 3
*Weight Change at the End of One Year, Given in Percents**

Weight Change	Professional Behavior Modification	Chapter Leaders Behavior Modification	Nutrition Education	TOPS Control
Gained five pounds	15	21	46	37
Lost five pounds	54	24	15	17
Gained ten pounds	5	6	23	21
Lost ten pounds	24	9	8	10
Gained 20 pounds	0	0	8	0
Lost 20 pounds	15	0	0	0

* The percents given here for weight changes are cumulative, in that the greater losses and gains are included in the lesser categories above them.

in their three previous years in TOPS.

The initial weight loss of subjects in the behavior modification program conducted by TOPS group leaders was not maintained during follow-up, and the subjects' weights returned to their pretreatment levels. However, these subjects did better than the control and nutrition education groups. Subjects in these two conditions actually gained 1.27 kg. (2.8 lb.) and 1.81 kg. (4.0 lb.) during the follow-up period.

In addition to the mean weight changes, we also examined the percentage of subjects gaining and losing certain amounts of weight. Table 3 shows the percentage of subjects in each experimental condition who attained three levels of weight change at the end of 12 months. The two behavior modification programs produced significantly greater rates of weight loss, and significantly lower rates of weight gain, at three criterion levels: 2.3 kg. (5 lb.) (x^2 = 39.69, p < .001), 4.5 kg. (10 lb.) (x^2 = 12.85, p < .05), and 9.1 kg. (20 lb.) (x^2 = 18.38, p < .01). In the professional-led behavior modification program, over 50 percent of the subjects lost more than five pounds, while only 15 percent gained that much weight. By contrast, in the TOPS control condition, 37 percent *gained* more than five pounds while only 17 percent of the subjects lost that amount of weight. Behavior modification by TOPS leaders was similar to the nutrition education condition in its rate of weight loss, but resulted in a far lower rate of weight gain.

A 9.1 kg. (20 lb.) criterion has often been used as a single measure of effectiveness. Only subjects in the professional-led behavior modification program achieved this degree of weight loss. The subjects who lost more than 9.1 kg. shared a striking similarity: all eight had been members of TOPS for more than two years and, during that time, all had gained weight! This criterion seemed an effective predictor of success in treatment. The mean weight loss of all subjects who met it was 8.35 kg. (18.4 lb.), and 88 percent of them lost more than 9.1 kg. These results contrast dramatically with the seven subjects who had been in TOPS for the same length of time but who had *lost* weight during that time. None of these lost more than 9.1 kg. and their mean weight loss was

only 0.54 kg. (1.2 lb.).

New Members

We analyzed separately the results of the small sample (N = 64) of new members. During the active treatment period the behavior modification program again produced lower attrition rates than did the control conditions: 11 percent for each of the behavioral conditions, 32 percent for nutrition education, and 20 percent for the TOPS control.

Mean weight losses during treatment followed the same pattern as that of longer-term members. The two behavior modification conditions achieved mean weight losses of 4.54 kg. (10 lb.) and 3.46 kg. (7.6 lb.) respectively. Subjects receiving nutrition education lost an average of 3.23 kg. (7.1 lb.), and those in the TOPS control condition 1.36 kg. (3.0 lb.). Because of the small sample size, differences among the groups did not reach statistical significance.

During the follow-up period, the dropout rates showed a different pattern from those of old members. Subjects in the three active treatment conditions dropped out at a *higher* rate than those in the TOPS control condition. Three months after termination of treatment, the attrition rates in the behavior modification conditions were 57 and 58 percent; in the nutrition education condition it was 52 percent. By contrast, the TOPS control showed a dropout rate of only 27 percent. At one year, 78 and 89 percent dropped out of the behavior modification groups, 73 percent out of the nutrition education condition, but only 53 percent from the TOPS control groups. Because of the small initial sample and the extremely high dropout rates in the active treatment conditions, not enough subjects remained in the treatment groups at one year to permit a comparison of final mean weight loss.

COMMENTS

The introduction of behavior modification techniques substantially improved the effectiveness of patient self-help groups on two interacting and critical measures of success. The program resulted in far lower dropout rates and in greater weight losses for those who remained in treatment, both during the treatment period and at follow-up.

The overall ineffectiveness of self-help groups for the obese was recently demonstrated in a two-year study of 485 TOPS members (1). Attrition rates were 47 percent in one year and 70 percent in two. Furthermore, attrition was not a result of successful weight reduction; members who dropped out were those who had lost less weight: "Although a small percentage of persons joining TOPS are able to lose substantial amounts of weight and to maintain the weight loss, for the vast majority of members, TOPS is a relatively ineffective method of weight control." The present investigation reaffirmed this conclusion; the four TOPS chapters that served as controls *gained* weight during the year of study.

The behavior modification program helped TOPS

members to lose weight. But the amount of weight lost was less than in other studies using similar treatment techniques (6–8). At least four factors may account for this difference.

1. TOPS members are older, less well-educated, and of lower socioeconomic status than were the subjects of previous behavior modification programs. Each of these factors may unfavorably influence the effectiveness of behavior modification.

2. The TOPS subjects had already lost weight (mean = 5.0 kg.), whereas other behavior modification studies used subjects new to treatment. A high percentage of obese persons lose weight at the outset of *any* weight reduction program.

3. Members who had reached or approximated their ideal weight before intervention were excluded from the data analysis. We thus started with a sample selected for their inability to lose weight.

4. Probably most important, each TOPS group was considerably larger than those in earlier studies, which had rarely exceeded eight members. By contrast, our chapters averaged 19 members. This larger size made it impossible to individualize treatment for each member.

In addition to these theoretical reasons, a recent study provides further empirical evidence that the performance of TOPS members is poorer than that of the subjects in earlier behavior modification research. A behavior modification program of individualized treatment for a small selected sample of TOPS members produced dropout rates and weight losses quite similar to ours (9).

Professional therapists achieved significantly greater weight losses in their subjects than TOPS chapter leaders, even though both used the same behavioral program. Equally important, subjects in the professional-led (but not TOPS leader-led) groups maintained their weight loss after the end of treatment. In one year, these subjects increased by one-half the weight loss they had attained in three previous years of TOPS membership. Moreover, only in the professional-led groups were there members who lost as much as 20 pounds.

We believe this is the clearest demonstration to date of the greater effectiveness of professional over non-professional therapeutic intervention. We have earlier shown that it is possible for a nonprofessional, carefully selected for successful weight reduction and leadership qualities, to promote substantial weight losses in a behavior modification group (10). But within the context of TOPS, a professional therapist was able to produce greater weight losses than were the TOPS group leaders using any of a variety of treatment approaches.

Neither investigators of obesity nor investigators of behavior modification have been able to predict an individual's response to treatment. The identification of even a small group who can predictably lose weight is thus of considerable theoretical importance. Further, the favorable response of persons whose motivation, unreinforced by weight loss, was high enough to stay in TOPS for two years is of practical importance. TOPS may be particularly useful in screening large numbers of obese persons to identify those with a good prognosis for weight loss. This would permit the more effective deployment of limited professional treatment resources.

REFERENCES

1. Garb J, Stunkard A: A further assessment of the effectiveness of TOPS in the control of obesity, in Proceedings of the Fogarty International Center Conference on Obesity. Edited by Bray G. Washington, DC, US Government Printing Office (in press)
2. Stuart RB, Davis B: Slim Chance in a Fat World: Behavioral Control of Obesity. Champaign, Ill, Research Press, 1972
3. Stunkard A, Levine H, Fox S: The management of obesity: patient self-help and medical treatment. Arch Intern Med 125:1067–1072, 1970
4. Stunkard A, McLaren-Hume M: The results of treatment of obesity. Arch Intern Med 103:79–85, 1959
5. Seaton DA, Rose K: Defaulters from a weight reduction clinic. J Chronic Dis 18:1007–1011, 1965
6. Stuart RB: Behavioral control of overeating. Behav Res Ther 5:357–365, 1967
7. Penick SB, Filion R, Fox S, et al: Behavior modification in the treatment of obesity. Psychosom Med 33:49–55, 1971
8. Stunkard AJ: New therapies for the eating disorders: behavior modification of obesity and anorexia nervosa. Arch Gen Psychiatry 26:391–398, 1972
9. Hall SM: Self-control and therapist control in the behavioral treatment of overweight women. Behav Res Ther 10:59–68, 1972
10. Jordan HA, Levitz LS: Behavior modification in a self-help group. J Am Diet Assoc 62:27–29, 1973

Overeaters Anonymous—
Report on a Self-help Group

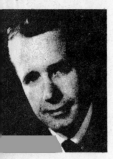

Peter G. Lindner, M.D.

Nothing is more frustrating in a bariatric practice than trying to help an obese patient who will not cooperate. Yet, the very fact that he has consulted a physician indicates that, at least on a subconscious level, he is willing to accept help, even though on a conscious level, he may try to undermine therapy.

Since our primary motive is the well-being of the patient, it behooves us to investigate all avenues which may benefit him. Consequently, I was pleased to be invited, as a representative of the American Society of Bariatric Physicians, to attend annual conventions of Overeaters Anonymous for the past two years. Since then, I have attended a local group meeting and on two separate occasions, have observed members of this group eating.

The Organization

Overeaters Anonymous (OA) is a nonprofit, self-help organization which is patterned after Alcoholics Anonymous (AA). It was founded approximately 14 years ago in Los Angeles and now has over 800 groups throughout the world, with more than 400 located in California.

OA's basic concept is that compulsive overeating is a

Address reprint requests to: 12132 Garfield Ave., South Gate, California 90280.

The author

Peter G. Lindner, M.D., practices bariatric medicine in South Gate, California. He is a member of the American Society of Bariatric Physicians and a diplomate of the American Board of Bariatric Medicine. Dr. Lindner is also a member of the editorial advisory board for *Obesity & Bariatric Medicine*.

disease which affects the person on three levels—physical, spiritual, and emotional. Members of OA feel that, like alcoholics, they are unable to control their compulsion permanently by unaided willpower.

The Members

Most individuals who join OA have completely lost faith in life and in themselves. The hand of understanding and strength which is extended by those who have suffered the same compulsion, and who are now examples that there is an answer, probably explains OA's success with the "hopeless" obese person who has repeatedly failed with the usual methods of weight control. Extreme friendliness and even love between members is easily observable at meetings.

Although the disciplines of the program are very strict, there is no coercion. Greater reliance is placed on the individual's wish to adhere. The spirit of cooperation is positively reinforced throughout meeting proceedings.

Brief talks, given before the group by individuals telling their experiences, seem to be one of the strongest motivating forces. When they recall their former complete hopelessness, feelings of futility and inadequacy, and then tell how they overcame these feelings by following OA precepts, they make a very dramatic and lasting impression on newcomers. The impact of this must be seen and experienced to appreciate its powerful influence on all those present. There are frequent spontaneous outbursts of applause to indicate approbation of the group. Once the individual can abstain from compulsive eating, he helps to maintain his recovery "one day at a time" by sponsoring others.

There are no dues or fees for OA membership, although they do pass the basket at meetings in order to fund local and world services. Each local group is self-supporting through their own contributions and they do not accept outside financial assistance.

Many OA members are former participants (and

dropouts) from commercial weight control groups. I observed a number of individuals who had been unsuccessful in the commercial organizations, but who had reached and maintained normal weight for a number of years after having joined OA. On being asked why they switched organizations, they were quick to inform me that the continual preparation of "free foods" and general preoccupation with food, as sometimes expounded, only kept their food compulsion alive.

The Program

Two types of dietary programs are offered. One is a low carbohydrate diet consisting of three regular meals a day with only sugar-free drinks between meals. The diet allows no refined sugars or starches, and no foods high in natural carbohydrates. All foods are weighed and measured. Protein allowances are usually four ounces per portion. Vegetable and fresh fruit portions are either one-half or one cup, depending on carbohydrate content. The other program is an alternate eating plan founded on the basic four food groups. Variations are perfectly acceptable, as in the case of patients with hypoglycemia. Most important, from the physician's standpoint, is that the "see your doctor" rule is adhered to. Eating slowly, taking small bites, eating meals sitting down, no second helpings at meals, no skipping of meals, and weighing only once monthly are also part of the plan. The admonition, "Call (your food sponsor) *BEFORE* you take your first bite" is also a prominent aspect of the program.

Personal—The 12 Steps

AA's 12 steps of recovery have been adapted to the compulsive eater and provide a means for members to grow spiritually and emotionally so that they do not need or want excess food (See Table 1).

Essentially five tools are used in OA's recovery program.
1) Abstinence from compulsive overeating. This requires adherence to the dietary program.
2) Sponsorship. When a newcomer enters the group, he asks someone to be his food sponsor. A qualified sponsor has established recovery from compulsive overeating and has maintained his own current state of abstinence, having been led through the steps of the recovery program by another qualified person.
3) Telephone calls. They are the lifeline between meetings and are the method of daily contact among members—particularly between sponsor and newcomer.
4) Anonymity. It is the spiritual foundation of the fellowship. What is said in the meeting room remains there. Anonymity is never to be broken at the level of press, radio, or television, and the individual who is still overeating is urged not to break his anonymity so as not to hurt the reputation of OA.
5) Printed materials. Literature is for sale at cost after meetings. Various sheets and pamphlets are distributed free of charge. Purchase and study of AA books is encouraged.
"Food" and "Compulsive Overeaters" are substituted for

Table 1: The Twelve Steps

1. We admitted we were powerless over food—that our lives had become unmanageable.

2. Came to believe that a Power greater than ourselves could restore us to sanity.

3. Made a decision to turn our will and our lives over to the care of God *as we understood Him.*

4. Made a searching and fearless moral inventory of ourselves.

5. Admitted to God, to ourselves and to another human being the exact nature of our wrongs.

6. Were entirely ready to have God remove all these defects of character.

7. Humbly asked Him to remove our shortcomings.

8. Made a list of all persons we had harmed, and became willing to make amends to them all.

9. Made direct amends to such people wherever possible, except when to do so would injure them or others.

10. Continued to take personal inventory and when we were wrong, promptly admitted it.

11. Sought through prayer and meditation to improve our conscious contact with God *as we understood Him,* praying only for knowledge of His will for us and the power to carry that out.

12. Having had a spiritual awakening as the result of these steps, we tried to carry this message to compulsive overeaters and to practice these principles in all our affairs.

the words "Alcohol" and "Alcoholics" and the identic principles of recovery are applied to the overeate problems.

Underlying Concepts

1) *A Power greater than ourselves.* When a compulsi overeater realizes that he cannot control his eating behavic he needs to accept and depend upon another Power— Power acknowledged to be greater than himself. T interpretation of this Power is left to the individual. M members of OA, of course, adopt the concept of God. But newcomer is merely asked to keep an open mind on th subject and, usually, he finds it is not too difficult to wo out a solution to this very personal problem, even if he is atheist or agnostic.

Psychologically, the obese individual is to attain a sen of reality and nearness of a greater Power which replaces egocentric nature. Then his point of view and outlook w take on a spiritual coloring. Hence, he no longer needs maintain his defiant individuality, but can live in peace a

rmony with his environment, sharing and participating
ely, especially with other members of the group. This is a
eat therapeutic weapon that we physicians need to fully
preciate. The obese individual no longer defies, but
cepts help, guidance, and control from the outside. As he
inquishes his negative, aggressive feelings towards himself
d towards life, he finds himself overwhelmed by positive
elings of love, friendliness, tranquility, and a pervading
ntentment. These latter feelings were evident among the
oups that I attended.

Surrender. A word frequently heard in OA groups, it can
st be described as "letting go." The individual gives up his
idities, he relaxes and admits that he is "licked" by his
mpulsive eating habit. The source of this feeling is almost
ways despair, which is so prevalent in newcomers to the
oup. It is all part of a crisis experience with an overload of
pelessness. When the individual surrenders, he is not just
ing up. He accepts a Power greater than himself, reduces
own ego, and admits the need for outside help. The "ego
duction" can be very profitable to the personality makeup
this individual.

It is important to differentiate between submission and
rrender. In submission, an individual accepts reality
nsciously, but not subconsciously. He accepts that he
nnot, at the moment, conquer reality but lurking in his
bconscious, is the feeling that "there will come a day when
vill be able to handle my problem on my own." Submission
plies no real acceptance of one's own inadequacy and
monstrates conclusively that the struggle is still going on.
bmission is, at best, a superficial yielding, with the inner
sions still present. When the individual accepts, on a
bconscious level, the reality of not being able to handle the
mpulsive overeating, there is no residual battle. Relaxation
sues with a freedom from strain and conflict. This freedom
the aim of the OA groups and complete surrender is
nifested by the considerable degree of relaxation which is
dent in the behavior of those who have achieved it.

Once he surrenders at the subconscious level, his
mpliance with the disciplines of the program should not
sen with time and lead to the inevitable regaining of
ight. He continues to get messages from his subconscious
it the need for outside help will remain for a prolonged, if
t indefinite, period. His wholehearted cooperation is then
thcoming and constructive action takes the place of skin-
ep assurances that he will merely "comply" temporarily
til the memory of his suffering and self-pity weakens and
need for compliance lessens. Surrender, then, is a
bconscious event. It is not willed by the patient. It can
cur only when he becomes involved with his subconscious
nd in a set of circumstances which signal the undeniable
ed for an external greater Power. The definition of
rrender can be understood only when all its subconscious
nifications and true inner meaning are glimpsed.
inically it is manifested by an inner calm and "live and let
e" attitude.

ganizational—The 12 Traditions

ain patterned after AA, the organization is guided by the
traditions (Table II).
Basically, there are three predominant concepts: unity,

Table 2: The Twelve Traditions

1. Our common welfare should come first; personal recovery depends upon O.A. unity.

2. For our group purpose there is but one ultimate authority—a loving God as He may express Himself in our group conscience. Our leaders are but trusted servants; they do not govern.

3. The only requirement for O.A. membership is a desire to stop eating compulsively.

4. Each group should be autonomous except in matters affecting other groups or O.A. as a whole.

5. Each group has but one primary purpose—to carry its message to the compulsive overeater who still suffers.

6. An O.A. group ought never endorse, finance or lend the O.A. name to any related facility or outside enterprise, lest problems of money, property and prestige divert us from our primary purpose.

7. Every O.A. group ought to be fully self-supporting, declining outside contributions.

8. Overeaters Anonymous should remain forever non-professional, but our service centers may employ special workers.

9. O.A., as such, ought never be organized; but we may create service boards or committees directly responsible to those they serve.

10. Overeaters Anonymous has no opinion on outside issues; hence the O.A. name ought never be drawn into public controversy.

11. Our public relations policy is based on attraction rather than promotion; we need always maintain personal anonymity at the level of press, radio, films, television, and other public media of communication.

12. Anonymity is the spiritual foundation of all these traditions, ever reminding us to place principles before personalities.

group autonomy, and personal anonymity. Anonymity is
vital because, by its practice, members are assured that self-
glorification will not be the undoing of the OA fellowship. It
also guarantees the newcomer that his confidences will not
be revealed. In other words, principles are placed before
personalities. There is evidence of a pervading sense of
humility among the majority of members. The individual
gives up personal distinction for the common good and thus
preserves the unity of OA. The 12 traditions represent to the
groups what the 12 steps represent to the individual, and
observance of the principles helps to insure the survival and
growth of the groups which comprise OA.

A Hypothesis of OA's Mechanism

In analyzing this group, I have reached a number of
conclusions. There appears to be a deep shift in the

individual's emotional tone, the disappearance of one set of feelings, and the emergence of a very different set. The member moves from a negative state of mind to a positive one. This may have the earmarks of a spiritual conversion. Be that as it may, it is an effective transformation and essential for long-term success. By this I do not mean to imply that there are never any slipups. Indeed, there are. But, they are usually due to the overconfidence of the individual as he becomes successful in the program. He once again becomes too preoccupied with himself. As long as he attends the group meetings, help is immediately available which inspires him to return to practicing the 12 steps of recovery. Associating with others who suffer in a similar manner brings hope to the overeater. He is neither judged, laughed at because of his size, nor scolded. There are no "weigh-ins." He can share his past experiences, his present problems, and his hopes for the future with those who understand and support him and who speak his own language. Working with a sponsor, he converses with a person who has "been through it himself," thus the communication between these two is on the same level. When he becomes a sponsor for someone else, his loneliness is particularly aided. He is needed and accepted at last. This has a very potent, positive influence on weight maintenance.

Cooperation not Replacement

OA literature strongly urges that the newcomer visit his doctor to decide upon a plan of eating suited to both physical needs and family habits. I can verify that this was, indeed, the policy with a number of patients whom I have referred to this group.

OA is not concerned with the medical aspects of obesity, but with the compulsive nature of overeating itself; thus, it complements the physician's care.

It is my belief that OA, in certain specific cases, can be of valuable help to the bariatrician. I urge other bariatricians to contact OA. There are chapters throughout the country and a local group should be nearby. OA is willing to help your patients at all times. The empathy and attention patients will receive at meetings during trying times can be of great therapeutic value. In cooperation with the physician, OA can help individuals restore their faith in themselves and in others and give them hope for recovery.

Conclusion

To conclude this report, I quote the "Serenity Prayer" which is invariably heard at OA meetings. It states so well, in a few words, what OA's basic philosophy is:

"God grant me the serenity to accept the things that I cannot change, the courage to change the things that I can, and the wisdom to know the difference."

Both physical activity and food intake are important factors in the treatment of obesity. Obese persons generally are less active than persons of normal weight. They sit more, move less, and perform daily activities (such as standing, bending, walking) less vigorously Fewer muscles are contracted and contractions are slower. In some individuals, these sedentary habits can be changed by instruction and movements can be made more vigorous. This will help to increase energy expenditure.

The main approach to weight loss is reduction of food intake. The diet should entail a deficit of 500 cal daily if a weight loss of 1 lb per week is desired (or 1000 cal daily for a weekly weight loss of 2 lb). Some obese people do not know the caloric values of the foods they eat, and most cannot resist eating food high in calories even if they know its caloric content. All obese subjects must be educated and motivated.

Success in weight reduction depends on the patient's interest and motivation. The physician helps by stressing incentives such as "appearance" or "health and longevity." Seeing the patient frequently is a motivating force in itself, and this probably explains in large part the popularity and success of organizations such as Weight Watchers and TOPS (Take Off Pounds Sensibly). The practice of routine visits to an interested person or group influences the response. One well-controlled double-blind study showed that the presence or absence of group discussions determined the number of patients who would

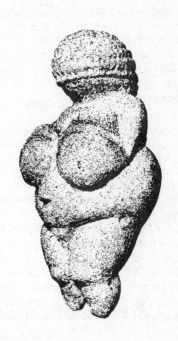

Use of Drugs in the Treatment of Obesity

Only a few of the various drugs used in the treatment of obesity have been shown to be more effective than placebos. Thyroid hormone has little effect on weight loss unless given to very obese, hospitalized patients on a restricted diet. In studies comparing a placebo with an amphetamine and with phentermine, weight loss was greater in the groups of patients receiving the latter agents than in the control groups.

HERBERT GERSHBERG, M.D.
New York University School of Medicine
New York

Table 1. Effects of an Amphetamine and of Phentermine* in Obese Subjects

Weight Loss (Pounds)

Agent	4 Weeks	8 Weeks	12 Weeks	16 Weeks
Placebo	4.8 (42)†	7.0 (38)	8.6 (26)	9.9 (25)
Amphetamine	8.8‡ (42)	13.6‡ (30)	15.5‡ (34)	17.0‡ (31)
Placebo	5.9 (31)	7.6 (28)	9.4 (20)	11.5 (16)
Phentermine	9.1‡ (31)	14.9‡ (26)	18.7‡ (21)	20.3‡ (21)

*Amphetamine: Biphetamine® '20'.
Phentermine: Ionamin® '30'.

†Figures in parentheses are the numbers of subjects.

‡Compared with placebo, p<0.02.

Table 2. Effects of Phentermine* in Obese Diabetics

Weight Loss (Pounds)

Agent	4 Weeks	8 Weeks	12 Weeks	16 Weeks
Placebo	5.6 (9)†	6.8 (6)	8.0 (6)	10.2 (6)
Phentermine	7.3 (6)	12.2‡ (6)	17.0‡ (6)	18.0‡ (6)

*Ionamin '30'.

†Figures in parentheses are the numbers of subjects.

‡Compared with placebo, p<0.02.

continue or who would drop out of a therapeutic program.

Many drugs have been used in attempts to promote weight loss. They include drugs producing anorexia, drugs causing nausea, drugs preventing gastrointestinal absorption, hormones increasing metabolism and lipolysis, tranquilizers and diuretics. None has been shown in properly controlled investigations to be more effective than a placebo when the diet is unrestricted. Thyroid hormone and the amphetamines have been documented to be more effective than a placebo when they are given in conjunction with a low-calorie diet.

Giving thyroid hormone to obese patients has been a common practice for many decades. The aim is to increase basal metabolism and energy output and theoretically to promote lipolysis by potentiating the effect of epinephrine. When it is given to patients in an office, clinic or outpatient setting as 1 to 3 gr of desiccated thyroid or its equivalent daily, it is not more effective than diet alone. Even 9 gr daily does not consistently induce more weight loss than diet alone.

In two situations, thyroid hormone has proved to be helpful. When 15 gr of desiccated thyroid was given daily to starved hospitalized patients, weight loss increased by

Table 3. Metabolic Changes Accompanying Weight Loss in Two Diabetics*

Weight (Pounds)	Blood Glucose (Milligrams per 100 Ml)						Serum Insulin (Microunits per Milliliter)						Serum Lipids (Milligrams per 100 Ml)	
	Minutes						Minutes							
	0	5	10	20	30	60	0	5	10	20	30	60	Cholesterol	Triglycerides
198	200	343	324	297	279	257	13	12	18	14	15	15	344	129
177 (two months)	139	294	252	243	143	195	8	11	10	7	29	12	204	33
161 (four months)	111	270	248	223	210	193	6	5	11	7	6	7	196	36
134	89	208	260	210	185	127	33	122	120	172	123	106	222	138
128 (two months)	92	256	244	200	145	82	21	46	86	72	92	39	190	91
122 (four months)	90	274	266	228	183	87	33	44	50	49	62	54	175	98

*Both patients were taking phentermine (Ionamin '30'). Glucose, 25 gm, was injected over two minutes at time 0, and blood levels of glucose and insulin were measured at the intervals listed.

38 percent. When massively obese (over 240 lb), hospitalized patients were given an 800 cal diet, the addition of 225 mcg of L-triiodothyronine daily induced weight losses of 29 lb in eight weeks and 37 lb in 12 weeks, compared with losses of 17 lb and 23 lb, respectively, with a placebo and diet. It is apparent that thyroid hormone has little effect on weight loss unless it is given to very obese subjects in a hospital and on a restricted diet.

The amphetamines and related sympathomimetic amines have been shown to be useful adjuncts to a restricted diet. They induce anorexia presumably by acting on the satiety centers of the hypothalamus. Their other actions, those of increasing physical activity and stimulating lipolysis, may contribute to their effectiveness, but the extent of these contributions has not yet been carefully measured.

The effectiveness of an amphetamine and of a sympathomimetic amine, phentermine (IONAMIN®), is being evaluated in a careful double-blind, randomized study of nonhospitalized patients.* The diets prescribed for

HERBERT GERSHBERG

Dr. Gershberg is associate professor of clinical medicine, New York University School of Medicine, and attending physician, New York University and Bellevue hospitals, New York.

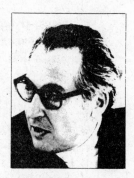

Obesity is common in maturity-onset diabetes, and weight loss is perhaps even more important in this group of patients than in other obese subjects. We have been studying the effect of drugs and diet in inducing weight loss in obese nonhospitalized diabetics given a 1000 cal diet and either a placebo or a drug in a double-blind, randomized fashion. The results, shown in table 2, indicate a significant drug effect. Weight loss is remarkably similar to that obtained in obese nondiabetics with the same drug and with Biphetamine '20', and the differences between the placebo-treated and drug-treated patients

---

Some of the metabolic abnormalities associated with obesity (elevated serum lipids, impaired glucose tolerance) may revert toward normal as weight is lost.

---

these patients provide 60 percent of the calories necessary to maintain ideal body weight. The effectiveness of the drugs as compared with a placebo is shown in table 1. The greater weight loss in the drug-treated group was apparent in four weeks and was maintained for 16 weeks.

*The amphetamine used is BIPHETAMINE® '20', containing 10 mg each of dextroamphetamine and amphetamine. The preparation of phentermine used is Ionamin '30', containing 30 mg phentermine as the cation exchange resin. Dosage of each is 1 capsule daily.

are much the same at eight weeks and at 16 weeks, indicating that obese subjects respond similarly to drugs and diet regardless of the presence or absence of diabetes.

What are the benefits of weight loss? Anesthesia risks increase with obesity. Life insurance statistics show an increase in the death rate from coronary disease and hypertension with increasing obesity. It is hoped that normalization of weight will reduce this higher morbidity and mortality. Some of the metabolic abnormalities associated with obesity (elevated serum lipids, impaired glucose tolerance) may revert toward normal as weight is lost. In overweight individuals, fasting serum insulin levels are elevated and insulin secretion in response to glucose is increased. When weight is lost, insulin levels decrease and glucose tolerance improves, indicating return of insulin sensitivity.

I have seen striking metabolic changes occur with relatively little weight change over a short period. In table 3 are data on two diabetic subjects who were part of the study mentioned previously. The first of these was a man weighing 33 percent more than his ideal body weight. When given a 1000 cal diet, the patient lost 21 lb, or 11 percent of his original weight, in two months. Glucose tolerance improved, insulin level decreased, and elevated serum cholesterol and triglyceride levels decreased. The second subject was a woman with mild diabetes who weighed 20 percent more than her ideal body weight. With a loss of only 5 percent of body weight in two months, she had a decrease in insulin level and in serum cholesterol and triglyceride levels.

The goal of treatment of obesity is to produce a permanent change in eating habits and physical activity, resulting in maintenance of normal weight. This can be accomplished in some individuals. Our efforts should be directed toward increasing the number of successes.

REFERENCES

1. Hollingsworth DR, Amatruda DT Jr, Scheig R: Quantitative and qualitative effects of L-triiodothyronine in massive obesity. Metabolism 19:934, 1970
2. Kalkhoff RK, Kim HJ, Ferrou CA: Metabolic effects of weight loss in obese subjects. Diabetes 20:83, 1971
3. London AM, Schreiber ED: A control study of the effects of group discussions and an anorexiant in outpatient treatment of obesity. Ann Intern Med 65:80, 1966
4. Sims EAH, Goldman RF, Gluck CM, et al: Experimental obesity in man. Trans Assoc Am Physicians 81:153, 1968

JEJUNO-ILEAL SURGERY: WHICH PATIENTS QUALIFY?

HENRY BUCHWALD, M.D., Ph.D.

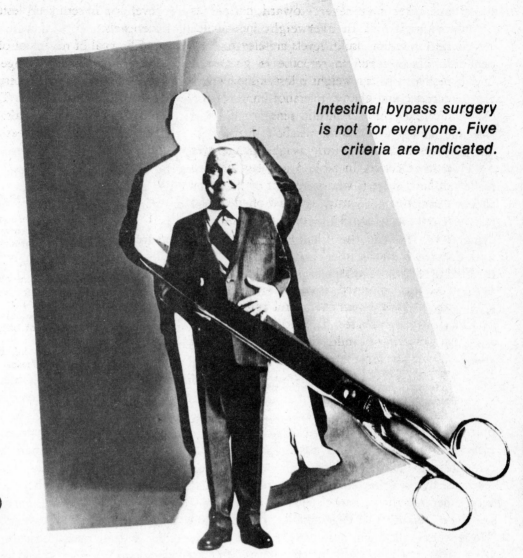

Intestinal bypass surgery is not for everyone. Five criteria are indicated.

In mid-July we performed a jejuno-ileal bypass on a 350-pound man. He was the third obese patient to undergo the procedure at our institution that week, the 188th in our series at the University of Minnesota.

He was neither the heaviest nor the lightest of our jejuno-ileal bypass patients. He was fairly typical —an emotionally stable, intellectually competent patient on whom all non-surgical modes of treatment had failed.

His liver was fatty, his lipids were high and his blood pressure far above normal. His personal life was miserable, his self-image low. He and his physician had tried for more than five years to get his weight under control. We could find no correctable metabolic cause for his obesity.

Only a few hours before the anesthesia was administered we told him that he could call off the surgery with no feelings of guilt whatsoever. "No, go ahead," he said.

His obesity posed a greater risk to his health and life than our surgical procedure and its potential side-effects and complications.

Make no mistake about it. There are considerable risks for the patient in association with the jejuno-ileal bypass for obesity. This is in sharp contrast to the rather minimal risks we have seen to be associated with the far less extensive partial ileal bypass for hyperlipidemia.

Dr. Richard L. Varco and I have made sure in our series that every patient clearly understands the risks. We tell them their chance of dying is two percent, the risk of liver damage is five percent, and the risk of diarrhea 100 percent. We try to have a relative present during the explanation of risks so the patients can be subsequently reminded of the situation they are about to accept.

Second Thoughts

We do about three of these procedures every week. Each week from six to eight patients pass through the initial screening to reach us. By then they are usually very eager for the operation and we try to temper that eagerness. We let them talk to our postoperative patients who are still in the hospital. We enforce a waiting period so they can decline the operation if they have second thoughts.

We are not certain how many patients drop out before reaching us, but some are discouraged when our surgical secretary explains our rather restrictive guidelines. But of those who reach us, 75 percent are accepted for surgery.

Every center involved in intestinal-bypass surgery for obesity has its own admission guidelines. There are, however, many similarities. Ours might serve clinicians as a rough checklist for considering patients for referral to one of the major centers doing this type of bypass.

We consider no one for the procedure unless he or she is:

• More than 100 pounds overweight, based on standard insurance tables.

• Able to document at least five years of effort to lose weight by dietary means, often including experience in group therapy such as TOPS (Take Off Pounds Sensibly), or other such organizations.

• Of sufficient intelligence and emotional stability to understand the implications of the side-effects and the potential complications of this procedure. We use psychiatric consultation to help determine stability.

• Afflicted with no known correctable metabolic or endocrine dysfunction.

• Committed to avoiding all alcoholic beverages for at least two years after the operation. We reject patients who have a history of alcohol abuse or who feel they must have a drink once a day.

Now we would like to mention that there are, of course, a number of different methods of performing the operation.

Our procedure involves the anastomosis of the proximal 40 centimeters of the jejunum, end-to-end, to the distal 4 centimeters of

ileum, with closure of the proximal end of the intervening bypassed bowel and anastomosis of the distal end of the bypassed loop, end-to-side, to the cecum for drainage. Our immediate postoperative morbidity includes a two percent wound infection rate, a seven percent urinary tract infection rate, two percent incidence of pulmonary emboli and a one percent incidence of postoperative pneumonia.

Our procedure, we believe, eliminates the potential for reflux. It also means we do everything in the right lower quadrant so if postoperative problems should develop, we generally know where they are localized.

Similar Procedures

Other, similar procedures have been developed over the years, all following a general principle that bypassing a sufficient length of small intestine can engender an absorptive caloric deficit, bringing about a weight loss.

Early in the development of bypass procedures, Payne and his associates in Los Angeles achieved a rapid and marked weight reduction by bypassing more than 90 percent of the small intestine, the right colon and half the transverse colon, with bowel continuity restored by end-to-side anastomosis of the proximal 15 inches of jejunum to the mid transverse colon. Payne conceived a need for a second operation to restore additional bowel length when ideal weight was obtained.

Subsequently Payne and De-Wind rejected that procedure and changed to the more moderate "14+4" procedure in which the proximal 14 inches of jejunum are anastomosed, end-to-side, to the terminal ileum four inches proximal to the ileocecal valve.

Modifications on the 14+4 jejuno-ileostomy have been advanced in recent years, primarily by converting the end-to-side anastomosis to an obligatory end-to-end restoration of bowel continuity. Salmon and Scott prefer to drain the

passes on 100 pigs. He divided them into five groups of 20 pigs and he is doing a different procedure on each group of 20.

We are testing the pigs for fecal output, fecal water content, B12 absorptive capacity, lipid levels, electrolyte balance, caloric absorption and weight loss. Hopefully we will be able to say in a year or two which procedures offer the best chance of success in the treatment of obesity.

Our patients usually undergo three days of workup before sur-

We also manage prophylactically for electrolyte problems, but some develop hypocalcemia and/or hypokalemia anyway. We have seen symptomatic hypocalcemia with episodes of tetany in three patients. We were unable to control the problem in one with oral supplements so we reoperated and restored two feet of intestine to the functioning bowel.

We do not admit patients to our program if they are unlikely to understand the necessity of returning at regular, frequent intervals for monitoring even though they may feel well. We believe we should continue seeing a patient for at least two years after surgery to watch for complications and side-effects. The patients must understand that they will require B12 injections every six months for life.

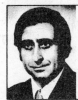

Henry Buchwald, M.D., Ph.D. (*Columbia Univ. College of Physicians and Surgeons, 1957*), *is Associate Professor of Surgery at the Univ. of Minnesota School of Medicine. He also holds a Ph.D. in Surgery from the Univ. of Minnesota and is a Fellow of the American College of Surgeons.*

bypassed segment more distally to the colon than we have. Scott recently advocated end-to-end anastomosis, preserving essentially identical 20 centimeter portions of the jejunum and ileum.

Scott's procedure incorporates more ileum into the functioning small intestine. This would be expected to increase the absorption of bile salts, reducing the cathartic effect of the salts on the colon. He and his associates also feel that Vitamin B12 supplementation will not be necessary if 20 centimeters of the distal ileum is preserved.

We are not certain which bypass procedure is superior, but we hope to find out. Dr. John Coyle, one of our surgical residents, has started a series of intestinal by-

gery and are discharged six days postoperatively. In nearly all patients the long-term side-effects consist of diarrhea, possible electrolyte imbalance and impaired B12 absorption, all of which usually respond to treatment.

Diarrhea is the problem which patients find most annoying. We treat for it prophylactically with Lomotil and calcium carbonate. Nearly all refractory diarrhea can be regulated by restricting the patients' diets to cottage cheese, cheddar cheese, skim milk, peanut butter and bananas for a few days. If this doesn't work, we use judicious doses of paregoric or Librax. If the diarrhea is intolerable to the patient, bowel continuity may have to be restored.

Liver Biopsy

They return two weeks immediately postoperatively, then every six weeks for six months, then every six months. They enter the hospital for a complete status evaluation and percutaneous liver biopsy at one year.

We stress that they include large amounts of protein, some carbohydrate and limited fats in their diets, not for weight reduction but for the same reason we outlaw all alcoholic beverages—to protect the liver as much as possible. The protein can also alleviate the self-limited problem of hair loss which occurs, albeit infrequently, in some of our patients.

The liver is an important problem. Three-fourths of our obese patients arrive with fatty livers. The rapid weight loss sometimes makes matters worse. It may be a year or two until the liver situation turns around and improvement can be noted. In less than five percent of the patients, liver decompensation can be progressive and it may be necessary to intervene and reestablish bowel continuity.

We have dwelled long enough, we believe, on the negative aspects of the bypass, long enough to make it clear that we don't think surgery is the answer for every obese patient. Intelligence, mental and emotional stability, determination and a willingness to follow directions and tolerate the discomfort are imperative.

From the literature, it appears that the jejuno-colic bypass results in an average weight loss of 41 percent, and the jejuno-ileal bypass an average weight loss of 35 percent. Salmon reported that two-thirds of his patients were within 20 pounds of ideal weight one to three years after surgery.

In our series of end-to-end bypass procedures, all patients have lost weight, 90 percent to within 50 pounds of their ideal weight within two years. The mean weight loss has been 33 percent below the preoperative baseline. A 500-pound individual loses more than a 250-pounder, of course.

The major weight loss occurs during the first year. A plateau is reached between the second and third year when the patient levels off, usually on the somewhat chubby side. Any further weight loss must be achieved by dietary means.

All of our patients have had a marked reduction in serum cholesterol and serum triglycerides, even those whose lipids were low prior to surgery. The average drop in lipid levels ranged from 40 to 50 percent.

Seventy-five percent of our patients were hypertensive, with a systolic blood pressure greater than 140 mm Hg or a diastolic above 90 mm Hg. Nearly all had significant blood pressure reductions after bypass and many became normotensive.

Eight percent of our patients arrived with adult-onset diabetes. With weight loss, their insulin requirements diminished and we were able to convert some of them to dietary control.

There has been a definite lessening of symptomatic extremity varicosities after substantial weight

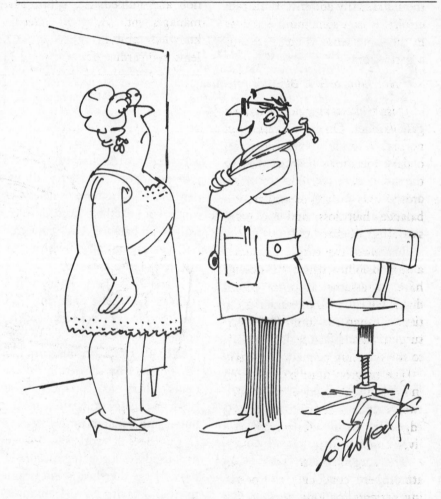

"The three squares a day I'm referring to are crackers."

loss. Four of our patients obtained relief from symptomatic spine and knee pathology.

Improved life-expectancy of these patients has been documented. It is logical to assume that the reversal or mitigation of obesity, hypertension, hyperlipidemia and overt diabetes is likely to prolong life.

We are often asked who should be performing intestinal bypass surgery.

We do not think a surgeon should casually add this to his repertoire. It isn't something one does in the same sense as one performs a gastrectomy.

Not Like a Gall Bladder

It isn't like taking out a diseased gall bladder. One is operating on normal intestines to achieve a secondary metabolic change, placing on the patient the potential hazards of liver failure, electrolyte imbalance, hair loss, and the main side-effect of diarrhea.

Therefore the surgeon assumes a responsibility which he doesn't have to assume in other procedures. He can't simply take the patient through the immediate post-surgical period and send him back to the referring primary physician.

The surgeon must be interested in following the patient for at least two years and he must be knowledgeable about electrolytes and liver abnormalities.

The surgeon must work in an atmosphere conducive to following patients for long periods. We doubt that a surgeon who moves from hospital to hospital, with no fixed focal point, can provide the necessary follow-up.

He must also be in an environment where excellent assistance is available. Postoperative care is almost comparable to that needed for an open heart surgery patient. Skilled assistants must be available to see the patient night and day.

The surgeon also needs a good anesthesiology department, especially for the preoperative evaluation and immediate postoperative management. A good internist knowledgeable in metabolic problems and cardiac disease should be available. The surgeon should have a relationship with a psychiatrist who has experience in dealing with obese patients and their problems. One also needs a radiology staff capable of dealing with the difficult arteriography sometimes required for these patients.

It would be risky, we think, for a surgeon or institution to perform intestinal bypass surgery on a now-and-then basis. To minimize postoperative complications it is necessary to have an experienced staff cognizant of warning signals and capable of averting hazards. A staff will not become experienced with an occasional case.   END

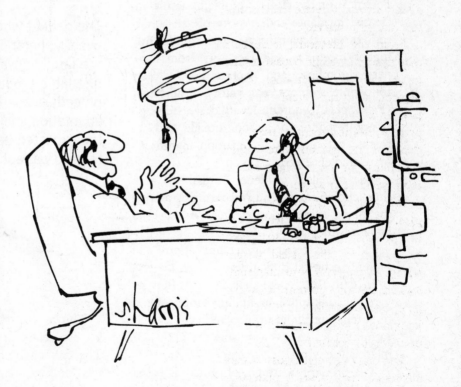

"But you can't sue me for malpractice. I'm not a doctor!"

A century or two ago obesity was a status symbol—a visible sign of affluence—and proof of a well-functioning digestive tract. Today obesity is considered a form of malnutrition caused by an imbalance in the intake and expenditure of calories. Estimates are that 30% of the people in the United States are 20% or more overweight. In more than 99% of cases, obesity is caused by overeating, induced by psychologic, social, and perhaps ethnic factors; only rarely is it caused by endocrine dysfunction.

Whatever the cause may be, obesity of significant proportions presents a complex of clinical, socioeconomic, and psychologic problems to the patient and to his physician. Foremost of the clinical problems is the increased incidence and severity of arteriosclerotic cardiovascular disease, with significantly higher morbidity and mortality from coronary thrombosis and hypertension. Closely following is chronic respiratory insufficiency (Pickwickian syndrome), with decreased respiratory response to carbon dioxide and increased carbon dioxide retention manifested by somnolence and lassitude.

The increased incidence of diabetes mellitus, cholelithiasis, and osteoarthritis among the obese is well documented. As surgical patients, they carry a high risk of cardiovascular and respiratory complications and present technical difficulties.

In daily life, obese persons are often severely handicapped in finding employment, in purchasing life insurance, and even in performing routine tasks at work, at home, or in social activities.

The primary treatment of obesity is based on a comprehensive program of restricted caloric intake, exercise, and medication linked together with psychologic motivation and support.[1] Unfortunately, results are often poor and the recurrence rate is higher than in many forms of cancer. In extreme cases of obesity, surgery may be used as a last resort.

Intestinal Bypass Operation for Massive Obesity

The patient who has had an intestinal bypass operation may seek help from the family physician for a related or unrelated problem. Knowledge of the procedure itself, the postoperative adaptation and clinical problems, and the expected benefits are essential to good patient care.

JEROME E. BLEICHER, MD
MIECZYSLAW CEGIELSKI, MD
JOSE A. SAPORTA, MD
Creighton University School of Medicine
Omaha

This article describes our experience with 50 consecutive intestinal bypass operations. The first operation was done in 1970, and the longest follow-up period among this group has been more than three years.

Surgical Criteria

The criteria used to select patients for intestinal bypass surgery are as follows:

1. Obesity of massive degree—at least double the ideal weight for height, age, and sex—and of at least five years' duration.

Figure 1. Intestinal bypass operation for obesity reduces digesting and absorbing surface of jejunum and ileum by about 90%. Bypassed small intestine is closed at proximal end.

a. Procedure of Payne and DeWind:[2] End-to-side anastomosis between proximal 14 inches of jejunum and distal 4 inches of ileum.

b. Procedure of Scott and co-workers:[3] End-to-end anastomosis between proximal 10 inches of jejunum and distal 10 inches of ileum. Distal end is anastomosed end-to-side to colon for drainage of mucus and enteric secretions.

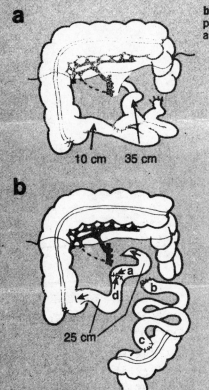

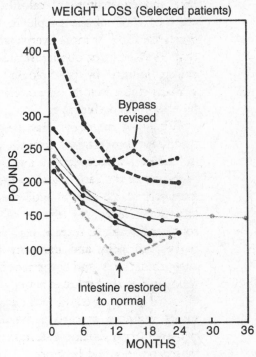

WEIGHT LOSS (Selected patients)

Figure 2. Weight loss in selected obese patients after intestinal bypass operation. Expected weight loss is 30% the first year and 10% the second year. Thereafter, loss levels off but attained weight remains stable indefinitely with only minor fluctuations.

Revision of bypass by converting from end-to-side to end-to-end anastomosis did not help one patient (arrow, top) who lost only 15% of his preoperative weight. Another patient (arrow, bottom) lost excessive weight and required restoration of intestine to normal.

2. Well-documented evidence of failure to reduce and to maintain reduced weight by ordinary methods like diet, appetite-suppressing drugs, and participation in TOPS, Weight-Watchers, or similar groups.

3. Reasonable emotional stability.

4. Absence of any correctable endocrinopathy, such as hypothyroidism or Cushing's syndrome, that may be the cause of obesity.

5. Absence of any other unrelated significant disease that might increase operative risk.

6. Presence of certain complications that may be corrected by significant weight reduction, such as Pickwickian syndrome, hypertension, or maturity-onset diabetes mellitus.

7. Informed consent for surgery.

Prospective candidates for an intestinal shunt should be aware of the inherent risk and should be prepared to bear with unpleasant side effects and to cooperate in a regular follow-up program. Whenever possible, we arrange a personal interview between a prospective candidate and a bypass patient of similar age and socioeconomic background.

Surgical Procedures

The surgical methods of Payne and De-Wind[2] and Scott and co-workers[3] (figure 1) are based on bypassing a major portion of the small intestine and thereby reducing the digesting and absorbing surface by about 90%. The simpler method of Payne and DeWind consists of end-to-side anastomosis between the proximal 14 inches of the jejunum and the distal 4 inches of the ileum. The method of Scott and associates involves end-to-end anastomosis between the proximal 10 inches of the jejunum and the distal 10 inches of the ileum. The bypassed mass of

TABLE 1. WEIGHT LOSS IN 50 OBESE PATIENTS AFTER INTESTINAL BYPASS OPERATION*

Time After Operation	No. of Patients	Weight Loss (% of Preoperative Weight)	Weight Status
3 yr	1 1 1	35 38 39	Stabilized
2½ yr	1 1 1	17 26 39	
2 yr	11 1	30 to 50 15†	
1½ yr	6	20 to 46	Continued slow loss
1 yr	9	22 to 47	
6 mo	9	18 to 26	Continued rapid loss
Less than 6 mo	8	—	

*Weight loss of less than 20% is considered inadequate.

†Revision of bypass from an end-to-side anastomosis to an end-to-end variant did not help this patient.

small intestine is closed at its proximal end, and in Scott and associates' variant, the distal end is anastomosed end-to-side to the colon to provide drainage of mucus and enteric secretions.

Since Payne and DeWind's first report, Salmon,[4] Weismann,[5] Wills,[6] and others have published articles describing a series of these operations. Almost a thousand cases have been published, and a reasonable estimate of the total number of intestinal bypass operations performed in the United States is several times this figure.

In our practice, we use the end-to-side procedure presented by Payne and DeWind[2] in their original paper.

Postoperative Adaptation Period

The intestinal bypass operation creates a controlled short-bowel syndrome with an adaptation period of one to two years. During this period, the patient loses weight fairly rapidly and undergoes several metabolic changes. Some are fortuitous, others are adverse; some are transient, others are permanent and irreversible.

After the first several months, weight loss tapers off and eventually stabilizes at a somewhat higher than ideal weight (figure 2). The expected loss is 30% during the first year and an additional 10% during the second year. When adaptation has taken place, weight loss levels off, but the attained weight remains stable indefinitely with only minor fluctuations, while the patients enjoy all the food they can afford and ingest.

Three of our 50 patients have passed the three-year mark with a weight loss of 35%, 38%, and 39%, respectively, and they are well and free of undesirable side-effects. The progress of all the patients is shown in table 1. Weight loss of less than 20% is considered inadequate. Revision of the bypass by conversion from an end-to-side anastomosis to an end-to-end variant did not help one patient who lost only 15% of his preoperative weight. Inadequate loss of weight may be expected in 5% to 10% of all bypass operations; however, weight gain is arrested in all cases.

Five of our patients had mild to moderate maturity-onset diabetes mellitus before surgery; none of them required insulin. Reduced carbohydrate absorption after a bypass operation is sufficient to maintain low to normal blood glucose levels without special diet or medication.

Serum cholesterol levels were within normal range in all of our patients before surgery. After surgery, the levels promptly dropped to the lower limit of normal or slightly below.

Postoperative Clinical Problems

A number of clinical problems are related to intestinal bypass surgery. The most common of these is diarrhea and the most serious is liver damage.

Diarrhea—The earliest and certainly the most frequent postoperative problem is diarrhea. It occurred in 48 of our 50 patients. Diarrhea begins with the first bowel movement after the operation and usually continues for three to six months. Some patients have 20 to 30 liquid, explosive eliminations daily; others have at most 6 to 12 stools daily. Severe diarrhea and related problems, such as perianal skin irritation, proctitis, hemorrhoids, and anal fissures, heavily tax the patient's endurance. Most patients have a difficult three-month period. They suffer a great deal, and their attitude varies from disenchantment to frank hostility; but as the diarrhea gradually relents and they begin losing weight, their mood improves.

During this difficult period, the family physician may help his patient by introducing him to the details of an antidiarrheal diet (bland, fat-free foods; no raw vegetables or other roughage; liquids between meals); by judicious prescription of codeine, opium preparations, or diphenoxylate hydrochloride with atropine sulfate (Lomotil); and by instruction in proper perianal skin care, including meticulous cleanliness, tender handling, frequent sitz baths, and the use of baby powder or sprays containing steroids.[7]

After the diarrhea tapers off, the patient may expect to have two or three formed stools each day, with only occasional bouts of diarrhea precipitated by dietary indiscretions. Steatorrhea with highly malodorous stools occurs rarely and creates more of a social problem than a clinical one.

Abdominal pain—Some patients have cramping abdominal pain of variable intensity and duration. This occurred in 18 of our patients. The pain usually responds well to codeine preparations or Percodan and eventually subsides completely.

Gastrointestinal bleeding—Three of our patients reported passing moderate amounts of clotted blood by rectum on several occasions. This did not affect their well-being and did not require any specific treatment. We could not determine the source of the bleeding.

Electrolyte imbalance—In the early postoperative period, sodium, chloride, and potassium values react as they do after any other major abdominal operation. Six of our patients had electrolyte imbalance. Later, serum sodium and chloride levels concentrated at the upper level of normal or slightly above, which does not create clinical problems. Serum potassium and calcium usually remain within normal limits, but occasionally drop slightly below the lower limit of normal without causing symptoms. Rarely is the hypocalcemia of significant degree to cause tetany. Calcium deficiency can be corrected by means of intravenous and later oral

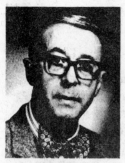

JOSEPH E.
BLEICHER

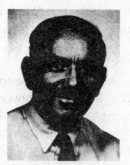

MIECZYSLAW
CEGIELSKI

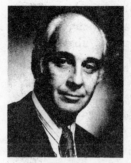

JOSE A.
SAPORTA

Dr. Bleicher is assistant
clinical professor of surgery,
Dr. Cegielski is associate
clinical professor of surgery,
and Dr. Saporta is clinical
instructor in surgery, Creighton
University School of Medicine,
Omaha.

administration of calcium preparations.

Only two of our patients had hypokalemia that was severe enough to manifest itself as muscle weakness and required hospital care. Both patients responded to potassium-salt supplements. These aberrations occurred during the early period of active weight loss and did not persist beyond the first year after surgery.

Serum iron levels tend to drop below normal. Because iron is absorbed in the duodenum and the first portion of the jejunum, oral administration of iron preparations corrects this deficiency. The hemoglobin and hematocrit values remained normal in all our patients.

Liver damage—Impaired liver function is probably the most serious and most difficult problem. It occurred in two of our patients. The histologic studies of Shibata and co-workers[8] and others have shown that even before bypass surgery, a variable degree of fatty infiltration of the liver occurs in obese patients. After surgery, these histologic changes may temporarily increase in severity; they usually decrease later but sometimes remain unchanged. In the early postoperative period, elevated hepatocellular enzyme values indicated certain degrees of liver damage in several patients, but these values gradually returned to normal.

Hypoalbuminemia with oncotic peripheral edema developed in four of our patients. This is another indication of liver damage, and it occurs rarely. Hypoalbuminemia alone, however, is quite common.

Excessive weight loss—Three of our patients lost excessive weight. The complex of excessive weight loss, peripheral edema, muscle weakness, and anorexia associated with hypoalbuminemia, hypokalemia, and hypocalcemia requires vigorous in-hospital treatment, sometimes with parenteral alimentation, and it may necessitate revision of the bypass operation. We were forced to revise the bypass or to restore the intestine to preoperative status in two of our patients about a year after the original operation (figure 2).

Vitamin deficiency—Impaired absorption of vitamin B_{12} and fat-soluble vitamins A, D, and K should be anticipated. As is routine with several other surgeons, we give our bypass patients injections of these vitamins at regular intervals during their follow-up visits. None of our patients have had vitamin deficiency. Some clinicians consider such vitamin therapy unnecessary.

Impaired absorption of certain drugs—Experience has taught us that intestinal absorption of orally given drugs and medications, especially in the popular enteric-coated or time-release form, is unreliable. Oral contraceptives have unpredictable results in bypass patients, and the use of other methods of contraception is advisable. We could not achieve adequate anticoagulation with bishydroxycoumarin (Dicumarol) when deep-vein thrombosis developed in one patient. Three of our 50 patients had impaired absorption of certain drugs.

Benefits of Operation

Benefits of intestinal bypass operation are (1) irreversible weight loss, (2) freedom from dieting and use of amphetamines and similar drugs, (3) improved cardiovascular and respiratory status, (4) low serum cholesterol levels, (5) self-limitation of diabetes mellitus, (6) regulation of the menstrual cycle, and (7) elimination of socioeconomic handicaps.

Our first patient was a 20-year-old woman. Before her operation in 1970, she was 168 cm (5 ft 6 in) tall, weighed 119.0 kg (262 lb), and was unemployed, on welfare, and unhappy. She now weighs 72.6 kg (160 lb), is steadily employed as a junior executive, and is happily married.

Comment

Surgeons who perform a jejunoileal bypass and family physicians caring for these patients must realize that the main goal of significant and irreversible loss of weight is accomplished by marked reduction of the absorptive and digestive surface of the intestine, with associated shifts in body metabolism. Many of these changes may be unknown at present and could appear several years hence. Careful, systematic follow-up is therefore essential in every case, both for the safety of the patient and for our better understanding of metabolic intestinal surgery.

Address reprint requests to Dr. Mieczyslaw Cegielski, Prairie Medical Clinic, Inc, 2602 "J" Street, Omaha, NE 68107.

REFERENCES

1. Braunstein JJ: Management of the obese patient. Med Clin North Am 55:391, 1971
2. Payne JH, DeWind LT: Surgical treatment of obesity. Am J Surg 118:141, 1969
3. Scott HW Jr, Law DH IV, Sandstead HH, et al: Jejunoileal shunt in surgical treatment of morbid obesity. Ann Surg 171:770, 1970
4. Salmon PA: The results of small intestine bypass operations for the treatment of obesity. Surg Gynecol Obstet 132:965, 1971
5. Weismann RE: Surgical palliation of massive and severe obesity. Am J Surg 125:437, 1973
6. Wills CE Jr: Jejunoileostomy for obesity. J Med Assoc Ga 58:456, 1969
7. LeVeen HH, Borek B, Axelrod DR, et al: Cause and treatment of diarrhea following resection of the small intestine. Surg Gynecol Obstet 124:766, 1967
8. Shibata HR, Mackenzie JR, Huang S: Morphologic changes of the liver following small intestinal bypass for obesity. Arch Surg 103:229, 1971

In obesity surgery, problems are the rule

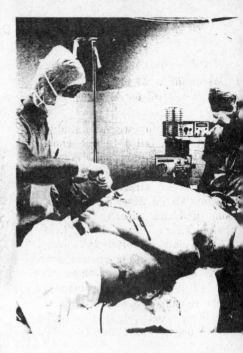

The concept of surgery for morbid obesity has always been beset by controversy and doubt. Obviously the procedure, which bypasses a large part of the intestinal tract, is a desperate measure fraught with extreme risk to the patient, to be used only when he cannot survive long without intervention. Now a new study from the University of Florida department of surgery suggests greater caution than ever before trying it.

At first glance such an operative detour, creating an artificial malabsorption syndrome, looked to early investigators like an attractive approach when ordinary methods failed to reduce a patient's caloric intake. Bypassing part of his digestive tract, they hoped, would also bypass his inability to stop gorging himself. And this should help head off such life-threatening complications of extreme overweight as cardiovascular or cardiopulmonary difficulties, obesity-induced diabetes, and liver disease.

But those hopes are largely shattered by the new study, done by Dr. J. Patrick O'Leary and his department chief at Gainesville, Dr. Edward R. Woodward. Their study of the outcome of surgery for obesity shows that a variety of disastrous sequelae appear to be the rule rather than the exception. Among disconcertingly frequent untoward results:
- Infections and other postoperative problems;
- Biochemical derangements of varying severity;
- Urinary tract oxalate stones;
- Liver failure, too often irreversible.

And a number of patients have required emergency removal of the shunt, restoring intestinal continuity, to save their lives.

"Since it is clear that the control of obesity by surgical bypass is still entirely experimental," Dr. O'Leary says, "we feel it mandatory to shorten the bowel in such a way as to make re-establishment of normal bowel function and anatomy possible should the need arise—as it has several times in our experience."

The Florida group has done some 40 jejunoileal bypasses to date, selected according to criteria very closely in agreement with those of Dr. H. William Scott Jr. of Vanderbilt University School of Medicine in Nashville, Tenn., one of the pioneers of bypass surgery. Patients must be massively obese, weighting two or three times normal, for at least five years. The heaviest patient treated at Gainesville weighed 500 lb; most were between 320 lb and 450 lb. (A man weighing some 800 lb was recently admitted to the Medical College of Virginia for intestinal bypass.)

In any event, most lose only about a third of their original weight after the operation, though six recent patients have lost about half.

Dr. O'Leary and gastroenterologist James J. Cerda, also of the University of Florida, have suggested that perhaps morbidly obese people process their food more efficiently than normal people do. At any rate, they seem to have two or three times the normal disaccharidase level in their small intestines. Dr. Cerda, after some follow-up studies, is not now entirely certain whether this is a concomitant of morbid obesity or of the diabetes so many of these patients suffer. The researchers studied 22 diabetics, normal and overweight, and found that those who were of normal weight, or were receiving adequate amounts of insulin, did not have such high disaccharidase activity.

Regardless of how much weight they lose, all bypass patients have persistent diarrhea, at least temporarily, if indeed there are no more serious complications. Much essential nutrient material, including proteins, carbohydrates, and electrolytes, is not passively absorbed but requires active transport across the intestinal epithelium. When only a short segment of it is left, there isn't much of a transport system available. Poor lipid absorp-

tion gives rise to steatorrhea; and removal of the selective area of the ileum where bile-salt absorption takes place depletes the recirculating bile-salt pool for dissolving fat. The unabsorbed long-chain fatty acids and bile salts irritate colonic mucusa; this alone may cause diarrhea.

Along with the loss of active transport systems, basic foods are not hydrolized fast enough for absorption in the short space available. One such transport system has been located for bile salts and vitamin B_{12}; and there is evidence that there are preferential sites equipped with specific enzymes for the solute transport of other specific nutrients. When these sites are removed those nutrients are not absorbed. Cholesterol, vitamin B_{12}, and bile salts are actively absorbed only from the terminal ileum, but the rest of the small intestine can adapt to the absorption of electrolytes, vitamins, and nutrients.

Gastric hypersecretion is another difficult problem that follows the operation, not only because of the acidic diarrhea it causes, but also because it may lead to gastroduodenal ulcers and all their complications. Acid hypersecretion seems to be proportional to the amount of bowel removed. Preserving the ileocecal valve seems to minimize excess motility.

In the end, patients apparently adapt to their interrupted intestines. They stop losing weight and stabilize, still vastly overweight but not necessarily morbidly so. This is because the remaining bowel segment hyper-

At Gainesville a 47-year-old, 375-lb diabetic is readied for bowel bypass.

trophies. And investigators studying patients who failed to lose enough weight found reflux of nutritive chyme into the bypassed ileum.

"It was not surprising that obese patients should develop many metabolic problems directly related to their surgery," says Dr. O'Leary. "While diarrhea, electrolyte imbalance, intussusception, anemia, ortho static hypotension and others have yielded to clinical improvements, there remain two major difficulties now being intensively studied: formation of urinary tract calculi and liver failure."

Since 1970 the Gainesville group has been trying to determine not only the incidence of stones but the stone type and the pathophysiology of stone production. "We now feel, as a result of our findings since then, that while poorly soluble oxalate excretion is probably the major factor promoting the formation of oxalate stones, loss of the solubilizing effect of citrate and magnesium may also contribute to stone formation," Dr. Leary says.

Because they can't predict which bypass patient is likely to develop them, the investigators presume they're all potential stone-formers. They try to reduce additional stone formation in those who already have some by correcting their acidosis, reducing caloric intake, and counseling them to avoid excessive amounts of liquids that contain soluble oxalate—especially tea and fruit juices.

But liver failure is obviously a far more serious matter. Nearly all severely obese people have fatty metamorphosis of the liver, even before surgery or other weight-reduction methods. They also have transient elevation of bromsulphalein (BSP) retention and bilirubin during fasting or near-fasting. "These facts might lead one to believe that the lipid-filled liver and associated chemical abnormalities in our surgically treated patients represent simply a continuation of the pre-shunt process," says Dr. O'Leary, "or perhaps that the patient has exchanged the fatty liver of hyperphagia for that of starvation. Yet a number of studies have shown

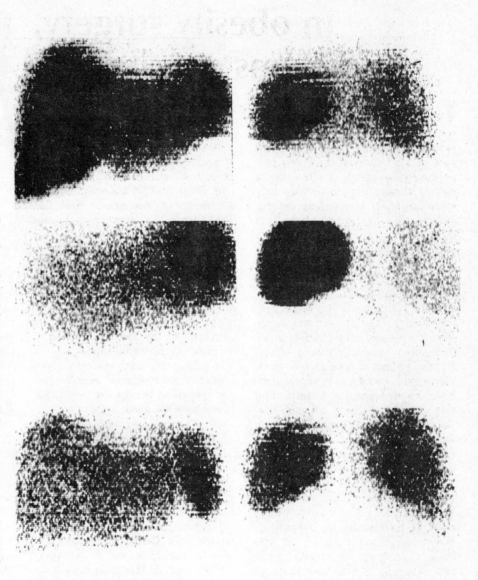

A Gainesville patient's liver scan is normal preoperatively (top), then indicates liver failure (center), improves after bypass removal (above).

this is not so. It has been demonstrated clearly that the fatty liver of obesity clears with fasting or near-fasting. In nonobese people, on the other hand, starvation *induces* a fatty liver."

At the University of Minnesota Hospital in Minneapolis, where Dr. Henry Buchwald and his associates do jejunoileal bypass operations for obesity and hypercholesteremia, needle biopsies at the time of operation show 61% to 98% of the patients to have fatty livers. The fatty changes appear to be more prevalent in men than in women, the Minnesota sur-

geons say, and the amount of fatty infiltration correlates with the amount of overweight. And Dr. Scott reports that all but five or six of the 91 patients he has done bypasses on had fatty livers before surgery.

At Gainesville, 20 of 21 patients who had liver biopsies at the time of surgery showed fatty metamorphosis. Two had micronodular cirrhosis, but one had already had a bypass associated with liver failure. Diabetes seemed to have no effect on the incidence of preoperative fatty liver, or on postoperative chemical abnormality of the liver.

Liver problems seem to appear in a regular sequence, say the Florida investigators. The earliest detectable functional abnormality is decrease in uptake of technetium sulfur colloid—the liver-scan tracer—by the Kupffer cells. Next BSP dye retention develops, followed by hypoalbuminemia and hypokalemia, and sometimes by mild rises in SGOT, SGPT and alkaline phosphatase. Along with these, patients are likely to go into fluid retention with weight gain, peripheral edema, and often ascites. Next comes hyperbilirubinemia of the conjugate type, perhaps with mild hypoprothrombinemia. Though this series of events seems inevitable, not all patients necessarily go through the whole sequence, the investigators say.

A research team at Los Angeles' VA Center and the UCLA department of medicine recently reported an investigation of obesity treated by fasting, reducing diets, or small-bowel bypass. They found that all their patients, except those treated by surgery, eventually had histologically normal livers after losing 100 lb or more. "But bypass surgery was followed variously by massive fatty changes, cholestasis, polynuclear inflammatory infiltrates, diffuse fibrosis, bile-duct proliferation, and fatal hepatic necrosis," they said. "Follow-up biopsy examinations are the only reliable means of judging whether a bypass procedure is causing progressive parenchymal damage."

With increasing understanding of such risks, criteria for the obesity operation have been made increasingly strict at Gainesville and elsewhere, and patients are selected only if they are prepared to accept a long clinical and metabolic follow-up study.

"Under no circumstances should bypass be undertaken without detailed preoperative tests and examinations, including liver biopsy and a battery of biochemical analyses," says Dr. O'Leary. "Here we prefer to operate only when the patient may be faced with untimely death because of enormous weight. There is no place whatever, we feel, for bypass as a cosmetic procedure." ∎

INDEX

A

Accident prone, 14

Acetone, 334

Acetylcoenzyme A, 163, 316

Acidosis, 96, 159, 166, 320

ACTH, 66, 317

Activity. See Exercise

Addiction, 89, 95, 101. See also Food, addict

Adenosine monophosphate, 317

Adenyl cyclase, 317

Adipocyte. See Fat cells

Adipose cells. See Fat cells

Adipose tissue, 1, 2-3, 7, 8, 11, 21-22, 29, 43, 48-51, 59, 66-67, 140, 162, 209, 211, 216-17, 255, 257, 268, 296, 311, 316, 329, 334

Adolescence, 23, 43, 50, 86-88, 110, 113, 117, 125, 197-264 (Part IV)

Adrenal cortex, 66

Adrenal gland, 194, 221-22

Adrenal medulla, 317

Adult-onset diabetes. See Diabetes

Adult-onset obesity. See Obesity

Advertisements, 149, 173. See also Media, Television

Aerobics, 292, 312, 349

Age of onset. See Obesity

Air Force diet, 162, 182, 189, 269. See also Diet

Albumen, 264

Albumin, 317

Alcohol, 83, 90, 97, 100-101, 149-50, 163, 189, 193, 390

Alcoholism. See Alcohol

Alimentary lipidemia. See Lipidemia

Allopurinal, 335

Alpha-glycerophosphate, 316-17

AMA (American Medical Association), 173 (address), 182, 323, 332, 335

American Diabetic Association's Food Exchange System. See Food, Exchange System

American Heart Association, 213, 301

American Medical Association. See AMA

Amino acids, 326

Amphetamines, 121, 196, 224, 282, 301, 386-87 399.

Anabolism, 257

Anapax, 172-73

Anemia, 159, 188, 207, 237, 401

Anger, 362

Angina pectoris, 168, 267

Anexoria, 46, 52, 67, 88, 92, 104, 107, 140, 184, 252, 281, 319, 326-27, 334-35, 386, 398

Anorexiant, 303, 307, 313

Anterior pituitary hormone. See Lipotropin

Anxiety, 40, 99, 287, 335, 356, 362; caloric, 40, 181

Apathy, 160, 181, 184

Aphagia, 64, 66

Appetite, 60-61, 200; suppressants, 32, 192, 282, 325, 330 (see also Diet, pills)

Ascorbic acid, 338. See also Vitamins, vitamin C

Asthma, 326

Arcus. See Corneal arcus

Arteries, hardening of. See Atherosclerosis

Arteriography, 320

Arthritic diseases, 112, 156, 192, 213

Arthritis. See Arthritic diseases

Asynchronism, 125

Atheromatous plaques. See Plaques

Atherosclerosis, 12, 43, 140, 184, 213-14, 230, 278, 320-21, 327, 332

Atherosclerotic plaques. See Plaques

Atkins' diet, 159-60, 168-71, 180, 182, 183-84, 319-330, 332-34

ATP, 272-73

A-V differences (arterial-venous), 66

B

Babies. See Childhood, Infancy

Baby food, 205-30

Balanced diet. See Diet

Basic Food Groups. See Four Basic Food Groups

B-complex vitamins. See Vitamins

Beauty, standard of, 146-47

Behavioral-control program, 351-52

Behavioral therapy, 298, 353-54, 355-59

Bel-Doxin, 173

Benzocaine, 172, 178

Better Business Bureau. See Council of Better Business Bureaus

Bile salts, 400

Bilirubin, 401

Binge-eating syndrome, 95, 223, 287, 341

Birth weight, 248

Blood: cholesterol (see Cholesterol); glucose, 65 (see also Glucose); lipids (see Cholesterol, Lipid, Triglycerides); -lipid test, 228; pressure, 228, 297, 305, 389, 392; sugar, 307, 335 (see also Glucose)

BMR (basal metabolic rate), 53-55, 243. See
   also Metabolism
Body: chemistry, 161; density, 33, 216; enve-
   lope method, 116; image, 23, 69, 86-87,
   120, 123, 213, 233, 251, 256; type (see
   Somatotype)
Boredom, 356, 362, 377
Breast feeding, 200, 203, 229-30
BSP (bromsulphalein), 401
Bypass. See Jejunoileal bypass, Intestinal bypass

C

Caffein, 83
Calcium, 187, 243, 264, 338, 397; depletion,
   160, 181, 184, 215
Calorie-activity chart, 348, 350
Caloric anxiety. See Anxiety
Caloric requirement. See Recommended
   Dietary Allowances
Calorimetric chamber, 344
Cancer, 186, 200, 394
Carbohydrates (few selected references), 31, 103,
   162-63, 183-84, 194. See also Diet
Cardiac arrhythmias, 160, 184, 320, 326, 335
Cardiac irregularity. See Cardiac arrhythmias
Cardiopulmonary syndrome. See Pickwickian
   syndrome
Cardiovascular disease, 78, 112, 181, 184, 192,
   214, 278, 286, 289, 394
Catecholamines, 334
Causes of obesity. See Obesity, etiology
Cecum, 264, 390
Cellular hypertrophy. See Hypertrophy
Cerebral hemorrhage, 158
Cerebral insufficiency, 320
Chest pain, 97. See also Angina pectoris
Child psychiatrist. See Psychiatrist
Cholelithiasis, 278
Cholesterol, 12, 43, 126, 167, 181, 184, 190,
   213-14, 231, 264-65, 319-23, 327-28,
   334-35, 346-47, 386, 397, 399
Chorionic gonadotropin. See Gonadotropin
Cigarette smoking, 214
Cirrhosis, 286, 401. See also Liver
Civilization, disease of. See Disease of civili-
   zation
Classification of obesities. See Obesity
Coffee, 83
Collagenase, 269
Colon, 264
Complications of obesity, 278. See also Ather-
   osclerosis, Diabetes, Heart disease, Hyper-
   tension, Obesity

Compulsive eating, 110. See also Obsessive-
   complusive syndrome
Congestive heart failure. See Heart failure
Conservation of energy. See Energy
Consumer Protection Bureau, 177
Control systems, 64-65
Coronary. See Heart disease
Coronary arteriography. See Arteriography
Coronary artery disease, 184, 214, 223, 368.
   See also Cardiovascular disease
Coronary insufficiency, 320
Coronary thrombosis, 394
Corneal arcus, 213
Corticosteroids, 221
Cortisol, 310, 317
Council of Better Business Bureaus, 173 (address)
Council on Foods and Nutrition, 182, 183, 332
Crash diet. See Diet, Fad diets
Craving for sweets. See Sweets
Creatinine, 264, 268
Criminal behavior, 97
Critical period (for weight development).
   See Obesity, development; Obesity, peak
   periods
Cult of youthfulness, 147, 150
Cushing's disease, 264, 309, 395

D

Daily caloric requirement. See Recommended
   Dietary Allowances
Depression, 99, 103-4, 110, 287, 290, 356, 363
Dermatological disorder, 178
Dehydration, 64, 66, 160, 184, 188
Density, body. See Body
Diarrhea, 264, 391, 393, 397, 400
Diabetes, 14, 30, 41-43, 65, 78, 97, 102, 140,
   156, 158, 180, 192, 195, 220, 223, 278, 281,
   308, 320, 326, 332, 335, 386, 392-93, 395,
   400; labile, 281; maturity-onset, 30, 42, 65,
   286, 387, 395
Diagnosis of obesity. See Obesity
Diet, 31, 46, 69-72, 78, 86, 97-100, 104, 106,
   109-111, 113, 115-128, 157-196 (Part III), 215,
   237-39, 265-402 (Part V); doctors, 121; pills,
   121-22, 178, 196 (see also Amphetamines,
   Diuretic); kinds: balanced, 161-62, 182, 290,
   322, 329, 333; crash, 162, 222 (see also
   Fad diets); high-protein, 123; macrobiotic,
   159, 166, 184; nibbling, 196, 281; "prudent,"
   213; sex, 175, 181; "unbalanced," 46. See
   also Air Force diet, Atkins' diet, Drinking
   man's diet, Fad diets, Grapefruit, Management, Mayo diets, Recommended regimen,
   Stillman's diet, Taller's diet, Treatment

404

Diet doctors. See Diet
Dietician, 168, 232. See also Nutrition
Diet Kitchen, 269
Diet pills. See Diet, Diuretic, Drugs
Diet Revolution. See Atkins' diet
Diet Workshop, 269
Digestive disease, 78, 158
Digitalis, 121, 196
Disease, obesity as. See Obesity
Disease of civilization, 62
Distention, 250
Diuretic, 131, 163, 196, 282, 386
Dizziness, 320, 326
DNA, 51
Drinking man's diet, 162, 169, 189, 269, 332
Drugs, 223, 307, 313, 385-88, 399; food as,
    103; psychotropic, 232. See also Amphet-
    amines; Anorexiant; Diet, pills; Tran-
    quilizers
Dyspnea, 97

E

Eating: addict (see Food, addict); patterns, 245;
    social significance of, 102
Edema, 328, 398
Eggs, 181, 335
Ego stability, 78, 293
Electrocardiagram, 320
Electrolyte, 264, 391, 393, 397-98, 400-401
Electrolyte imbalance. See Electrolyte
Encephalitis, 95
Endocrine disorders, 218, 309, 390
Endocrine Society, 335
Endomorphy, 37-38, 113, 199, 248. See also
    Somatotype
Energy: balance, 3-5, 15, 286, 297; conser-
    vation, 162, 315; for the brain, 163. See
    also First law of thermodynamics
Energy balance. See Energy, Equilibrium,
    First law of thermodynamics
Energy conservation. See Energy, First law of
    thermodynamics
Enzymes, 316-17; defects, 222
Epinephrine, 65, 221, 317, 386
Equilibrium, 3-5. See also Energy, balance
Euphoria, 281, 320, 326
Exercise, 31-32, 60, 67, 104, 106, 176, 178-79,
    190, 191, 193, 194, 196, 201, 208, 212, 235-
    37, 249, 265-402 (Part V)
Exercise chart. See Calorie-activity chart

F

Fad diets, types, 159-60, 162, 166, 188-90. See
    also Diet
Fainting, 160
Fantasy, 251, 260
Fashion, 124
Fatigue, 109-110, 181, 320, 326, 329, 334, 377
Fat cells, 5, 7, 8, 21, 29, 44-45, 59, 140, 155,
    160, 200, 203, 209-211, 215, 218, 228-29,
    269-70. See also Adipose tissue
Fat measurement, 33-35. See also Skinfold
    thickness, Triceps skinfold
Fats. See Cholesterol, Lipids, Saturated fats,
    Unsaturated fats
FDA (Food and Drug Administration), xiii, 173
    (address), 178, 187
Feeding machine, 9-10
Ferropenia, 230
Fetal damage, 170, 184
First law of thermodynamics, 162, 170, 315, 321,
    332
FMH ("fat mobilizing hormone"), 183, 334
Folic acid. See Vitamins
Food: addict, 89, 103 (see also Addiction);
    exchange, 292; Exchange System, 167;
    shopping (see Shopping); solid (see Solid
    foods)
Food and Drug Administration. See FDA
Formulas. See Infant formulas
Four Basic Food Groups, 162, 322
Fraud, 172-73, 189
Frustration, 362
FTC (Federal Trade Commission), 173 (address),
    176-78

G

Gall bladder, 112, 192, 286, 393
Gastric contractions, 65
Gastrointestinal tract, 64, 178
Genitourinary infections, 326
Gestation, 50. See also Pregnancy
Glands, 194. See also Adrenal cortex, Adrenal
    gland, Hypothalamus, Pituitary
Glucagon, 65, 317
Glucocorticoids, 66
Gluconeogenesis, 163, 316, 326
Glucoreceptors, 58
Glucose, 30, 58-59, 65, 211, 218, 220-21,
    257, 264, 312, 316, 326, 334, 386

Glucostatic mechanism, 59
Glucostatic theory, 65-66
Gluttony, 78, 118, 195
Glycerol, 221, 326
Glycerophosphate cycle, 272-73
Glycogen, 65, 211, 257, 316
Glycosis, 317
Gonadotropins, 32, 173-74, 215, 301
Gonads, 317
Gout, 184, 192
Gouty diathesis, 334
Grapefruit, 174, 181, 189, 193, 196, 269. See also Mayo diets
Group weight control, 126-27, 299, 301, 312, 351, 362, 367-84. See also TOPS, Weight Watchers
Growth hormone, 30, 66, 215, 221, 317, 334
Growth rate, 248
Gynecological disorder, 178

H

Habituation, 95, 100-101
Hardening of the arteries. See Atherosclerosis
Heart: attacks, 12, 168, 301, 304; disease, 14, 17, 41-42, 47, 102, 112, 126, 158, 160, 166, 188, 213, 214, 267, 278, 301, 320-21, 327, 335; failure, 178, 181, 279, 320; muscle, 31; palpitations, 320
Heat stroke, 65
Hemoglobin, 211, 230, 249
Hepatic necrosis. See Necrosis
Heptomegaly, 264
Height-weight charts. See Weight-height tables
Heredity, 15, 36, 60, 195. See also Obesity, genetic factors
Hernia, 178
Heterozygote, 213
Hidden sugar, 344
High-protein diets. See Diet
Hip joint disease, 278
Holiday eating, 297
Homeostasis, 63
Homeotherms, 65
Homogenization, 187
Homozygote, 213
Hormones, 32, 58, 65-66, 173-74, 183, 215, 272, 286, 313, 316-17. See also FMH, Growth hormone, Lipotropin
Hostility, 287
Hunger: awareness, 87-88, 100, 249, 329; definitions of, 20, 56, 81-85
Hyperadrenalcorticism, 277

Hypercellularity, 220-22, 229. See also Hyperplasia
Hypercholesterolemia, 46, 213-14, 230, 334, 368, 401
Hyperglycemia, 65-66, 316
Hyperinsulinemia, 30, 220-21, 310
Hyperinsulinism, 327
Hyperlipidemia, 43, 160, 184, 213-14, 328, 334, 390, 393
Hyperlipogenesis, 316
Hyperlipoproteinemia, 230
Hyperphagia, 52, 56, 64-65, 66, 95, 249, 252, 256, 401
Hyperplasia, 5, 7, 21, 22, 44, 48, 209, 211
Hypertension, 97, 156, 192, 214, 223, 230, 257, 328, 367-68, 393, 394
Hyperthyroidism, 170, 334
Hypertriglyceridemia, 214, 334
Hypertrophy, 7, 48, 140, 209, 211
Hyperuricemia, 160, 319, 334, 335
Hypnosis, 223
Hypoalbuminemia, 398, 402
Hypocalcemia, 391, 398
Hypoglycemia, 65, 66, 221, 332, 335, 382
Hypogonadism, 277
Hypokalemia, 391, 398
Hypophagia, 52
Hypoprothrombinemia, 402
Hypotension, 180, 320, 326, 334, 401
Hypothalamus, 30, 56-58, 164-65, 200, 209, 250, 286, 309, 322, 387; disease of, 277; lesions of, 21, 56, 64, 66-67; POAH (preoptic anterior hypothalamus), 65; ventromedial areas, 56, 64-65
Hypothyroidism, 264, 273, 277, 395

I

Ideal weight. See Weight
Ideopathic edema. See Edema
Ileum, 264, 390, 395, 400
Infancy, 22, 140, 317. See also Obesity, childhood
Infant formulas, 207
Inositol, 185
Insomnia, 252
Insulin, 30, 65, 220-21, 316-17, 325, 330, 334, 386
Insulinoma, 277
Intestinal bypass, 343, 394-99. See also Jejunoileal bypass
Intussusception, 401
IQ, 119
Iron, 192, 205, 207, 224, 230, 237, 243, 249, 301

J

Jejunoileal bypass, 264, 314, 342, 389-93, 400-402
Jejunoileal shunting. See Jejunoileal bypass
Jejuno-ileostomy. See Jejunoileal bypass
Jejunum, 264, 398-93, 395
Jogging, 349-50
Juvenile-onset obesity. See Obesity

K

Ketone bodies, 316-17, 332-33. See also Ketosis
Ketonemia, 296
Ketonuria, 329, 334
Ketosis, 46, 160, 163, 170, 180, 183-84, 188, 204, 224, 296, 319-23, 325, 334
Kidneys, 187, 333; damage, 188; disorders, 178; failure, 160; stones, 184; trouble, 181. See also Renal diseases
Kleptomania, 92

L

Lactic acidosis. See Acidosis
Law of thermodynamics. See First law of thermodynamics
Laxatives, 121
Lean body mass, 224, 238, 248, 257, 268, 317
Lean tissue, 163, 315
Lesions, 21, 43, 49, 56, 64, 66-67, 209, 218. See also Hypothalamus, lesions
Linoleic acid, 334-35
Lipemia, 334-35
Lipids, 167, 181, 182, 230, 311, 386, 391, 400. See also Cholesterol, Triglycerides
Lipogenesis, 162, 220, 312, 315-17
Lipolysis, 221, 313, 315-17, 387
Lipophelia, 45
Lipostatic hypothesis, 66
Lipotropin, 317
Liver, 66, 188, 211, 264, 281, 286, 316, 389, 391, 398, 400-402
Loneliness, 362
Love, food and, 107, 110, 195, 287
Lung conditions, 126

M

Macrobiotic diet. See Diet, kinds
Magnesium, 186, 264

Malnutrition, 110, 164, 320
Management, 278-84. See also Diet, Exercise, Treatment
Massage, 193, 300
Maturation rate, 248
Maturity-onset diabetes. See Diabetes
Maturity-onset obesity. See Obesity, adult-onset
Mayo diets, 162, 181, 189, 269
Measurement. See Fat measurement, Skinfold thickness, Triceps skinfold
Media, 149. See also Advertisements, Television
Menstrual cycle, 399
Mesomorphy, 37-38, 113, 119. See also Somato-type
Metabolism, 32, 52, 195, 218, 220, 257, 272, 278, 286-87, 311, 326, 386
Methyl cellulose, 172, 178
Microcytosis, 230
Migraine, 326
Minerals, 188, 237
Mood, 81-85
Morphologic characteristics. See Somatotype
Mortality rate, 14, 41, 192
Motivation, 68, 95, 304
Multiple sclerosis, 178
Muscular disorder, 178, 185
Muscular dystrophy, 185
Myocardial infarction, 320

N

NADPH, 316
Nausea, 160, 170, 184, 250, 320, 326, 334, 335, 386
Necrosis, 402
Negative mood. See Mood
Negative protein balance, 163
Nephrosis, 187
Nervousness, 329
Neurological disorders, 178
Neurosis, 252
Niacin, 185. See also Vitamins
Nibbling diet. See Diet, kinds
Night-eating syndrome, 95, 195, 252, 287, 328, 341
Nitrogen, 163, 184, 215, 257, 264
Norepinephrine, 317
Nutrition, 29-30, 158, 169, 164, 166, 167, 181, 185-87, 191, 194, 229, 232, 242, 245, 259, 324, 338, 341. See also Council on Foods and Nutrition
Nutrionists. See Nutrition

O

Obestiy: adult-onset, 22, 30, 43-44, 120, 125, 140, 204; age of onset, 45, 248, 263, 279; childhood, 22, 43, 61, 87, 110, 120, 126, 140, 192, 197-264 (Part IV); classification of, 45; definition of, 13-14, 112, 216, 315-16; development of (critical periods), 217, 228; diagnosis, 1-68 (Part I), 69-156 (Part II), 275-76; as disease, 164, 308; environmental factors, 16, 19, 36, 60, 101, 152, 212, 251, 277, 353; etiology (cause), 1, 15, 101, 1-68 (Part I), 69-156 (Part II), 287, 309-10, 315-18; familial component, 15, 296, 358; genetic factors, 15, 28, 36-38, 43, 49, 59, 152, 195, 205, 209-11, 212, 222, 249, 277, 286; growth-onset, 22, 30, 43; juvenile-onset, 22, 23, 48, 125, 140, 197-264 (Part IV), 310; metabolic, 7, 16, 45, 59; paradoxical, 87; peak periods, 212-13; prevalence of, 14, 113, 217, 267, 275; prognostic factors (tables), 283; psychological factors, 223, 248 250-52, 277, 287, 341; "pull" theory, 7-8; "push" theory, 7-8; racial differences in, 113-117; "regulatory," 7, 16, 45, 59; sex differences in, 113-14, 117, 123, 138, 256, 287. See also Overweight
Obsessive-compulsive syndrome, 90-93, 99
Oral agression, 145
Oral area, 90
Oral sensations, 64
Oral stages, 145, 267
Oriental dinner, 170
Organic foods, 187
Orthopedic disorder, 178
Overeaters Anonymous, 381-85
Overweight: definition of, 13-14, 112, 216, 267; prevalence of, 94, 158, 194, 199, 203. See also Obesity
Oxalate stones, 264, 400-401

P

Pancreas, 65, 194
Paranoia, 98
Passivity, 69, 79, 197, 251
Pasteurization, 187
Pathogenesis, 1
Peer group attitude, 152
Pemmican, 334
Peripheral edema. See Edema
Pharmacologic therapy. See Drugs

Phentermine, 386
Pickwickian syndrome, 223, 278, 297, 394, 395
Pinch test, 196, 307
Pituitary, 30, 66, 194
Plaques, 213, 214, 217
POAH. See Hypothalamus
Postural hypotension. See Hypotension
Positive mood. See Mood
Potassium, 221, 268, 397
Potassium chloride, 187
Pregnancy, 102, 155, 192, 212, 232, 281, 287
President's Commission on Youth Fitness, 300
Prodromal condition, 164
Prognostic factors in obesity. See Obesity
"Prudent diet." See Diet, kinds
Psychiatrist, 247, 264, 342, 360
Psychological factors in obesity. See Obesity
Psychotropic drugs. See Drugs
"Pull" theory of obesity. See Obesity
"Push" theory of obesity. See Obesity

Q

QQF theory, 315-18
Quackery, 167, 172, 177-78, 293
Quick Weight Loss Diet, 269. See also Stillman's diet

R

Radio-immunoassay, 30
Recommended Dietary Allowances, 161, 215
Recommended regimen, 318
Reducing devices, 176-79. See also Relaxacizer, Tone-O-Matic, Vibrating devices
Reducing rate. See Weight-loss rate
Rejection, 69, 79
Relaxacizer, 177
Religious practices, 135, 137, 144-45
Renal diseases, 78, 159, 166, 184, 286, 320
Respiratory diseases, 112. See also Pickwickian syndrome
Riboflavin, 172-73, 338.

"Roller coaster effect," 190, 362

S

Safflower oil, 171, 188
Salad oils, 193. See also Safflower oil, Vegetable oil
Salt, 230, 282, 322

Satiety, 58, 66, 81-84, 200, 249-50, 287, 298, 322, 339
Saturated fats, 301, 334-45. See also Cholesterol
Sauna Belt, 179
Scopolamine aminoxide, 173
Scale-weight loss. See Weight
Schizophrenia, 88
School weight control programs. See Weight
Scurvy, 159, 166, 181
Sedentary living, 214, 236, 343
Select Committee on Nutrition and Human Needs, 160, 181
Self-concept, 78, 79, 80, 86-87, 107, 111, 119-20, 122
Self-control. See Self-discipline
Self-discipline, 161, 288, 292, 330, 374
Self-help organizations. See Group weight control
Self-image. See Self-concept
Serum cholesterol levels. See Cholesterol
Serum insulin. See Insulin
Serum lipids. See Lipids
Set point, 66
Sex diet. See Diet
Sexuality, 97, 103, 147, 251, 287, 303
Shopping, 290-91
Skinfold thickness, 35, 116, 137-38, 153, 216, 231, 233, 241, 256, 258, 276, 368. See also Fat measurement, Pinch test, Triceps
Sleepiness, 97
Sloth, 118
Snacking, 245, 261, 353
Social class, 17-19, 30, 77, 113, 115, 126, 131-36, 137-42, 153, 287
Social mobility, 131-36, 148, 287
Socioeconomic groups, 368, 380. See also Social class
Sodium, 333. See also Salt
Solid foods, time for starting, 200-201, 204
Somatotype, 35, 37-38, 112-13, 248-49
Spinal fusion, 178
Spine disease, 278
Sports, 348
Spot reduction, 179, 192
Starvation, 70, 95-100, 174, 184, 211, 320
Steam baths, 193
Steatorrhea, 397, 400
Stereotypes, 118-19
Stigma, 77-79
Stillman's diet, 169, 182, 188, 323, 332
Stress, 97, 103
Stroke, 215. See also Heat stroke
Surgery, 192, 264, 278, 321, 360. See also Intestinal bypass, Jejunoileal bypass

Sweets, craving for, 320, 327
Sympatho-adrenomedullary discharge, 317
Syncope, 320, 326

T

Tables. See Weight-height tables
Tachycardia, 320, 326
Taller's diet, 169, 171, 189, 323, 332
Television, 199, 201, 207, 297, 298
Teenagers. See Adolescence
Thermodynamics, 240. See also First law of thermodynamics
Thermogenesis, 316
Thiamine, 172-73, 243, 335, 338.
Thyroid, 194, 222, 272-73; extract, 121, 196, 215, 282, 313; hormone, 386; stimulating hormone, 317
Thyroxine, 317
Tissue. See Adipose tissue, Lean tissue
Tone-O-Matic, 176-77
TOPS, xiii, 25, 168, 269, 283, 301, 371-75, 376-80, 385, 390, 395
Tranquilizers, 232, 386
Trauma, 15, 87, 320, 323
Triceps fatfold, 211. See also Skinfold thickness
Triglycerides, 7, 43-44, 181, 184, 214, 220, 264, 313, 315-17, 321-23, 327-28, 334-35, 386
Tubo-ovarian abcess, 178
TV. See Television

U

Ulcers, 178, 200
"Unbalanced" diet. See Diet, kinds
Unemployment, 97
United States Postal Service, 173 (address), 178
Unsaturated fats, 301
Urea, 159, 173, 264
Urinary tract, 264
U. S. Food and Drug Administration. See FDA

V

Vagus nerve, 56, 59
Varicose veins, 178
Vascular complications, 43, 178, 184, 335
Vasopressin, 317
Vegetable oil, 301. See also Salad oils
Ventromedial areas. See Hypothalamus
Vibrating devices, 193, 196, 300. See also Reducing devices

Vinegar, 193
Virilization, 257
Vitamins, 186, 188, 192, 207, 211, 237, 335;
    vitamin A, 185, 244, 348; vitamin B1, 173;
    vitamin B_2, 173; vitamin B_{12}, 187, 391, 398,
    400; vitamin C, 187, 244, 335 (see also
    Ascorbic acid); vitamin D, 187, 398; vitamin
    E, 185, 186-87, 335; vitamin K, 398; B-com-
    plex, 335, folic acid, 338; niacin, 185
Volvulus, 159, 166
Vomiting, 320, 326, 334

W

Walking, 350
Waltzing gene, 61
Water: balance, 163; weight loss, 190; reten-
    tion, 332-33
Weakness, 160, 184, 329
Weight: control programs, 127-28; ideal, 36,
    153, 245; illusionary loss of, 163; loss rate
    (see Weight-loss rate); methods of loss, 120;
    minimum body, 39; scale, 162; tables (see
    Weight-height tables)
Weight control. See Diet; Weight, control
    programs
Weight-height tables, 78, 115, 131, 153, 196
Weight-loss rate, 16, 166, 175, 191, 280, 296,
    322, 328, 334, 364; deviations by age, 114
Weight Watchers, xiii, 80, 124, 127, 168, 269,
    283, 301, 368, 371, 385, 395
Withdrawal, 69, 79, 197-98, 251

X

Xanthelasma, 213
Xanthoma, 213
Xylose, 264

Y

Youthfulness, cult of. See Cult of Youthfulness